The SAGES Manual of Physiologic Evaluation of Foregut Diseases

Ankit D. Patel • Amir Aryaie
Jayleen Grams • Leena Khaitan
Editors

The SAGES Manual of Physiologic Evaluation of Foregut Diseases

Springer

Editors
Ankit D. Patel
Department of Surgery
Emory University School of Medicine
Atlanta, GA, USA

Jayleen Grams
Department of Surgery
University of Alabama at Birmingham and Birmingham VA Health Care System
Birmingham, AL, USA

Amir Aryaie
BMI Surgical Institute
Atlanta, GA, USA

Leena Khaitan
Department of Surgery
University Hospitals, Cleveland Medical Center
Cleveland, OH, USA

ISBN 978-3-031-39198-9 ISBN 978-3-031-39199-6 (eBook)
https://doi.org/10.1007/978-3-031-39199-6

This Springer imprint is published by the registered company Springer Nature Switzerland AG
The registered company address is: Gewerbestrasse 11, 6330 Cham, Switzerland

Paper in this product is recyclable.

Contents

Part V Pathology/Symptom Based

Contributors

Mujjahid Abbas, MD New Jersey Bariatric Center, Hackettstown, NJ, USA

University Hospitals Cleveland Medical Center, Cleveland, OH, USA

Case Western University School of Medicine, Cleveland, OH, USA

Stuart A. Abel, MD Division of Upper GI and General Surgery, Department of Surgery, Keck Medical Center of USC, University of Southern California, Los Angeles, CA, USA

Emily Adams, MD Department of Surgery, The University of Utah, Salt Lake City, UT, USA

Ali M. Ahmed, MD Division of Gastroenterology and Hepatology, University of Alabama at Birmingham, Birmingham, AL, USA

Mohsen Alhashemi, MD, MSc, FRCSC Department of Surgery, College of Health Sciences, Kuwait University, Kuwait, QC, Kuwait

Abdulaziz Karam Ali, MD Department of Surgery, McGill University, Montreal, QC, Canada

Montreal General Hospital, Montreal, QC, Canada

Department of Surgery, College of Health Sciences, Kuwait University, Kuwait, QC, Kuwait

Mohammed Al Mahroos, MD, FRCSC Department of Surgery, St Mary's Hospital, McGill University, Montreal, QC, Canada

Edward Auyang, MD, MS, FACS Department of Surgery, University of New Mexico School of Medicine, Albuquerque, NM, USA

Alexander L. Ayzengart Department of Surgery, University of Florida Health, Gainesville, FL, USA

Amy Banks-Venegoni, MD, FACS Spectrum Health Medical Group and Corewell Health West-Department of Surgery, Michigan State School of Medicine, East Lansing, MI, USA

Nikolai A. Bildzukewicz University of Southern California, Los Angeles, CA, USA

Shaoxu Bing, MD Department of Surgery, UF Health Jacksonville, Jacksonville, FL, USA

Jenna Borys, DO Department of Surgery, Grant Medical Center, Columbus, OH, USA

Joseph R. Broucek, MD Division of General Surgery, Department of Surgery, Vanderbilt University Medical Center, Nashville, TN, USA

Andrew M. Brown, MD Department of Surgery, St. Luke's University Hospital, Bethlehem, PA, USA

J. Christian Brown Department of Surgery, University of Florida Health, Gainesville, FL, USA

Francis P. Buckley III Dell Medical School, University of Texas at Austin, Austin, TX, USA

Michelle Campbell, MD University of Chicago Medical Center, Chicago, IL, USA

Jennwood Chen Division of Gastroesophageal and Bariatric Surgery, University of Utah, Salt Lake City, UT, USA

Paul D. Colavita Division of Gastrointestinal Surgery, Department of Surgery, Carolinas Medical Center, Charlotte, NC, USA

Tanuja Damani, MD, FACS NYU Grossman School of Medicine, New York, NY, USA

Center for Esophageal Health, NYU Langone Health, New York, NY, USA

S. Scott Davis Jr., MD, FACS Emory Endosurgery Unit, Department of Surgery, Emory University, Atlanta, GA, USA

D'Artagnan DeBow, MD Division of Minimally Invasive and Bariatric Surgery, Zucker School of Medicine at Hofstra/Northwell, Lenox Hill Hospital, New York, NY, USA

Gabriel Diaz Del Gobbo, MD Cleveland Clinic Abu Dhabi, Abu Dhabi, UAE

Cleveland Clinic Lerner College of Medicine, Cleveland, Ohio, USA

Abdul-Rahman Fadi Diab, MD Division of Gastrointestinal Surgery, Department of Surgery, University of South Florida Morsani College of Medicine, Tampa, FL, USA

Maggie L. Diller, MD Division of General and GI Surgery, Department of Surgery, Emory University, Atlanta, GA, USA

Stephanie Doggett Dell Medical School, University of Texas at Austin, Austin, TX, USA

Rodrigo Duarte-Chavez, MD Department of Gastroenterology, St. Luke's University Hospital, Bethlehem, PA, USA

Christopher DuCoin, MD, MPH, FACS Division of Gastrointestinal Surgery, Department of Surgery, University of South Florida Morsani College of Medicine, Tampa, FL, USA

Justin Eagleston, MD, MHA Trihealth Good Samaritan Hospital, Cincinnati, OH, USA

Carolinas Medical Center, Charlotte, NC, USA

Sofiane El Djouzi Barijuve Surgical, Darien, IL, USA

Michael T. Fastiggi, MD New Jersey Bariatric Center, Hackettstown, NJ, USA

University Hospitals Cleveland Medical Center, Cleveland, OH, USA

Case Western University School of Medicine, Cleveland, OH, USA

Filippo Filicori, MD Division of Minimally Invasive and Bariatric Surgery, Zucker School of Medicine at Hofstra/Northwell, Lenox Hill Hospital, New York, NY, USA

Fermin Fontan, MD University of Iowa Carver College of Medicine, Iowa City, IA, USA

Meredith Freeman, MD Tulane University, School of Medicine, New Orleans, LA, USA

Gregory Fritz, MD Corewell Health General Surgery Residency, Michigan State School of Medicine, East Lansing, MI, USA

Elisa J. Furay, MD Dell Medical School, University of Texas at Austin, Austin, TX, USA

Carlos Galvani, MD, FACS, FASMBS Division of Minimally Invasive Surgery and Bariatric, Department of Surgery, Tulane University, School of Medicine, New Orleans, LA, USA

Meredith A. Harrison, MD Department of Surgery, St. Luke's University Hospital, Bethlehem, PA, USA

Alison Y. Haruta, MD Department of Surgery, University of Washington, Seattle, WA, USA

Ivy N. Haskins, MD Esophageal Swallowing Center, MIS/Bariatric, Foregut, and Hernia Surgery, Omaha, NE, USA

Justin Henning, MD Center for Esophageal Health, NYU Langone Health, New York, NY, USA

NYU Langone Health, New York, NY, USA

Kelly M. Herremans Department of Surgery, University of Florida Health, Gainesville, FL, USA

Charles Hill, MD Dell Medical School, University of Texas at Austin, Austin, TX, USA

Justin Hsu, MD Corewell Health General Surgery Residency, Michigan State School of Medicine, East Lansing, MI, USA

Anna Ibele, MD, FACS Department of Surgery, The University of Utah, Salt Lake City, UT, USA

Hope T. Jackson, MD Department of Surgery, The George Washington University School of Medicine and Health Sciences, Washington, DC, USA

Tayler J. James University of Southern California, Los Angeles, CA, USA

Bora Kahramangil, MD Cleveland Clinic Florida, Department of General Surgery, Bariatric and Metabolic Institute, Weston, FL, USA

Kshitij Kakar, MD, FACS Trihealth Bethesda North Hospital, Cincinnati, OH, USA

Umashankkar Kannan, MD Institute for Bariatric and Minimally Invasive Surgery, Mount Sinai Morningside Medical Center, New York, NY, USA

Angela M. Kao Division of Gastrointestinal Surgery, Department of Surgery, Carolinas Medical Center, Charlotte, NC, USA

Abdulaziz Ali Karam Department of Surgery, St Mary's Hospital, McGill University, Montreal, QC, Canada

Subhash Kini, MD Institute for Bariatric and Minimally Invasive Surgery, Mount Sinai Morningside Medical Center, New York, NY, USA

Isaac R. Kriley, MD Department of Surgery, UF Health Jacksonville, Jacksonville, FL, USA

Matthew Kroh, MD Cleveland Clinic Abu Dhabi, Abu Dhabi, UAE

Cleveland Clinic Lerner College of Medicine, Cleveland, Ohio, USA

James Kurtz, DO, FACOS Valley Forge Surgical Associates, Phoenixville, PA, USA

Danuel Laan, MD Division of Minimally Invasive Surgery and Bariatric, Department of Surgery, Tulane University, School of Medicine, New Orleans, LA, USA

Ryan Lamm, MD Department of SurgeryThomas Jefferson University Hospital, Philadelphia, PA, USA

Megan Lundgren, MD Department of Surgery, Penn Highlands Healthcare, Dubois, PA, USA

Emanuele Lo Menzo, MD, PhD, FACS, FASMBS Cleveland Clinic Florida, Department of General Surgery, Bariatric and Metabolic Institute, Weston, FL, USA

Ronak Modi, MD Department of Gastroenterology, St. Luke's University Hospital, Bethlehem, PA, USA

Peter Nau, MD, MS, FACS University of Iowa Carver College of Medicine, Iowa City, IA, USA

Krzystof M. Nowak, MD ENT and Allergy Associates, Yonkers, NY, USA

Dmitry Oleynikov, MD Department of Surgery, Monmouth Medical Center, Long Branch, NJ, USA

Francesco Palazzo, MD, FACS Department of Surgery, Thomas Jefferson University Hospital, Philadelphia, PA, USA

Abhishek D. Parmar, MD Department of Surgery, University of Alabama at Birmingham, Birmingham, AL, USA

Kyle A. Perry Division of General and Gastrointestinal Surgery, Ohio State University, Columbus, OH, USA

Jennifer F. Preston, MD College of Medicine Phoenix, University of Arizona, Phoenix, AZ, USA

Ruchir Puri, MD, FACS Department of Surgery, UF Health Jacksonville, Jacksonville, FL, USA

Joel Richter, MD, FACP, MACG Division of Gastrointestinal Surgery, Department of Surgery, University of South Florida Morsani College of Medicine, Tampa, FL, USA

Matthew W. Romine, MD Department of Surgery, East Carolina University Hospital System, Greenville, NC, USA

Raul Rosenthal, MD, FACS, FASMBS Cleveland Clinic Florida, Department of General Surgery, Bariatric and Metabolic Institute, Weston, FL, USA

Ramses A. Saavedra, MD, MS Department of Surgery, University of New Mexico School of Medicine, Albuquerque, NM, USA

Sarah Samreen, MD University of Texas Medical Branch, Galveston, TX, USA

Stefan Scholz, MD, PhD, FACS, FAAP Department of Surgery, University of Pittsburgh School of Medicine, Pittsburgh, PA, USA

Division of Pediatric General and Thoracic Surgery, UPMC Children's Hospital of Pittsburgh, Pittsburgh, PA, USA

Luis Serrano, MD, FACS HCA Florida Osceola Surgical Care Specialists, Kissimmee, FL, USA

Federico Serrot, MD Department of Surgery, Emory University, Atlanta, GA, USA

Elizabeth Sharbaugh, MD Department of Surgery, University of Pittsburgh Medical Center, Pittsburgh, PA, USA

Lindsey C. Shipley, MD Division of Gastroenterology and Hepatology, University of Alabama at Birmingham, Birmingham, AL, USA

Daniel Shouhed, MD Cedars Sinai Medical Center, Los Angeles, CA, USA

Vibha Sood, MD Department of Pediatrics, University of Pittsburgh School of Medicine, Pittsburgh, PA, USA

Division of Pediatric Gastroenterology, Hepatology, and Nutrition, UPMC Children's Hospital of Pittsburgh, Pittsburgh, PA, USA

Nathaniel J. Soper, MD College of Medicine Phoenix, University of Arizona, Phoenix, AZ, USA

Joseph Sujka, MD Department of Surgery, University of South Florida Morsani College of Medicine, Tampa, FL, USA

Samuel Szomstein, MD, FACS, FASMBS Cleveland Clinic Florida, Department of General Surgery, Bariatric and Metabolic Institute, Weston, FL, USA

Oscar Talledo, MD University of Iowa Carver College of Medicine, Iowa City, IA, USA

Talar Tatarian, MD Department of Surgery, Thomas Jefferson University Hospital, Philadelphia, PA, USA

Jeffrey Thomas, DO, MPH Department of Surgery, Doctors Hospital, Columbus, OH, USA

Michael Ujiki, MD NorthShore University HealthSystem, Evanston, IL, USA

Natacha Wathieu, MD Tulane University, School of Medicine, New Orleans, LA, USA

Michael L. Williford, MD WakeMed Health and Hospitals, Raleigh, NC, USA

Andrew S. Wright, MD Department of Surgery, University of Washington, Seattle, WA, USA

Lauren Yoder, MD Trihealth Good Samaritan Hospital, Cincinnati, OH, USA

Mohanad R. Youssef, MD Division of Minimally Invasive Surgery and Bariatric, Department of Surgery, Tulane University, School of Medicine, New Orleans, LA, USA

Part I

Understanding Anatomy and Physiology

Anatomy and Physiology of the Esophagus

1

Jeffrey Thomas and James Kurtz

Anatomy

Topography of the Cervical, Thoracic, and Abdominal Esophageal Segments

Topographically, the cervical portion of the esophagus extends from the pharynx to the suprasternal notch, with an average distance of approximately 5 centimeters. In this region, the esophagus is bordered posteriorly by the vertebral column, laterally by the carotid sheaths, and anteriorly by the trachea. The cervical esophagus is adherent to the posterior trachea and the vertebral column via loose connective tissue (anteriorly) and the prevertebral fascia (posteriorly). The thoracic duct is also found to the left of the sixth cervical vertebra in close proximity to the esophagus.

J. Thomas
Department of Surgery, Doctors Hospital, Columbus, OH, USA
e-mail: Jeffrey.Thomas@ohiohealth.com

J. Kurtz (✉)
Valley Forge Surgical Associates, Phoenixville, PA, USA
e-mail: James.Kurtz@towerhealth.org

A. D. Patel et al. (eds.), *The SAGES Manual of Physiologic Evaluation of Foregut Diseases*,
https://doi.org/10.1007/978-3-031-39199-6_1

The primary source of arterial inflow to the cervical esophagus is derived from the inferior thyroid arteries, branches of the subclavian artery on the right, and the thyrocervical trunk on the left.

The cervical esophagus is notable for its composition of striated muscle, making it distinct from the muscular composition of the remaining 2/3 of the esophagus, which is primarily smooth muscle. The upper esophageal sphincter (UES) is an important high-pressure zone at the inlet of the esophagus that allows bolus passage and protection of the airway during swallowing. The high, constant resting tone (mean 60 mmHg) of the UES is accomplished by the cricopharyngeus muscle, the inferior pharyngeal constrictor, and the musculature of the cervical esophagus (which are arranged in a horizontal orientation). The cricopharyngeus muscle is thought to be the main contributor to the UES and also marks the most proximal of three narrowing points in the esophagus that contribute to its hourglass shape. In contrast, the opening of the UES is accomplished by contraction of the suprahyoid superiorly and the thyrohyoid musculature inferiorly, which act together to pull the hyoid bone anterior and inferior to its native position, ultimately displacing the laryngeal complex anteriorly and opening the UES. Posterior musculature including the stylopharyngeus, palatopharyngeus, and pterygopharyngeus acts to stabilize the posterior aspect of the UES and increase its diameter on opening.

Also, within the cervical esophagus is an area of relative weakness in the wall of the esophagus known eponymously as Killian's triangle. This triangle represents a common site for the diverticula of the esophagus. This anatomic triangle is formed by the transversely oriented fibers of the cricopharyngeus and by the obliquely oriented inferior pharyngeal constrictor muscles. The weakest point of this triangle wherein diverticula may be found is known as Killian's dehiscence and is characterized by its lack of posterior esophageal muscularis. In addition to being a frequent site of diverticular formation, this area is subject to iatrogenic injury in routine procedures including esophagogastroduodenoscopy (EGD) secondary to its ease of penetration.

The thoracic portion of the esophagus extends from the suprasternal notch to the level of the diaphragmatic hiatus. It is in this region that the esophagus encounters a number of important intrathoracic structures including the trachea, the mainstem bronchi, and the aortic arch. The esophagus deviates slightly to the left of the trachea at the thoracic inlet, shifts to the right at the carina to accommodate the aortic arch, and turns left again posterior to the left mainstem bronchus before entering the diaphragmatic hiatus at the level of the 11th thoracic vertebra. The two remaining narrowing points of the esophagus occur at this bronchoaortic constriction near the fourth vertebra and at the diaphragmatic hiatus. The majority of the arterial flow is supplied to the thoracic portion of the esophagus via the bronchial arteries and the four to six esophageal branches of the aorta. This blood supply is supplemented by descending branches from the inferior thyroid arteries and intercostal arteries and ascending branches of the paired inferior phrenic arteries.

The final segment of the esophagus is the abdominal portion, a short segment extending from the entry of the esophagus into the esophageal hiatus of the diaphragm until its smooth transition into the cardia of the stomach. Within the abdomen, after passing through the esophageal hiatus, the esophagus lies in a shallow groove of the posterior aspect of the left lobe of the liver, formally referred to as the esophageal groove. Blood supply to this region of the esophagus is generally provided by an ascending branch of the left gastric artery and from both the left and right inferior phrenic arteries.

The lower esophageal sphincter (LES) is a zone of high pressure (mean, 24 mmHg) measuring approximately 3 centimeters with intrathoracic and intra-abdominal components. This marks the exit point of the esophagus and is at the level of the gastroesophageal junction. The LES acts in conjunction with gastric sling fibers and the crural diaphragm to protect the epithelium of the esophagus from injury related to refluxed gastric contents (Fig. 1.1). While it does not have a truly identifiable landmark, the LES can be identified as a pressure gradient, which is higher than

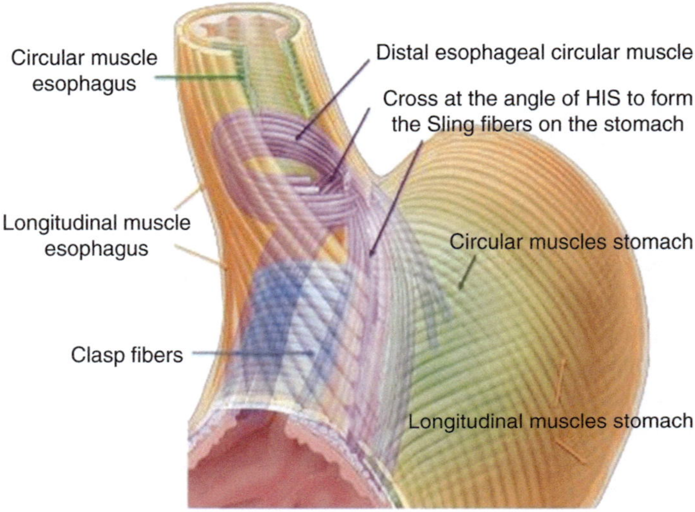

Fig. 1.1 Schematic of the microscopic myoarchitecture of the circular and longitudinal muscle layers of the lower esophageal sphincter and stomach. (From Zifan, A., Kumar, D. Cheng, L.K. et al. Three-Dimensional Myoarchitecture of the Lower Esophageal Sphincter and Esophageal Hiatus Using Optical Sectioning Microscopy. Scientific Reports 7, Article number: 13188 (2017))

the normal gastric pressure on manometry or at the squamocolumnar epithelial junction on endoscopy. Externally, one could say that the LES rests under the gastroesophageal fat pad or where the circular muscular fibers of the esophagus join the oblique fibers of the stomach (the collar of Helvetius).

The wall of the esophagus in its entirety is composed of mucosa, submucosa, and a muscularis propria. In contrast to the remainder of the gut, the esophagus lacks a serosal outer layer and instead is invested by a thin layer of loose connective tissue. The muscularis propria is furthermore divided into two distinct muscular layers—an inner circular layer and an outer longitudinal layer. Histologically, the mucosa is characterized by the presence of a stratified squamous epithelium through the majority of its course through the cervical and thoracic portions; however, there is seen a distal, 1 to 2 cm transition to a gastric columnar epithelium, more suited to tolerate repeated insults from gastric contents refluxed into the lumen of the esophagus.

Physiology

The Normal Swallowing Mechanism

The completion of a single swallow involves precise movement and function of approximately 30 muscles and nerves [1]. These neuromuscular groups are not only vital for the complete passage of food from the mouth to the stomach, but also for airway protection during the passage of a food or liquid bolus. Commonly divided into the oral, pharyngeal, and esophageal phases, swallowing dysfunction can lead to a variety of complications including dysphagia, regurgitation, and aspiration. Primary motor disturbances, abnormal upper or lower esophageal sphincters, and collagen vascular diseases can also lead to diverticula, gastroesophageal reflux, stricture, or even malignancies of the esophagus.

Swallowing: Oral Phase

Further subdivided into the oral preparatory and propulsive stages, the oral phase functions to ready a bolus of food or liquid for passage from the oral cavity to the pharynx. A contrast exists between the oral phase of liquid swallowing versus solid food swallowing, characterized in the oral preparatory with sealing of the posterior pharynx by the tongue and soft palate during swallowing of liquids, whereas the cyclical movement of the jaw and palate during chewing requires an open passage between the mouth and pharynx. In the propulsive stage of the oral swallowing mechanism, in the case of liquids, the tongue lifts to meet the hard palate, while the posterior aspect of the tongue simultaneously lowers away from the soft palate propelling the bolus posteriorly into the pharynx.

Solid food boluses are better described via a staged transport model in the oral phase, termed the "Process Model of Feeding" [2]. In stage 1 of this model, the tongue carries the food to the surface of the lower teeth for food processing via mastication, a process which requires cyclical motion of the jaw, tongue, palate, and hyoid bone in a coordinated fashion in order to adequately process the bolus [3]. Stage 2 transport is initiated by the anterior tongue meeting the hard palate and propelling the bolus posteriorly to the pharynx, mirroring the propulsive stage for liquids. Importantly, dysfunction/discoordination in the oral phase of both solids (uncoordinated movement of the jaw and tongue) and liquids (inability to form an adequate seal between the posterior tongue and soft palate) can lead to premature entry of a food bolus in the pharynx leading to complications such as choking, regurgitation, and aspiration.

Swallowing: Pharyngeal Phase and Function of the Upper Esophageal Sphincter

The pharyngeal phase is a short, coordinated phase, which generally is complete within a single-second timeframe. This phase involves both food passage through the pharynx and the upper esophageal sphincter and functions to protect the airway as the bolus passes through the pharynx. During this phase, as the food or liquid bolus meets the pharynx, the soft palate elevates to cover the nasal passages and prevent entry into the nose. Simultaneously, the posterior tongue retracts to force the bolus against the structure of the pharynx, while the pharyngeal musculature contracts in a superior to inferior sequence to drive the bolus downward. Dysfunction in this phase of swallowing carries a risk for aspiration secondary to inadequate bolus passage through the pharynx and insufficient protection of the airway during this process.

Important to a discussion of esophageal physiology, this phase also includes the opening of the upper esophageal sphincter, which remains closed at rest [4]. There are three distinct factors, which impact the adequate relaxation and opening of the upper esophageal sphincter including relaxation of the cricopharyngeus, contraction of suprahyoid and thyrohyoid musculature (allowing the laryngeal complex to be pulled anteriorly), and sufficient pressure from the incoming bolus. The relaxation of the upper esophageal sphincter is unique as it requires active opening via contraction of the suprahyoid and relaxation of the thyrohyoid musculature rather than a passive opening process [5].

Swallowing: Esophageal Phase and the Lower Esophageal Sphincter

The esophageal phase is characterized by the passage of a food bolus along the length of the esophagus toward the gastroesophageal junction. In contrast to the pharyngeal phase, the esophageal phase of swallowing is a process of peristalsis, wherein control is regulated by the function of the autonomic nervous system. This difference in the function of swallowing is mirrored in anatomic changes via changes in the muscular composition of the esophagus— the pharyngeal phase takes place primarily in the pharynx and cervical esophagus, which is primarily striated muscle (under conscious control), whereas the thoracic esophagus demonstrates a transition to smooth muscle (under autonomic control). After a bolus is passed through the upper esophageal sphincter, a peristaltic wave is ultimately responsible for carrying the bolus through the esophagus to the lower esophageal sphincter, at which time the food bolus finally passes into the stomach, terminating the swallowing mechanism.

Peristaltic contractions can be categorized as either primary (initiated by a swallow) or secondary (initiated by distension of the esophagus). Tertiary contractions have also been described as nonprogressive, nonperistaltic, monophasic, or multiphasic, simultaneous waves. These represent uncoordinated contractions of smooth muscle responsible for esophageal spasm. It is believed that both the circular and longitudinal layers of the muscularis propria play distinct roles in peristalsis. While the circular musculature serves to contract and force the food bolus toward the stomach, it is hypothesized that the longitudinal layer serves to shorten the esophagus and increase the diameter of the esophagus ahead of an oncoming bolus [6]. Immediately following relaxation of the upper esophageal sphincter, the lower esophageal sphincter relaxes and a contraction wave is generated sequentially along the esophageal body until it reaches the lower esophageal sphincter. Complex neuronal interactions along the length of the esophagus are responsible for this contraction. The amplitude and frequency of contractions are modified by a number of factors including temperature, bolus size, and viscosity. Additionally, in well-spaced swallows, the esophageal contraction responds in a 1:1 ratio, whereas swallows taken in rapid succession will inhibit contraction until the final swallow in a sequence. It is believed that these modifications are mediated by vasovagal and neuromuscular reflexes.

The lower esophageal sphincter (LES) marks an important limiting factor in the speed and completeness of the esophageal phase of swallowing and representing an important pathophysiologic landmark in foregut disorders including gastroesophageal reflux and achalasia. The LES, composed of portions of the esophagus, stomach, and diaphragmatic crura, has a resting pressure, which ranges between 15 and 35 mmHg. Peristaltic waves alone do not generate enough force to open the LES. Vagal-mediated relaxation of the LES occurs in increments of approximately 5 to 10 s to allow passage of a food bolus, starting at the initiation of the peristaltic wave and remaining in the relaxed position for several seconds following passage of a bolus; however, there are also spontaneous relaxations of the LES, which occur intermittently and remain a common cause of gastroesophageal reflux disease [7].

Complex Innervation and Neuronal Control of the Esophagus and Esophageal Peristalsis

As previously discussed, the upper esophageal sphincter is composed of striated muscle fibers stemming from both the cricopharyngeus muscles and the esophagus. This sphincter complex receives its innervation from the glossopharyngeal nerve, branches of the vagus nerve, portions of the ansa cervicalis, and sympathetic innervation from a portion of the cervical ganglion. Motor function of the upper esophageal sphincter is primarily derived from the vagus nerve, with lower motor neurons located in the nucleus ambiguus, via the superior laryngeal and recurrent laryngeal nerve branches [8]. It is the swallow mechanism and introduction of a food bolus (swallow-induced peristalsis), which activates the lower motor neuron of the nucleus ambiguus of the brainstem, which allows for peristalsis of the striated muscle of the upper esophagus and the function of the upper esophageal sphincter [9]. While a number of neuropeptides have been shown to be present at the endplate of these motor neurons, acetylcholine acting on nicotinic receptors is thought to predominate the motor function of the sphincter [10].

Esophageal peristalsis is regulated by autonomic nerves located in the intramural enteric nervous system. Derived from both vagal motor efferent fibers and sympathetic inputs, this plexus is located between the inner circular and outer longitudinal smooth muscle layers of the esophagus. It is widely accepted that this plexus contains both excitatory and inhibitory neurons, which result in either the synchronized contraction, or relaxation, of the esophageal body. Both the excitatory contractile and inhibitory neurons in this plexus do appear to be innervated by separate sets of preganglionic vagal fibers [11]. Peristalsis of the esophagus is the result of precise, coordinated movement between the inner circular and outer longitudinal muscular layers of the esophagus controlled by these neural inputs.

The LES, located at the distal end of the thoracic esophagus, is innervated by both vagal parasympathetic and splanchnic sympathetic nerve fibers. It is important to note that it is the vagal input that is vital for the reflexive relaxation required for the passage of a bolus through the sphincter [12]. Based on several studies into the neuronal control of the LES, it has become apparent that the resting tone of the LES is primarily myogenic in nature with excitatory input from the vagus nerve. However, the vagus nerve also provides an inhibitory effect on the sphincter eliciting relaxation. This has been supported by studies demonstrating that vagotomy results in contraction of the LES, while stimulation of vagal efferents results in LES relaxation [13].

References

1. Matsuo K, Palmer J. Coordination of mastication, swallowing and breathing. Jpn Dent Sci Rev. 2009;45:31–40.
2. Palmer J, Rudin N, Lara G, Crompton A. Coordination of mastication and swallowing. Dysphagia. 1992;7:187–200.
3. Hiiemae K, Palmer J. Food transport and bolus formation during complete feeding sequences on foods of different initial consistency. Dysphagia. 1999;14:31–42.
4. Cook I, Dodds W, Dantas R, Massey B, Kern M, Lang I, et al. Opening mechanisms of the human upper esophageal sphincter. Am J Physiol. 1989;257:G748–59.
5. Shaw D, Cook I, Gabb M, Holloway R, Simula M, Panagopoulos V, Dent J. Influence of normal aging on oral-pharyngeal and upper esophageal sphincter function during swallowing. Am J Physiol. 1995;268:389–96.
6. Wood J. Physiology of the enteric nervous system. In: Physiology of the gastrointestinal tract; 1987. p. 67–109.
7. Allaix M, Patti M. The esophagus from pathophysiology to treatment. In: Reference module in biomedical sciences. Elsevier; 2014.
8. Mittal RK. Motor function of the pharynx, esophagus, and its sphincters. San Rafael, CA: Morgan & Claypool Life Sciences; 2011.
9. Goyal RK, Chaudhury A. Physiology of normal esophageal motility. J Clin Gastroenterol. 2008;42:610–9.
10. Sivarao D, Goyal R. Functional anatomy and physiology of the upper esophageal sphincter. Am J Med. 2000;108:27S–37S.
11. Mittal RK. Regulation and dysregulation of esophageal peristalsis by the integrated function of circular and longitudinal muscle layers in health and disease. Am J Physiol. 2016;311:431–43.
12. Hornby P, Abrahams T. Central control of lower esophageal sphincter relaxation. Am J Med. 2000;108:90–8.
13. Goyal R, Rattan S. Nature of the vagal inhibitory innervation to the lower esophageal sphincter. J Clin Investig. 1975;55:1119–26.

Anatomy and Physiology of the Stomach

2

Jenna Borys and James Kurtz

Anatomy

The stomach is the most proximal abdominal organ of the alimentary tract. It is fixed proximally at the GE junction and distally by the retroperitoneal attachments of the proximal duodenum [1]. Many surgeons divide the stomach into two units: proximal and distal gastric units. The proximal unit includes the distal esophagus, esophageal hiatus, and the proximal stomach—all of which incorporate the gastroesophageal junction and lie at the level of the 11th or 12th thoracic vertebra. The distal gastric unit contains the gastric antrum, pylorus, and first portion of the duodenum [2].

The stomach is composed of several anatomic divisions, as shown in Fig. 2.1. The gastric cardia is the portion of the stomach

J. Borys
Department of Surgery, Grant Medical Center, Columbus, OH, USA
e-mail: Jenna.Borys@Ohiohealth.com

J. Kurtz (✉)
Valley Forge Surgical Associates, Phoenixville, PA, USA
e-mail: James.Kurtz@towerhealth.org

A. D. Patel et al. (eds.), *The SAGES Manual of Physiologic Evaluation of Foregut Diseases*,
https://doi.org/10.1007/978-3-031-39199-6_2

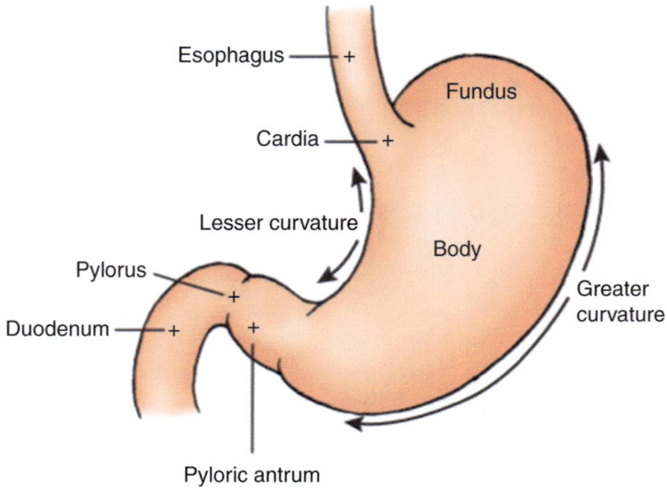

Fig. 2.1 Divisions of the stomach. (From Yeo C: Shackelford's surgery of the alimentary tract, ed. 8, Philadelphia, 2019, Elsevier)

that extends just distal to the gastroesophageal junction. The fundus is the portion of the stomach above and to the left of the GE junction. As the esophagus enters the abdomen at an oblique angle, the position of the fundus creates an acute "angle of His." This forms an internal flap valve that helps prevent reflux at the lower esophageal sphincter. The corpus or body of the stomach lies between the fundus and the antrum. The antrum transitions into the thicker-walled pylorus, which then transitions distally to the smooth, thin-walled first portion of the duodenum.

Despite the surgical and physiologic relevance, there are no obvious external landmarks to delineate the boundaries between each portion of the stomach. Of important surgical relevance is determining the junction between the body and the antrum, as complete antrectomy is essential for acid-reducing surgery in patients with peptic ulcer disease. Combining techniques from multiple sources best describes the boundary as 2/5 of the distance from the pylorus to the cardia along the lesser curve and 1/8 of the distance from the pylorus to the cardia along the greater curvature [3]. The antrum can also be described as the portion from the angularis incisura (seen as a notch on the lesser curve where the stomach makes a sharp angle to the right) to pylorus. Histologically, the antrum can be confirmed by the lack of chief and parietal cells.

The superior aspect of the stomach is lined by the lesser omentum, a double layer of peritoneum. This omentum extends from the porta hepatis along the lesser curve of the stomach and upward to contribute to the ventral mesentery of the abdominal esophagus. The superior aspect of the lesser omentum makes up the gastrohepatic ligament, containing the left gastric artery and vein, hepatic division of the anterior vagal trunk, anterior and posterior gastric divisions of the vagal trunks (nerves of Laterjet), and lymph nodes [3]. An aberrant left hepatic artery can also be found in the gastrohepatic ligament as it arises from the left gastric artery. The lateral, or dextral, portion of the lesser omentum becomes the hepatoduodenal ligament, which contains the hepatic artery, portal vein, and common bile duct—otherwise known as the portal triad. The medial (left) portion of the lesser omentum gives rise to the gastrophrenic ligament. The pars flaccida is an avascular portion of the gastrohepatic ligament overlying the caudate lobe of the liver that can be entered to expose the right crus of the diaphragm. This allows for posterior dissection and passage of a penrose drain around the distal esophagus to aid in retraction.

The greater omentum is a larger fold of visceral peritoneum that hangs from the greater curvature of the stomach, overlying the anterior surface of the small intestines, and then returns to ascend to the transverse colon. Since it is folded on itself, it contains four layers of visceral peritoneum. The greater omentum contains the left and right epiploic arteries along the greater curvature of the stomach. Division of the avascular plane between the greater omentum and transverse mesocolon permits entrance into the lesser sac and visualization of the posterior surface of the stomach and anterior surface of the pancreatic body and tail.

Complete visualization of the posterior surface of the stomach often requires the division of short gastric arteries to aid in mobilization.

The outermost portion of the stomach is covered by the peritoneum, which forms the serosa of the stomach. Moving internally, the next layer of the stomach is the muscularis propria or muscularis externa, which is composed of three layers of smooth muscle, an outer longitudinal, middle circular, and inner oblique layer. The middle circular layer is noted to be the only complete muscle layer of the stomach wall. The Auerbach myenteric nerve plexus lies within the layers of the muscularis externa. The submucosa overlies the muscularis externa and is a collagen-rich layer of connective tissue. Within the submucosa is a rich blood supply with extensive anastomosis and collateral circulation in addition to the Meissner plexus of autonomic nerves. The submucosa is the strength layer of the gastric wall. The mucosa of the stomach is comprised of surface epithelium, lamina propria, and muscularis mucosa. It is this histologic layer that marks the microscopic boundary between invasive and noninvasive gastric carcinoma.

The microscopic anatomy of the stomach helps delineate the functionality of the stomach. The mucosa of the stomach is lined by simple columnar glandular epithelium composed of surface mucous cells. The luminal surface contains gastric pits, which further contain the gastric glands that are responsible for the physiologic functions of the stomach. Within gastric pits, there are three types of glands: cardiac, parietal, and antral glands.

Cardiac glands are found adjacent to the esophagus and contain mucous, endocrine, and undifferentiated cells, but do not contain parietal or chief cells. Parietal glands are found within the fundus and the body of the stomach and contain parietal cells, which are the sites of hydrochloric acid production. Parietal glands also contain chief cells, which represent the site of pepsinogen synthesis and secretion. Antral glands occupy the mucosa of the distal stomach and pylorus. The presence of gastrin cells is the distinguishing feature of antral glands.

Blood Supply, Lymphatics, and Innervation

Blood Supply

The stomach is richly vascularized with extensive collateralization from the four main arteries: left and right gastric arteries and left and right gastroepiploic arteries, depicted in Fig. 2.2. The left gastric artery is the first major branch, origi-

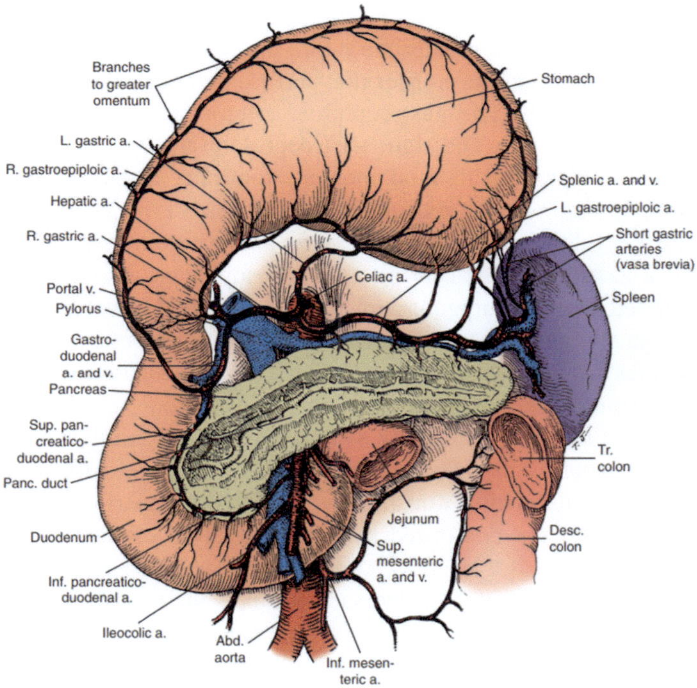

Fig. 2.2 Vascular supply of the foregut. The stomach is shown reflected cephalad and the pancreatic duct is exposed. (From Yeo C: Shackelford's surgery of the alimentary tract, ed. 8, Philadelphia, 2019, Elsevier)

nating from the celiac trunk in approximately 90% of individuals. The left gastric artery travels along the lesser curve of the stomach, providing 1–3 esophageal branches as it travels to the gastric cardia [4]. The right gastric artery most commonly branches off the proper hepatic artery, but, alternatively, may branch off the left hepatic artery or common hepatic artery. The right gastric artery also travels along the lesser curvature of the stomach and eventually anastomosis with the left gastric artery. Traveling along the greater curvature, the left gastroepiploic artery typically branches from the splenic artery and the right gastroepiploic artery most commonly branches from the gastroduodenal artery. The right gastroepiploic artery anastomoses along the greater curvature and each epiploic artery supplies short gastric arteries that perfuse the greater curvature of the stomach. The gastroepiploic arteries also supply the greater omentum. The right gastroepiploic artery deserves a special mention for its fundamental importance in foregut surgery. In settings of total or near-total gastrectomy, the right gastroepiploic artery will often serve as the sole blood supply for a gastric conduit serving as a neoesophagus. It is recommended that all surgeons aim to preserve this vessel during foregut surgery of any kind. The extensive vascular supply ensures a rich collateral network that allows adequate stomach perfusion, even with ligation of three out of four vessels [5]. This fact has led to the study of ischemic conditioning prior to esophagectomy to improve the neovascularization of the new conduit. This also, unfortunately, means that gastric hemorrhage cannot be controlled by simple ligation of the gastric artery.

Venous drainage of the stomach parallels the arterial flow in most cases, with the left and right gastric arteries draining into the portal vein, the right gastroepiploic artery draining into the superior mesenteric vein, and the left gastroepiploic draining into the splenic vein.

Lymphatics

Lymphatics of the stomach are divided into four zones, as noted below [2]. Zone III, the superior gastric zone, is the largest area of drainage. Despite the described zones, it should be noted that gastric cancers may metastasize to any of the four nodal groups, regardless of the location of the cancer. Nodal metastasis is the most important prognostic factor regarding curable gastric cancer and is the best predictor of recurrence and overall survival [6]. The extent of lymphadenectomy varies between Eastern and Western countries, but given the important prognostic implications, this topic is subject to ongoing research.

Zone I: Inferior gastric → drains into subpyloric and omental nodes.

Zone II: Splenic → drains into pancreaticosplenic nodes.

Zone III: Superior gastric → drains into superior gastric nodes.

Zone IV: Hepatic → drains into suprapyloric nodes.

Innervation

The stomach receives both parasympathetic and sympathetic innervations. The sympathetic innervation originates from the T5–T10 thoracic splanchnic nerves that reach the celiac plexus. This innervation conducts afferent impulses that mediate sensation and pain.

Parasympathetic innervation is provided by the vagus nerve. As the vagus nerve descends inferiorly through the thorax, the left and right vagal nerves travel parallel with the esophagus. Both trunks divide into several branches around the esophagus, several centimeters distal to the tracheal bifurcation. These branches then coalesce above the esophagus hiatus, forming a periesophageal plexus. From this plexus, the left and right vagal trunks divide as they pass through the esophageal hiatus. The left vagus nerve is found along the anterior surface of the esophagus, and the right vagus nerve travels posteriorly, lying between the esophagus and the aorta. This anatomic arrangement is often remembered with the acronym "LARP" (left anterior, right posterior). A truncal vagotomy is when both the right and left vagus nerves are divided above the level of the GE junction.

Most often at the level of the abdominal esophagus, the left vagus nerve gives off a hepatic branch to the liver, which travels within the lesser omentum and innervates the liver and biliary tract. The remaining left vagal fibers travel along the lesser curve of the stomach as the anterior nerve of Latarjet, typically identified 0.5–1.0 cm from the lesser curvature. Anywhere from 2 to 12 branches supply the anterior stomach wall.

The right, or posterior, vagal nerve branches into the celiac division and innervates the posterior surface of the stomach. The criminal nerve of Grassi is the first branch from the right/posterior nerve and is known for being a potential cause of recurrent ulcers when left undivided in vagotomies. Division of right and left vagus nerves distal to the celiac and hepatic branches is described as a selective vagotomy. Highly selective vagotomy is accomplished by selective division of the vagus nerves, known as the crow's feet, which supply the corpus and fundus while maintaining more proximal innervation.

Physiology

The functionality of the stomach is dependent on the various peptides that are released from specialized cells. Gastrin is produced by G cells, located in the gastric antrum. Gastrin is the major hormonal regulator of the gastric phase of acid secretion. Secretion of gastrin has trophic effects on the parietal cells and gastric enterochromaffin cells. Parietal cells, which produce hydrochloric acid, are stimulated by gastrin, acetylcholine from the vagus nerve, and histamine from enterochromaffin-like cells. Therefore, via different mechanisms, acid secretion can be decreased by surgical removal of G cells with antrectomy, vagotomy, and/or medications.

As food enters the stomach, the resultant gastric distention activates cholinergic neurons and stimulates gastrin release. As the food bolus empties through the pylorus, gastric distention decreases. This leads to the cessation of cholinergic stimulation, and the gastrin stimulates the production of somatostatin, which, when released, provides negative feedback for gastrin release.

Gastrin is inhibited in environments of pH less than 3. A gastric pH greater than 3 will lead to hypergastrinemia. This is seen in patients with pernicious anemia in the setting of chronic achlorhydria, which leads to increased gastrin release. While the mechanism has not been definitively elucidated, chronic gastric infection with *Helico pylori* infection has been shown to cause increased gastrin release. It is thought that the presence of proinflammatory cytokines has been shown to stimulate gastrin release. Hypergastrinemia can also be seen in patients being treated with acid-reducing agents such as proton pump inhibitors due to the lack of negative feedback on gastrin release by luminal acid. The lack of acid leads to a lack of somatostatin, which leads to a lack of inhibition of G cells and increased, uninhibited gastrin release. Hypergastrinemia can also be seen in patients with retained gastric antrum or Zollinger–Ellison syndrome.

Somatostatin is considered an inhibitor of gastric peptides. Somatostatin is produced by D cells located in the fundus and antrum. Somatostatin release is stimulated by antral acidification. Somatostatin has an inhibitory effect on the secretion of acid from parietal cells. Somatostatin release is inhibited by acetylcholine from vagal fibers.

Histamine is stored in the acidic granules of enterochromaffin cells and stimulates parietal cells to release hydrochloric acid.

Pepsinogen is a precursor to pepsin, a proteolytic enzyme secreted by chief cells and functions to initiate protein digestion.

Intrinsic factor is produced by the parietal cells within the gastric mucosa. The release of intrinsic factor is necessary for the absorption of cobalamin (vitamin B12) from the ileal mucosa. This is of clinical relevance, as total gastrectomy can lead to cobalamin malabsorption due to loss of intrinsic factor. Atrophic gastritis can lead to similar effects due to a lack of intrinsic factor production by the gastric mucosa.

Gastric bicarbonate is produced by the surface mucus cells that line the gastric lumen.

Gastric acid secretion is ultimately regulated by acetylcholine, gastrin, and histamine. Receptors for each of these are located along the basolateral membrane of the parietal cell. Ultimately, stimulation of any of these receptors activates that parietal cell proton pump, an H+/K+-ATPase that exchanges cytosolic hydrogen ions (H+) for luminal potassium cations (K+). Parietal cells also have receptors for somatostatin, which serves to inhibit acid secretion. Gastric acid production can be prevented by receptor antagonist for each of the three primary stimulants listed above.

There are three phases of gastric acid secretion: the cephalic, gastric, and intestinal phases.

The gastric phase begins with the sight, smell, thought, or taste of food, which triggers the release of acetylcholine. This phase accounts for approximately 20% of gastric acid secretion. The release of acetylcholine also stimulates histamine release from enterochromaffin cells, HCl release from parietal cells, and gastrin release from the G cells. The gastric phase starts when food enters the gastric lumen, and the antral distension triggers gastrin release. This phase accounts for 30–40% of the acid production. The intestinal phase is activated when a food bolus enters the small intestine. This phase accounts for 10% of the secretory response to a meal. Eventually, luminal acidification will incite D cells to produce somatostatin and begin the inhibitory effect on acid secretion.

References

1. Teitelbaum EN, Hungness ES, Mahvi DM. Stomach. In: Townsend CM, editor. Sabiston textbook of surgery. 20th ed. Pennsylvania: Elsevier; 2016. p. 1188–201.
2. Skandalakis LJ, et al. Surgical anatomy and technique. New York: Springer; 2009. p. 285–94.
3. Brenkman HJF, van der Wielen N, Ruurda JP, et al. Surgical anatomy of the omental bursa and the stomach based on a minimally invasive

approach: different approaches and technical steps to resection and lymphadenectomy. J Thorac Dis. 2017;9(Suppl 8):S809–16.
4. Mirilas P, Loukas M, Skandalakis LJ. Anatomic considerations in gastroduodenal surgery. In: Fisher JE, editor. Fisher's mastery of surgery. 7th ed. Pennsylvania: Wolters Kluwer; 2017. p. 44136–5042.
5. Mulholland MW. Gastric anatomy. In: Mulholland MW, editor. Greenfield's surgery scientific principles and practice. 6th ed. Pennsylvania: Wolters Kluwer; 2017. p. 36715–7164.
6. Lirosi M, Biondi A, Ricci R. Surgical anatomy of gastric lymphatic drainage. Transl Gastroenterol Hepatol. 2017;2:14. https://doi.org/10.21037/tgh.2016.12.06.

Effect of Obesity on Foregut Physiology

3

Ryan Lamm and Francesco Palazzo

Introduction

Obesity has reached epidemic proportions and affects the health of children and adults throughout the world. It is defined as a body mass index (BMI) > 30 kg/m^2 for adults or greater than the 95th percentile of BMI according to the 2000 Centers for Disease Control and Prevention growth charts [1]. The prevalence of obesity has been on the rise during the last two decades, with 40% of the adult population in the United States and 13% of the adult population worldwide currently considered obese [1, 2]. Obesity is a predisposing risk factor for several morbid conditions, and research is accumulating on the pathways that link chronic weight gain to the onset of several pathological states. The cost of said comorbidities has been estimated to have an impact on the US annual healthcare cost of $147–210 billion [2].

Obesity has an impact on several aspects of human physiology that are critical to the normal functioning of the GI tract. Several

R. Lamm · F. Palazzo (✉)
Department of Surgery, Thomas Jefferson University Hospital, Philadelphia, PA, USA
e-mail: Ryan.lamm@jefferson.edu; Francesco.palazzo@jefferson.edu

A. D. Patel et al. (eds.), *The SAGES Manual of Physiologic Evaluation of Foregut Diseases*,
https://doi.org/10.1007/978-3-031-39199-6_3

factors are suspected to be implicated in these changes, including but not limited to proportion of visceral body fat, intra-abdominal pressure, dietary composition (high-fat diet), changes in gastrointestinal hormonal levels (leptin, ghrelin, GLP-1), and diabetes mellitus [3, 4]. Changes in the microbiome are also being studied for their potential role in altered function of the GI tract in obese patients, but appear to play a more significant role in the distal portions [5]. In this chapter, we will focus on these interactions as it pertains to the anatomic and physiologic integrity of the esophagus and stomach.

Esophagus

Esophageal peristalsis and functionality of the lower esophageal sphincter (LES) have been suspected to be altered in obese and morbidly obese patients for several years [6]. Kuper et al. in 2009, using traditional manometric testing, identified morbidly obese patients as having dysfunction of the LES and altered esophageal motility, even in the absence of GERD symptoms [6].

The advent of high-resolution manometry (HRM) and the methodological classification of esophageal dysmotility disorders with the Chicago Classification allow for more reliable findings with reproducible/consistent nomenclature [3].

Esophageal Dysmotility

While there are numerous factors responsible for the onset of dysmotility disorders, obesity has been implicated in the dysfunction at numerous critical portions of normal esophageal peristalsis (see Fig. 3.1).

Esophageal dysmotility is common in morbidly obese patients. Utilizing HRM, Kristo et al. found that the prevalence of esophageal motility disorders, as classified by the Chicago algorithm, was 34% among obese patients [7]. In this study, a significant proportion of the disorders were outflow obstruction and a novel hypercontractile disorder, which they referred to as jackhammer esophagus. These findings mirrored previous studies, which found

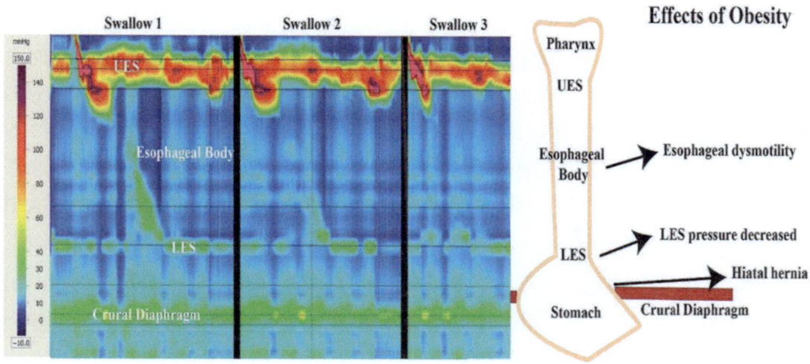

Fig. 3.1 High-resolution manometry (HRM) and the effects of morbid obesity. *UES* upper esophageal sphincter, *LES* lower esophageal sphincter

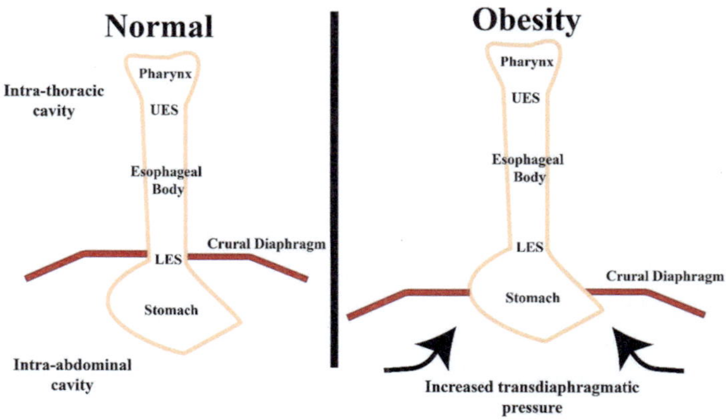

Fig. 3.2 Increased transdiaphragmatic pressure causing hiatal hernia. *UES* upper esophageal sphincter, *LES* lower esophageal sphincter

high rates of dysmotility, specifically hypercontractile abnormalities, in obese patients [8, 9].

The presumed mechanism of esophageal dysmotility arises from the increased pressure from excess adipose tissue characteristic of obese patients [7]. This creates a gradient, which exceeds the normal force from the intra-abdominal cavity and intra-thoracic cavity, a phenomenon referred to as increased transdiaphragmatic pressure (TP) (see Fig. 3.2). The increased pressure opposes the forward-flowing peristalsis, which may cause compensatory increases in contractile forces resulting in dysmotility or simply disrupting the natural peristalsis. More evidence needs to be elucidated for the exact mechanism. However, some speculate esophageal motility derangements are secondary to the measurable changes in LES pressure, presence of hiatal hernias, and increased gastric pressure, all of which are discussed later in this chapter.

The increasing use of bariatric surgery with the potential impact that some of the more common procedures (sleeve gastrectomy) may have on esophageal motility makes it critically important for clinicians and patients to have a better understanding of esophageal motility of morbidly obese patients at baseline.

There is evidence that a variety of dysmotility disorders can occur after or as a result of bariatric surgical procedures [10]. These are described in dedicated chapters later in this manual (Chaps. 27, 29, 41, and 42).

Integrity of the Lower Esophageal Sphincter (LES)

Perhaps the most profound of the effects of obesity is its alteration of the lower esophageal sphincter (LES) and the implications of those alterations. Normal resting pressure at the LES is 10–26 mmHg [11]. During swallowing, LES pressure initially rises to 45 mmHg and then slowly relaxes to the resting pressure over 2–3 s [11]. LES length, defined as the distance between the upper and lower borders of LES, is usually in the range of 3–4 cm in healthy adults [12]. This pressure and length are adequate to protect the esophagus from refluxing acid produced in the stomach.

In obese patients, due largely to the increased transdiaphragmatic pressure, LES resting pressure and length are both significantly decreased. HRM LES resting pressures in obese patients are significantly decreased, measuring $\leq$6 mmHg [13–18]. Jung et al. showed that obesity also contributes to LES length shortening to $\leq$1 cm [19]. Both of these contribute to the breakdown of protection from esophageal reflux from the stomach, resulting in gastroesophageal reflux disease (GERD) and its sequelae. This problem is so prevalent in the obese patient population that when studied Klaus et al. found that patients with obesity were twice as likely to have mechanically defective LES complexes as compared to healthy adults [13]. Besides resting LES pressures, one study found that there were independently increased LES relaxations in obese patients during the postprandial phase [6]. Consequently, the prevalence of LES disruption is evident in the obese patient population.

Integrity of the Hiatal Crura

As alluded to earlier, obesity increases transdiaphragmatic pressure (TP) both at rest and during strain. We have described in the previous section the impact this has on the contractility of the esophagus. In addition, chronically increased TP can result in macroscopic anatomic changes to the diaphragmatic crura resulting in the development of a hiatal hernia. A hiatal hernia is defined as the migration of the LES and/or stomach and, in some cases, additional intra-abdominal organs, normally located below the diaphragm through the hiatus in the diaphragm and above the diaphragm [20].

Rates of hiatal hernias in patients having a BMI ≥ 30 vary based on the modality of diagnosis with up to 23% being diagnosed on esophagogastroduodenoscopy (EGD) [20] and 40% on upper gastrointestinal (UGI) contrast studies [21]. Data from preoperative bariatric EGD studies have found hiatal hernias in up to 52% of patients with BMI ≥ 30 [22, 23]. Evidence shows that higher TP is directly correlated with increasing BMI and waist circumference [13, 24]. Most current data illustrate correlative data between obesity and hiatal hernia occurrence. However, recent models in dogs show that the presence of increased abdominal pressure increased the diameter of the hiatal opening in the diaphragm, and esophageal shortening can disrupt the integrity of the LES/crura and force the foregut into the chest causing the migration or hernia [25] (see Fig. 3.2).

Stomach

Some of the obesity-related factors that play a key role in inducing changes to the esophageal function—TP—also have an impact on the stomach. Higher intra-abdominal pressure increases intragastric pressure, which contributes to gastric contents physically crossing the EGJ [14, 26] and contributes to the propulsion of the stomach from the intra-abdominal cavity into the intra-thoracic cavity [21]. However, there are a few stomach-specific pathophysiologic changes worth noting in the obese population.

Regulation of Appetite

Ghrelin is an orexigenic hormone produced by endocrine cells in the stomach after stimulation by the vagus nerve causing an increase in appetite [27]. Obesity has been shown to be correlated with higher levels of ghrelin, proposed to be the result of altered stimulation from the vagus nerve in obese patients [27–29]. The overall effect is appetite stimulation, increased intake, and weight gain. This is supported by the fact that, in most bariatric procedures, the exclusion of the fundus results in decreased ghrelin secretion, which contributes to weight loss [29]. In addition, studies have shown decreased satiety and feelings of fullness correlated with altered appetite-regulating hormone pathways, which include feedback from the stomach in obese patients [30].

Gastric Size and Motility

Obesity also affects the size and function of the stomach itself. One large study involving >500 patients showed that obese patients had larger fasting gastric volume [31]. In addition, some studies have shown that patients with obesity have larger stomachs on ultrasound, CT scan, and at direct visualization at the time of surgery [32]. These data were correlated with a delayed feeling of satiety, as well as increased levels of hunger leading to higher consumption [31].

Gastric motility appears to be altered in obesity as well. The overall effect of obesity on motility is controversial and likely multifactorial. On one hand, some studies have observed increased gastric emptying times in obese patients, which is believed to contribute to late satiety [31] and could very well predispose to increase gastroesophageal reflux. On the other hand, diabetes mellitus (DM) contributes to decreased contractility via gastroparesis, which is thought to arise from damage to the vagus nerve [33]. Krishnasamy et al. found that 20–50% of diabetic patients suffer from gastroparesis [34]. Likely, both of these pathologic states exist simultaneously and the overall effect is different for each patient. To complicate things further, evidence exists to suggest an even stronger role of hormonal regulation on motility than previously thought [35].

Obesity as a Risk Factor for Defined Pathologic States

Gastroesophageal Reflux Disease (GERD)

All of the aforementioned alterations in anatomy and physiology help contribute to an overall increased acid/alkaline exposure of the esophagus in the obese patient. Herbella et al. showed that BMI was independently associated with the severity of GERD and that in most morbidly obese patients with GERD, reflux occurred despite normal or hypertensive esophageal motility [36]. Obese patients have a threefold increase in total acid exposure events (defined as a number of times at which $pH < 4$ at LES) [37, 38]. This relationship has also been shown to be reversible with weight loss both via lifestyle modifications and bariatric surgery [39]. In other words, a portion of GERD in obese patients can be attributed to increased transdiaphragmatic pressure; however, the majority of obese patients have a pathophysiology completely independent of isolated LES dysfunction (which argues against traditional anti-reflux surgery being effective in this patient population). The pathologic effect of GERD is exacerbated by the fact that esophageal dysmotility, present in many obese patients, is associated with decreased acid clearance, which increases total acid exposure time [24].

Barrett's Esophagus (BE)

Linked to higher rates of GERD, perhaps the most consequential physiologic change IN the foregut associated with obesity is Barrett's esophagus (BE). BE is the metaplastic change in mucosal cells lining the lower portion of the esophagus from stratified squamous to simple columnar epithelium, a premalignant condition [40].

Studies have shown that while the rate of BE in the non-obese population is close to 1.2%, it can reach as high as 9% in obese patients [40, 41]. Other studies have shown that in obese women, every 5 kg/m^2 increase in BMI leads to a 35% increase in the incidence of BE [39].

While all of the aforementioned mechanisms of increased acid exposure contribute to this higher incidence of BE in obese patients, other theories including decreased sensitivity to acid exposure in obese patients leading to longer exposure times have been proposed, also called silent reflux [42].

Esophageal Adenocarcinoma (EAC)

With increased levels of BE reported in the obese population, it is no surprise that higher levels of esophageal adenocarcinoma (EAC) also exist as BE is a significant risk factor for the development of EAC [43, 44] and cancers of the esophageal body and stomach cardia [39].

Recent studies have also proposed that the local microbiome of the foregut created by obesity and the hormonal changes it creates could be a contributing factor leading to EAC; however, more research into the topic is required [5].

Conclusion

As the prevalence and incidence of obesity continue to steadily increase, consideration of the effects of this disease on the anatomy and physiology of the foregut will become essential in health care going forward. Clinicians caring for these patients will need to be able to utilize a broader set of diagnostic tools and consider more complex pathophysiologic pathways than those that are accepted for non-obese patients. While preventive care for obesity, in the form of lifestyle modifications, remains the gold standard for treating physicians, bariatric surgery to treat obesity and reverse the pathophysiology discussed above is increasing in popularity.

Foregut surgeons who want to properly and comprehensively care for this patient population will need to embrace the importance of bariatric surgical options in the care of some of the disorders traditionally approached with standard—and likely ineffective in obese patients—anti-reflux procedures.

References

1. Hales CM, et al. Prevalence of obesity among adults and youth: United States, 2015-2016. NCHS Data Brief. 2017;288:1–8.
2. Nau P, et al. Surgical management of gastroesophageal reflux disease in the obese patient. Surg Endosc. 2020;34(1):450–7.
3. Mushref MA, Srinivasan S. Effect of high fat-diet and obesity on gastrointestinal motility. Ann Transl Med. 2013;1(2):14.
4. Cote-Daigneault J, et al. Plasma leptin concentrations and esophageal hypomotility in obese patients. Can J Gastroenterol Hepatol. 2015;29(1):49–51.
5. Kaakoush NO, Morris MJ. The oesophageal microbiome: an unexplored link in obesity-associated oesophageal adenocarcinoma. FEMS Microbiol Ecol. 2016;92(10):fiw161.
6. Kuper MA, et al. Dysfunction of the lower esophageal sphincter and dysmotility of the tubular esophagus in morbidly obese patients. Obes Surg. 2009;19(8):1143–9.
7. Kristo I, et al. Modern esophageal function testing and gastroesophageal reflux disease in morbidly obese patients. Obes Surg. 2019;29(11):3536–41.

8. Hong D, et al. Manometric abnormalities and gastroesophageal reflux disease in the morbidly obese. Obes Surg. 2004;14(6):744–9.
9. Suter M, et al. Gastro-esophageal reflux and esophageal motility disorders in morbidly obese patients. Obes Surg. 2004;14(7):959–66.
10. Boules M, et al. Achalasia after bariatric surgery. J Laparoendosc Adv Surg Tech A. 2016;26(6):428–32.
11. Ayazi S, et al. Obesity and gastroesophageal reflux: quantifying the association between body mass index, esophageal acid exposure, and lower esophageal sphincter status in a large series of patients with reflux symptoms. J Gastrointest Surg. 2009;13(8):1440–7.
12. Marshall RE, et al. Esophageal body length, lower esophageal sphincter length, position and pressure in health and disease. Dis Esophagus. 1999;12(4):297–302.
13. Klaus A, Weiss H. Is preoperative manometry in restrictive bariatric procedures necessary? Obes Surg. 2008;18(8):1039–42.
14. Friedenberg FK, et al. The association between gastroesophageal reflux disease and obesity. Am J Gastroenterol. 2008;103(8):2111–22.
15. Schneider JH, et al. Transient lower esophageal sphincter relaxation in morbid obesity. Obes Surg. 2009;19(5):595–600.
16. Tanaka Y, et al. Clinical characteristics associated with esophageal motility function. J Gastroenterol Hepatol. 2016;31(6):1133–40.
17. Burgerhart JS, et al. Nocturnal and daytime esophageal acid exposure in normal-weight, overweight, and obese patients with reflux symptoms. Eur J Gastroenterol Hepatol. 2014;26(1):6–10.
18. Fornari F, et al. Obese patients have stronger peristalsis and increased acid exposure in the esophagus. Dig Dis Sci. 2011;56(5):1420–6.
19. Jung HS, et al. Obesity is associated with increasing esophageal acid exposure in korean patients with gastroesophageal reflux disease symptoms. J Neurogastroenterol Motil. 2013;19(3):338–43.
20. Makiewicz K, et al. Prevalence of upper gastrointestinal pathology in patients with obesity on preoperative endoscopy. JSLS. 2020;24(2):e2020.00021.
21. Che F, et al. Prevalence of hiatal hernia in the morbidly obese. Surg Obes Relat Dis. 2013;9(6):920–4.
22. D'Silva M, et al. High-percentage pathological findings in obese patients suggest that Esophago-gastro-duodenoscopy should be made mandatory prior to bariatric surgery. Obes Surg. 2018;28(9):2753–9.
23. Csendes A, et al. Endoscopic and histologic findings of the foregut in 426 patients with morbid obesity. Obes Surg. 2007;17(1):28–34.
24. Tack J, Pandolfino JE. Pathophysiology of gastroesophageal reflux disease. Gastroenterology. 2018;154(2):277–88.
25. Sivacolundhu RK, Read RA, Marchevsky AM. Hiatal hernia controversies--a review of pathophysiology and treatment options. Aust Vet J. 2002;80(1–2):48–53.

26. Nam SY. Obesity-related digestive diseases and their pathophysiology. Gut Liver. 2017;11(3):323–34.
27. Hunt RH, et al. The stomach in health and disease. Gut. 2015;64(10):1650–68.
28. Swidnicka-Siergiejko AK, et al. Esophageal pH and impedance reflux parameters in relation to body mass index, obesity-related hormones, and bariatric procedures. Pol Arch Intern Med. 2018;128(10):594–603.
29. Browning KN, Fortna SR, Hajnal A. Roux-en-Y gastric bypass reverses the effects of diet-induced obesity to inhibit the responsiveness of central vagal motoneurones. J Physiol. 2013;591(9):2357–72.
30. Delgado-Aros S, et al. Independent influences of body mass and gastric volumes on satiation in humans. Gastroenterology. 2004;126(2):432–40.
31. Acosta A, et al. Quantitative gastrointestinal and psychological traits associated with obesity and response to weight-loss therapy. Gastroenterology. 2015;148(3):537–546 e4.
32. Xing J, Chen JD. Alterations of gastrointestinal motility in obesity. Obes Res. 2004;12(11):1723–32.
33. Miron I, Dumitrascu DL. Gastrointestinal motility disorders in obesity. Acta Endocrinol (Buchar). 2019;15(4):497–504.
34. Krishnasamy S, Abell TL. Diabetic gastroparesis: principles and current trends in management. Diabetes Ther. 2018;9(Suppl 1):1–42.
35. Park MI, Camilleri M. Gastric motor and sensory functions in obesity. Obes Res. 2005;13(3):491–500.
36. Herbella FA, et al. Gastroesophageal reflux disease and obesity. Pathophysiology and implications for treatment. J Gastrointest Surg. 2007;11(3):286–90.
37. El-Serag HB, et al. Obesity is an independent risk factor for GERD symptoms and erosive esophagitis. Am J Gastroenterol. 2005;100(6):1243–50.
38. El-Serag HB, et al. Obesity increases oesophageal acid exposure. Gut. 2007;56(6):749–55.
39. Valezi AC, et al. Gastroesophageal reflux disease in obese patients. J Laparoendosc Adv Surg Tech A. 2018;28(8):949–52.
40. Gorodner V, et al. Gastroesophageal reflux disease and morbid obesity: evaluation and treatment. Updat Surg. 2018;70(3):331–7.
41. Braghetto I, et al. Laparoscopic treatment of obese patients with gastroesophageal reflux disease and Barrett's esophagus: a prospective study. Obes Surg. 2012;22(5):764–72.
42. Ortiz V, et al. Decreased esophageal sensitivity to acid in morbidly obese patients: a cause for concern? Gut Liver. 2017;11(3):358–62.
43. Feakins RM. Obesity and metabolic syndrome: pathological effects on the gastrointestinal tract. Histopathology. 2016;68(5):630–40.
44. Braghetto I, Csendes A. Patients having bariatric surgery: surgical options in morbidly obese patients with Barrett's esophagus. Obes Surg. 2016;26(7):1622–6.

Further Reading

Kristo I, et al. Modern esophageal function testing and gastroesophageal reflux disease in morbidly obese patients. Obes Surg. 2019;29(11):3536–41.

Nam SY. Obesity-related digestive diseases and their pathophysiology. Gut Liver. 2017;11(3):323–34.

Tack J, Pandolfino JE. Pathophysiology of gastroesophageal reflux disease. Gastroenterology. 2018;154(2):277–88.

Valezi AC, et al. Gastroesophageal reflux disease in obese patients. J Laparoendosc Adv Surg Tech A. 2018;28(8):949–52.

Xing J, Chen JD. Alterations of gastrointestinal motility in obesity. Obes Res. 2004;12(11):1723–32.

Part II

Diagnostic Testing: Diagnostic Imaging

4 Esophagram

Elisa J. Furay, Stephanie Doggett, and Francis P. Buckley III

Introduction

Diagnostic investigation of esophageal disorders commonly utilizes pH studies, endoscopy, and high-resolution manometry. The barium esophagram is another important diagnostic tool that tends to be underutilized and misused by surgeons and gastroenterologists. An esophagram combines both static and dynamic imaging techniques to allow for the evaluation of both structural and functional abnormalities within the esophagus and stomach. With specialized protocols, trained clinicians are able to gather important data on esophageal anatomy and even esophageal motility with the correct protocol. This study has the benefit of being noninvasive, inexpensive, and readily available, and it does not require sedation.

In order for this study to have the greatest utility, the radiologist performing it should be trained on standard techniques and protocols, as well as familiar with the imaging findings of varying esophageal diseases. An esophagram combines both single- and

E. J. Furay (✉) · S. Doggett · F. P. BuckleyIII
Dell Medical School, University of Texas at Austin, Austin, TX, USA

A. D. Patel et al. (eds.), *The SAGES Manual of Physiologic Evaluation of Foregut Diseases*,
https://doi.org/10.1007/978-3-031-39199-6_4

double-contrast techniques to give the most comprehensive evaluation of the esophagus. The single-contrast load aids in the dilation of the esophagus and reveals structural abnormalities including masses, strictures, and diverticula. The double-contrast technique utilizes an effervescent agent after ingesting barium, which allows radiologists to see subtle irregularities in esophageal mucosa and improves the diagnostic yield of the study [1–3]. The study also utilizes both single-frame X-rays and fluoroscopy. Fluoroscopy is the more dynamic portion of the study and allows for the evaluation of esophageal motility by taking continuous X-ray images, while the patient performs multiple swallows using different contrast loads with varying consistencies [4]. The most commonly used contrast medium is barium sulfate as it provides improved mucosal detail compared with water-soluble contrasts [5]. There are certain situations in which you would want to evaluate the esophagus with a water-soluble contrast medium and those are discussed later.

How to Perform an Esophagram and Variations in Technique

An esophagram is a multiphasic study, which generally starts with a single-contrast bolus followed by a spot film captured in the upright position 1 min following barium ingestion. This assesses the emptying of the esophagus into the stomach. If the barium has not emptied from the esophagus after 1 minute, then subsequent 2- and 5-min films are taken and compared with the 1-min film. A normal esophagus should empty approximately 250 mL of low-density barium within seconds [6]. If there is significant liquid dysphagia, then the study should conclude the study to prevent patient aspiration. If there is no significant liquid dysphagia, then the radiologist should proceed with the upright double-contrast (also known as air contrast) phase of the study. In this portion, the patient is given an effervescent medium allowing air to fill the lumen of the esophagus and enhance the visualization of the mucosa, which has been coated with barium. This technique improves the sensitivity for detecting subtle mucosal irregularities [7, 8]. This is then followed by the motility portion of the study, where the patient is placed in a semi-prone position and asked to swallow barium. The radiologist images multiple swallows using fluoroscopy and focuses on the end of the barium column to evaluate bolus transit through the esophagus. Previous studies have compared esophageal motility findings on barium esophagram to manometric findings and have shown concordance between a normal manometry and five normal swallows on a properly performed barium esophagram [9, 10]. The next step of the esophagram is a distended esophageal phase, in which the patient drinks a larger bolus of barium in order to distend the esophagus and identify any subtle narrowing along the esophagus. This is again performed in a semi-prone position and is typically evaluated by using fluoroscopy. The patient is then positioned supine and upright until the barium has cleared the esophagus. In order to completely clear the barium from the esophagus, the patient may need to take a few swallows of water. The patient is then again placed horizontally and the esophagus is evaluated with fluoroscopy. If barium is seen in the distal esophagus, then a reflux episode can be inferred. If no barium is seen, some centers perform provocative maneuvers to try and elicit a reflux event [6]. Performing these maneuvers increases the sensitivity of identifying clinically significant reflux [11]. Following evaluation for reflux, the solid food phase of the esophagram begins. The patient ingests a barium tablet, and its movement through the esophagus and into the stomach is evaluated. Stomach emptying is also commonly observed at this time, although much of this interpretation is subjective and should be evaluated formally with a gastric emptying study if specific pathology is suspected.

There have been several slight modifications to the solid food phase of the esophagram to improve the evaluation of esophageal function. Using alternatives to the barium tablet, such as marshmallow or hamburger-impregnated mediums, has been shown to better assess esophageal motility and bolus transport abnormalities [12]. The addition of an alternative solid bolus more accurately assesses esophageal motility because the contraction amplitude of the esophagus is highly dependent on the size and consistency of the bolus [13]. About 14% of patients who demonstrate abnormal transit of liquids will show normal transit of a solid bolus, supporting the need for more viscous mediums in the evaluation of esophageal function [14]. This modification to the classic esophagram has been adopted at many large institutions to better establish esophageal function during the routine workup of foregut disorders, particularly in the evaluation of motility in patients undergoing antireflux surgery.

D'Alessio et al. evaluated patients with esophageal dysmotility demonstrated on manometry who in addition had either GERD and/or symptomatic hiatal hernias. Their group evaluated these patients with specialized esophagography to determine their ability to clear food boluses of different consistencies. This technique observes esophageal peristalsis and emptying in both the prone horizontal and prone slight Trendelenburg position. Patients consumed a single large bolus swallow of barium and were subsequently examined for uninterrupted progression of the contraction wave and complete emptying of the esophagus with two or fewer stripping waves. Each patient was then challenged with a food bolus using a marshmallow followed by a bite of bagel food bolus. Again, normal clearance was defined as the passage of the food bolus with two or fewer stripping motions. In this study, patients with findings of esophageal dysmotility on manometry but normal esophageal clearance on food boluses on esophagography underwent laparoscopic Nissen fundoplication. These patients' outcomes were then compared to patients with normal esophageal motility in manometry who underwent laparoscopic Nissen fundoplication. They found that these two groups had functionally similar outcomes, which suggests that preoperative solid challenge esophagrams can be utilized as a predictor of positive postoperative outcomes in antireflux surgery patients [15].

Diagnostic Implications

GERD

An esophagram is an excellent initial test for patients with a wide variety of esophageal complaints. As the name implies, gastroesophageal reflux disease (GERD) results from the retrograde reflux of caustic gastric juices into the esophagus. These reflux events are able to be captured on an esophagram, and radiologists commonly report gastroesophageal reflux as findings on an esophagram. Serna-Gallegos et al. looked at patients found to have reflux on the esophagram and investigated if they had objective evidence of reflux on pH study. They showed a very poor correlation between reflux reported on the esophagram and objective evidence of acid reflux on pH studies [16]. It is important to remember that the diagnosis of GERD must be made using objective evidence of acid reflux in the form of positive pH study or significant endoscopy findings.

Mucosal Irregularities

Patients with chronic reflux can develop reflux esophagitis, which is irritation of the esophageal mucosa from caustic juices of the stomach leading to mucosal edema and inflammation. This can be identified best on the double-contrast phase of the barium esophagram because of the fine mucosal detail provided. Figure 4.1 demonstrates the grainy appearance of the proximal esophagus seen on an esophagram secondary to edema and inflammation [17].

Peptic strictures are caused by chronic reflux and are most commonly located in the distal esophagus and often above a hiatal hernia. On an esophagram, strictures are best seen during the esophageal distention portion of the study. Ott et al. were able to show that the addition of the esophageal distention phase to the esophagram improved the accuracy of detecting peptic strictures to a nearly 95% sensitivity rate [18]. Some studies suggest that, when performed properly, esophagrams can be as effective as endoscopy for diagnosing peptic strictures or rings [18] (Fig. 4.2).

Barrett's esophagus is a condition in which cells of the distal esophagus undergo metaplastic changes from stratified squamous epithelium to simple columnar epithelium-containing goblet cells. These metaplastic changes increase patients' risk of undergoing dysplastic changes and ultimately developing esophageal adenocarcinoma. The diagnosis of Barrett's esophagus is based on a tissue sampling obtained during endoscopy, but esophagography may be able to identify patients at higher risk for Barrett's esophagus. Gilchrist et al. were able to demonstrate that patients with a high esophageal stricture, ulcer, or reticular mucosal pattern had a 90% chance of having Barrett's mucosa at endoscopy [19]. Although we do not advocate for this as a screening method for intestinal metaplasia, we do recognize that some esophagram

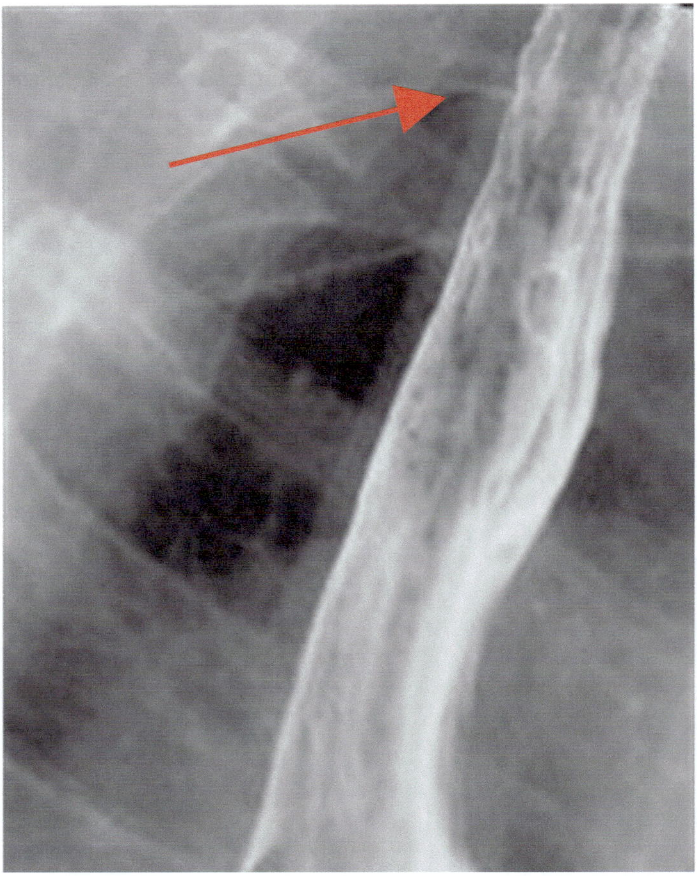

Fig. 4.1 Esophagitis. The red arrow demonstrates the grainy appearance of esophagitis on an esophagram

findings may be suggestive of Barrett's esophagus and may warrant endoscopic evaluation.

Eosinophilic esophagitis (EoE) is a relatively new diagnosis in esophageal pathology. It is characterized by symptoms similar to GERD in association with mucosal biopsy demonstrating 15 eosinophils/HPF in one or more biopsy specimens, absence of pathologic GERD on pH study, and lack of response to high dose PPI therapy [20]. Like Barrett's esophagus, a diagnosis of EoE is

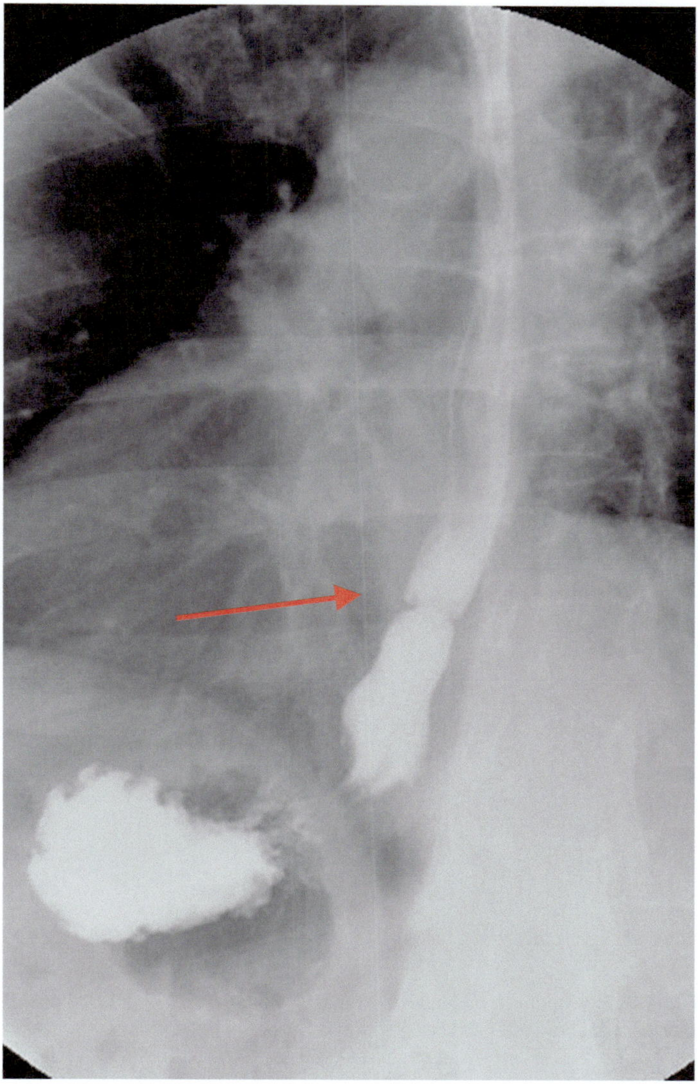

Fig. 4.2 Stricture. Seen here as an abrupt narrowing in the distal esophagus

heavily reliant on tissue sample, but there are some features on an esophagram, which can suggest the presence of EoE. Radiologic features of EoE include the presence of fixed rings, sometimes

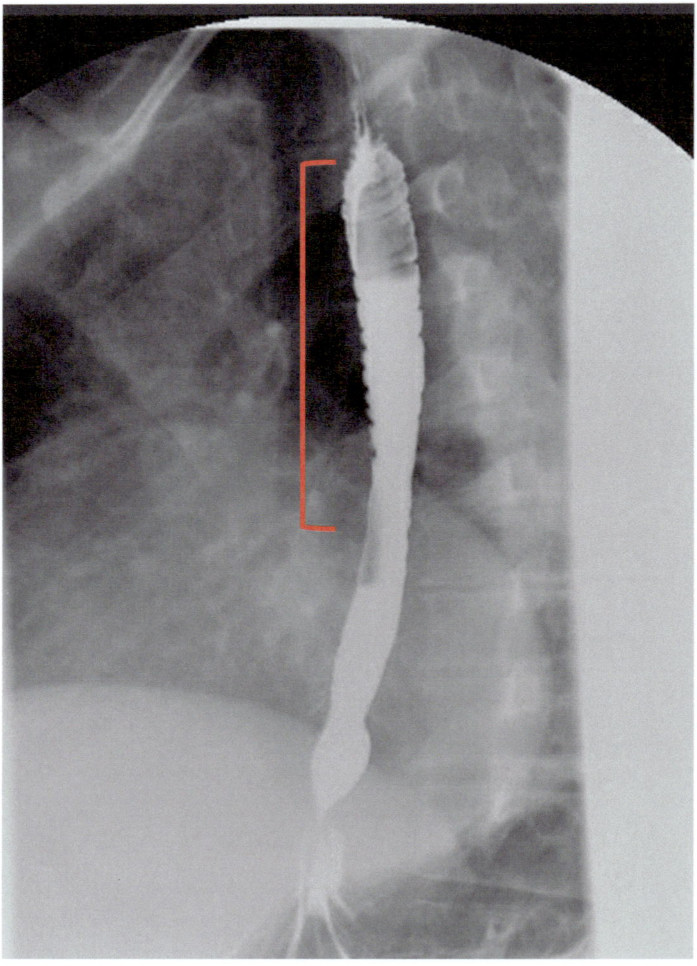

Fig. 4.3 Eosinophilic esophagitis. You can see the "stack of coins" appearance shown in the red bracket

described as a "stack of coins" (Fig. 4.3), either diffusely throughout the esophagus or at fixed segments and strictures [21]. These findings should be further investigated with endoscopy and biopsies.

Hiatal Hernias

Patients with GERD often are found to have hiatal hernias, which can be identified on the barium esophagram. There are four types of hiatal hernias. A type I hernia is also referred to as a sliding hernia and involves displacement of the gastroesophageal junction (GEJ) above the diaphragm. A type II hernia is characterized by the GEJ fixed below the diaphragm with herniation of the gastric fundus above the diaphragm. A type III hernia involves both the GEJ and gastric fundus herniating above the diaphragm and a type IV hiatal hernia involves both gastric and non-gastric viscera herniating above the diaphragmatic hiatus [22]. Hiatal hernias can be identified on esophagography when the gastric rugal folds or a gastric bubble is noted to be above the level of the diaphragmatic hiatus (Fig. 4.4). Esophagography has superiority over endoscopy in identifying hiatal hernias, especially type I sliding hernias. The improved identification of sliding hiatal hernias is a result of increased intraabdominal pressure while being in the prone position causing the hernia to be more apparent than when the stomach is insufflated with air [23]. Identification of hiatal hernias in the workup of foregut disorders is very important as their identification can alter the therapeutic plan for patients. Radiologists should be discouraged from characterizing hiatal hernias as small, medium, or large as no such standard exists. Rather, they should be described in terms of axial and transverse length, as well as relative positioning of the LES, fundus, and give information regarding evidence of organo-axial or meso-axial volvulus.

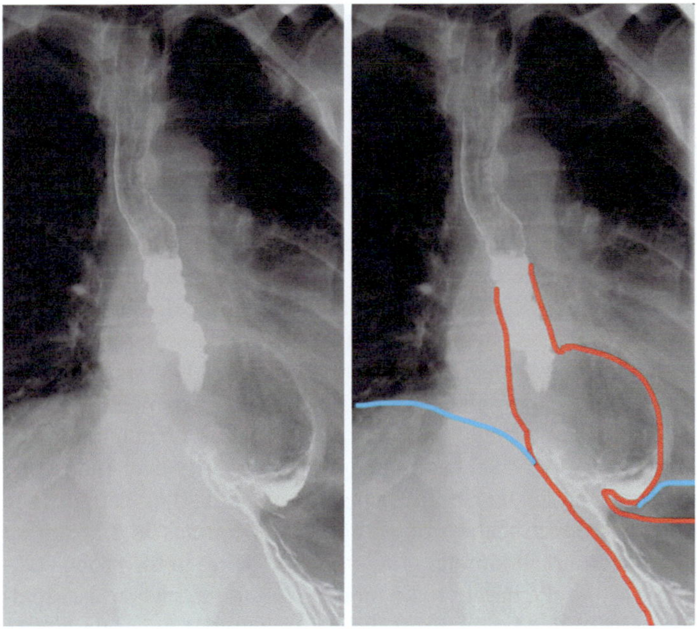

Fig. 4.4 Type III paraesophageal hernia. The red line represents the outline of a type III paraesophageal hernia. The blue line represents the diaphragm

Esophageal Diverticula

The esophagus can develop multiple types of diverticula, such as Zenker's, pulsion, and traction diverticula. A Zenker's diverticulum is an acquired outpouching of mucosa and submucosal layers between the cricopharyngeal and the inferior pharyngeal constrictor muscles resulting in a false diverticulum [24]. On esophagography, the diverticulum usually arises from the midline of the posterior wall and is best identified on the lateral view of the esophagram (Fig. 4.5) [25]. Pulsion diverticula typically occur in the distal esophagus and are usually associated with motility disorders of the esophagus. They do not contain the muscular layer of the esophagus, thus making them a false diverticulum. On the esophagram, they appear as broad-based contrast-filled outpouchings and typically retain barium after the esophagus has emptied [26, 27]. In

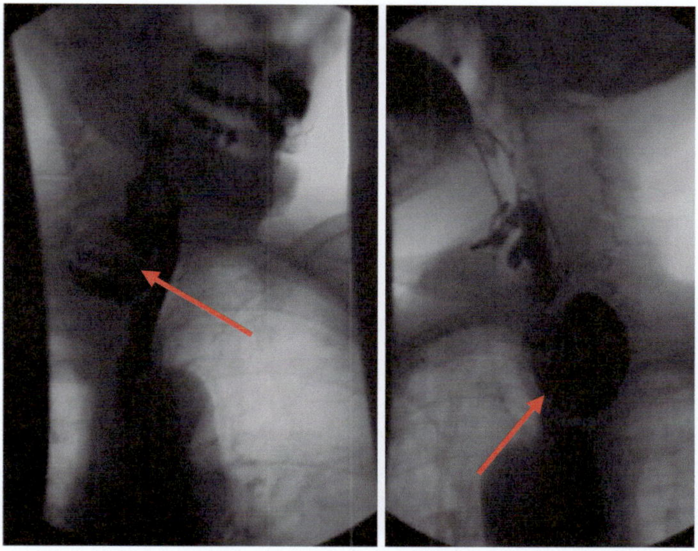

Fig. 4.5 Zenker's diverticulum

contrast, traction diverticula are typically seen in the mid-esophagus and contain all the layers of the esophagus and thus are considered a true diverticulum. They are caused by mediastinal scarring secondary to infectious processes, leading to traction on the adjacent esophagus [27]. On barium swallow, traction diverticula tend to have a triangular and tented appearance [27, 28]. Esophagram allows for safe identification of this diverticulum and in some cases is enough workup to warrant operative intervention.

Neoplasms

Other structural abnormalities such as malignant and nonmalignant tumors are able to be identified on an esophagram. These present as crescent-shaped filling defects. More benign tumors are characterized by smooth edges without irregularity or ulceration, whereas more malignant tumors commonly result in irregular luminal narrowing and ulcerations (Fig. 4.6) [29]. It is important to note that these findings and alarm symptoms for malignancy must be further evaluated using endoscopy.

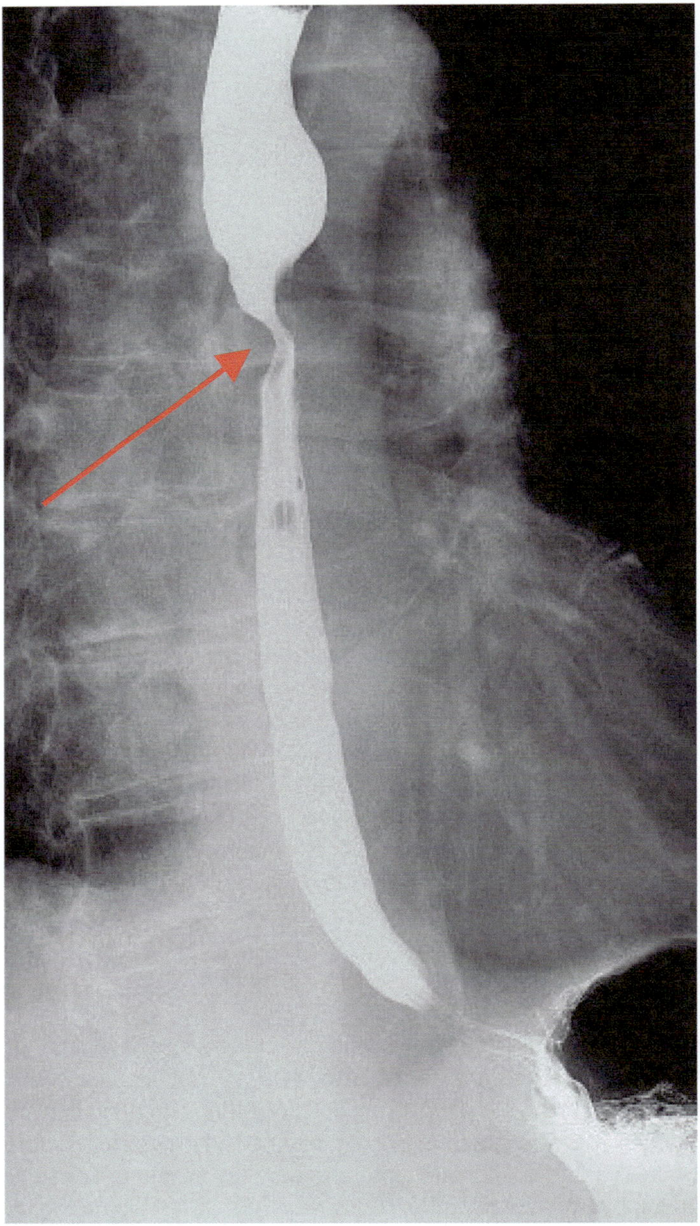

Fig. 4.6 Mid-esophageal tumor seen as a crescent-shaped filling defect on the esophagram

Perforation

Iatrogenic, spontaneous, and traumatic esophageal perforations may have different management strategies, but their diagnostic approach remains fairly similar. In an unstable patient with a high index of suspicion for esophageal perforation, regardless of etiology, operative intervention should not be delayed. In those patients who are stable and further workup is reasonable, utilizing esophagography is useful. Although we commonly advocate using barium for most esophagrams, when investigating for a perforation we advocate for the initial use of a water-soluble contrast because barium extravasation into the mediastinum carries a risk of mediastinitis/pleuritis and is harder to washout during surgical exploration [30]. If no perforation is identified using water-soluble contrast, further evaluation using barium should be considered if there is a high clinical suspicion for perforation. The identification of contrast extravasation from the esophageal lumen confirms the diagnosis of esophageal perforation.

Motility Disorders

Esophageal motility disorders are commonly seen in patients with GERD, with some sources quoting esophageal dysmotility in up to 44% of patients with GERD [31]. Schima et al. reported that esophagram has about a 79% sensitivity rate for identifying dysmotility in patients with dysphagia [32]. During an esophagram, a radiologist not only assesses structural abnormalities, but also evaluate the esophagus for functional disorders. In a normal esophagus, the primary peristaltic wave and occasionally a secondary peristaltic wave are able to clear a contrast bolus [13]. For a radiologist to consider clearance of the contrast bolus to be normal, the patient should clear the bolus in two or fewer strippings from the esophagus [12]. Tertiary contractions are one of the findings suggestive of disordered esophageal motility, but when patients with tertiary contractions were further evaluated with high-resolution manometry (HRM), only about 47% had confirmed dysmotility [33].

In addition to minor motility disorders, barium esophagrams can be useful in diagnosing more severe forms of motility disorders such as achalasia and diffuse esophageal spasm. While high-resolution manometry remains the gold standard for these diagnoses, barium esophagrams have proven to be a practical and beneficial initial diagnostic test.

Achalasia is a condition associated with the loss of myenteric plexus ganglion cells in the distal esophagus and lower esophageal sphincter (LES) leading to impaired relaxation of the LES and aperistalsis in the esophageal body. On the esophagram, the most diagnostic finding is a dilated esophageal body and distal narrowing at the LES creating the classic “bird’s beak” appearance (Fig. 4.7). Patients with achalasia will demonstrate bolus retention in the distal esophagus [34]. Blonski et al. examined different characteristics of the barium esophagram in patients with achalasia and proposed that a barium column height of >2 cm at 5 min from ingestion of barium be used as a cutoff point for identifying patients with achalasia [35]. When findings on the esophagram suggest achalasia, the diagnosis should be confirmed and categorized using HRM.

Diffuse esophageal spasms (DES) are characterized by abnormal esophageal peristalsis with multiple simultaneous non-peristaltic contractions [36], often leading to chest pain and dysphagia This disorder is classically seen with a distinct “corkscrew appearance” caused by intermittent bouts of nonpropulsive contractions causing alternating areas of narrowing and normal esophageal diameter [36]. Similar to achalasia, esophagography findings suggestive of DES should be confirmed with HRM prior to initiating therapy.

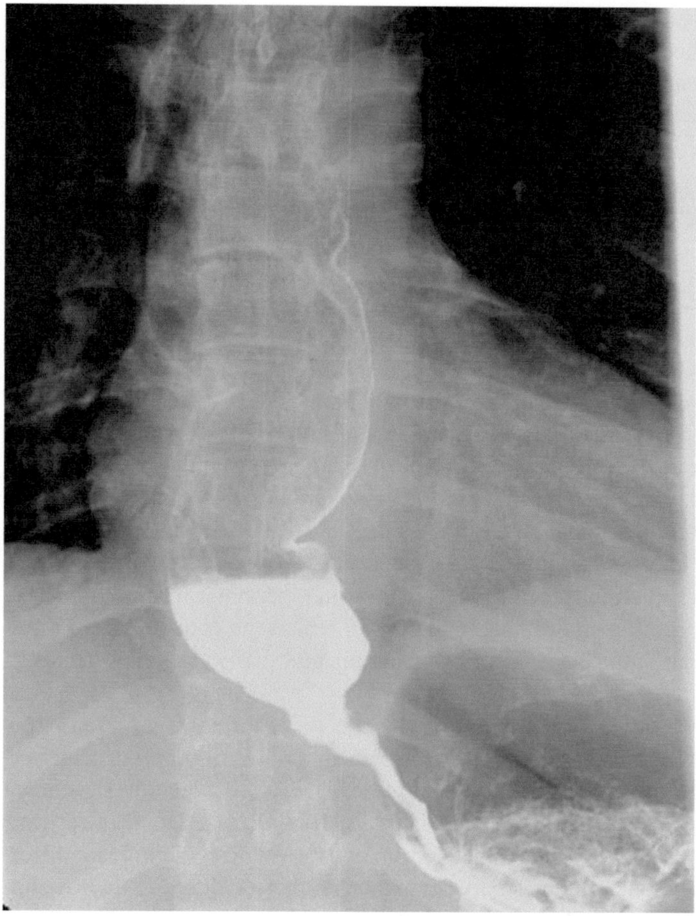

Fig. 4.7 Typical bird's beak appearance in a patient with achalasia

Utilization in Pre- and Post-surgical Management

The esophagram plays an important role in surgical planning for patients undergoing antireflux surgery (ARS). During the upright double-contrast phase of an esophagram, the radiologist is sometimes able to identify a foreshortened esophagus. This becomes important in surgical planning as patients with significant esophageal foreshortening occasionally require esophageal lengthening procedures such as a Collis gastroplasty. The knowledge of this prior to the operation can prepare the surgeon for this possibility or refer to a provider with the knowledge and skill in performing esophageal lengthening procedures [37].

Although a small sample size, Kahrilas and colleagues were able to show a correlation between normal esophageal motility in barium studies and normal peristalsis on manometry [38]. Alicuben et al. also demonstrated that an esophagram is a good screening tool for esophageal motility disorders. They were able to show that a normal esophagram, which they defined as stasis of liquid barium on less than three of five swallows, can reliably rule out the presence of clinically significant esophageal dysmotility in preoperative patients [39]. Overall, we do not recommend omitting manometry in the workup of a patient undergoing antireflux surgery, but there is a select subset of patients who are unable to tolerate catheter placement during manometric studies or have a large paraesophageal hernia in which the catheter may coil in the stomach, and an esophagram may aid in surgical decision-making.

Esophageal dysmotility has been suggested as a reason many surgeons avoid complete Nissen fundoplication and instead perform partial fundoplications because of the fear of significant postoperative dysphagia. Two small randomized controlled trials were able to refute this notion, both showing no significant difference in outcomes between patient surgery tailored to their preoperative esophageal motor function compared with those whose surgery was not tailored to their esophageal function [40, 41]. Baigrie et al. advocated that laparoscopic Nissen fundoplication (LNF) should not be considered a contraindication in patients with disordered peristalsis as they were able to show similar satisfaction between those with and those without disordered esophageal peristalsis after LNF [42].

After ARS, esophagrams are extremely valuable in assessing dysphagia or recurrent GERD symptoms. They are able to evaluate the integrity and positioning of a fundoplication, confirm the

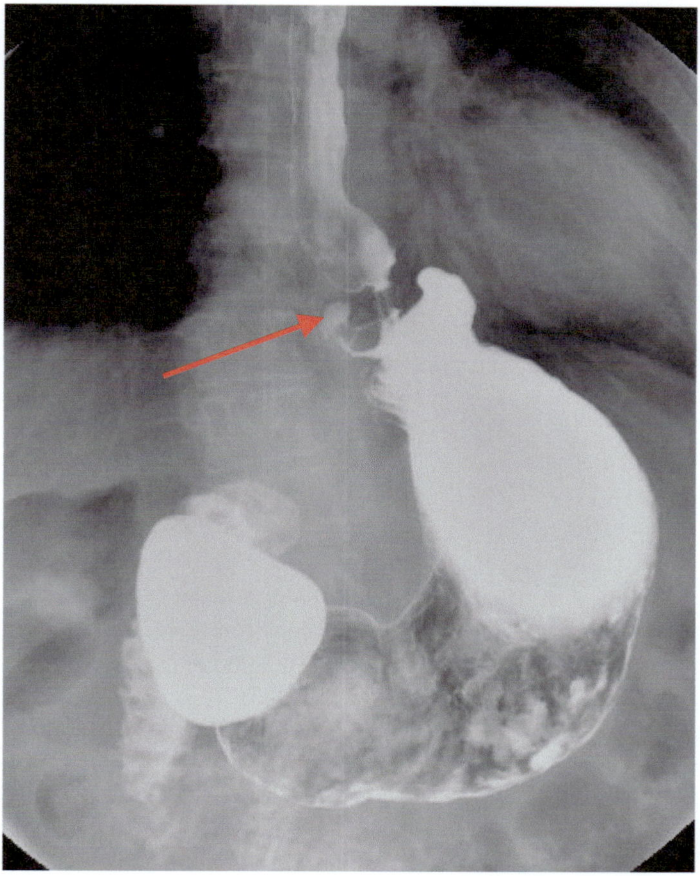

Fig. 4.8 Recurrent hernia after previous Nissen fundoplication

adequate position of a magnetic sphincter augmentation device, and can identify recurrent hiatal hernias (Figs. 4.8 and 4.9). During the double-contrast portion of the esophagram positioning, the patient supine or in a slight Trendelenburg position can allow contrast to reflux into the fundoplication and assess its position and ensure its integrity [37]. A form of secondary achalasia can develop in patients whose fundoplication was created too tightly and an esophagram may show the characteristic findings of

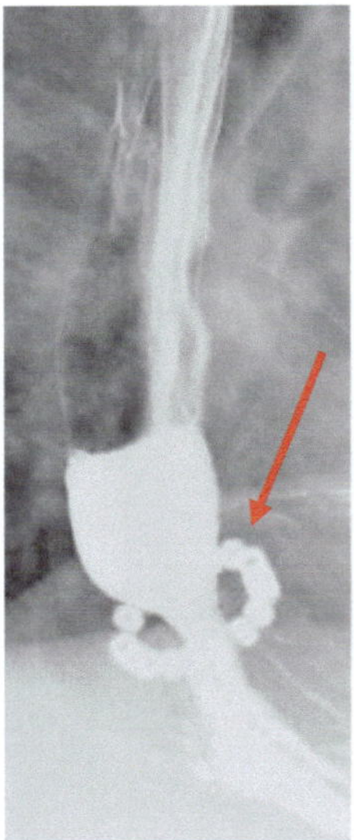

Fig. 4.9 Well-positioned magnetic sphincter augmentation device on the distal esophagus below the hiatus

a patient with achalasia without the associated dilation of the more proximal esophagus [43]. Diagnosis of this early is important as treatment for this may involve dilation of the wrap or even surgical revision of the fundoplication [43].

Conclusion

The humble esophagram is an excellent initial imaging modality for the evaluation of suspected esophageal diseases or to evaluate postoperative complications in ARS. It provides excellent structural detail and gives insight into esophageal function. When properly utilized and interpreted by the foregut surgeon, the esophagram is integral in the evaluation of patients with diseases of the esophagus and stomach.

Author Contributions EF involved in the literature review; EF wrote the study; and EF, SD, and FPB involved in critical revision.

Acknowledgements None.

Conflicts of Interest There are no conflicts of interest to disclose and no funding for this study.

References

1. Gelfand DW. High density, low viscosity barium for fine mucosal detail on double-contrast upper gastrointestinal examinations. AJR Am J Roentgenol. 1978;130:831–3.
2. Rubesin SE, Jessurun J, Robertson D, Jones B, Bosma JF, Donner MW. Lines of the pharynx. Radiographics. 1987;7:217–37.
3. Rubesin SE, Laufer I. Pictorial review: principles of double-contrast pharyngography. Dysphagia. 1991;6:170–8.
4. Katzka DA. The role of barium Esophagography in an endoscopy world. Gastrointest Endosc Clin N Am. 2014;24:563–80.
5. ACR Committee on Drugs and Contrast Media. ACR manual on contrast media-version 10.3. 2018.
6. Baker ME, Einstein DM. Barium esophagram: does it have a role in gastroesophageal reflux disease? Gastroenterol Clin N Am. 2014;43:47–68.
7. Koehler RE, Weyman PJ, Oakley HF. Single- and double-contrast techniques in esophagitis. AJR Am J Roentgenol. 1980;135:15–9.
8. Creteur V, Thoeni RF, Federle MP, Cello JP, Moss AA, Ominsky SH, Goldberg HI, Axel L. The role of single and double-contrast radiography in the diagnosis of reflux esophagitis. Radiology. 1983;147:71–5.
9. Hewson EG, Ott DJ, Dalton CB, Chen YM, Wu WC, Richter JE. Manometry and radiology. Complementary studies in the assessment of esophageal motility disorders. Gastroenterology. 1990;98:626–32.
10. Ott DJ, Chen YM, Hewson EG, Richter JE, Dalton CB, Gelfand DW, Wu WC. Esophageal motility: assessment with synchronous video tape fluoroscopy and manometry. Radiology. 1989;173:419–22.
11. Thompson JK, Koehler RE, Richter JE. Detection of gastroesophageal reflux: value of barium studies compared with 24-hr pH monitoring. AJR Am J Roentgenol. 1994;162:621–6.
12. Peters JH. Modern imaging for the assessment of gastroesophageal reflux disease begins with the barium esophagram. J Gastrointest Surg. 2000;4:346–7.
13. Chen J-H. Ineffective esophageal motility and the vagus: current challenges and future prospects. Clin Exp Gastroenterol. 2016;9:291–9.
14. Tutuian R, Castell DO. Clarification of the esophageal function defect in patients with manometric ineffective esophageal motility: studies using

combined impedance-manometry. Clin Gastroenterol Hepatol. 2004;2:230–6.
15. D'Alessio MJ, Rakita S, Bloomston M, Chambers CM, Zervos EE, Goldin SB, Poklepovic J, Boyce HW, Rosemurgy AS. Esophagography predicts favorable outcomes after laparoscopic Nissen fundoplication for patients with esophageal dysmotility. J Am Coll Surg. 2005;201:335–42.
16. Serna-Gallegos D, Basseri B, Bairamian V, Pimentel M, Soukiasian HJ. Gastroesophageal reflux reported on esophagram does not correlate with pH monitoring and high-resolution esophageal manometry. Am Surg. 2014;80:1026–9.
17. Levine MS, Rubesin SE. History and evolution of the barium swallow for evaluation of the pharynx and esophagus. Dysphagia. 2017;32:55–72.
18. Ott DJ, Chen YM, Wu WC, Gelfand DW. Endoscopic sensitivity in the detection of esophageal strictures. J Clin Gastroenterol. 1985;7:121–5.
19. Gilchrist AM, Levine MS, Carr RF, Saul SH, Katzka DA, Herlinger H, Laufer I. Barrett's esophagus: diagnosis by double-contrast esophagography. Am J Roentgenol. 1988;150:97–102.
20. Furuta GT, Liacouras CA, Collins MH, et al. Eosinophilic esophagitis in children and adults: a systematic review and consensus recommendations for diagnosis and treatment. Gastroenterology. 2007;133:1342–63.
21. Alexander JA. Endoscopic and radiologic findings in eosinophilic esophagitis. Gastrointest Endosc Clin N Am. 2018;28:47–57.
22. Siegal SR, Dolan JP, Hunter JG. Modern diagnosis and treatment of hiatal hernias. Langenbeck's Arch Surg. 2017;402:1145–51.
23. Katzka DA. A gastroenterologist's perspective on the role of barium esophagography in gastroesophageal reflux disease. Abdomin Radiol. 2018;43:1319–22.
24. Siddiq MA. Pharyngeal pouch (Zenker's diverticulum). Postgrad Med J. 2001;77:506–11.
25. Balfe DM, Heiken JP. Contrast evaluation of structural lesions of the pharynx. Curr Probl Diagn Radiol. 1986;15:73–160.
26. Levine MS. Miscellaneous abnormalities of the esophagus. In: Textbook of gastrointestinal radiology; 2008. p. 465–93.
27. Debi U, Sharma M, Singh L, Sinha A. Barium esophagogram in various esophageal diseases: a pictorial essay. Indian J Radiol Imag. 2019;29:141–54.
28. Hartman T. Pearls and pitfalls in thoracic imaging: variants and other difficult diagnoses. Cambridge University Press; 2011.
29. Lewis RB, Mehrotra AK, Rodriguez P, Levine MS. From the radiologic pathology archives: esophageal neoplasms: radiologic-pathologic correlation. Radiographics. 2013;33:1083–108.
30. Chen A, Tafti D, Tuma F. Barium swallow. StatPearls [Internet]; 2020.
31. Diener U. Esophageal dysmotility and gastroesophageal reflux disease. J Gastrointest Surg. 2001;5:260–5.

32. Schima W, Stacher G, Pokieser P, Uranitsch K, Nekahm D, Schober E, Moser G, Tscholakoff D. Esophageal motor disorders: videofluoroscopic and manometric evaluation--prospective study in 88 symptomatic patients. Radiology. 1992;185:487–91.
33. O'Rourke AK, Lazar A, Murphy B, Castell DO, Martin-Harris B. Utility of esophagram versus high-resolution manometry in the detection of esophageal dysmotility. Otolaryngol Head Neck Surg. 2016;154:888–91.
34. Pandolfino JE, Gawron AJ. Achalasia: a systematic review. JAMA. 2015;313:1841–52.
35. Blonski W, Kumar A, Feldman J, Richter JE. Timed barium swallow: diagnostic role and predictive value in untreated achalasia, esophagogastric junction outflow obstruction, and non-achalasia dysphagia. Am J Gastroenterol. 2018;113:196–203.
36. Levine MS, Rubesin SE, Laufer I. Barium esophagography: a study for all seasons. Clin Gastroenterol Hepatol. 2008;6:11–25.
37. Baker ME, Einstein DM, Herts BR, Remer EM, Motta-Ramirez GA, Ehrenwald E, Rice TW, Richter JE. Gastroesophageal reflux disease: integrating the barium esophagram before and after antireflux surgery. Radiology. 2007;243:329–39.
38. Kahrilas PJ, Dodds WJ, Hogan WJ. Effect of peristaltic dysfunction on esophageal volume clearance. Gastroenterology. 1988;94:73–80.
39. Alicuben ET, Bildzukewicz N, Samakar K, Katkhouda N, Dobrowolsky A, Sandhu K, Lipham JC. Routine esophageal manometry is not useful in patients with normal videoesophagram. Surg Endosc. 2019;33:1650–3.
40. Rydberg L, Ruth M, Abrahamsson H, Lundell L. Tailoring antireflux surgery: a randomized clinical trial. World J Surg. 1999;23:612–8.
41. Fibbe C, Layer P, Keller J, Strate U, Emmermann A, Zornig C. Esophageal motility in reflux disease before and after fundoplication: a prospective, randomized, clinical, and manometric study. Gastroenterology. 2001;121:5–14.
42. Baigrie RJ, Watson DI, Myers JC, Jamieson GG. Outcome of laparoscopic Nissen fundoplication in patients with disordered preoperative peristalsis. Gut. 1997;40:381–5.
43. Wehrli NE, Levine MS, Rubesin SE, Katzka DA, Laufer I. Secondary achalasia and other esophageal motility disorders after laparoscopic Nissen fundoplication for gastroesophageal reflux disease. AJR Am J Roentgenol. 2007;189:1464–8.

The Upper GI Series

5

Emily Adams and Anna Ibele

An upper gastrointestinal study (UGIS) is a fluoroscopic study, which evaluates the contrast-filled esophagus, stomach, gastric outlet, and proximal duodenum. It is useful in establishing or further defining pathology at the gastroesophageal junction, pathology related to the gastric outlet and duodenum, and post-surgical anatomy and related pathology. The upper GI series (UGIS) classically involves the patient ingesting contrast, while under fluoroscopic and spot radiographic imaging so that the movement of contrast through the esophagus, gastroesophageal junction, stomach, and first portion of the duodenum may be visualized and recorded in real time. Classically, the study is performed with barium sulfate as an oral contrast medium. Some radiologists prefer to initiate the study with water-soluble contrast if there is clinical concern for a leak (historically gastrografin although, this has fallen out of favor due to concerns for the risk of aspiration pneumonitis) The American College of Radiology states that the upper GI examination can be helpful in the diagnosis of peptic ulcer

E. Adams · A. Ibele (✉)
Department of Surgery, The University of Utah,
Salt Lake City, UT, USA
e-mail: emily.adams@hsc.utah.edu; anna.ibele@hsc.utah.edu

A. D. Patel et al. (eds.), *The SAGES Manual of Physiologic Evaluation of Foregut Diseases*,
https://doi.org/10.1007/978-3-031-39199-6_5

disease, hiatal hernia (HH), varices, neoplasm, gastric outlet obstruction, gastric or duodenal mass, and varices [1]. In practicality, many of these entities such as ulcers, masses, and varices are best and most safely diagnosed endoscopically.

UGIS in Conventional Anti-Reflux Surgery

Although not a sensitive or specific test for pathologic reflux, UGIS can be helpful in the assessment for hiatal hernia as a potential anatomic contributing factor to reflux symptoms or dysphagia and is also sometimes useful for the evaluation of postoperative dysphagia, regurgitation, or vomiting after an anti-reflux operation. Barium esophagram and/or upper GI X-rays were historically recommended as a screening test for GERD, but are no longer part of the diagnostic algorithm to confirm or refute pathologic reflux. In a study of 125 patients, Johnson et al. compared esophageal pH monitoring and barium esophagram/upper GI to assess the accuracy of barium screening as a predictor of pathologic reflux. The sensitivity and specificity of barium study to identify pathologic reflux were insufficient [2], and objective testing with upper endoscopy and esophageal pH monitoring is now the gold standard for diagnosis of pathologic GERD.

The upper GI X-ray is useful in the initial evaluation of dysphagia and reflux symptoms when there is clinical suspicion of distal esophageal pathology or abnormal postoperative anatomy [3]. In the patient presenting for consideration of anti-reflux surgery who has undergone minimal objective evaluation, an UGIS can also help to further define the presence, type, and size of a hiatal hernia, which can guide further diagnostic maneuvers and operative planning [4]. For example, an upper GI X-ray, which demonstrates anatomy conducive to obstructive symptoms such as a type III paraesophageal hernia with delay in the flow of contrast on cine images, may indicate to the ordering physician that anatomic obstruction is the likely etiology for symptoms of regurgitation and dysphagia. Based on such imaging, the aforementioned patient may not require physiologic pH testing prior to anti-reflux surgery, while a patient experiencing heartburn with a small type I hiatal hernia will likely require this additional testing to clarify whether the symptoms are truly from pathologic GERD (Fig. 5.1). In patients with dysphagia, an upper GI is a quick and relatively well-tolerated examination that may give the clinician an early suspicion of achalasia of the esophagus; the classic finding for achalasia on a UGIS is a markedly dilated and tortuous esophagus with characteristic "bird's beak" tapering at the lower esophageal sphincter. There is often an air-fluid level visualized within the esophagus, which can correspond with the degree of resistance imposed by the non-relaxing sphincter. (This diagnosis is then confirmed and further classified via high-resolution manometry.) An upper GI X-ray may also demonstrate evidence of esophageal stricture or foreshortened esophagus and may allow the surgeon to anticipate the need for an esophageal dilation or esophageal lengthening procedure during an anti-reflux operation.

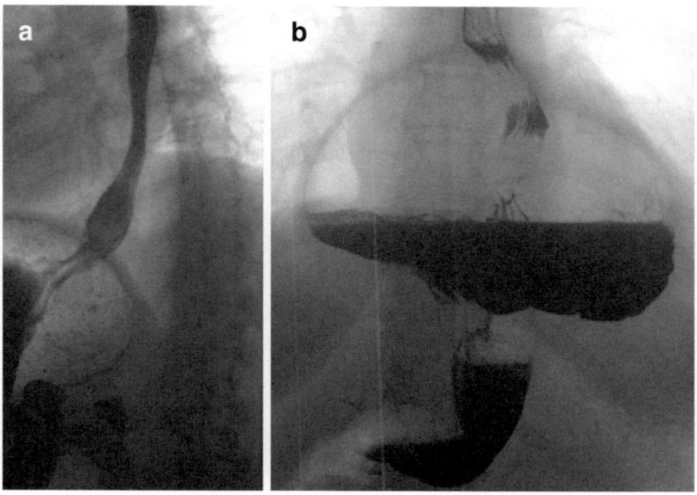

Fig. 5.1 Upper GI series in two patients presenting with reflux and dysphagia. The patient in (**a**) has a small hiatal hernia and underwent esophageal manometry, which was consistent with type 2 achalasia. The patient in (**b**) has a large type 3 paraesophageal hernia with esophageal compression of the esophagus by the herniated stomach, which is an anatomic explanation for her dysphagia

It should be noted that while UGIS provides a useful initial evaluation of anatomy in a patient presenting with reflux, regurgitation, or dysphagia, endoscopy has been shown to be more specific for preoperative assessment of hernia type when used solely as a tool for assessment of the nature of a hiatal hernia. Linke et al. prospectively evaluated 40 consecutive patients who were tested with preoperative barium upper GI and endoscopy before laparoscopic surgery for gastroesophageal reflux disease and/or symptomatic hiatal hernia. The presence and the type of hiatal hernia found by UGI and endoscopy were correlated with the intraoperative finding as the reference standard. A barium study and endoscopy allowed the diagnosis of hiatal hernia in 75% and 97.5%, respectively ($p = 0.003$). The correct classification of hiatal hernia was confirmed in 50% by barium swallow and 80% by endoscopy ($p = 0.005$) [2].

UGIS in Conventional Bariatric Surgery

In many bariatric practices, UGIS is done prior to surgery to assess for hiatal hernia (HH) with the anticipation that this might require concurrent repair as part of a bariatric operation. In a 2009 study, Fornari et al. compared the efficacy of endoscopy and UGIS in the diagnosis of type I hiatal hernia prior to bariatric surgery. Endoscopy was found to have low sensitivity (40%) and high specificity (94%) in the diagnosis of type I hiatal hernia compared to UGIS [5]. However, additional groups have found that preoperative UGIS is unlikely to change the operative course for the patient. A study by Ghassemian et al. showed similar findings after they retrospectively reviewed 817 charts of obese patients who underwent gastric bypass surgery. Of these patients, 80.7% of them had undergone UGIS screening prior to surgery. Of this group, 40.2% had abnormal findings (most commonly hiatal hernia, 62%), none of which resulted in cancelation or delay of surgery; however, the authors did not comment on whether the finding of hiatal hernia led to a modification in type of surgery or operative approach [6]. In 2004, Sharaf et al. conducted a retrospective study in which the records of 171 patients with obesity who underwent UGIS prior to bariatric surgery were reviewed. Although 48% of patients had an abnormal finding on UGIS, only 5.1% of patients had a clinically relevant finding, which delayed surgery or changed the surgical approach, most commonly being a crural repair for a hiatal hernia (18.7%) [7]. It should be noted that both of these studies, however, were published before the advent of laparoscopic sleeve gastrectomy (LSG). In 2019, Mizrahi et al. reviewed the cases of 1810 patients who underwent routine UGIS prior to LSG for the radiographic and intraoperative presence of hiatal hernia, Considering the intraoperative identification of HH the gold standard for diagnosis, the sensitivity and specificity of preoperative UGI fluoroscopy for HH detection were 32% (66/201) and 94% (1512/1609), respectively. The median operative time was significantly longer when concomitant LSG and HH repair was performed compared to LSG alone (76 min vs. 55 min, $p < 0.001$, respectively). The foreknowledge of HH had no influence on the median operative times (77 min vs. 75 min, predicted vs. incidental, respectively, $p = 1.34$) [8].

In the early days of laparoscopic bariatric surgery, many groups routinely obtained postoperative upper GI X-rays to evaluate for leak prior to patient discharge. Subsequent research has shown that routine postoperative UGIS is not useful in detecting or predicting leaks after bariatric surgery and therefore not indicated unless the patient shows clinical signs of leak [9–11]. Brockmeyer et al. and Csendes et al. both published studies demonstrating that UGIS on post-op days 1–3 after RYGB might show a mechanical defect in the staple or suture line, but was unlikely to demonstrate leaks from other, more common, causes of leaks such as ischemia, or tension/traction on the staple line, all of which classically manifest later in the postoperative course [11, 12]. In 2014, Quartararo et al. performed a systematic review including 22 studies and 19,389 patients who underwent Roux-en-Y gastric bypass. Based on their review of the extant data, the group argued that selective UGIS based on clinical presentation is preferable to routine screening [13] However, the effectiveness of UGIS in confirming a clinically suspected leak may be inferior to that of a CT scan with IV and oral contrast. Bingham et al. showed that CT scan had a 95% sensitivity (95% CI 81.8–99.1%) and a 100% specificity

(95% CI 93.1–100%) compared to a 79.4% sensitivity (95% CI 61.6–90%) and 95% specificity (95% CI 85.2–98.7%) of UGIS in detecting anastomotic leaks in patients who underwent RYGB [14]. Arteaga-González et al. found data to support this conclusion in a study that included patients who underwent RYGB and sleeve gastrectomy. In their study, 15% of abdominal CT scans had false negativity for leak versus 28.6% for intraoperative oral methylene blue and 33.3% for UGIS [15]. Based on the above literature, the practice at our institution is to obtain a CT abdomen with IV and oral contrast in patients that show clinical signs of anastomotic leak [9–11, 14].

The UGIS plays a more important role in establishing the diagnosis in a patient who presents with a late or chronic complication of bariatric surgery. For example, in patients presenting with weight regain and epigastric pain after non-divided gastric bypass or vertical banded gastroplasty, gastro-gastric fistula is often a concern. Carrodeguas et al. found that the UGIS was the most sensitive test for gastro-gastric fistula following gastric bypass when compared with CT scan and upper GI endoscopy [16]. Brethauer et al. showed that UGIS was complementary to an EGD in diagnosing gastro-gastric fistulae and that when these tests were combined, all gastro-gastric fistulae were successfully diagnosed in their patient population [17]. In a small series by Gumbs et al., the use of UGIS to detect a gastro-gastric fistula combined with a confirmatory EDG was their diagnostic method of choice [18].

UGIS can also be helpful in the diagnostic evaluation of reflux following sleeve gastrectomy. The study can demonstrate de novo or recurrent hiatal hernia, dilation of the fundus, and incisural narrowing, all of which may contribute to acute or chronic reflux and regurgitation following sleeve (Fig. 5.2). However, if incisural narrowing is suspected, some have advocated for proceeding directly with endoscopy as opposed to obtaining imaging studies. In a recent study of 30 consecutive patients with nausea, vomiting, and obstructive symptoms following the sleeve, Bhalla et al. reviewed the positive and negative predictive value of upper GI X-ray in assessing stenosis of the gastric sleeve. Twenty-two (73.3%) patients underwent UGIS prior to EGD. On diagnostic

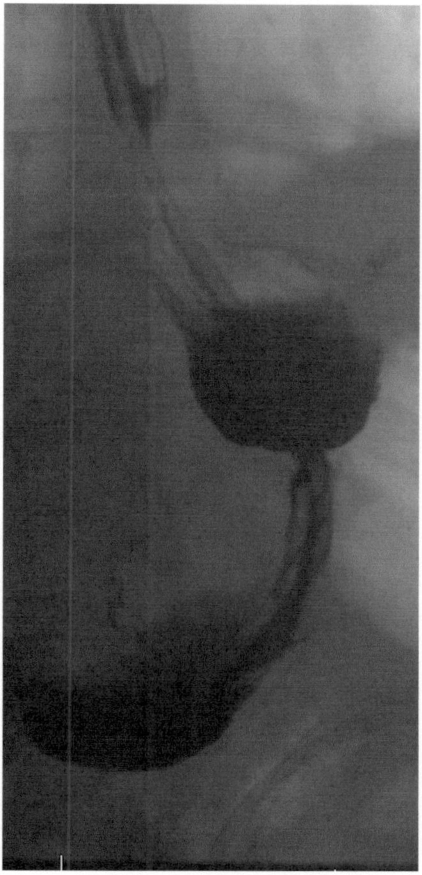

Fig. 5.2 Upper GI series demonstrating incisural narrowing and subsequent dilation of retained gastric fundus in a patient with refractory reflux and regurgitation following laparoscopic sleeve gastrectomy

EGD, 27 (87.1%) patients were diagnosed with gastric sleeve stenosis (GSS). The sensitivity and negative predictive value of UGIS to detect GSS were 30.0% and 12.5%, respectively. All six patients with GSS on UGIS also had incisural stenosis on endoscopic evaluation (specificity = 100% and PPV = 100%), leading the authors to suggest proceeding directly with endoscopy if incisural stenosis is suspected in the early postoperative period [19].

In summary, the UGIS is a useful adjunct in the evaluation and diagnosis of many upper gastrointestinal disorders including esophageal stricture, achalasia, hiatal and paraesophageal hernias, post-bariatric surgical pathology, and other conditions in which the surgeon wishes to illuminate the patient's precise upper GI anatomy. There is typically no role for this study in preoperative workup or routine postoperative evaluation of a bariatric patient. Although upper GI X-ray is often effective in diagnosing most anastomotic leaks, the CT scan has a higher sensitivity and specificity for this condition. This test has been most useful at our institution as an initial first study to guide further management of patients presenting with dysphagia and reflux or to evaluate post-surgical anatomy in patients presenting with complications of prior gastric surgery.

References

1. American College of Radiology. Practice parameter for the performance of esophograms and upper gastrointestinal examinations in adults. 2019.
2. Johnston BT, Troshinsky MB, Castell JA, Castell DO. Comparison of barium radiology with esophageal pH monitoring in the diagnosis of gastroesophageal reflux disease. Am J Gastroenterol. 1996;91(6):1181–5.
3. Dempsey DT. Barium upper GI series in adults: a surgeon's perspective. Abdom Radiol. 2018;43(6):1323–8.
4. Jobe BA, Richter JE, Hoppo T, et al. Preoperative diagnostic workup before antireflux surgery: an evidence and experience-based consensus of the esophageal diagnostic advisory panel. J Am Coll Surg. 2013;217(4):586–97.
5. Fornari F, Gurski RR, Navarini D, Thiesen V, Mestriner LHB, Madalosso CAS. Clinical utility of endoscopy and barium swallow X-ray in the diagnosis of sliding hiatal hernia in morbidly obese patients: a study before and after gastric bypass. Obes Surg. 2009;20(6):702–8.
6. Ghassemian AJ, MacDonald K, Cunningham PG, et al. The workup for bariatric surgery does not require a routine upper gastrointestinal series. Obes Surg. 1997;7(1):16–8.
7. Sharaf RN, Weinshel EH, Bini EJ, Rosenberg J, Ren CJ. Radiologic assessment of the upper gastrointestinal tract: does it play an important preoperative role in bariatric surgery? Obes Surg. 2004;14(3):313–7.
8. Mizrahi I, Abubeih A, Rachmuth J, et al. Routine upper gastrointestinal fluoroscopy before laparoscopic sleeve gastrectomy: is it necessary? Obes Surg. 2019;29(6):1704–8.

9. Dallal RM, Bailey L, Nahmias N. Back to basics – clinical diagnosis in bariatric surgery. Routine drains and upper GI series are unnecessary. Surg Endosc. 2007;21(12):2268–71.
10. Singh R, Fisher BL. Sensitivity and specificity of postoperative upper GI series following gastric bypass. Obes Surg. 2003;13(1):73–5.
11. Brockmeyer JR, Simon T, Jacob RK, Husain F, Choi Y. Upper gastrointestinal swallow study following bariatric surgery: institutional review and review of the literature. Obes Surg. 2012;22(7):1039–43.
12. Csendes A, Burgos A, Braghetto I. Classification and management of leaks after gastric bypass for patients with morbid obesity: a prospective study of 60 patients. Obes Surg. 2012;22(6):855–62.
13. Quartararo G, Facchiano E, Scaringi S, Liscia G, Lucchese M. Upper gastrointestinal series after Roux-en-Y gastric bypass for morbid obesity: effectiveness in leakage detection. A systematic review of the literature. Obes Surg. 2014;24(7):1096–101.
14. Bingham J, Shawhan R, Parker R, Wigboldy J, Sohn V. Computed tomography scan versus upper gastrointestinal fluoroscopy for diagnosis of staple line leak following bariatric surgery. Am J Surg. 2015;209(5):810–4.
15. Arteaga-González I, Martín-Malagón A, Martín-Pérez J, Carrillo-Pallarés A. Usefulness of clinical signs and diagnostic tests for suspected leaks in bariatric surgery. Obes Surg. 2015;25(9):1680–4.
16. Carrodeguas L, Szomstein S, Soto F, et al. Management of gastrogastric fistulas after divided Roux-en-Y gastric bypass surgery for morbid obesity: analysis of 1292 consecutive patients and review of literature. Surg Obes Relat Dis. 2005;1(5):467–74.
17. Brethauer SA, Nfonsam V, Sherman V, Udomsawaengsup S, Schauer PR, Chand B. Endoscopy and upper gastrointestinal contrast studies are complementary in evaluation of weight regain after bariatric surgery. Surg Obes Relat Dis. 2006;2(6):643–8.
18. Gumbs A, Duffy A, Bell R. Management of gastrogastric fistula after laparoscopic Roux-en-Y gastric bypass. Surg Obes Relat Dis. 2006;2(2):117–21.
19. Bhalla S, Yu JX, Varban OA, et al. Upper gastrointestinal series after sleeve gastrectomy is unnecessary to evaluate for gastric sleeve stenosis. Surg Endosc. 2021;35(2):631–5.

6 Timed Barium Swallow in Foregut Disease

Joseph Sujka, Joel Richter, and Christopher DuCoin

Case Presentation

A 50-year-old male presents to the office with progressive dysphagia to solids. His symptoms began 3 months ago and have worsened over time. Foods that exacerbate his symptoms the most are bread and steak. He reports a 15-pound weight loss in the past 3 months. His primary care physician ordered a timed barium swallow (TBS) that showed the normal passage of contrast at 1 and 5 min (Image 6.1). The 13 mm barium tablet failed to pass and remained lodged above the gastroesophageal junction. What is the differential diagnosis? What is the next step in the workup of this patient?

J. Sujka (✉)
Department of Surgery, University of South Florida Morsani College of Medicine, Tampa, FL, USA
e-mail: josephsujka@usf.edu

C. DuCoin · J. Richter
Division of Gastrointestinal Surgery, Department of Surgery, University of South Florida Morsani College of Medicine, Tampa, FL, USA

A. D. Patel et al. (eds.), *The SAGES Manual of Physiologic Evaluation of Foregut Diseases*,
https://doi.org/10.1007/978-3-031-39199-6_6

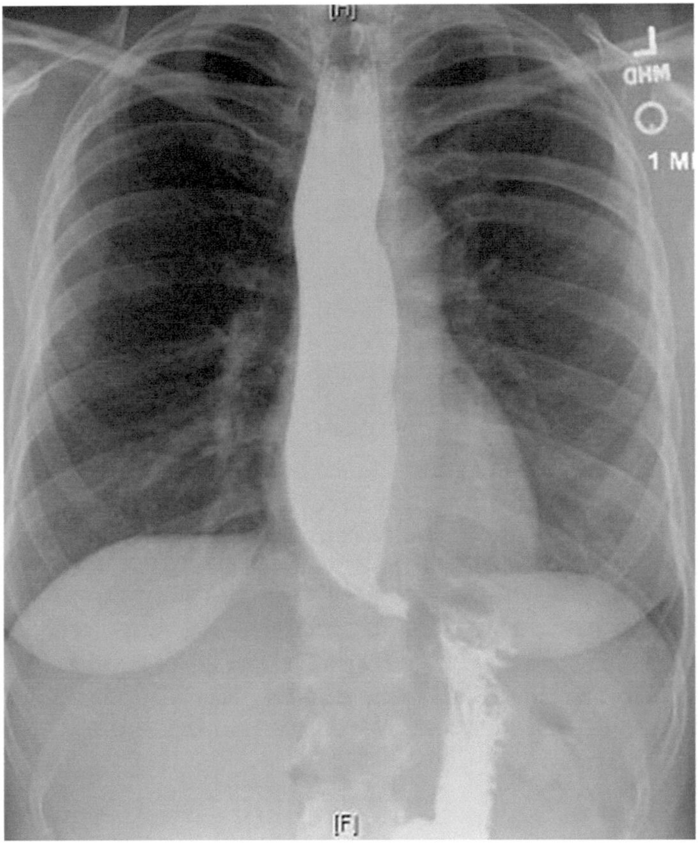

Image 6.1 Timed Barium Swallow showing classic Type 2 Achalasia with a large column of retained barium and "bird's beak" sign at the distal esophagus

Introduction

Timed barium swallow (TBS) was described in the late 1990s by de Oliveira at the Cleveland Clinic. It was developed as an inexpensive test that was easy to perform while additionally having the benefit of being noninvasive, well-tolerated, and utilizing minimal radiation. It is applied in the diagnosis and evaluation of esophageal pathology while also having a value in the postoperative period to assess the success of therapy [1].

TBS and barium swallow can aid in the diagnosis of upper gastrointestinal pathology, such as; achalasia and other esophageal motility disorders, esophageal strictures, gastroesophageal reflux disease (GERD), hiatal hernias, and esophageal cancer [2]. TBS originally started as a modification to existing methods of documenting esophageal emptying in patients with achalasia after treatment. Various volumes of barium were tried in an effort to create a protocol [3]. TBS has now been standardized and consists of administering 8 oz. of low-density barium in the upright position and obtaining a spot film at 1 and 5 min to assess for evacuation of the barium from the esophagus. After this initial evaluation, the esophagus is rinsed with a drink of water, and subsequently, a 13 mm barium pill is administered. Another film is obtained to assess the passage of the tablet out of the esophagus at 5 min. Results are considered abnormal when the initial barium column at 1 and 5 min is greater than 5 cm and 2 cm, respectively. Failure to clear the barium tablet at 5 min is also considered an abnormal result [1, 4].

The 13 mm barium tablet is a key component of a TBS because it can increase the test's diagnostic accuracy. The 13 mm size is used in TBS specifically because it has been shown to be the threshold of dysphagia and discomfort in patients with esophageal strictures smaller than 13 mm. On the other hand, strictures that are larger than 13 mm will likely be asymptomatic [3]. The barium tablet helps delineate strictures in the esophagus that are not evident with liquid barium alone. These strictures are typically not tight and will allow passage of the liquid barium, but the pill will get trapped in the area of narrowing, which is usually the esophagogastric junction [3].

There are limitations to TBS, such as if a patient has retained food or liquid in the esophagus, this can lead to misinterpretation of the barium column [3]. Another limitation is in patients with type III or vigorous achalasia, powerful esophageal contractions can make interpreting the films difficult. When obtaining a TBS in patients with high-amplitude esophageal spasms, the imaging must be taken once esophageal spasms resolve [3].

Use as a Diagnostic Tool

TBS was initially used for the diagnosis of achalasia and the assessment of treatment. However, it can be used to delineate the anatomy of the esophagus and other spastic esophageal motility disorders and esophageal strictures. It can also be used in the diagnosis and preoperative workup of other benign and malignant esophageal disorders, such as hiatal hernias and cancer [1].

Achalasia

Achalasia is an uncommon esophageal motility disorder where the ability of the lower esophageal sphincter (LES) to relax is impaired. In addition, there is a component of aperistalsis in the body of the esophagus. The most common presentation is dysphagia; however, chest pain, regurgitation, weight loss, and aspiration are also part of the clinical picture. The diagnosis of achalasia is made with a combination of endoscopy, high-resolution manometry (HRM), and TBS [5]. HRM can be challenging to obtain because it is invasive and at times not tolerated by the patient. However, HRM is 93% accurate in making the diagnosis of achalasia [6].

TBS can be helpful in delineating esophageal anatomy and function as part of the workup for achalasia. Retention of contrast on TBS correlates closely to the distensibility of the esophagogastric Junction (EGJ) [6]. However, approximately 20% of the patients with achalasia can have a non-diagnostic liquid barium test. Hold up of the 13 mm tablet improves the diagnostic accuracy to 100% [1]. In the case scenario above, TBS and HRM are used together in making the diagnosis of achalasia [1]. TBS can also function as a substitute for HRM in patients that are not able to tolerate the catheter or where there is no access to manometry.

Despite its usefulness, TBS does not always present a uniform picture of achalasia and can at times have different image results. For example, type I achalasia has a dilated esophagus that is frequently distorted with a tapering at the end of the GE junction creating the classic "birds' beak" appearance. On the other hand, type II achalasia will have a dilated esophagus as seen in type I; however, the esophagus remains straight. The classic single point of obstruction at the GE junction is again seen in type II. Type III achalasia, also called vigorous achalasia, can have a characteristic image on TBS with multiple areas of narrowing in a normal-diameter esophagus with multiple tertiary contractions along the length of the esophagus. All of these images are affected by the skill of the proceduralist to both perform and interpret the results.

Due to this difference in achalasia presentation, TBS has been examined for reproducibility and inter-observer reliability. Kostic et al. compared the TBS studies of healthy individuals, achalasia patients pretreatment, and achalasia patients post-treatment. They found that healthy patients uniformly emptied their esophagus by 2 min; however, achalasia patients had variable findings depending on the severity of their disease state. More importantly, the TBS studies had excellent intra- and inter-observer reliability with good reproducibility [7]. This suggests that even with the variable presentation of achalasia TBS represents a consistent and repeatable study to monitor patients.

The Use of TBS in Non-achalasia

Esophagogastric junction outlet obstruction (EGJOO) is similar to achalasia and is defined as an elevated LES pressure with failure of the relaxation mechanism, with normal body peristalsis on HRM. What differentiates EGJOO from achalasia is that the esophagus has normal body peristalsis, while in achalasia there is aperistalsis. Like with achalasia, the highest yield in making the diagnosis of EGJOO is when TBS is used in combination with HRM [8]. In situations where esophageal peristalsis is maintained, the TBS can have varying results. The most common pattern is barium retention at 1 min with complete emptying by 5 min due to generally intact peristalsis. Often, the columns of barium are within normal limits at 1 and 5 min. This is believed to be the result of the maintained contractile force of the esophagus that can push the food bolus; in this case, liquid barium down past the strictured or pathologic area. However, the 13 mm barium tablet will fail to pass 50% of the time in EGJOO [1]. While TBS can help suggest EGJOO along with HRM, it is unable to differentiate between anatomic obstruction and functional EGJOO [9].

TBS is a valuable tool for both the foregut and bariatric surgeon. The foregut surgeon can use the TBS for the perioperative workup of a hiatal hernia. A barium study will provide important information regarding the type of hernia, its size, and the approximate length of the esophagus, thus helping the surgeon plan the procedure. In the postoperative period, barium studies can be used to assess for appropriate hernia repair and function of the fundoplication. TBS can also evaluate patients with postoperative complications like recurrence, slipped Nissen, or a crura repair that is too tight.

For the bariatric surgeon, TBS may be used preoperatively to delineate the anatomy before surgical intervention and in certain instances can replace preoperative endoscopy. TBS can also be used in the immediate postoperative period to rule out complications such as a leak in Bariatric surgery. In the late postoperative period, TBS can be used to evaluate patient anatomy or help diagnose a marginal ulcer or anastomotic strictures [2]. Finally, barium studies can evaluate patients with a slipped gastric band.

TBS Uses in Evaluating Treatment Efficacy

TBS is not only diagnostic for various esophageal pathologies but can also be used in the postoperative period as an objective measure to evaluate the effectiveness of various treatments. In the reported series on patients with achalasia undergoing pneumatic dilation, there is a 73% correlation between a postoperative resolution of symptoms and clearance of barium on TBS. When performing a post-dilation TBS evaluation, there can be concordant or discordant findings between symptomatic relief and improvement of TBS. Vaezi et al. defined improvement of TBS after pneumatic dilation when there was an objective decrease in at least 50% of the barium column length compared to pre-procedure images. In this study, they found that 77% of patients that had concordant findings, meaning improvement in both TBS and symptoms, will remain symptom-free at 6 years. On the other hand, 90% of patients with discordant findings, in this case symptomatic improvement with a change less significant than 50% on TBS, had a recurrence of symptoms before 12 months [10]. Longer-term follow-up corroborated these findings showing patients with concordant findings have better long-term outcomes and symptom relief [11].

Another study by Kostic et al. examined the success of surgical myotomy with TBS. The study evaluated 45 patients both pre- and post-myotomy with a TBS. They examined the height and width of the barium columns and compared these changes to related symptoms. The authors found a decrease in barium height after myotomy, correlated with symptom improvement. Prior to treatment, patients with a higher column had more regurgitation and those with little change in height over 5 min had more dysphagia [12].

Andersson et al. also examined whether or not TBS could be used to monitor treatment efficacy in the context of a randomized controlled trial. They randomized patients into two groups, pneumatic dilation or laparoscopic myotomy with TBS performed both before and after treatment. There was a median interval of 6 months between the TBS in both groups with follow-up for 18 months. Comparing the TBS from both groups, there was no significant difference in TBS findings. However, the height of the barium column at 1 min and symptom scores had a significant correlation with dysphagia for liquids, chest pain, and dysphagia. Patient's with less than 50% improvement in their height at 1 min had a 40% risk of treatment failure in follow-up [13]. This study lends additional data that TBS can be used both in a diagnostic setting but also to check for treatment efficacy.

Some have questioned whether or not other measures besides barium column height may better define success after achalasia treatment. Blonski et al. identified 81 consecutive patients who were treatment naïve for achalasia that underwent either pneumatic dilation, Heller myotomy, or POEM between 1/2012 and 7/2017. They assessed the accuracy of percent change in pre- and post-myotomy barium height at 5 min versus an absolute <5 cm cutoff for assessing treatment response. They concluded that a 3% improvement in barium height at 5 min was more accurate than an absolute cutoff value of <5 cm on post-treatment TBS [14]. Similarly, Sangapalli et al. examined a single cohort of 24 patients who underwent treatment for achalasia and their TBS findings. They compared post-therapy residual barium absolute height, residual height, and surface area. They also found that other measures, in this case change in barium surface area, were superior to the conventional barium height in defining objective response to achalasia therapy [15].

Achalasia and other esophageal motility disorders are lifelong diseases that have no definitive cure. Treatment is geared toward the improvement of symptoms, and this must be clear when discussing both the diagnosis and treatment options. TBS is often used in the workup of patients that had treatment and present with persistent or recurrence of symptoms of these conditions. Ideally, patients will have a postoperative TBS, which can be used to objectively compare it with the symptoms [16].

Conclusion

TBS is a low-cost and easily reproducible test that can aid in the diagnosis of achalasia and other foregut diseases. It can be interpreted with ease by radiologists, gastroenterologists, and surgeons with similar results. It can be used as a standalone diagnostic tool, or in combination with HRM, for the diagnosis of achalasia. It can similarly be used in the early postoperative period to assess for successful treatment, as well as in the late postoperative period and during follow-up. Lastly, it is useful in the evaluation and workup of patients that have postoperative recurrence of symptoms after either endoscopic or surgical treatment of foregut disorders.

References

1. Blonski W, Kumar A, Feldman J, Richter JE. Timed barium swallow: diagnostic role and predictive value in untreated achalasia, Esophagogastric junction outflow obstruction, and non-achalasia dysphagia. Am J Gastroenterol. 2018;113(2):196–203.
2. Dempsey DT. Barium upper GI series in adults: a surgeon's perspective. Abdom Radiol N Y. 2018;43(6):1323–8.
3. de Oliveira JM, Birgisson S, Doinoff C, Einstein D, Herts B, Davros W, et al. Timed barium swallow: a simple technique for evaluating esophageal emptying in patients with achalasia. AJR Am J Roentgenol. 1997;169(2):473–9.
4. Neyaz Z, Gupta M, Ghoshal UC. How to perform and interpret timed barium esophagogram. J Neurogastroenterol Motil. 2013;19(2):251–6.
5. Schlottmann F, Neto RML, Herbella FAM, Patti MG. Esophageal achalasia: pathophysiology, clinical presentation, and diagnostic evaluation. Am Surg. 2018;84(4):467–72.
6. Richter JE. Tailoring therapy for achalasia. Gastroenterol Hepatol. 2020;16(5):249–57.
7. Kostic S, Andersson M, Hellström M, Lönroth H, Lundell L. Timed barium esophagogram in the assessment of patients with achalasia: reproducibility and observer variation. Dis Esophagus Off J Int Soc Dis Esophagus. 2005;18(2):96–103.
8. Richter JE, Clayton SB. Diagnosis and management of esophagogastric junction outflow obstruction. Am J Gastroenterol. 2019;114(4):544–7.
9. Clayton SB, Patel R, Richter JE. Functional and anatomic esophagogastric junction outflow obstruction: manometry, timed barium Esophagram findings, and treatment outcomes. Clin Gastroenterol Hepatol Off Clin Pract J Am Gastroenterol Assoc. 2016;14(6):907–11.
10. Vaezi MF, Baker ME, Richter JE. Assessment of esophageal emptying post-pneumatic dilation: use of the timed barium esophagram. Am J Gastroenterol. 1999;94(7):1802–7.
11. Vaezi MF, Baker ME, Achkar E, Richter JE. Timed barium oesophagram: better predictor of long term success after pneumatic dilation in achalasia than symptom assessment. Gut. 2002;50(6):765–70.
12. Kostic SV, Rice TW, Baker ME, Decamp MM, Murthy SC, Rybicki LA, et al. Timed barium esophagogram: a simple physiologic assessment for achalasia. J Thorac Cardiovasc Surg. 2000;120(5):935–43.
13. Andersson M, Lundell L, Kostic S, Ruth M, Lönroth H, Kjellin A, et al. Evaluation of the response to treatment in patients with idiopathic achalasia by the timed barium esophagogram: results from a randomized clinical trial. Dis Esophagus Off J Int Soc Dis Esophagus. 2009;22(3):264–73.

14. Blonski W, Kumar A, Feldman J, Richter JE. Timed barium swallow for assessing long-term treatment response in patients with achalasia: absolute cutoff versus percent change - a cross-sectional analytic study. Neurogastroenterol Motil Off J Eur Gastrointest Motil Soc. 2020;33:e14005.
15. Sanagapalli S, Plumb A, Maynard J, Leong RW, Sweis R. The timed barium swallow and its relationship to symptoms in achalasia: analysis of surface area and emptying rate. Neurogastroenterol Motil Off J Eur Gastrointest Motil Soc. 2020;32(12):e13928.
16. Swanström LL. Achalasia: treatment, current status and future advances. Korean J Intern Med. 2019;34(6):1173–80.

7 Role of CT Imaging in Foregut Physiology and Benign Pathology

Maggie L. Diller and Daniel Shouhed

Introduction

Computed tomography (CT) is an important diagnostic tool utilized throughout the perioperative period and helps guide clinical decision-making. While the functional or dynamic information provided by CT is limited, several studies support its role in the evaluation of both benign and malignant pathologies of the upper gastrointestinal (GI) tract. CT imaging demonstrates both the organ or system of interest and more distant regions—a unique feature when compared to other imaging modalities and an important adjunct to direct mucosal visualization via endoscopy. Recent advances in CT technology, in particular the routine use of multidetector computed tomography (MDCT), have further enhanced our ability to evaluate the upper GI tract [1]. While traditional single-section spiral CT was limited by a relatively large section thickness, MDCT uses thin col-

M. L. Diller (✉)
Division of General and GI Surgery, Department of Surgery, Emory University, Atlanta, GA, USA
e-mail: maggie.l.diller@kp.org

D. Shouhed
Cedars Sinai Medical Center, Los Angeles, CA, USA

A. D. Patel et al. (eds.), *The SAGES Manual of Physiologic Evaluation of Foregut Diseases*,
https://doi.org/10.1007/978-3-031-39199-6_7

limation and is able to cover a large volume in a very short scan time [2]. This creates high-quality, multiplanar reformation and allows for three-dimensional visualization, significantly improving the diagnostic capability of CT imaging [1]. In this chapter, we will focus on the role of CT imaging in the diagnosis and evaluation of benign foregut pathology, including gastroesophageal reflux disease, hiatal hernias, achalasia, and its specific applications in the postoperative period.

CT Technique

High spatial resolution with proper distension of the esophagus, stomach, and small bowel is necessary for optimum CT technique. Proper timing of intravenous (IV) contrast media injection is especially important with MDCT imaging given short scan times. Administration of IV contrast 30 s prior to image acquisition will capture the arterial phase and further detail the mucosa and gastroesophageal junction (GEJ) wall. When evaluating for mass or tumor, images obtained during the portal venous phase of the entire abdomen will be useful in the detection of distant disease (60-s delay between administration of IV contrast and image acquisition). Additionally, distension of the upper GI tract with oral contrast facilitates the detection of subtle changes within the esophageal/gastric/intestinal wall.

In general, recommendations for imaging of the upper GI tract include a fasted state for at least 6 h followed by administration of 1000–1500 mL of oral contrast [1, 2]. Positioning the patient prone or in a lateral decubitus position while ingesting contrast has also been shown to improve image acquisition of the esophagus and stomach [1, 2]. Over time, acquired expertise in specific pathologies has led to the refinement of these generalized recommendations. Nuances in CT technique specific to a certain disease will be discussed in more detail below. Ideally, CT examinations will be performed on either a 16- or 64-detector row scanner with a 0.5-s tube rotation. For diagnostic viewing, reconstruction of 3–4-mm-thick axial sections should be obtained along with 3–5-mm-thick coronal and sagittal sections along the length of the esophagus, stomach, and proximal small bowel [1, 2]. Multiplanar reformation is optional but may be useful when diagnostic questions remain unresolved.

Gastroesophageal Reflux Disease (GERD) and Hiatal Hernias

Gastroesophageal reflux disease (GERD) is associated with a broad spectrum of symptoms and significantly impacts the quality of life. Prolonged reflux has been associated with changes in the esophageal squamous epithelium leading to Barrett's esophagus and increased risk of esophageal adenocarcinoma. While the gold standard for evaluating reflux esophagitis is endoscopy, contrasted CT plays an important role in the initial evaluation of these patients, particularly as GERD is a common cause of non-cardiac chest pain [3]. The most common CT findings for esophagitis, irrespective of etiology, are circumferential esophageal wall thickening, submucosal edema, and mucosal enhancement [3]. A distal esophageal wall thickness of 5.0 mm or greater predicts the presence of esophagitis on endoscopy with a specificity of 88% and sensitivity of 56% [4]. Additional CT findings associated with reflux esophagitis include the presence of a target sign (ring enhancement) and peri-esophageal lymphadenopathy; however, these findings are nonspecific [4].

Compared to upper endoscopy, CT imaging identifies approximately 50–60% of sliding-type hiatal hernias [4]. Sliding-type hiatal hernias predispose one to gastroesophageal reflux due to displacement of the proximal stomach and GE junction into the posterior mediastinum with the resulting compromise of the lower esophageal sphincter. While endoscopy is more sensitive, even small sliding-type hiatal hernias may be seen on CT with Valsalva or colonic distension.

Esophageal hiatal hernias comprise three types: sliding-type hiatal hernia, paraesophageal hernia, and combined hernia. Sliding hiatal hernia was described above and constitutes more than 90% of esophageal hiatal hernias (HH). Type II paraesophageal hernias involve herniation of all or part of the stomach into the chest, while the gastroesophageal junction remains below the diaphragm. It accounts for less than 10% of HH [5]. Typically, the gastroesophageal sphincter mechanism functions normally in this setting and gastroesophageal reflux does not typically occur [5]. Instead, hemorrhage, incarceration, obstruction, and strangulation of the stomach and intestines are the most common complications. Axial herniation of the stomach results in a retrocardiac mass as the cardia is displaced into the thoracic cavity. With CT, there is a demonstration of gastric folds in this retrocardiac space, which is pathognomonic [5]. While most paraesophageal hernias are associated with fixation of the gastric cardia and a portion of the stomach herniated alongside the esophagus, an extreme form of herniation can occur in which all of the stomach is found within the thoracic cavity and no such portions identified below the diaphragm [5]. This finding on CT is termed "upside down stomach" [5].

Surgical repair is frequently necessary; therefore, preoperative imaging is crucial for the delineation of the hernia's nature, the extent of defect, and to identify obstruction or strangulation, which would necessitate emergent intervention. Multi-slice CT with sagittal, coronal, and 3D reformatted images has significantly improved the diagnostic sensitivity of CT imaging in the setting of all hiatal and diaphragmatic hernias [5]. CT scan often depicts diaphragmatic discontinuity, intrathoracic herniation of abdominal contents, and waist-like constriction of mesenteric folds (the "collar sign") [5]. If intestinal obstruction and strangulation occur, dilated intestinal segments with air–fluid levels will be seen within the thorax and abdomen. Omental vessels may be seen as funicular-shaped densities, running longitudinally in the superior to the inferior direction [5].

Gastric volvulus is a rare but potentially life-threatening condition that may occur in the setting of a hiatal or diaphragmatic hernia. Gastric volvulus refers to at least 180° rotation of the stomach and leads to gastric outlet obstruction, impairment of vascularity, and eventual ischemia. Patients may have a nonspecific clinical presentation, which typically prompts diagnostic imaging. CT scan is the initial examination of choice as it is both sensitive and specific with an overall accuracy of 90% [6]. There are two main gastric volvulus subtypes—organoaxial and mesenteroaxial. Each has unique features on CT scan.

Organoaxial rotation involves rotation of the stomach along its long axis passing through the gastroesophageal junction and pylorus resulting in gastric obstruction. This is the most common subtype and is associated with paraesophageal hernia and diaphragmatic hernia [6]. On CT, the inverted stomach has a horizontal lie with the greater curvature superior to the lesser curvature. Mesenteroaxial rotation of the stomach occurs along its short axis, perpendicular to the long axis. The stomach has a vertical lie, and the antro-pyloric junction is displaced above the gastroesophageal junction.

Additional CT features with high sensitivity and specificity for gastric volvulus include a transition point at the pylorus and stenosis at the hernia neck [6]. CT findings indicative of overt ischemia include gastric wall edema, poor gastric wall enhancement, perigastric fluid, pneumatosis, pleural effusion, and pneumoperitoneum; while they occur infrequently, the findings are highly specific for gastric volvulus [6]. Of these, perigastric fluid and the presence of a pleural effusion have the highest sensitivities (30–47% and 27–37%, respectively) for gastric volvulus [6].

CT Imaging Pre- and Post-fundoplication

GERD refractory to medical therapy requires surgical intervention. Anti-reflux operations aim to accomplish the following three key steps: (1) reduction in any hiatal hernia by returning the LES to the abdomen, (2) construction of a gastric wrap or fundoplication around the distal esophagus, and (3) re-approximation of the diaphragmatic crura. Preoperative imaging is imperative prior to anti-reflux surgery. Traditionally, endoscopy and fluoroscopy-based upper GI series (UGI) are performed and provide sufficient anatomic and functional detail. CT can be performed prior to surgery and may be helpful in the setting of large hiatal or paraesophageal hernias and in determining esophageal length and predicting the need for an esophageal lengthening procedure. The 5-year success rate for anti-reflux operations is approximately 90%;

however, early and late complications do occur with nearly 3% of patients requiring redo fundoplication [7]. In cases of failed fundoplication, UGI or CT assist in the identification of the mechanism of failure and its functional consequences, the need for and timing of additional surgery, and help to guide the choice of surgical repair [7].

MDCT with oral contrast is the preferred method of CT imaging for the evaluation of post-fundoplication anatomy. Positioning the patient in the right anterior oblique position for image acquisition increases intra-abdominal pressure and enhances visualization of hiatal hernias, while eliminating the effect of gravity on esophageal emptying [8]. Multiplanar and volumetric reconstructions for a 3D image are especially valuable in visualizing the anatomical and spatial relationships between the esophagus, the fundoplication and the stomach, and the diaphragm [8].

Persistent or recurrent symptoms of reflux and/or persistent postoperative dysphagia are the most common indicators of fundoplication failure. Such failures are usually due to a wrap that is either too tight or too loose, a disrupted fundoplication, or an incorrectly positioned or herniated fundoplication. CT findings are suggestive of a tight fundoplication include a narrowing of the distal esophagus with proximal dilation [7]. A disruption of the fundoplication involves partial or complete breakdown of the wrap with a recurrent hiatal hernia, both of which are evident on CT [7]. Various findings on CT may indicate an incorrectly positioned or herniated wrap: The wrap may be intact and infra-diaphragmatic with herniation of only the proximal stomach into the chest, or there may be complete migration of the stomach into the chest. Hourglass deformities may also occur. For example, in transdiaphragmatic wrap herniation, an intact wrap and distal esophagus are visualized above the diaphragm on CT with the diaphragmatic hiatus compressing the stomach and creating an hourglass shape [7].

Achalasia

There are two types of achalasia— primary and secondary. Primary achalasia is a benign disease characterized by incomplete relaxation of the lower esophageal sphincter (LES) on swallowing and aperistalsis of the esophageal body. Secondary achalasia, or pseudoachalasia, mimics the symptoms of primary achalasia but typically results from submucosal infiltration of the lower esophagus or proximal stomach by adenocarcinoma. Fluoroscopic-based imaging with UGI is typically the initial imaging procedure when achalasia is suspected [9]. This provides a global assessment that includes swallowing function, esophageal and gastric morphology and motility, gastroesophageal reflux, and abnormalities of the gastric cardia and fundus. CT imaging is an important adjunct when initial diagnostic studies are either equivocal for primary versus secondary achalasia or worrisome for pseudoachalasia of malignancy [10]. CT findings of primary achalasia include long-segment dilation of the esophagus with little or no esophageal wall thickening [9–11]. In contrast, CT findings of secondary achalasia typically include asymmetric esophageal wall thickening (wall thickness > 5 mm), irregular narrowing, or a soft-tissue mass at the gastroesophageal junction [9–11].

CT Imaging Post-myotomy

CT has been used in some centers as part of the initial diagnostic evaluation for post-myotomy adverse events [12]. Compared to fluoroscopic-based studies, CT esophagrams appear more sensitive in detecting post-procedure contrast extravasation and have the added benefit of feasibility—CT imaging can be performed at any time without the direct involvement of a radiologist [12]. To improve sensitivity in detecting small leaks, patients may be given both thin and thick liquid contrast medium. Patients should drink sequentially 3/4 of the thin and thick liquid contrast media followed by ingestion of the last 1/4 immediately prior to the post-oral contrast scan [12]. Image reformation should be done in the coronal and sagittal planes with 10-mm thickness and 5-mm spacing.

The main CT findings post-myotomy can be divided into frequent and reversible sequelae, such as pneumomediastinum, pneumoperitoneum, and subcutaneous emphysema, and potential adverse events, including pneumothorax, pleural effusion, pneumonitis, and focal atelectasis [12–14]. While there is a plethora of abnormal CT findings following surgical or endoscopic myotomy, less than 1% of patients typically require intervention based on clinical symptoms. As such, routine chest CT for achalasia patients is probably not warranted post-myotomy [13, 14].

CT Imaging Versus UGI in the Postoperative Setting

In the assessment of postoperative complications, surgeons typically rely on one of two studies—fluoroscopic-based UGI or CT scan. There is increasing evidence to suggest that CT imaging is the preferred modality in the postoperative period, particularly for the detection of leaks. While UGI is very specific, its sensitivity is lower than that of CT imaging, even with the use of thin barium following a non-diagnostic study [15]. CT with the use of water-soluble contrast along with the evaluation of mediastinal gas has been shown to significantly raise the sensitivity and negative predictive value of CT in the detection of leaks following esophageal surgery [15]. Studies evaluating the role of CT in the detection of leaks following bariatric surgery support this modality as a more sensitive and specific tool in the evaluation of postoperative complications [16]. Nevertheless, it has been suggested that real-time images acquired during an UGI may offer a more accurate depiction of the magnitude and anatomic origin of a leak [17]. As such, UGI remains a useful tool in guiding management decisions, especially once a leak has been identified [16].

There are some additional advantages of CT imaging that should be noted. CT will detect acute processes that may be missed by UGI, i.e., abscess, ileus, early postoperative obstruction, and remnant/duodenal stump or staple line disruption [16]. As mentioned above, UGI is operator-dependent and requires the presence of an expert radiologist both at the time of the study and in the interpretation of results [16]. UGI is also more time-intensive for both the radiologist and the patient, and it requires that the patient be able to tolerate standing upright, whereas a CT scan may be performed entirely with the patient in the supine position. Total radiation exposure is a consideration when deciding between the two studies. An UGI is a dynamic study, and therefore, the total dose of radiation varies, while the dose with CT is more constant. While the overall dose delivered to tissues is less with UGI, the total effective dose is relatively low for both studies. Typical values for an adult patient average 6 and 10 mSv for UGI and CT, respectively [16].

Conclusions

Advances in technology and technique have significantly improved the sensitivity and specificity of CT in the diagnosis and evaluation of upper GI tract pathology. While CT imaging is predominantly an anatomic study with limited functional capability, it may serve as the primary diagnostic tool or as an adjunct to other modalities such as UGI, manometry, and endoscopy. Modern-day surgeons will benefit from a basic understanding of the methods of image acquisition to expedite accurate diagnoses. Thorough knowledge of the appearance of normal and surgically altered anatomy and findings specific to disease processes will be imperative in the interpretation of results and guiding clinical decision-making.

References

1. Ba-Ssalamah A, et al. Dedicated multidetector CT of the stomach: spectrum of diseases. Radiographics. 2003;23(3):625–44.
2. Ba-Ssalamah A, et al. Dedicated multi-detector CT of the esophagus: spectrum of diseases. Abdom Imaging. 2009;34(1):3–18.
3. Young CA, et al. CT features of esophageal emergencies. Radiographics. 2008;28(6):1541–53.
4. Lambert L, et al. The predictive value of computed tomography in the detection of reflux esophagitis in patients undergoing upper endoscopy. Clin Imaging. 2018;49:97–100.
5. Eren S, Ciriş F. Diaphragmatic hernia: diagnostic approaches with review of the literature. Eur J Radiol. 2005;54(3):448–59.
6. Mazaheri P, et al. CT of gastric volvulus: interobserver reliability, radiologists' accuracy, and imaging findings. Am J Roentgenol. 2018;212(1):103–8.

7. Carbo AI, et al. Imaging findings of successful and failed fundoplication. Radiographics. 2014;34(7):1873–84.
8. Rodríguez Carnero P, et al. Multislice computed tomography for the study of complications of gastric fundoplication. Radiología (English Edition). 2014;56(5):435–9.
9. Rabushka LS, Fishman EK, Kuhlman JE. CT evaluation of achalasia. J Comput Assist Tomogr. 1991;15(3):434.
10. Licurse MY, et al. Utility of chest CT for differentiating primary and secondary achalasia. Clin Radiol. 2014;69(10):1019–26.
11. Carter MD, Robert C, Smith RC, Burrell MI, Traube M. Differentiation of achalasia from pseudoachalasia by computed tomography. Am J Gastroenterol. 1997;92(4):624–8.
12. Pannu D, et al. Prospective evaluation of CT esophagram findings after peroral endoscopic myotomy. Gastrointest Endosc. 2016;84(3):408–15.
13. Cai M-Y, et al. Thoracic CT after peroral endoscopic myotomy for the treatment of achalasia. Gastrointest Endosc. 2014;80(6):1046–55.
14. Reddy CA, et al. The clinical impact of routine esophagram after peroral endoscopic myotomy. Gastrointest Endosc. 2021;93(1):102–6.
15. Strauss C, et al. Computed tomography versus water-soluble contrast swallow in the detection of intrathoracic anastomotic leak complicating esophagogastrectomy (Ivor Lewis): a prospective study in 97 patients. Ann Surg. 2010;251(4):647.
16. Bingham J, et al. Computed tomography scan versus upper gastrointestinal fluoroscopy for diagnosis of staple line leak following bariatric surgery. Am J Surg. 2015;209(5):810–4.
17. de Aretxabala X, et al. Gastric leak after sleeve gastrectomy: analysis of its management. Obes Surg. 2011;21(8):1232–7.

3D Modeling with CT

8

Angela M. Kao and Paul D. Colavita

Introduction

Effective treatment of benign and malignant diseases of the esophagus and stomach often requires a combination of diagnostic tests to adequately evaluate the anatomy and physiologic function of the esophagus and stomach. The role of conventional computed tomographic (CT) imaging in the diagnostic evaluation of foregut disease is often an adjunct test; however, it remains a mainstay of preoperative staging of esophageal and gastric malignancies. In patients who undergo foregut surgery, CT imaging is commonly obtained to detect postoperative failures or complications such as esophageal leak.

In recent years, advancements in technology, such as the multidetector CT scanner, have enabled three-dimensional (3D) reconstruction using methods such as multiplanar reformation and volume rendering. Following these advances, 3D CT has gained renewed interest in its use during preoperative

A. M. Kao · P. D. Colavita (✉)
Division of Gastrointestinal Surgery, Department of Surgery, Carolinas Medical Center, Charlotte, NC, USA
e-mail: Paul.D.Colavita@atriumhealth.org

A. D. Patel et al. (eds.), *The SAGES Manual of Physiologic Evaluation of Foregut Diseases*,
https://doi.org/10.1007/978-3-031-39199-6_8

evaluation and surgical planning. While the clinical value of 3D CT reconstruction has been extensively reported in other fields such as maxillofacial surgery and orthopedic surgery, similar widespread use has been slower to gain traction in abdominal surgery due to the complexity in image processing of various abdominal soft tissues, compared to bones or vessels [1]. The adoption of 3D CT modeling in abdominal surgery has progressively increased over the past decade, with newer clinical applications of 3D reconstruction for the esophagus and stomach.

Multidetector CT imaging of the esophagus and stomach with 3D reconstruction offers many advantages, including improved diagnosis of pathologic anatomy and increased staging accuracy of malignancies. The diagnostic yield of traditional CT imaging has been limited by the collapsed lumen of the esophagus which prevents accurate evaluation of esophageal wall thickening and detection of endoluminal masses. Compared to two-dimensional imaging, 3D visualization of a lesion in multiple planes enhances the viewer's perspective and depth perception, allowing for improved characterization of morphologic features and relation to adjacent structures [2]. Optimal visualization of the esophagus and accurate characterization of pathologic lesions can be facilitated by adequate distention of the esophageal lumen with air or liquid, as well as obtaining images with the patient in prone and supine positions [3].

Esophageal Injuries

Initial evaluation of esophageal injuries often begins with a contrast swallow study using water-soluble contrast followed by thin barium; however, CT has been increasingly used due to its widespread availability and ability to rapidly obtain high-resolution images. In patients with a negative contrast swallow study, CT is a valuable noninvasive diagnostic test that can detect esophageal perforation with high sensitivity. CT findings suggestive of esophageal perforation include contrast extravasation, as well as indirect signs, such as mediastinal inflammation, subcutaneous or muscular emphysema of the neck and/or chest, widened mediastinum, pneumomediastinum, pneumopericardium, left-sided pleural effusion, or pneumothorax [4].

Achalasia

Although CT is not routinely indicated in the evaluation and workup of achalasia, it can serve as a useful adjunct in complicated cases by detecting atypical features that may indicate the presence of malignancy or other esophageal pathology [4]. Neoplastic infiltration of the submucosa layer in the distal esophagus can result in pseudoachalasia, with symptoms that mimic idiopathic achalasia. In advanced achalasia, CT shows uniform dilatation of a long esophageal segment, with normal-appearing boundaries surrounded by mediastinal fat. In contrast, patients with pseudoachalasia often demonstrate CT findings of a mass or wall thickening at the site of esophageal narrowing, with asymmetric or marked wall thickening >10 mm being highly suggestive of pseudoachalasia.

3D CT modeling has also been used for surgical planning of achalasia with complex anatomy. Based on a patient's CT scan demonstrating a markedly tortuous aorta, Marano et al. printed a 3D model of the esophagogastric junction that allowed the surgeon to measure the position of the esophagus relative to the thoracic aorta [5]. Demonstration of the interspatial relationship of the esophagus with critical surrounding structures using 3D CT modeling enabled preoperative discussion of optimal surgical approaches and facilitated the ability to plan possible critical maneuvers.

Hiatal Hernia

Hiatal hernias refer to herniation of the stomach into the thoracic cavity and can cause reflux, epigastric, or retrosternal pain, respiratory symptoms, or can be incidentally detected in asymptomatic patients. Types of hiatal hernia are typically grouped into four types. Type I hernias are also labeled sliding type, with the displacement of the gastroesophageal junction (GEJ) upward into the posterior mediastinum, with no aspect of the stomach superior to the GEJ and no other herniated organs. Type II hernias are paraesophageal hernias, where the stomach herniates into the thoracic cavity with a non-displaced gastroesophageal junction. Type III hernias are also paraesophageal hernias and are defined by herniation of the stomach superior to an also herniated GEJ. Type IV hernias involve the herniation of other abdominal contents into the thoracic cavity. On CT imaging, the demonstration of gastric folds in the chest is pathognomonic and frequently visualized, particularly with adequate distention of the stomach and esophagus [4]. Surrogate markers of the GEJ, such as the angle of His and abrupt change in tubular contour, visualized more than 2 cm above the level of the diaphragm also indicate the presence of a hiatal hernia [6]. Sliding hiatal hernias appear as axial herniation of the stomach as a retrocardiac mass with displacement of the cardia into the thoracic cavity, while type II hernias are associated with fixation of the gastric cardia.

The potential clinical application of 3D CT imaging has recently been described for hiatal hernias. Kavic et al. describe using surface modeling techniques to create 3D models of the various types of hiatal hernias [7]. The ability to appreciate relevant anatomy from different viewpoints enables a more comprehensive understanding of spatial relationships and facilitates preoperative planning, particularly in laparoscopic surgery, where strategic port placement is critical [8]. Recent interest in tailoring hiatal closure techniques to the size of the hiatal defect has also led to CT measurements of esophageal hiatus surface area (HSA) using 3D imaging. Ouyang et al. described a significantly larger mean HSA of 6.9 cm^2 and 11.5 cm^2 in patients with type I and type III hiatal hernias, respectively, compared to those without hiatal hernia [6]. Similarly, 3D CT volumetric measurements can be utilized for surgical planning of paraesophageal hernia repair. In a retrospective analysis, the authors of this chapter demonstrated a significant correlation between increases in HSA and hernia sac volume with emergent case status and operative findings of gastric volvulus and incarceration [9]. Furthermore, preoperative 3D CT measurements predicted the inability to perform primary cruroplasty and the need for salvage gastropexy and relaxing incisions [9].

Esophageal Stenosis

The use of multidetector CT is noninvasive and a valuable alternative diagnostic tool for evaluating patients with esophageal stenosis that may not be amenable to endoscopic evaluation. In these patients, 3D CT can accurately determine the location and length of the stricture, as well as visualize the esophagus and stomach distal to the stenosis [3]. Findings of esophageal wall thickening, obliteration of surrounding fat planes, and mediastinal adenopathy can distinguish between benign and malignant etiologies of esophageal stenosis. Benign esophageal strictures, such as those caused by peptic ulcer disease, are often characterized by diffuse, regular, or concentric wall thickening and uninvolved surrounding fat planes. In contrast, irregular asymmetric wall thickening, obliteration of the fat planes between the esophagus and adjacent structures, and presence of mediastinal adenopathies point to malignant etiologies of stenosis. The use of post-image processing also enables virtual endoscopic assessment of intraluminal, mural, and extraluminal pathology; however, limitations of CT include the inability to obtain histologic biopsy or to treat stenosis using dilation and other endoscopic techniques.

Placement of a self-expandable stent in patients with an unresectable neoplasm causing esophageal stenosis can palliate symptoms of dysphagia; however, radial forces exerted by the stent can cause mass effect on adjacent mediastinal structures, potentially leading to compression of the tracheobronchial tree and airway compromise [10]. CT assessment of the area of stenosis and degree of compression on adjacent structures facilitates pretreatment planning, including choice of size and type of stent. The use of 3D CT offers potential advantages over traditional axial CT, including the ability to obtain internal images of the upper airways and esophagus, allowing for easier measurement of the stenosis caliber and length, as well as potentially preventing risky maneuvers [11].

Esophageal Malignancy

Preoperative staging of esophageal cancer currently remains the most important indication for MDCT of the esophagus. In addition to upper endoscopy, CT is an important test in the workup and staging of esophageal cancer, particularly in the detection of regional nodal spread and distant metastases to the liver and lung.

Compared to enhanced 2D CT imaging, which is limited in its evaluation of the spatial location and overall length of esophageal tumors and understages tumor depth in 40% of patients, 3D CT imaging provides additional information regarding endoluminal morphology and longitudinal extent of tumors that previously was obtained using conventional barium study [12]. Furthermore, 3D CT provides a large advantage in the evaluation of tumor response to neoadjuvant chemotherapy and radiation.

Esophageal malignancy is best represented on 3D CT imaging by asymmetric wall thickening of the esophagus with increased heterogeneous enhancement compared to adjacent mucosa; however, diffuse symmetric thickening greater than 3 mm should also raise suspicion for malignant pathology. In their 3D CT protocol, Panebianco et al. identified pathologic wall thickening measuring between 3.0 and 30 mm in 97% of patients with neoplasia compared to normal esophageal wall thickness measuring less than 3 mm [13]. Eccentric lesions with intact overlying mucosa and smooth lobulated margins without obliteration of esophageal layers into the adjacent fat were characterized as submucosal tumors [12]. While CT poorly distinguishes between T1 and T2 diseases, imaging findings such as stranding or increased attenuation of the paraesophageal fat, ill-defined soft tissue density around the tumor, mucosal irregularities, or bulging of the outside border are suggestive of T3 disease, with tumor invasion into the adventitia and paraesophageal fat [13]. Similarly, invasion of adjacent structures evidenced by mass effect or loss of fat planes is consistent with the T4 stage. Correlation between 3D CT tumor staging and pathologic findings in patients who underwent demonstrated an overall sensitivity of 92% [13]. Cai et al. demonstrated that 3D CT reconstruction was superior to traditional gastroscopy in determining the location of pathologic changes and extent of disease, or tumor stage, with greater accuracy [14]. Accuracy of tumor staging by 3D CT is also higher than previously reported rates with axial CT imaging, demonstrating enhanced diagnostic capabilities using 3D reconstruction techniques.

3D CT reconstruction enables accurate assessment of the tumor location relative to adjacent structures and can aid in determining the surgical approach. The ability to characterize esophageal tumors using a noninvasive method is particularly advantageous in patients with malignant esophageal narrowing that is not amenable to endoscopy. In one-third of patients who were unable to undergo gastroscopy, the use of 3D reconstruction enabled accurate preoperative evaluation and planning of surgical treatment [14]. Wada et al. described the efficacy of 3D CT in delineating bronchial artery anatomy prior to esophagectomy, allowing for the identification of vascular anomalies and bronchial artery preservation, the latter of which has been shown to significantly reduce pulmonary complications and tracheal ischemia [15].

In addition, multidetector CT (MDCT) plays an important role in the evaluation of postoperative complications including the presence and severity of esophageal perforation. Furthermore, MDCT can detect tumor recurrence after esophagectomy with an accurate demonstration of locoregional recurrent esophageal tumor on MDCT. Furthermore, it is superior for the detection of distant metastatic disease and can also accurately delineate the neoesophagus and its surroundings [4].

Esophageal Atresia

Esophageal atresia (EA) with tracheoesophageal fistula (TEF) is a correctable congenital anomaly that occurs in up to 0.03% of neonates, with distal TEF being the most common type. Preoperative evaluation of EA-TEF patients has traditionally included chest radiographs, as well as invasive tests such as endoscopy and bronchoscopy. Recently, several have advocated for the role of CT imaging in the preoperative evaluation of EA-TEF patients, as it is a noninvasive test that can delineate the anatomy of the tracheobronchial tree, both esophageal pouches, and the exact location of the TEF. Importantly, the use of 3D images can demonstrate the spatial relationship between the proximal esophageal pouch and distal fistula and provide an accurate assessment of the interpouch gap, which is critical to planning the surgical approach, as well as risk stratification and prognosis [16]. Compared to rough assessment on chest radiographs that tend to underestimate the interpouch distance, several studies have reported the superiority of 3D CT in accurately assessing interpouch distance and fistula level, as well as the detection of concomitant mediastinal or thoracic anomalies [17, 18]. Mahalik et al. reported in their study of type C TEF (the most common type), the majority of patients had a short-to-intermediate interposition gap, and thus, preoperative CT evaluation did not change the surgical management [16]. Thus, the benefits are outweighed by the significant risk of exposure to ionizing radiation and the potential for future radiation-induced malignancies.

Gastric Diseases

CT is commonly used in the evaluation of gastric diseases; however, its sensitivity and specificity vary in different diseases. While endoscopy is often the initial diagnostic test in the evaluation of gastric lesions, it is an invasive test with limited ability, particularly with submucosal or extramural pathology. The use of stomach CT protocols that use effervescent granules to fill the gastric lumen with air and ensure the stomach is adequately distended can improve diagnostic sensitivity and specificity [19]. Recently, 3D CT imaging has also gained wide clinical application due to advances in post-image processing that have enabled virtual endoscopic assessment of gastric mucosa. Advantages of 3D CT over traditional endoscopy include the detection of mural and extramural gastric pathology, while the use of new reconstruction techniques such as volume rendering can be manipulated to orient the stomach, providing superior images compared to shaded surface display rendered images seen in early 3D imaging (CT gastroscopy). Additionally, visualization of lesions in multiple planes with 3D CT adds valuable perspective by enhancing depth perception and improving the characterization of lesion morphology and spatial relationship to adjacent structures [2].

Gastric Cancer

CT imaging, in combination with endoscopic ultrasound (EUS), is commonly utilized for the evaluation and staging of gastric cancers. While adequate stomach distention and the use of negative intraluminal contrast agents have increased the diagnostic accuracy of CT, detection of gastric cancers with CT varies with the stage of cancer, ranging between 90 and 100% for advanced gastric cancer [19]. In contrast, the accuracy of CT in diagnosing early gastric cancers or depressed, endophytic lesions ranges from 20% with portal venous phase CT scan to 88% with arterial phase imaging [19]. Additionally, both EUS and traditional CT scans have been shown to be inaccurate in restaging of gastric cancer after neoadjuvant chemotherapy.

The advantages of 3D CT can further improve the detection of both early and advanced gastric tumors, with a reported diagnostic accuracy of 96% and 100%, respectively [20]. In patients with early gastric cancer, studies have demonstrated a significantly higher detection rate (94%) with 3D CT imaging compared to axial images alone [21]. 3D CT has also demonstrated high accuracy, sensitivity, and specificity in the staging assessment of locoregional spread, nodal involvement, and distant metastases [2]. In advanced gastric cancer, the use of 3D CT demonstrated superior tumor staging accuracy over axial imaging alone [22]. While EUS has higher accuracy rates of T staging (87%), accurate assessment of N stage is equivalent to 3D CT, which has reported accuracy of 83% and 75% for tumor and nodal staging, respectively [20].

More recently, tumor volumetric studies have further broadened the potential clinical applications of 3D CT in gastric cancer. Tumor volume measurements on CT have demonstrated a strong correlation with pathologic T and N stages for gastric cancer, both in patients who have not received treatment and restaging following neoadjuvant chemotherapy [23, 24]. The utility of 3D CT volumetry was further investigated in advanced gastric cancer patients who underwent neoadjuvant chemotherapy. The study showed that the percentage volume reduction rate of the primary gastric tumor correlated highly with histopathologic tumor regression and can be used to predict tumor response to neoadjuvant chemotherapy [25].

Gastric Lymphoma

In patients with gastric lymphoma, CT scan remains the primary imaging modality for the evaluation and staging. On CT imaging, lymphomas can appear with nonspecific findings of diffuse gastric wall thickening, infiltrating lesions, or a polypoid mass. Preservation of gastric distensibility and nodular thickening of the gastric folds are features seen with lymphoma and can help differentiate them from adenocarcinoma. Other distinguishing features on CT imaging suggestive of lymphoma include lymphadenopathy below the renal hilum.

Gastrointestinal Stromal Tumors (GISTs)

CT scan is the preferred diagnostic test of choice for GISTs, due to the limited evaluation of submucosal pathology with traditional upper endoscopy. GISTs often appear on CT as exophytic submucosal lesions in the gastric body or antrum, however, can also present as an intraluminal mass. GISTs can grow to a large size, with tumors frequently ranging between 3 and 10 cm in size, and heterogeneous enhancement can be seen in larger tumors due to tumor necrosis. Similarly, mucosal ulceration can occur resulting in CT findings of extraluminal air or contrast within the lesion.

Gastrectomy: Preoperative and Postoperative Evaluation

The role of 3D CT in preoperative planning prior to gastric surgery has been described in patients with gastric cancer, as well as the bariatric patient population [26–28]. Laparoscopic-assisted gastrectomy is less invasive and now widely performed due to benefits in recovery time and quality of life; however, disadvantages of laparoscopy include the limited view of the entire stomach and increased operative time required to identify anatomic vasculature. Several studies evaluating the utility of preoperative 3D CT in laparoscopic gastric cancer surgery describe its efficacy in visualizing pertinent gastric vascular anatomy with 100% sensitivity in identifying the left and right gastric arteries [27]. 3D CT also allowed for preoperative assessment of individual variation in vasculature such as a replaced left hepatic artery, which can be unintentionally ligated if misidentified intraoperatively, resulting in postoperative liver dysfunction [26, 27]. In addition to vascular anatomy, 3D CT can be used in gastric cancer surgery to simulate the complex anatomical variations of the splenic hilum and assist with lymph node dissection. Comparative studies of surgical outcomes with and without preoperative 3D CT simulation reveal significantly reduced operative time and blood loss with 3D CT simulation, while other authors report a larger harvest of splenic hilum (station 10) lymph nodes. Additionally, identification of the caudal pancreatic artery or vein on 3D CT can increase the preservation of these vessels, which may prevent the development of postoperative pancreatic fistula [28].

CT is commonly obtained in the postoperative setting in patients who have undergone partial or total gastrectomy. In gastric cancer patients, CT plays a role in surveillance and is used to detect the presence of disease recurrence or progression to metastatic spread during the follow-up period. After bariatric surgery, CT imaging can be used to evaluate the anastomosis after gastric bypass and is frequently used to detect complications including bleeding, perforation, or internal hernia [19, 29]. Similarly, 3D CT after Roux-en-Y gastric bypass can be used to derive accurate measurements of pouch volume, a key component of weight loss after bariatric surgery [30]. In the acute postoperative setting, 3D CT allows for immediate assessment of the anastomosis and structural integrity of the pouch.

The clinical utility of multidetector CT may also include the prediction of post-surgical weight loss after bariatric surgery, as traditional methods of estimating gastric volume have been variable and often inaccurate. Multiple studies of 3D CT volumetry in patients undergoing sleeve gastrectomy describe the feasibility and accuracy of gastric volumetric measurements and have established their relationship with estimated weight loss [31, 32]. Pawanindra et al. used multidetector CT to calculate the volume of the resected stomach in patients undergoing sleeve gastrectomy and demonstrated a strong correlation with early postoperative weight loss. Similar findings were reported by Hanssen et al., who used 3D CT to measure the volume of the postoperative gastric remnant 6 months after surgery, showing a strong correlation between remnant gastric volume > 100 mL and poor estimated weight loss [31]. One recent study attempted to minimize the varying degrees of gastric distention seen with heterogeneous CT protocols showed gastric wall volume, rather than gastric luminal volume, was the key indicator of weight loss 1 year after sleeve gastrectomy [32].

References

1. Pietrabissa A, Marconi S, Negrello E, et al. An overview on 3D printing for abdominal surgery. Surg Endosc. 2020;34(1):1–13. https://doi.org/10.1007/s00464-019-07155-5.
2. Duan SY, Zhang DT, Lin QC, Wu YH. Clinical value of CT three-dimensional imaging in diagnosing gastrointestinal tract diseases. World J Gastroenterol. 2006;12(19):2945–8. https://doi.org/10.3748/wjg.v12.i18.2945.
3. Carrascosa P, Capuñay C, Martín López E, Salis G, Mazzadi S, Carrascosa J. Esophageal stenosis: three-dimensional multidetector CT and virtual endoscopy. Abdom Imaging. 2009;34(1):19–25. https://doi.org/10.1007/s00261-008-9435-1.

4. Ba-Ssalamah A, Zacherl J, Noebauer-Huhmann IM, et al. Dedicated multi-detector CT of the esophagus: spectrum of diseases. Abdom Imaging. 2009;34(1):3–18. https://doi.org/10.1007/s00261-007-9290-5.
5. Marano L, Ricci A, Savelli V, et al. From digital world to real life: a robotic approach to the esophagogastric junction with a 3D printed model. BMC Surg. 2019;19(1):1–6. https://doi.org/10.1186/s12893-019-0621-6.
6. Ouyang W, Dass C, Zhao H, Kim C, Criner G. Multiplanar MDCT measurement of esophageal hiatus surface area: association with hiatal hernia and GERD. Surg Endosc. 2016;30(6):2465–72. https://doi.org/10.1007/s00464-015-4499-9.
7. Kavic SM, Segan RD, George IM, Turner PL, Roth JS, Park A. Classification of hiatal hernias using dynamic three-dimensional reconstruction. Surg Innov. 2006;13(1):49–52. https://doi.org/10.1177/155335060601300108.
8. Mastrangelo MJ, Stich J, Hoskins JD, et al. Advancements in immersive virtual reality as a tool for preoperative planning for laparoscopic surgery. Stud Heal Technol Inf. 2002;85:274–9.
9. Kao AM, Ross SW, Otero J, et al. Use of computed tomography volumetric measurements to predict operative techniques in paraesophageal hernia repair. Surg Endosc. 2020;34(4):1785–94. https://doi.org/10.1007/s00464-019-06930-8.
10. Dasgupta A, Jain P, Sandur S, Dolmatch BL, Geisinger MA, Mehta AC. Airway complications of esophageal self-expandable metallic stent. Gastrointest Endosc. 1998;47(6):4–7.
11. Di Simone MP, Mattioli S, D'Ovidio F, Bassi F. Three-dimensional CT imaging and virtual endoscopy for the placement of self-expandable stents in oesophageal and tracheobronchial neoplastic stenoses. Eur J Cardio-thoracic Surg. 2003;23(1):106–8. https://doi.org/10.1016/S1010-7940(02)00620-6.
12. Kim SH, Lee JM, Han JK, et al. Three-dimensional MDCT imaging and CT esophagography for evaluation of esophageal tumors: preliminary study. Eur Radiol. 2006;16(11):2418–26. https://doi.org/10.1007/s00330-006-0337-8.
13. Panebianco V, Grazhdani H, Iafrate F, et al. 3D CT protocol in the assessment of the esophageal neoplastic lesions: can it improve TNM staging? Eur Radiol. 2006;16(2):414–21. https://doi.org/10.1007/s00330-005-2851-5.
14. Cai H, Wang R, Li Y, Yang X, Cui Y. Role of 3D reconstruction in the evaluation of patients with lower segment oesophageal cancer. J Thorac Dis. 2018;10(7):3940–7. https://doi.org/10.21037/jtd.2018.06.119.
15. Wada T, Takeuchi H, Kawakubo H, et al. Clinical utility of preoperative evaluation of bronchial arteries by three-dimensional computed tomographic angiography for esophageal cancer surgery. Dis Esophagus. 2013;26:616–22. https://doi.org/10.1111/dote.12012.

16. Mahalik SK, Sodhi KS, Narasimhan KL, Rao KLN. Role of preoperative 3D CT reconstruction for evaluation of patients with esophageal atresia and tracheoesophageal fistula. Pediatr Surg Int. 2012;28(10):961–6. https://doi.org/10.1007/s00383-012-3111-9.
17. Fitoz S, Atasoy C, Yagmurlu A, Akyar S, Erden A, Dindar H. Three-dimensional CT of congenital esophageal atresia and distal tracheoesophageal fistula in neonates: preliminary results. Am J Roentgenol. 2000;175(5):1403–7. https://doi.org/10.2214/ajr.175.5.1751403.
18. Lam WW, Tam PKH, Chan F, Chan K, Cheung W. Esophageal atresia and tracheal stenosis: use of three-dimensional CT and virtual bronchoscopy in neonates, infants, and children. Am J Roentgenol. 2000;174:1009–12.
19. Nagpal P, Prakash A, Pradhan G, et al. MDCT imaging of the stomach: advances and applications. Br J Radiol. 2017;90(1069):20160412. https://doi.org/10.1259/bjr.20160412.
20. Bhandari S, Shim CS, Kim JH, et al. Usefulness of three-dimensional, multidetector row CT (virtual gastroscopy and multiplanar reconstruction) in the evaluation of gastric cancer: a comparison with conventional endoscopy, EUS, and histopathology. Gastrointest Endosc. 2004;59(6):619–26. https://doi.org/10.1016/S0016-5107(04)00169-5.
21. Lee DH, Ko YT. Gastric lesions: evaluation with three-dimensional images using helical CT. Am J Roentgenol. 1997;169:787–9.
22. Lee DH, Ko YT. Advanced gastric carcinoma: the role of three-dimensional and axial imaging by spiral CT. Abdom Imaging. 1999;24(2):111–6. https://doi.org/10.1007/s002619900456.
23. Hallinan JTPD, Venkatesh SK, Peter L, Makmur A, Yong WP, So JBY. CT volumetry for gastric carcinoma: association with TNM stage. Eur Radiol. 2014;24:3105–14. https://doi.org/10.1007/s00330-014-3316-5.
24. Wang ZC, Wang C, Ding Y, Ji Y, Zeng MS, Rao SX. CT volumetry can potentially predict the local stage for gastric cancer after chemotherapy. Diagnostic Interv Radiol. 2017;23(4):257–62. https://doi.org/10.5152/dir.2017.16517.
25. Lee SM, Kim SH, Lee JM, et al. Usefulness of CT volumetry for primary gastric lesions in predicting pathologic response to neoadjuvant chemotherapy in advanced gastric cancer. Abdom Imaging. 2009;34(4):430–40. https://doi.org/10.1007/s00261-008-9420-8.
26. Lee SW, Shinohara H, Matsuki M, et al. Preoperative simulation of vascular anatomy by three-dimensional computed tomography imaging in laparoscopic gastric cancer surgery. J Am Coll Surg. 2003;197(6):927–36. https://doi.org/10.1016/j.jamcollsurg.2003.07.021.
27. Matsuki M, Kani H, Tatsugami F, et al. Preoperative assessment of vascular anatomy around the stomach by 3D imaging using MDCT before laparoscopy-assisted gastrectomy. Am J Roentgenol. 2004;183(1):145–51. https://doi.org/10.2214/ajr.183.1.1830145.
28. Sunagawa H, Kinoshita T. Three-dimensional computed tomography simulation for laparoscopic lymph node dissection in the treatment of

proximal gastric cancer. Transl Gastroenterol Hepatol. 2017;2(54):54. https://doi.org/10.21037/tgh.2017.04.10.
29. Guniganti P, Bradenham CH, Raptis C, Menias CO, Mellnick VM. CT of gastric emergencies. Radiographics. 2015;35(7):1909–21.
30. Alva S, Eisenberg D, Duffy A, Roberts K, Israel G, Bell R. Virtual three-dimensional computed tomography assessment of the gastric pouch following laparoscopic roux-Y gastric bypass. Obes Surg. 2008;18(4):364–6. https://doi.org/10.1007/s11695-008-9438-6.
31. Hanssen A, Plotnikov S, Acosta G, et al. 3D volumetry and its correlation between postoperative gastric volume and excess weight loss after sleeve gastrectomy. Obes Surg. 2018;28(3):775–80. https://doi.org/10.1007/s11695-017-2927-8.
32. Lin CH, Hsu Y, Chen CL, et al. Impact of 3D-CT-based gastric wall volume on weight loss after laparoscopic sleeve gastrectomy. Obes Surg. 2020;30:4226. https://doi.org/10.1007/s11695-020-04783-y.

Role of the Gastric Emptying Study

9

Michael L. Williford and S. Scott Davis Jr.

Role of a Gastric Emptying Study

A gastric emptying study is a noninvasive method of obtaining an objective measure of the rate of gastric emptying. The study can be performed pre- or postoperatively and provides useful information that will help guide clinical decision-making. A nuclear medicine study to describe gastric emptying was first reported in 1966 [1]. Over time, the technology has evolved, and the study is currently ordered to evaluate for both delayed and rapid gastric emptying. A joint consensus statement was released in 2008 by the Society of Nuclear Medicine and the American Neurogastroenterology and Motility Society that provides the following framework for the performance and interpretation of a gastric emptying study [2].

M. L. Williford
WakeMed Health and Hospitals, Raleigh, NC, USA

S. S. Davis Jr. (✉)
Emory Endosurgery Unit, Department of Surgery, Emory University, Atlanta, GA, USA
e-mail: sdavisj@emory.edu

A. D. Patel et al. (eds.), *The SAGES Manual of Physiologic Evaluation of Foregut Diseases*,
https://doi.org/10.1007/978-3-031-39199-6_9

Patients are asked to discontinue medications that could affect gastric motility, including prokinetic agents (e.g., metoclopramide), anticholinergics, and opioids. The patients are then kept without eating for 6 h prior to the study. They are asked to eat a meal consisting of a low-fat solid (typically Tc-99 radiolabeled egg whites), and this is often accompanied by specific volumes of toast, jam, and water. Radiolabeled solids are most often used if there is a concern for delayed gastric emptying, as emptying of liquids may be preserved in this condition. The meal must be finished within 10 min. A gamma camera is then used to obtain anterior and posterior images of the stomach at the 0-, 1-, 2-, and 4-h time points. It is important to reach the 4-h time point if the results are indeterminate, as a patient may have the appearance of normal gastric emptying initially, but the results at the later time points may be abnormal.

Delayed gastric emptying is consistent with >90% of the radiotracer present in the stomach at 1 h, >60% at 2 h, and >10% at 4 h. Rapid gastric emptying is consistent with <70% of the radiotracer present in the stomach at 30 min or <30% at 1 h [3]. These normal values were determined by analyzing the results of asymptomatic volunteers.

Interpretation of Results

The radiotracer counts will be analyzed and graphed over time. A typical radiologist interpretation includes a calculated half-time (the time at which 50% of the tracer has exited the stomach) and the percentages of the tracer remaining at the 0-, 1-, 2-, and 4-h time points. The following are actual patient vignettes with the associated gastric emptying study images and interpretation based on the above criteria.

Normal Gastric Emptying

Patient 1 is a 36-year-old woman with gastroparesis who originally underwent gastric stimulator placement in 2012. Her ability to tolerate PO intake improved for several years, but in 2019 she

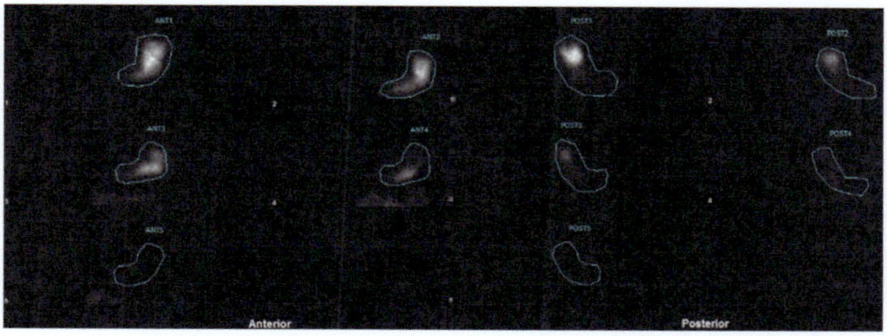

Fig. 9.1 Anterior and posterior projections of the radiotracer within the stomach at various time points [4]

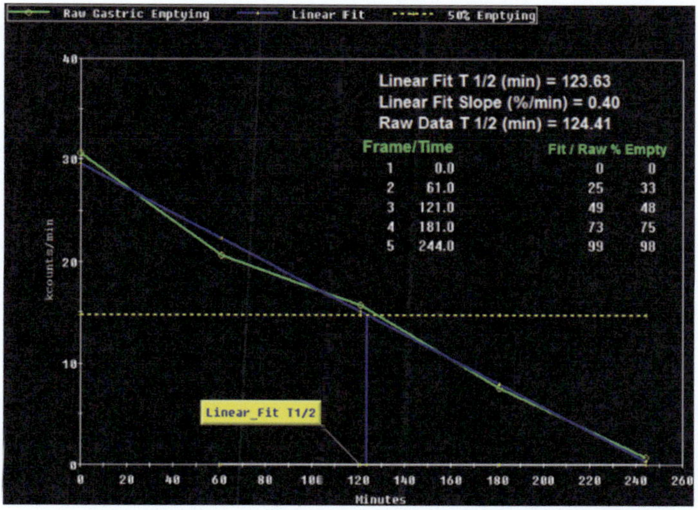

Fig. 9.2 Amount of radiotracer remaining in the stomach over time

developed recurrent symptoms. Interrogation of her battery revealed the need for replacement. She underwent battery replacement in January 2020, and the following images were obtained in March 2020 (Fig. 9.1).

The raw percentage empty values in the right upper corner of the image (Fig. 9.2) correspond with the 0-, 1-, 2-, and 4-h time points. When compared to the normal values listed above, each of these values remains within the expected range. Therefore, this study is interpreted as normal gastric emptying. This example underscores the importance of evaluating the percentage empty (or conversely the percentage remaining) at each time point instead of focusing solely on the half-time. The half-time value is potentially less representative of the overall clinical picture, especially if the study is stopped short of 4 h.

Rapid Gastric Emptying

Patient 2 is a 56-year-old woman who underwent Nissen fundoplication in 2007. She then developed a paraesophageal hernia with symptoms of dysphagia and reflux. Given her prior foregut surgery, the following gastric emptying study was obtained prior to paraesophageal hernia repair to evaluate the gastric function and ensure that a concurrent gastric emptying procedure was not indicated (Fig. 9.3).

At the 30-min mark, approximately 50% of the tracer had exited the stomach based on the raw percentage empty. At the 1-h

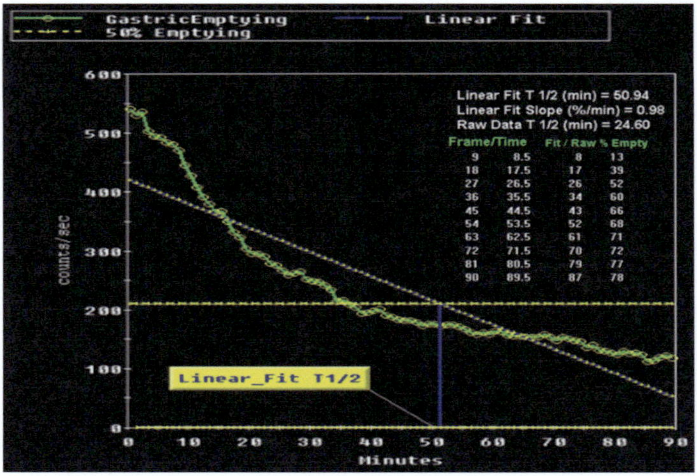

Fig. 9.3 Gastric emptying study in patient status post-Nissen fundoplication, rapid emptying

mark, approximately 70% of the tracer had exited the stomach. Therefore, this study is interpreted as rapid gastric emptying. This example represents an appropriate preoperative use of the study. The surgeon wanted to ensure that the patient did not have delayed gastric emptying. If that were the case, a gastric emptying procedure such as a pyloroplasty may have also been performed. Instead, because the patient's emptying was rapid, no additional procedures were indicated and she proceeded with paraesophageal hernia repair.

Delayed Gastric Emptying

Patient 3 is a 55-year-old woman with a history of gastric atony who underwent partial gastrectomy with gastrojejunostomy. She developed severe reflux and recurrent episodes of aspiration pneumonia, and her nutrition declined to the point where she was TPN-dependent. The following gastric emptying study was obtained prior to further surgical intervention (Fig. 9.4).

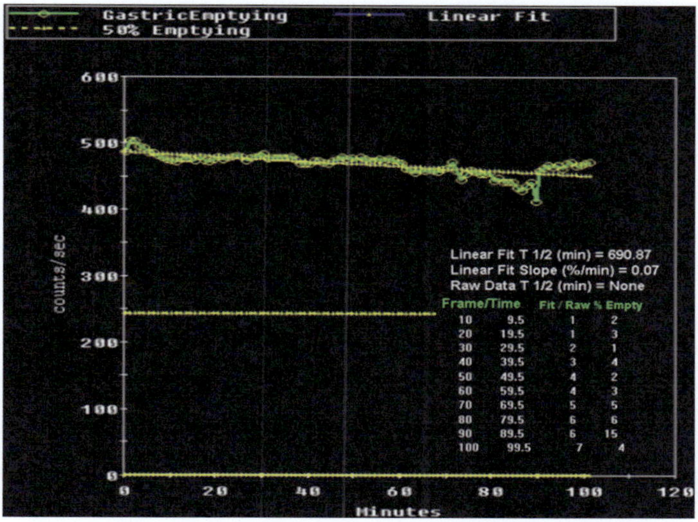

Fig. 9.4 Severe delayed gastric emptying

At the 1-h mark, 97% of the tracer remained in the stomach, and at the 1.5-h mark, 85% of the tracer remained in the stomach. This study was interpreted as delayed gastric emptying, and the study was terminated prior to the 4-h mark. These findings were relatively worse when compared to a previous study, and the patient proceeded to undergo a completion gastrectomy.

Borderline Delayed Gastric Emptying

The final example is again of patient 1, the 36-year-old woman with gastroparesis who originally underwent gastric stimulator placement in 2012. Her symptoms returned in 2019, and the following gastric emptying study was obtained (Fig. 9.5).

This example again underscores the importance of continuing the study to the 4-h mark, as well as understanding the clinical indication. The raw percentage empty is within normal limits at the 1-h and 2-h time points, but the rate of emptying slows to the point at which the percentage of tracer remaining in the stomach at the 4-h time point is abnormal. These findings are not nearly as pronounced as the delayed gastric emptying seen in Patient 3, but

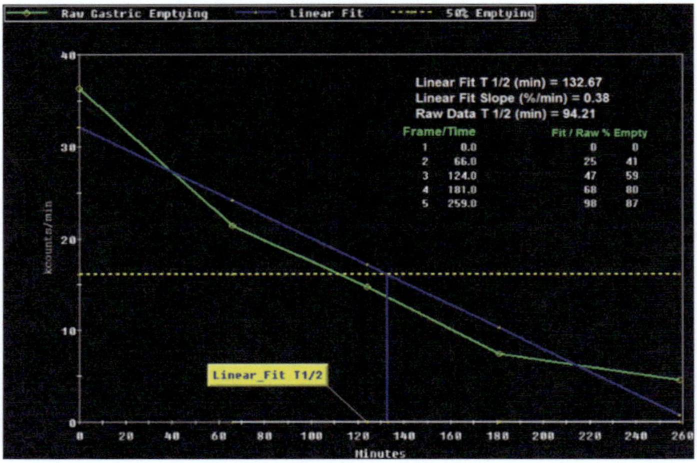

Fig. 9.5 Delayed emptying in 4-h study

given this patient's clinical course the findings were indicative that the gastric stimulator warranted interrogation. This patient proceeded to undergo gastric stimulator battery replacement.

Clinical Applications

Understanding the principles of a gastric emptying study will allow a clinician to better understand how this test can be used to prevent postoperative failures and complications. The result may affect the surgeon's operative plan, particularly if the patient has undergone previous foregut surgery or has atypical symptoms.

The following examples represent clinical scenarios in which a preoperative gastric emptying study would be useful.

1. A patient with gastroparesis prior to placement of a gastric pacemaker or pyloroplasty. It is important to document gastric emptying preoperatively as a baseline study for later comparison.
2. A patient who has previously undergone foregut surgery who develops symptoms concerning delayed gastric emptying when considering further surgical intervention.
3. Prior to performing a paraesophageal hernia repair to determine if any concurrent gastric emptying procedure should be performed.
4. A patient who has previously undergone partial gastrectomy, now with symptoms of either delayed or rapid gastric emptying prior to any further surgical intervention.

The following examples represent clinical scenarios in which a postoperative gastric emptying study would be useful.

1. Following gastric pacemaker insertion or pyloroplasty to document function relative to preoperative values.
2. Prior to removing a gastrostomy tube following paraesophageal hernia repair to ensure that the stomach is emptying adequately.

Conclusion

When ordering a gastric emptying study, it is important to have a defined clinical question and consider how the results will affect the operative plan. Knowing how the study is performed and having a basic framework for interpretation will ultimately allow for improved clinical decision-making.

References

1. Griffith GA, Owen GM, Kirkman S, et al. Measurement of the rate of gastric emptying using chromium-51. Lancet. 1966;1:1244–5.
2. Abell TL, Camilleri M, Donohoe K, et al. Consensus recommendations for gastric emptying scintigraphy: a joint report of the American Neurogastroenterology and Motility Society and the Society of Nuclear Medicine. J Nucl Med Technol. 2008;36:44–54.
3. Tougas G, Eaker EY, Abell TL, et al. Assessment of gastric emptying using a low fat meal: establishment of international control values. Am J Gastroenterol. 2000;95:1456–62.
4. Davis, S. Nuclear medicine gastric emptying study. Atlanta, GA: Emory University School of Medicine. 2020.

Endoscopic Ultrasound 10

Lindsey C. Shipley and Ali M. Ahmed

Introduction to EUS

In the 1980s, flexible endoscopy and ultrasound merged to form endoscopic ultrasound (EUS) [1]. EUS enables the visualization of structures located inside and outside of the luminal gastrointestinal tract such as lymph nodes and pancreatic lesions without the interference of other organs, bowel gas, fat, or bone [2]. Ultrasound utilizes absorptive, reflective, refractive, and scatter properties to construct a representative image of tissue structure [3]. With the creation of endoscopic ultrasound fine-needle aspiration (EUS-FNA) in 1991 and recent advancements, both the diagnostic and therapeutic capacities of EUS have expanded tremendously [1]. EUS now assists with the diagnosis and staging of malignancies via EUS-FNA, EUS elastography, and contrast-enhanced EUS. Therapeutically, EUS has been used for celiac

A. M. Ahmed (✉) · L. C. Shipley
Division of Gastroenterology and Hepatology, University of Alabama at Birmingham, Birmingham, AL, USA
e-mail: amahmed@uabmc.edu

A. D. Patel et al. (eds.), *The SAGES Manual of Physiologic Evaluation of Foregut Diseases*,
https://doi.org/10.1007/978-3-031-39199-6_10

plexus neurolysis, pseudocyst drainage, pancreaticogastrostomy, brachytherapy, and gene or cellular therapy. Moreover, its diagnostic and therapeutic potentials can span across organ systems and include the lung, liver, pancreas, and surrounding lymph nodes [4].

Application for Foregut Anatomy and Physiology

The primitive gut tube develops during weeks 3–4 and is divided into three distinct sections: foregut, midgut, and hindgut. The foregut is supplied by the celiac artery and consists of the esophagus, stomach, first and second portions of the duodenum, liver, pancreas, biliary apparatus, and gallbladder [5]. Parasympathetic innervation is via the vagus nerve and sympathetic innervation is by the preganglionic thoracic splanchnic nerves and postganglionic cell bodies, such as the celiac ganglion [6]. The trachea separates from the esophagus by forming a ventricular diverticulum off the primitive pharynx. By weeks 4–5, the complete trans-esophageal septum is created separating the respiratory and digestive tracts. Failure of this separation can result in esophageal atresia or tracheoesophageal fistula [7]. The stomach develops via a fusiform dilation by week 4. The remainder of the foregut forms via budding organs using an abundant number of signaling pathways and transcription factors including Hnf1b, Hnf6, retinoic acid (RA), and Prox1 [8]. The first and second portions of the duodenum from the end of the foregut. As the stomach rotates, this portion of the duodenum rotates to the right to move into the retroperitoneal space. The liver and biliary tree appear around week 3 as an outgrowth from the most distal foregut, the future ampulla of Vater. The liver grows rapidly forming a large portion of the abdominal cavity, and its diverticulum then expands to form the gallbladder and the cystic duct. In week 5, the pancreas forms a ventral and dorsal bud off the duodenum. The dorsal bud forms the upper half of the pancreatic head, isthmus, body, and tail, while the ventral bud forms the uncinate process and inferior part of the head of the pancreas. As the pancreatic buds fuse, their ducts anastomose to form the main pancreatic duct. Foregut malformations can occur at any point during this process and include esophageal atresia, esophageal stenosis, pyloric stenosis, atresia of the gallbladder and bile ducts, liver malformations, accessory pancreatic tissue, Meckel's diverticulum, duplication cysts, and annular pancreas [9]. EUS is currently utilized to evaluate and occasionally treat many of these abnormalities.

Role of EUS in Evaluation and Diagnosis of Foregut Pathology

Pretreatment Staging for Esophageal, Gastric, and Pancreatic Cancer

EUS is a useful tool to assist with pretreatment staging in esophageal, gastric, and pancreatic malignancies. Accurate staging can prevent both inadequate and unnecessary treatments and assist with balancing benefits versus risks of morbidity related to treatment.

Esophageal Cancer

Once esophageal cancer is identified, usually via endoscopy, the next step staging studies include CT and PET. Occasionally, these imaging modalities do not demonstrate distant disease. In this case, EUS is the most accurate modality for locoregional staging and is recommended to determine the extent of the disease. EUS can provide more information on the degree of tumor invasion (T status) and lymph node involvement (N status) [10]. The EUS image below demonstrates tumor invasion into the adventitia suggesting T3 esophageal cancer (Fig. 10.1). Furthermore, in a study of 125 patients, EUS-FNA can increase the sensitivity and specificity of identification of lymph node as compared to EUS alone (87% vs. 74%, $p = 0.012$) [11]. Current guidelines recommend EUS with or without FNA in cases where it is likely to change management such as confidence in clinical staging and helping to guide appropriate management and avoid unnecessary treatment.

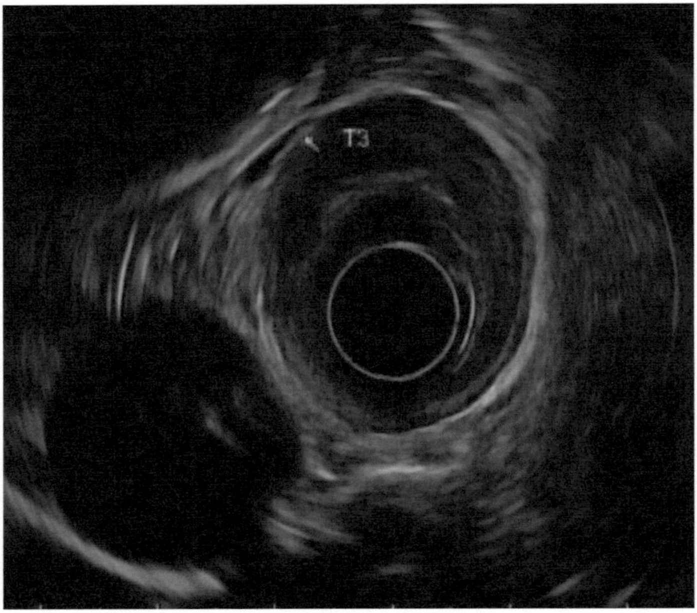

Fig. 10.1 Pretreatment esophageal cancer staging

The data on EUS elastography for esophageal cancer is limited; however, it may have a role in the future to reduce the need for FNA of lymph nodes. Contrast-enhanced EUS is limited in esophageal carcinoma as these tumors are not highly vascularized [12].

Gastric Cancer

EUS is a moderately accurate modality to determine staging for gastric cancer. In a meta-analysis of 22 articles, EUS-pooled accuracy T staging was 75%, with the highest accuracy for T3, followed by T4, T1, and T2. EUS-pooled accuracy for N staging was 64%, sensitivity 74%, and specificity 80% [2]. Another meta-analysis of 66 articles and 7747 patients with gastric cancer who were staged with EUS also found that performance is lower in diagnosing superficial tumors (T1a vs. T1b sensitivity 0.87 and specificity 0.75) and lymph node status (sensitivity 0.83, specificity 0.67). Further research is needed to determine its use in clinical practice [13].

Pancreatic Cancer

In one prospective study of 132 patients with suspected pancreatic tumor, sensitivity and specificity of EUS (99% and 100%) were found to be superior to US (67%, 40%) and CT (77%, 53%) and equal to ERCP (sensitivity 90%) in pancreatic tumor diagnosis. Further, EUS provides direct visualization of tumor size and shape, while ERCP only provides indirect evidence. However, EUS, similar to other modalities' accuracy for malignancy, was 76% and 46% for focal inflammation [14]. With the addition of fine-needle aspiration (EUS-FNA), the accuracy, sensitivity, and specificity for malignancy diagnosis rose to 86%, 84%, and 96%, respectively, in a study of 333 patients [15]. EUS has an important role in preoperative staging due to its accuracy of delineating location, size, lymph node metastasis (sensitivity 69%, specificity 81%), vascular invasion (85%, 91%) and to predict resectability. Further, no other modality can simultaneously assess atypical portocaval lymph nodes, ascitic fluid, peritoneal nodules, or suspected liver metastasis [16].

Evaluation and Diagnosis of Foregut Submucosal Nodules

Submucosal nodules, also known as submucosal tumors (SMT), are often asymptomatic and incidentally discovered during routine endoscopy. These lesions are best characterized by EUS both via ultrasound and biopsy, especially if the lesion is less than 0.5 cm. EUS can provide information regarding malignant potential, origination, and distinguishing solid versus cystic and extraluminal extension. Lesions commonly seen at EUS include leiomyoma, gastrointestinal stromal tumor (GIST), aberrant pancreas, lipoma, duplication cyst, and varices. The ability to use Doppler during EUS can discern varices from the remainder of the lesions and thus a safe target for tissue diagnosis [17]. EUS-FNA or EUS trucut biopsy (EUS-TCB) can be utilized for tissue diagnosis. In a small study of 19 patients comparing EUS-guided

FNA vs. TCB, EUS-TCB reduced the number of needle passes compared with EUS-FNA, potentially reducing the cost and time of the procedure [18].

Evaluation of Duplication Cysts and Childhood Congenital Abnormalities of the Esophagus

Duplication cysts arise from abnormal budding of the embryonic foregut at 5–8 weeks of gestation. They most commonly occur in the ileum, esophagus, and colon with 50–70% enterogenic and 7–15% bronchogenic. These cysts can either be found within the wall or extrinsic to the wall and usually present as an asymptomatic mediastinal mass with rare mass effect symptoms such as dysphagia. EUS is the diagnostic modality of choice as it can differentiate cystic versus solid lesions and location with regard to surrounding tissues [19]. EUS-FNA has been used to assist with diagnosis, however should be performed with caution given the increased risk of infection [20]. Definitive treatment is surgical removal; however, if asymptomatic, surveillance with EUS may be considered [21].

EUS has also proven to be effective in treating other types of esophageal congenital abnormalities such as esophageal stenosis [22]. Congenital esophageal stenosis is further classified into fibromuscular thickening (54%), tracheobronchial remnants (TBR) (30%), and membranous web (16%). Current management includes surgery and dilation, except for the TBR subtype. EUS can identify TBR subtype, and thus, EUS-guided case selection has been shown to be predictive of success rate (90% vs. 29%) and decreases the rate of perforation (7% vs 24%) [22, 23].

Walled-Off Pancreatic Necrosis

Walled-off pancreatic necrosis (WOPN) is associated with high morbidity and mortality. Interventions for both diagnosis and treatment have shifted toward a less-invasive strategy,

EUS-guided methods. EUS allows for better visualization of the contents, structure, and surrounding structures of the pseudocyst [24].

Evaluation and Diagnosis of the Liver

EUS can sample liver lesions suspected of metastatic disease for diagnosis and staging. An example is shown in the figure below (Fig. 10.2).

New developments in endoscopic ultrasound have expanded evaluation from sampling liver lesions and liver parenchyma for diagnosis to the measurement of portal pressure utilizing a novel catheter. The first EUS-guided liver biopsy was performed in 2007 utilizing the linear array echoendoscope. Since then, several

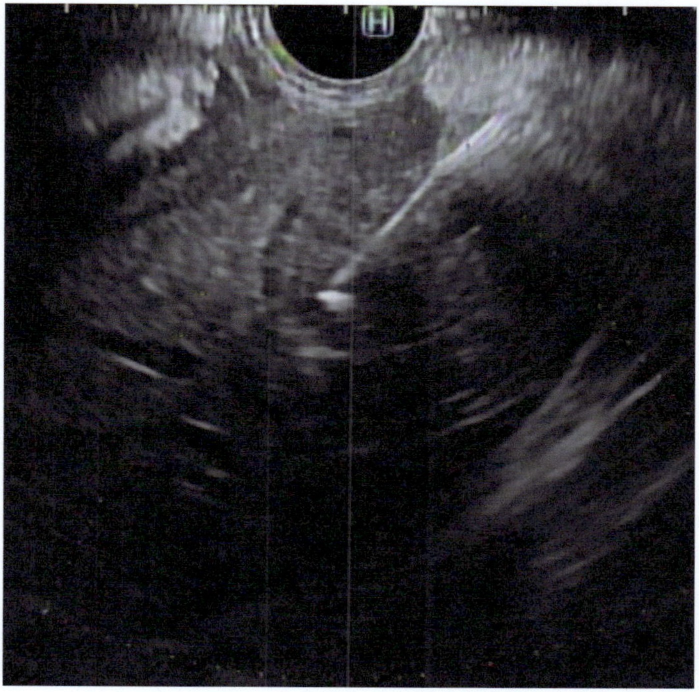

Fig. 10.2 Fine-needle biopsy of metastatic liver lesion

studies have demonstrated the efficacy of the technique with 93.9% diagnostic yield [25] and a comparative study between EUS-guided liver biopsy with percutaneous and transjugular techniques demonstrated lower complicates by EUS ($p = 0.03$) and increased specimen length by EUS ($p < 0.01$) but fewer complete portal tracts ($p < 0.01$). NASH can present sporadically in the liver, and sampling both the left and right hepatic lobes may better assess the disease. This is more easily accomplished by EUS with directed passes to the specific lobes. Additionally, patient recovery is faster than the traditional methods of liver biopsy [26].

A recently approved device has a manometer that attaches to a needle that can be placed through the EUS and directly into hepatic vessels. This permits EUS-guided portal pressure measurement. The fibrosis in cirrhosis manifests itself by portal hypertension, which is best measured by portal venous pressure. The field of EUS hepatology is novel with many advances expected in the coming years and includes EUS-guided portal vein embolization/thrombolysis, EUS-guided portal vein stent placement, EUS-guided therapy for liver lesions, and EUS-directed drainage of liver abscesses/cysts and bilomas [26].

Role of EUS in Foregut Treatment

Treatment of Esophageal, Gastric, and Pancreatic Cancer

Endoscopic ultrasound fine-needle injection (EUS-FNI) is currently used for palliative biliary drainage [27], palliative celiac plexus blockade, and precise submucosal injection prior to endoscopic mucosal resection of neoplasia or other lesions [28]. Research efforts are currently focused on EUS-FNI as treatment for cancer; however, they have not been successful thus far [29]. Ethanol, brachytherapy seeds, chemotherapeutic agents, immunomodulating cell cultures, and viral vectors have all been used in research efforts for anti-tumor therapy; however, this is largely limited to animal studies and a few small case series. Prospective studies are needed to determine the utility of EUS in cancer management [28].

Treatment of Duplications Cysts and Childhood Congenital Abnormalities of the Esophagus

Treatment of duplication cysts is typically via surgical enucleation in symptomatic cases, while asymptomatic cases are commonly observed. EUS-guided needle aspiration has been proposed for treatment but has only been used in a small number of case reports, primarily in colonic duplication cysts [19].

Treatment of Walled-Off Pancreatic Necrosis

In addition to the ability to better visualize the contents, structure, and surrounding structures of the pseudocyst, current EUS-guided strategies to treat WOPN include lumen-apposing metal stents (LAMS) and direct endoscopic necrosectomy (DEN) [24]. Further, EUS-guided drainage is safe, can be performed at a lower cost and decreases hospital stay, [30] and has a high success rate (Fig. 10.3). In a randomized control study of 60 patients with pseudocysts, EUS-guided drainage showed a higher rate of technical success when compared to conventional transmural drainage (CTD) (94% vs. 72%, $p = 0.039$); however, long-term outcomes showed no significant difference in EUD versus CTD (89% vs. 86%, $p = 0.696$) [31]. A recent multicenter randomized study compared endoscopic luminal drainage followed by endoscopic necrosectomy versus percutaneous drainage followed by minimally invasive surgical necrosectomy, if needed. The primary end point of mortality was equal in both groups, but the endoscopic group had fewer complications such as pancreatic fistulas (5% vs 32%, $p = 0.0011$) and a shorter mean length of hospitalization (53 days vs 69 days, $p = 0.014$) [32]. Larger prospective studies are needed to study long-term outcome,

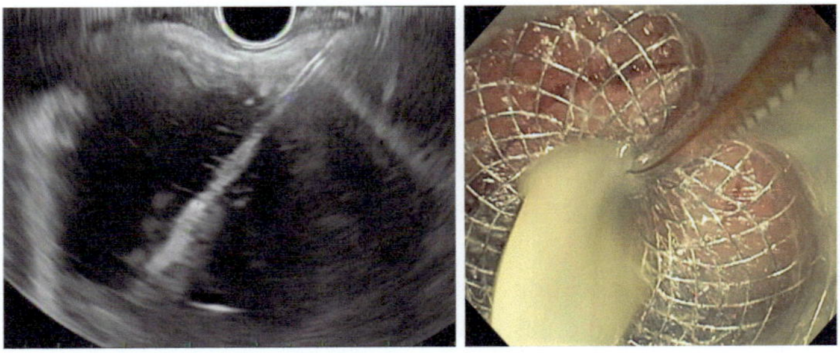

Fig. 10.3 Pseudocyst, walled-off necrosis drainage

but a paradigm shift toward endoscopic drainage is being seen in the treatment of these patients.

Conclusion

EUS is currently utilized to evaluate and occasionally treat many abnormalities of the foregut. It offers a safe, cost-effective, and accurate diagnosis of malignancies, cysts, and tissue previously not well-defined. There are exciting new frontiers for the advanced endoscopist with regard to the treatment of foregut pathology; however, further prospective studies are needed to evaluate more recent advancements.

References

1. Friedberg SR, Lachter J. Endoscopic ultrasound: current roles and future directions. World J Gastrointest Endosc. 2017;9(10):499–505.
2. Cardoso R, Coburn N, Seevaratnam R, Sutradhar R, Lourenco LG, Mahar A, et al. A systematic review and meta-analysis of the utility of EUS for preoperative staging for gastric cancer. Gastric Cancer. 2012;15(Suppl 1):S19–26.
3. Hawes R, Fockens P, Varadarajulu S. Endosonography. 3rd ed. Elsevier Saunders; 2015.
4. Giovannini M, Sun S. Welcome to your new journal: endoscopic ultrasound. Endosc Ultrasound. 2012;1(1):1.

5. San Roman AK, Shivdasani RA. Boundaries, junctions and transitions in the gastrointestinal tract. Exp Cell Res. 2011;317(19):2711–8.
6. Espinosa-Medina I, Jevans B, Boismoreau F, Chettouh Z, Enomoto H, Müller T, et al. Dual origin of enteric neurons in vagal Schwann cell precursors and the sympathetic neural crest. Proc Natl Acad Sci U S A. 2017;114(45):11980–5.
7. de Jong EM, Felix JF, de Klein A, Tibboel D. Etiology of esophageal atresia and tracheoesophageal fistula: "mind the gap". Curr Gastroenterol Rep. 2010;12(3):215–22.
8. McCracken KW, Wells JM. Mechanisms of embryonic stomach development. Semin Cell Dev Biol. 2017;66:36–42.
9. Pansky B. Review of medical embryology. New York: Macmillan; 1982.
10. Berry MF. Esophageal cancer: staging system and guidelines for staging and treatment. J Thorac Dis. 2014;6(Suppl 3):S289–97.
11. Vazquez-Sequeiros E, Wiersema MJ, Clain JE, Norton ID, Levy MJ, Romero Y, et al. Impact of lymph node staging on therapy of esophageal carcinoma. Gastroenterology. 2003;125(6):1626–35.
12. Thakkar S, Kaul V. Endoscopic ultrasound staging of esophageal cancer. Gastroenterol Hepatol. 2020;16(1):14–20.
13. Mocellin S, Pasquali S. Diagnostic accuracy of endoscopic ultrasonography (EUS) for the preoperative locoregional staging of primary gastric cancer. Cochrane Database Syst Rev. 2015;(2):CD009944.
14. Rösch T, Lorenz R, Braig C, Feuerbach S, Siewert JR, Schusdziarra V, et al. Endoscopic ultrasound in pancreatic tumor diagnosis. Gastrointest Endosc. 1991;37(3):347–52.
15. Williams DB, Sahai AV, Aabakken L, Penman ID, van Velse A, Webb J, et al. Endoscopic ultrasound guided fine needle aspiration biopsy: a large single Centre experience. Gut. 1999;44(5):720–6.
16. Moutinho-Ribeiro P, Iglesias-Garcia J, Gaspar R, Macedo G. Early pancreatic cancer - the role of endoscopic ultrasound with or without tissue acquisition in diagnosis and staging. Dig Liver Dis. 2019;51(1):4–9.
17. Guo J, Liu Z, Sun S, Wang S, Ge N, Liu X, et al. Endosonography-assisted diagnosis and therapy of gastrointestinal submucosal tumors. Endosc Ultrasound. 2013;2(3):125–33.
18. Levy MJ, Jondal ML, Clain J, Wiersema MJ. Preliminary experience with an EUS-guided trucut biopsy needle compared with EUS-guided FNA. Gastrointest Endosc. 2003;57(1):101–6.
19. Liu R, Adler DG. Duplication cysts: diagnosis, management, and the role of endoscopic ultrasound. Endosc Ultrasound. 2014;3(3):152–60.
20. Wildi SM, Hoda RS, Fickling W, Schmulewitz N, Varadarajulu S, Roberts SS, et al. Diagnosis of benign cysts of the mediastinum: the role and risks of EUS and FNA. Gastrointest Endosc. 2003;58(3):362–8.
21. Versleijen MW, Drenth JP, Nagengast FM. A case of esophageal duplication cyst with a 13-year follow-up period. Endoscopy. 2005;37(9):870–2.

22. Terui K, Saito T, Mitsunaga T, Nakata M, Yoshida H. Endoscopic management for congenital esophageal stenosis: a systematic review. World J Gastrointest Endosc. 2015;7(3):183–91.
23. Usui N, Kamata S, Kawahara H, Sawai T, Nakajima K, Soh H, et al. Usefulness of endoscopic ultrasonography in the diagnosis of congenital esophageal stenosis. J Pediatr Surg. 2002;37(12):1744–6.
24. Alali A, Mosko J, May G, Teshima C. Endoscopic ultrasound-guided management of pancreatic fluid collections: update and review of the literature. Clin Endosc. 2017;50(2):117–25.
25. Mohan BP, et al. Efficacy and safety of EUS-guided liver biopsy: a systemic review and meta analysis. Gastrointest Endosc. 2019;89:238–46.
26. Hashimoto R, Chang KJ. Endoscopic ultrasound guided hepatic interventions. Dig Endoscopy. 2021;33:54–65.
27. Giovannini M, Dotti M, Bories E, Moutardier V, Pesenti C, Danisi C, et al. Hepaticogastrostomy by echo-endoscopy as a palliative treatment in a patient with metastatic biliary obstruction. Endoscopy. 2003;35(12):1076–8.
28. Verna EC, Dhar V. Endoscopic ultrasound-guided fine needle injection for cancer therapy: the evolving role of therapeutic endoscopic ultrasound. Ther Adv Gastroenterol. 2008;1(2):103–9.
29. Faigel DO. The role of endoscopic ultrasound in esophageal cancer. Gastroenterol Hepatol (N Y). 2019;15(10):519–21.
30. Antillon MR, Shah RJ, Stiegmann G, Chen YK. Single-step EUS-guided transmural drainage of simple and complicated pancreatic pseudocysts. Gastrointest Endosc. 2006;63(6):797–803.
31. Park DH, Lee SS, Moon SH, Choi SY, Jung SW, Seo DW, et al. Endoscopic ultrasound-guided versus conventional transmural drainage for pancreatic pseudocysts: a prospective randomized trial. Endoscopy. 2009;41(10):842–8.
32. van Brunschot S, et al. Endoscopic or surgical step-up approach for infected necrotising pancreatitis: a multicentre randomised trial. Lancet. 2018;391:51–8.

Part III

Diagnostic Testing

High-Resolution Esophageal Manometry with and without Impedance: Understanding the "Chicago Classification"

11

Mohanad R. Youssef, Meredith Freeman, Natacha Wathieu, Danuel Laan, and Carlos Galvani

Introduction to High-Resolution Manometry (HRM) without Impedance

High-resolution manometry is an updated version of conventional manometry that provides a panoramic view of the proximal physiology of the gastrointestinal tract from the pharynx to the stomach. The modifications introduced in the 90's included decreasing pressure sensors spacing from 3 to 5 cm to 1-cm intervals, increasing the number of sensors and therefore lengthening the pressure sensing of the catheter from the pharynx to the stomach [1]. This allowed for simultaneous and continuous recording of motor

M. R. Youssef · D. Laan · C. Galvani (✉)
Division of Minimally Invasive Surgery and Bariatric, Department of Surgery, Tulane University, School of Medicine, New Orleans, LA, USA
e-mail: cgalvani@tulane.edu

M. Freeman · N. Wathieu
Tulane University, School of Medicine, New Orleans, LA, USA

A. D. Patel et al. (eds.), *The SAGES Manual of Physiologic Evaluation of Foregut Diseases*,
https://doi.org/10.1007/978-3-031-39199-6_11

activity along the entire esophageal length (UES to LES) with each swallow. In addition, as compared to conventional manometry, pull-through is not required, it is more comfortable and faster, shifts of position do not affect the reliability and reproducibility of pressure recordings, and it reduces inter-observer variability [2]. The uniqueness of this revolutionary method lies in its ability to convert pressure data onto a topographical plot [3]. The esophageal pressure topography plots (EPT) or "Clouse Plots" have the capacity to convert manometric pressure into a topographic (color contour) plot that illustrates the better spatial resolution of esophageal motor function [4].

Even though in its inception this work was only used for research, over time these remarkable advances have led to the development of new measurements and resulted in a new classification. The Chicago Classification (CC) of esophageal motility disorders was developed to enable an objective analysis of HRM metrics and topography, utilizing an algorithmic scheme to analyze clinical high-resolution manometry (HRM) studies [5]. The CC divides esophageal motility disorders according to the relaxation of the lower esophageal sphincter (LES) as characterized by the integrated relaxation pressure (IRP) and motility of the esophageal body. Once LES relaxation has been characterized, motility disorders may be further categorized by abnormalities of esophageal body peristalsis. The initial CC was modified [6], and the most recent revision of the Chicago Classification (v3.0) was published in 2015 [4].

As a result of these advances, today HRM is a diagnostic method that is considered the gold standard for the evaluation of esophageal motor function. HRM supplements endoscopy and radiologic studies not only to help elucidate numerous foregut symptoms, but also to guide different therapeutic options such as medical, endoscopic, surgical, and even behavioral therapy. The purpose of this chapter was to explore high-resolution manometry and the Chicago Classification v3.0 and its utilization in the characterization of esophageal motility disorders.

How Does HRM Work?

The combination of two fundamental developments revolutionized the diagnostic evaluation of esophageal motor function. The first one was the ability to measure pressures from the pharynx to the stomach simultaneously with a newly designed catheter. This was feasible due to the incorporation of multiple closely spaced pressure sensors within the catheter. Specifically, the catheter is a solid-state catheter 4 mm in diameter that contains 36 circumferential sensors, spaced 1 cm apart, covering a length of 35 cm. This enables simultaneous recording from all segments (UES to LES), without the need to reposition the catheter during the study (Fig. 11.1). This makes the procedure faster and more tolerable for patients.

Sensors are spaced at 1-cm intervals from center to center. This gives the catheter a recording segment of 35 cm. Each individual sensor (magnified at center) detects pressure from 12 loci (arrow) around its circumference. Computer processing of the signals coming from pressure sensing elements allows average

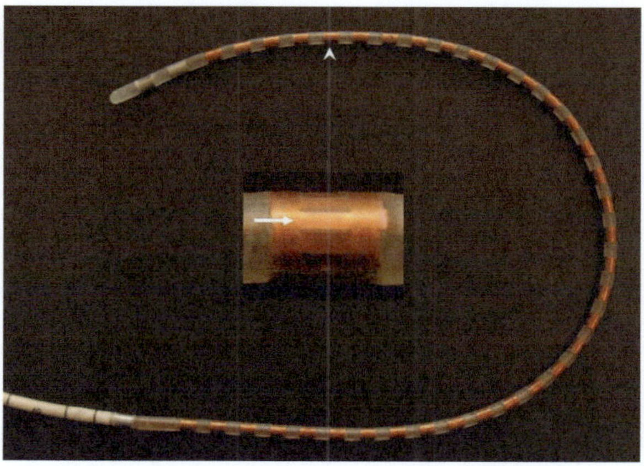

Fig. 11.1 High-resolution manometry catheter. The high-resolution manometry catheter pictured here is 4.2 mm in diameter and consists of 36 circumferential, solid-state, pressure sensors (copper-colored bands, arrowhead)

circumferential pressures over the entire 35-cm recording segment to be displayed in real time and recorded for subsequent analysis.

The second development was the computer software that allowed the conversion of the data acquired by HRM into a topographic (color contour) plot. The software analyzes the manometric pressures and provides color contours to illustrate the intraluminal pressures. Time and pressure contour lines are applied to the tracings with isobaric pressure lines at 5-mmHg intervals. Colors are assigned to pressures; therefore, cooler colors represent lower pressures, and warmer colors represent higher pressures [3]. The contour mode display is 2-dimensional in which the distance from the nose is on the y-axis, time is on the x-axis, and the pressure is presented by color (z-axis). (Fig. 11.2).

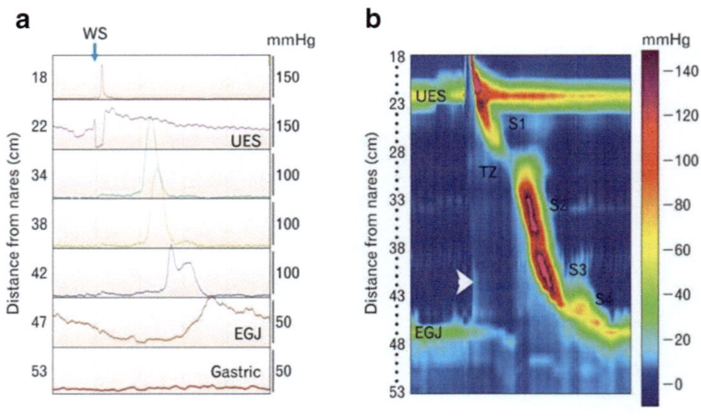

Fig. 11.2 Comparing conventional recordings of manometric pressure (**a**) with the Clouse plot or esophageal pressure topography EPT (**b**) In the latter, pressure in the swallowed bolus (intrabolus pressure) is represented by a small simultaneous rise in intraesophageal pressure seen as a simultaneous change to a lighter blue color (arrowhead). Notice that when the peristaltic wave passes, the color becomes a darker blue indicating bolus clearance. TZ, transition zone. (Copyright 2013 Korean Society of Neurogastroenterology and Motility)

How to Perform High-Resolution Esophageal Manometry?

The adequate diagnosis of esophageal motility disorders requires high-quality HRM studies. Understandably, the motility laboratory requires not only dedicated personnel (physicians, nurses, or technicians) but also adequate HRM equipment (catheters, acquisition software, and analysis software) [7]. Today, there are several companies in the market that offer HRM equipment. Yet, it is worth mentioning that the ManoScan™ ESO catheter (Medtronic Plc, Dublin, Ireland) was the catheter used for all the research studies performed for the development of the Chicago Classification. For that reason, if manometry is performed with a catheter other than the ManoScan™, the interpretation of the study should be based on normal values generated for those HRM systems [8].

Before performing the study, patients should be instructed to fast for at least 6 h for solids and 2 h for liquids prior to the procedure. In patients with obstructive symptoms and suspected achalasia, fasting times should be extended as per laboratory policies. Medications that affect esophageal motility should also be stopped for at least 3 days in preparation for the study. Some of these medications include calcium channel blockers, nitrates, prokinetics, loperamide, β-blockers, opioids, and anticholinergic agents. Patients should be given a detailed explanation of the procedure and informed consent should be obtained.

The motility catheter with 36 circumferential sensors is inserted transnasally after the application of topical anesthesia. The catheter is positioned so that at least two distal sensors are in the stomach and two proximal sensors are located above the UES. A 5-min acclimation period should be provided to the patient before starting the study. As an alternative for patients with known strictures or large hiatal hernias, the catheter can be placed endoscopically after routine calibration. The laboratory technician can perform the study after the patient recovers from anesthesia. The correct catheter placement is of key importance for the performance of a high-quality study and can be confirmed by identifying the pressure inversion point (PIP; negative intrathoracic pressure associated with inspiration inverts to positive intraabdominal pressure) by asking the patient to take several deep breaths. After the correct placement of the catheter is confirmed and the patient is acclimated to the catheter, the study begins. Figure 11.3 demonstrates the HRM of the esophagus at rest and the software tool that aids in identifying the diaphragm (PIP). It is important to mention that the PIP is not present in studies in which the catheter does not cross the EGJ and indicates a technically inadequate study.

The standard protocol that was used for the development of the Chicago Classification entails a 30-s swallow-free recording to obtain the resting pressures of the UES and EGJ (esophagogastric junction). This period is followed by 10 consecutive swallows of a 5-ml bolus in the supine position for patients without prior surgery affecting the esophagus or the EGJ [6]. Patients should be instructed to swallow only once per wet swallow, and swallows should be about 20–30 s apart. This allows for the LES pressure to return to its resting state and to prevent the deglutitive inhibition from hindering the motility of the esophagus. Figure 11.4 demonstrates a swallow.

The HRM can also be performed in the upright position; however, it should be recognized that pressures are lower in the upright position compared to supine and normal values are available for both situations [9]. Additionally, several motility experts have described the use of apple sauce, solid boluses, or multiple water swallows to challenge the esophagus and uncover motility disorders that otherwise would not be uncovered by the swallows of 5 ml of water [3].

How Is the Study Interpreted?

The manometry software provides an automated computer-generated analysis of the study; however, the computerized analysis is imperfect and unable to recognize areas where artifact could be distinguished from true peristaltic contractions. For that reason, an experienced clinician must review each swallow and

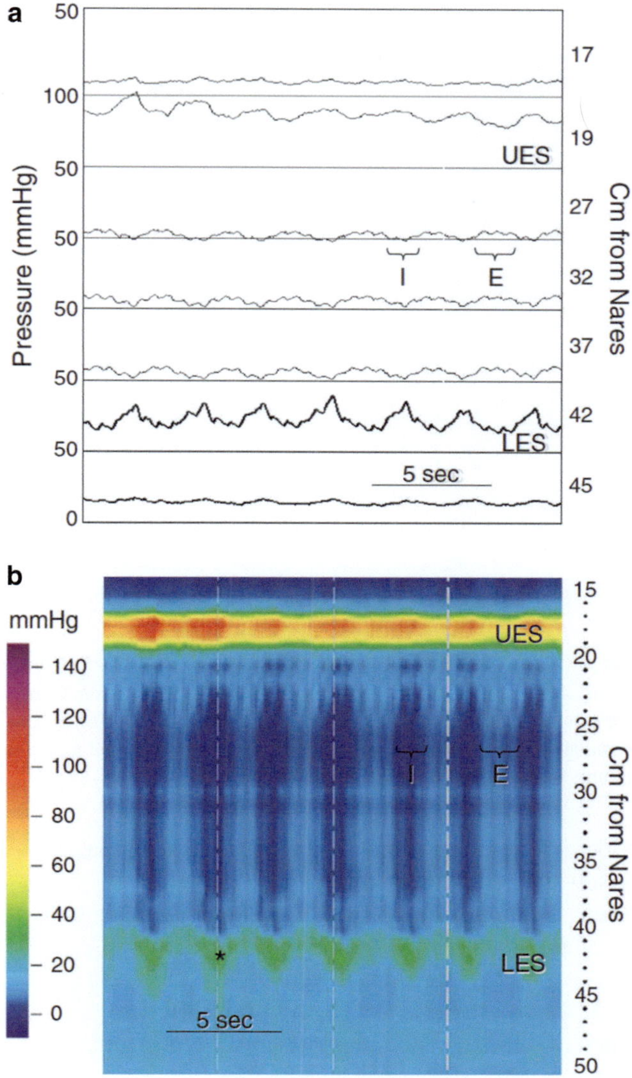

Fig. 11.3 High-resolution manometry of the esophagus at rest. (**a**) Demonstrates a typical recording of the esophagus at rest. The sensor at 17 cm from the nares is in the pharynx, the sensor at 19 cm is in the upper esophageal sphincter (UES), and the sensor at 24 cm is in the LES. Those at 27, 32, and 37 cm are in the esophagus, and the one at 45 cm is intragastric. (**b**) Inspiration is indicated by I and expiration by E

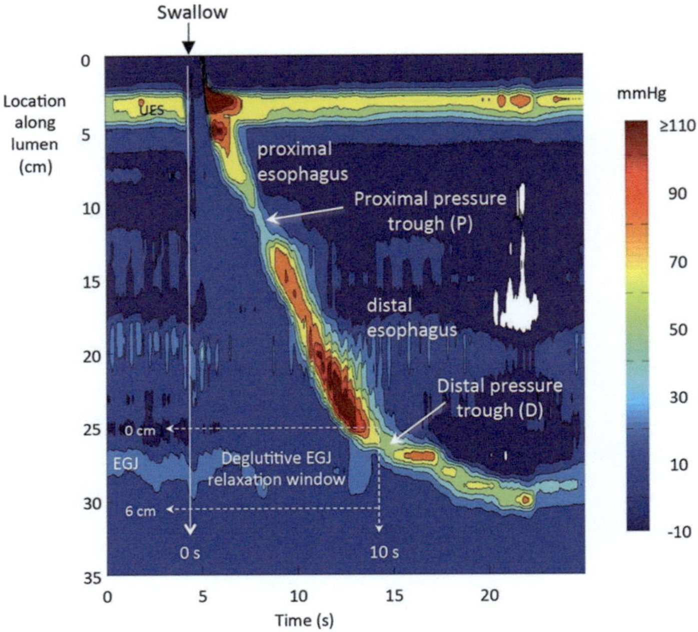

Fig. 11.4 Esophageal pressure topography [Clouse plot] illustrating a normal peristaltic contraction and key landmarks used in the Chicago Classification of esophageal motility. P is the proximal pressure trough separating the proximal and distal contractile segments; D is the trough separating the distal esophagus from the esophagogastric junction

provide a final interpretation since an inadequate diagnosis can adversely affect patient outcomes.

There are three main steps that make up the diagnostic algorithm of an esophageal HRM study:

Step 1: Assess the EGJ Anatomy and Function

- Main EGJ metrics (EGJ morphology, LES pressure, separation from the crural diaphragm and the LES)

This is a decisive step because disorders are separated at this point, determined by those with or without outflow obstruction at the EGJ. This portion begins with the evaluation of the LES rest-

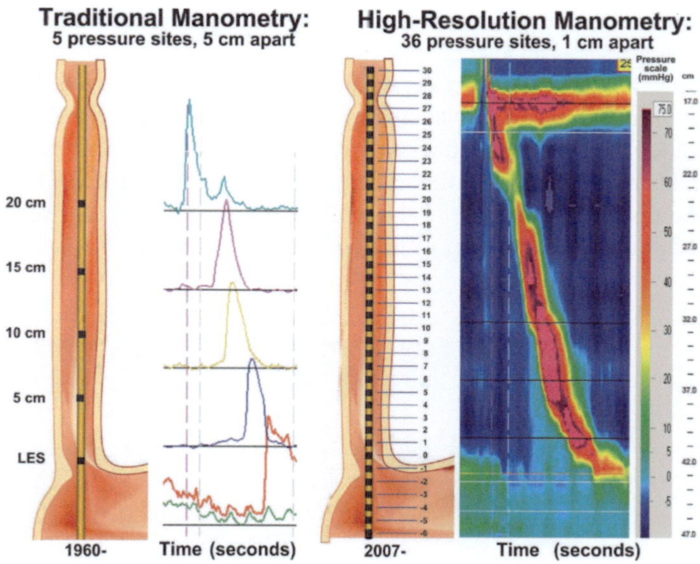

Fig. 11.5 Traditional and high-resolution manometry: comparison of the 2 esophageal manometry systems currently available. Traditional low-resolution manometry (left; 1960-present) is 5 line tracings derived from pressure sites located in the LES and 5, 10, 15, and 20 cm above the LES in the esophagus. In contrast, HRM (2007-present) is a color-based topographic plot extending from pharynx to stomach derived from sophisticated computer algorithms converting data from 36 pressure sites 1 cm apart into a topograph

ing pressures during the swallow-free period, the morphology of the EGJ (LES and diaphragmatic crura), and the presence or absence of a hiatal hernia. The morphology of the EGJ is classified into three types according to the level of separation that exists between the location of the LES and the PIP (which indicates the location of the crural diaphragm) (Fig. 11.5) [3, 4].

Type I: the LES and the crural diaphragm coincide.

Type II: small spatial separation of less than 2 cm between the crural diaphragm and the LES.

Type III: large spatial separation of more than 2 cm between the crural diaphragm and the LES.

Next, the LES pressure is assessed, as well as whether the EGJ is appropriately relaxed with swallowing. Even though the CC does not take into account the LES pressure, its assessment is recommended as an average of inspiratory and expiratory values for three normal respiratory cycles during a swallow-free period. The EGJ function during swallowing is determined by a measurement called the 4-s integrated relaxation pressure (IRP). The integrated relaxation pressure (IRP) measures the relaxation of the EGJ. It is expressed as a median of the ten test swallows in mm Hg with 15 mm Hg being the upper limit of normal (Fig. 11.6).

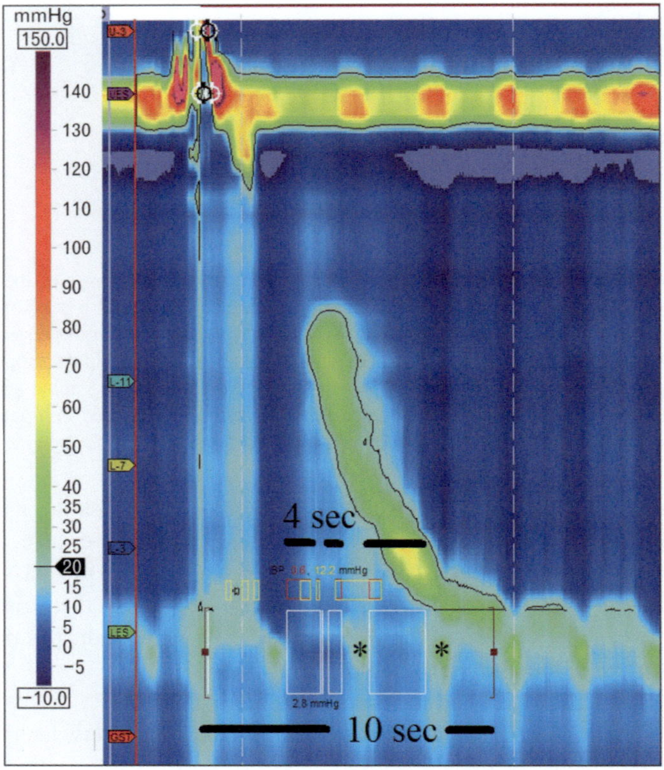

Fig. 11.6 Integrated relaxation pressure (IRP) corresponds to the mean pressure of 4 s of greatest post-deglutitive relaxation in a 10-s gap, triggered at the beginning of a swallow. Note diaphragmatic contraction pressure (*) during relaxation excluded from the analysis

Any mechanical or functional abnormality that creates an obstruction at the EGJ can elevate the IRP (achalasia, neoplasms, or strictures at the EGJ, hiatal hernias, and antireflux surgery.

Step 2: Assess Esophageal Body Function (Table 11.1) (Fig. 11.7)

- Main esophageal contractility metrics:

Contraction Vigor The DCI is a measure of the contractile (peristaltic) force of esophageal contraction (mm Hg/s/cm). Each swallow is defined based on the DCI as either normal (DCI >450, but <8000), failed (DCI < 100), weak (DCI >100, but <450 mm),

Table 11.1 Characteristics of deglutitive peristaltic function proposed for the Chicago Classification v3.0 (note that contraction pattern is not scored with failed or weak vigor)

Contractile vigor	
Failed	DCI < 100 mmHg-s-cm
Weak	DCI > 100 mmHg-s-cm, but <450 mmHg-s-cm
Ineffective	Failed or weak
Normal	DCI > 450 mmHg-s-cm but <8000 mmHg-s-cm
Hypercontractile	DCI ≥ 8000 mmHg-s-cm
Contraction pattern	
Premature	DL < 4.5 s
Fragmented	Large break (>5 cm) in the 20 mmHg isobaric contour, but not failed and DCI > 450 mmHg-s-cm
Intact	Not achieving the above diagnostic criteria
Intrabolus pressure pattern (30 mmHg isobaric contour referenced to atmospheric)	
Panesophageal pressurization	Uniform pressurization of >30 mmHg extending from the UES to the EGJ
Compartmentalized esophageal pressurization	Pressurization of >30 mmHg extending from the contractile front to the EGJ
EGJ pressurization	Pressurization restricted to zone between the LES and CD in conjunction with LES-CD separation
Normal	No bolus pressurization >30 mmHg

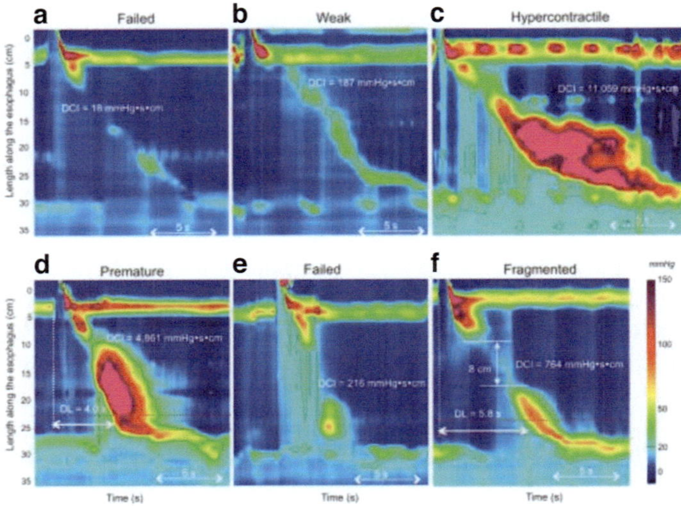

Fig. 11.7 Contractile vigor as assessed using the DCI and contraction pattern. A contraction with a DCI <100 mmHg-s-cm is failed (**a**); a contraction with a DCI > 100 but <450 mmHg-s-cm is weak (**b**); and a hypercontractile swallow is defined as a DCI >8000 mmHg-s-cm (**c**). Premature contraction is defined as a distal latency (DL) <4.5 s (**d**). A weak contraction (DCI < 450 mmHg-s-cm) with reduced distal latency is considered failed (**e**). A contraction with a normal DCI (450–8000 mmHg-s-cm) and a break >5 cm is a fragmented contraction (**f**)

ineffective (failed or weak), or hypercontractile (DCI $\geq$ 8000) using the 20-mmHg isobaric contour (IBC) tool (Fig. 11.8).

Contraction Pattern Distal latency (DL) is the time interval in seconds between the relaxation of the UES and the inflection point along the isobaric contour of 30 mm Hg where the velocity of propagation slows. DL is an indirect measure of swallowing inhibition and therefore of normal peristalsis (Fig. 11.9). A measurement of less than 4.5 s and a DCI > 450 define a premature contraction. Fragmented contractions are considered segmental defects (break in the 20-mmHg isobaric contour >5 cm) with normal contraction vigor.

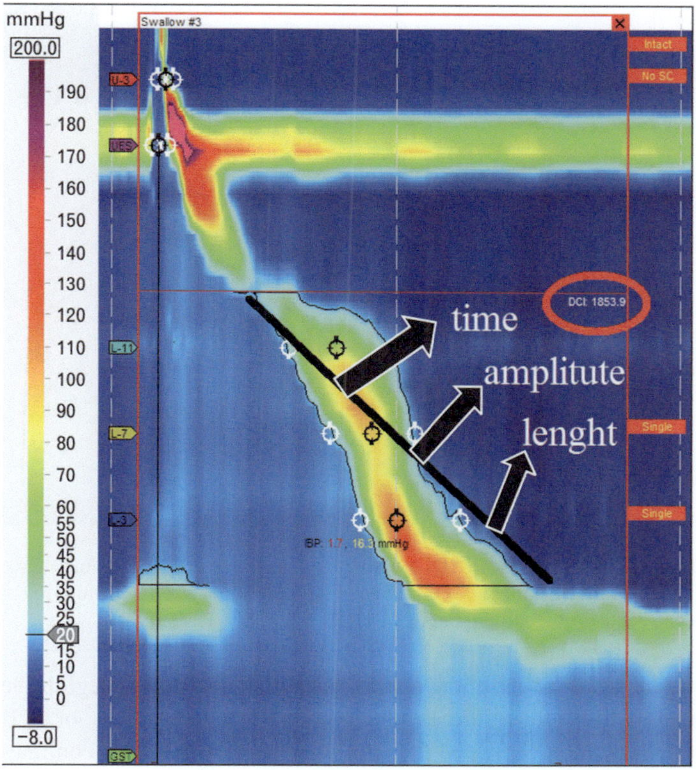

Fig. 11.8 Distal contractile integral (DCI). DCI value is calculated as the product of the mean amplitude of contraction in the distal esophagus (mmHg) times the duration of contraction (seconds) times the length of the distal oesophageal segment (cm) exceeding 20 mmHg for the region spanning from the transition zone to the proximal aspect of the lower esophageal sphincter

Step 3: Review Pressurization Patterns

Each swallow should be evaluated using the IBC (isobaric contour) tool to document isobaric pressurization >30 mmHg. Pressurization occurs when the swallowed liquid becomes trapped between two contracting segments of the esophagus and is identified by a vertical isobaric pressure band. Pressurization of >30 mmHg that spans from the UES to the EGJ is termed pane-

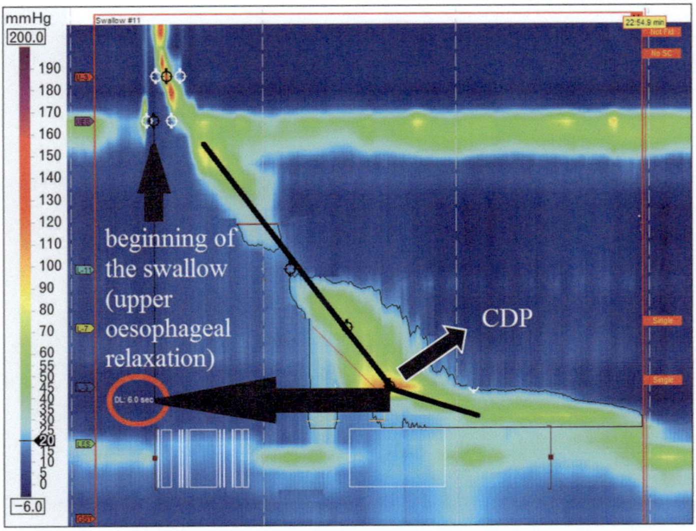

Fig. 11.9 Distal latency (DL) measures objectively the time frame of the wave from the beginning of the swallow (upper esophageal relaxation) to the contractile deceleration point (CDP)

sophageal pressurization, compartmentalized (from the deglutitive contractile front to the esophagogastric junction [EGJ]), or EGJ pressurization (between the LES and the diaphragm in conjunction with a hiatal hernia).

The Chicago Classification v3.0

The Chicago Classification (CC) was developed to standardize the interpretation of high-resolution esophageal manometry studies. The CC categorizes esophageal motility disorders utilizing high-resolution manometry (HRM) imaged with pressure topography plots. This classification is intended for patients with no previous surgeries compromising the esophagus or the EGJ. It utilizes a hierarchical approach, sequentially prioritizing (a) disorders of the esophagogastric junction (EGJ) outflow, (b) major disorders of peristalsis, and (c) minor disorders of peristalsis [4].

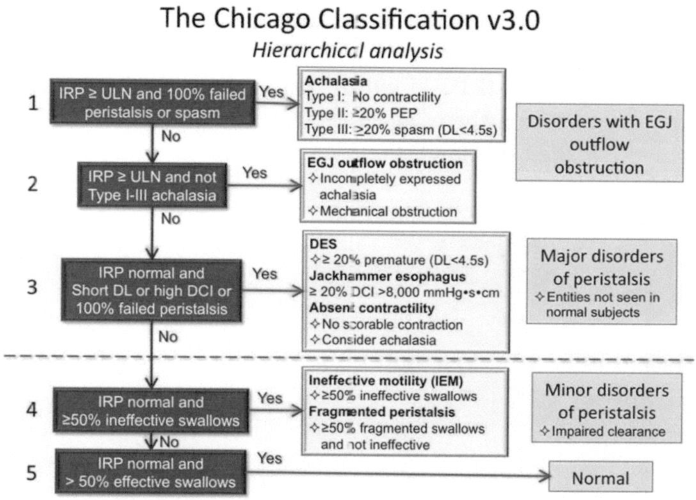

Fig. 11.10 Chicago Classification v3.0

It is worth it to remark that there are technology-specific normal and abnormal values, especially for the IRP. The practitioner analyzing the study should be aware of the cutoff values according to their device. For the purpose of this chapter, we will be focusing on the Medtronic technology.

After the detailed analysis of the 10 wet swallows, the Chicago Classification is utilized to analyze data from HRM to determine the manometric diagnosis. The presence or absence of outflow obstruction, represented by an IRP of >15-mmHg, is the initial assessment used in the hierarchical algorithm for the interpretation of HRM studies with the CC v3.0 (Fig. 11.10).

1. **Esophageal Motility Disorders with Elevated IRP**
   (a) Achalasia: It is a condition characterized by aperistalsis and failure of the LES to relax. The Chicago Classification has identified three subtypes of achalasia through esophageal HRM that are all associated with incomplete LES relaxation (IRP >15 mmHg) but with different pressurization patterns.

Type I: IRP >15 mmHg, and aperistalsis with no pressure waves recorded (Fig. 11.11).

Type II: IRP >15 mmHg, panesophageal pressurization >30 mmHg in at least 20% of swallows, and 100% failed swallows (Fig. 11.12).

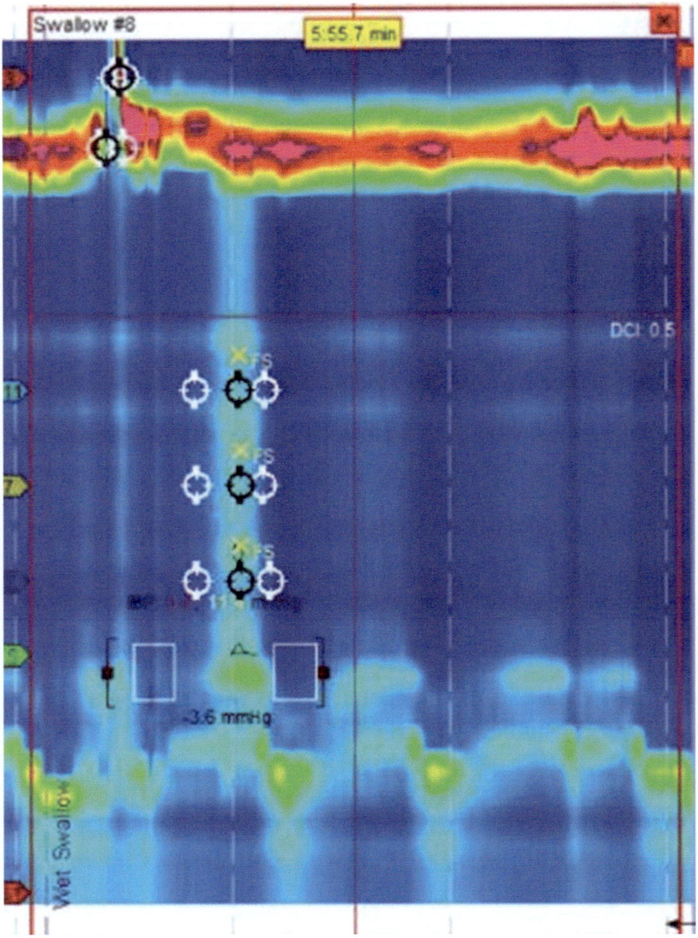

Fig. 11.11 Type 1 achalasia (classic achalasia) is diagnosed when there are 100% aperistalsis, elevated mean IRP (>15 mmHg Medtronic), and DCI less than 100 mHg-sec-cm. Even if aperistalsis is present and IRP is at the upper limit of normal, achalasia should still be taken into consideration as a potential diagnosis

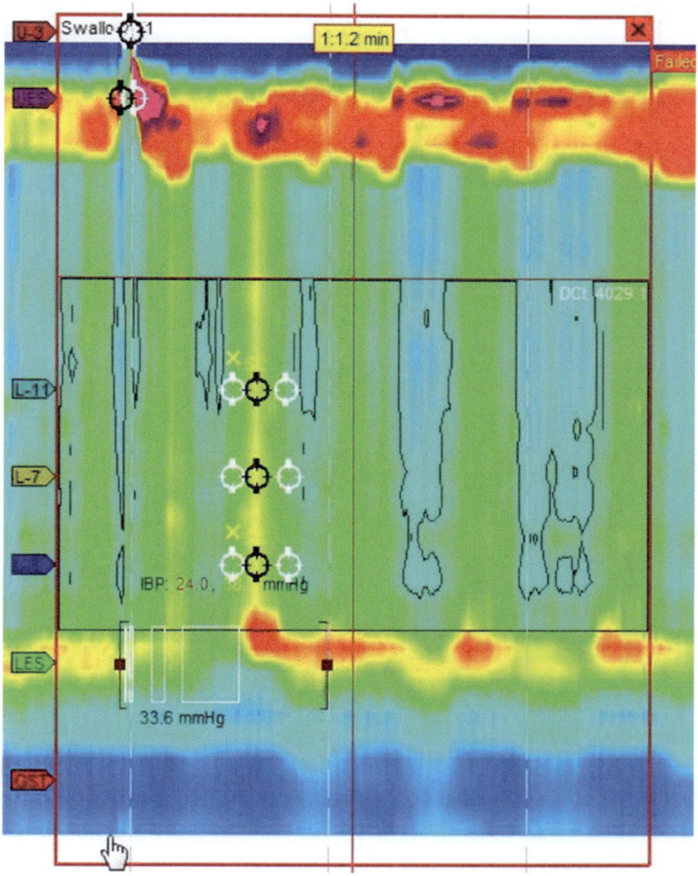

Fig. 11.12 Type 2 achalasia, elevated median IRP (>15 mmHg*), 100% failed peristalsis, and panesophageal pressurization with ≥20% of swallows. Contractions may be masked by esophageal pressurization and DCI should not be calculated

Type III: (spastic achalasia) It is associated with IRP ≥15 mmHg and premature (spastic) contractions with or without periods of compartmentalized pressurization in ≥20% of swallows (Fig. 11.13).

(b) EGJ Outflow Obstruction (EGJOO): It is defined as failure of the LES to relax (IRP >15 mmHg) with intact or weak

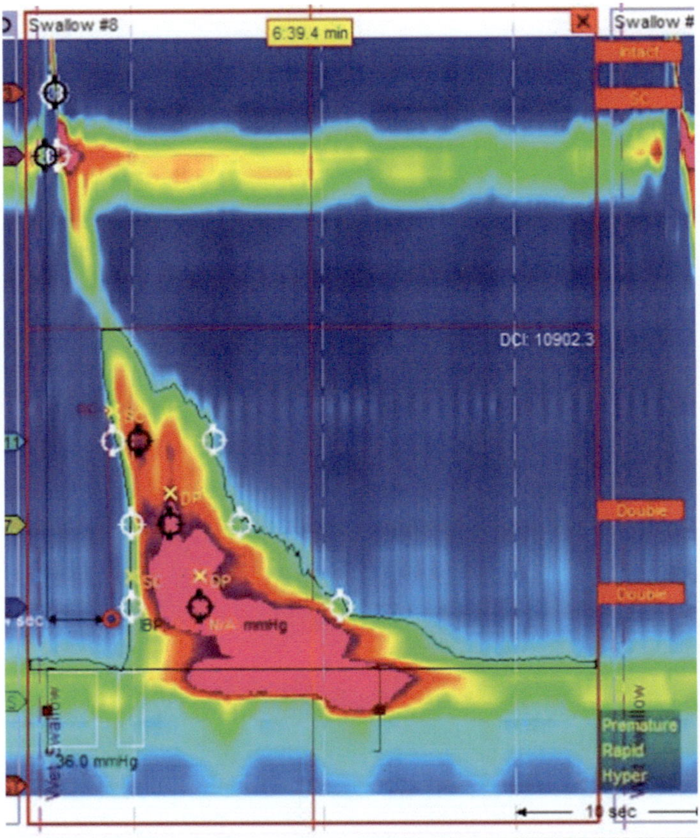

Fig. 11.13 Type 3 achalasia, elevated median IRP (>15 mmHg*), no normal peristalsis, premature (spastic) contractions with DCI > 450 mmHg-s-cm with ≥20% of swallows. May be mixed with panesophageal pressurization

peristalsis not meeting criteria for achalasia as being an EGJ outflow obstruction (Fig. 11.14). This is a heterogeneous diagnosis with a differential diagnosis that includes early, evolving, or incomplete achalasia, mechanical obstruction, hiatal hernia, and pressure artifacts. In this situation, patients will need additional diagnostic studies such as barium swallow and/or endoscopy.

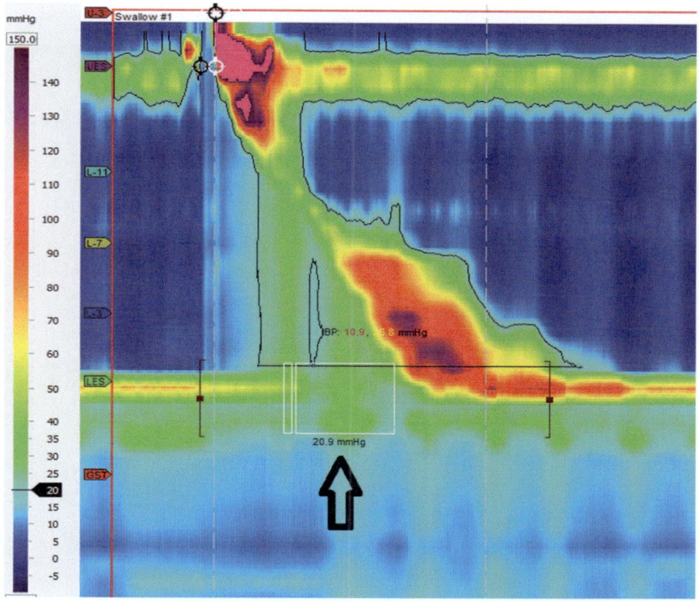

Fig. 11.14 EGJ obstruction is characterized by an altered IRP in the absence of other criteria for achalasia. Manometry in a patient with dysphagia after Nissen fundoplication

(c) **Esophageal Motility Disorders with Normal IRP**—major disorders of peristalsis (not encountered in normal subjects).

Diffuse Esophageal Spasm: ≥20% premature contractions (DL < 4.5 s) with DCI > 450, physiologically representing an impairment of deglutitive inhibition, thus showing incomplete inhibition in the esophageal body during multiple rapid swallows (MRS). Some normal peristalsis (segmental spasm) and normal EGJ relaxation may be present. Most patients with a distal latency of <4.5 are eventually diagnosed with distal esophageal spasm or type III achalasia (Fig. 11.15).

Hypercontractile Esophagus (Jackhammer esophagus): It is characterized by DCI > 8000 mmHg/sec/cm in at

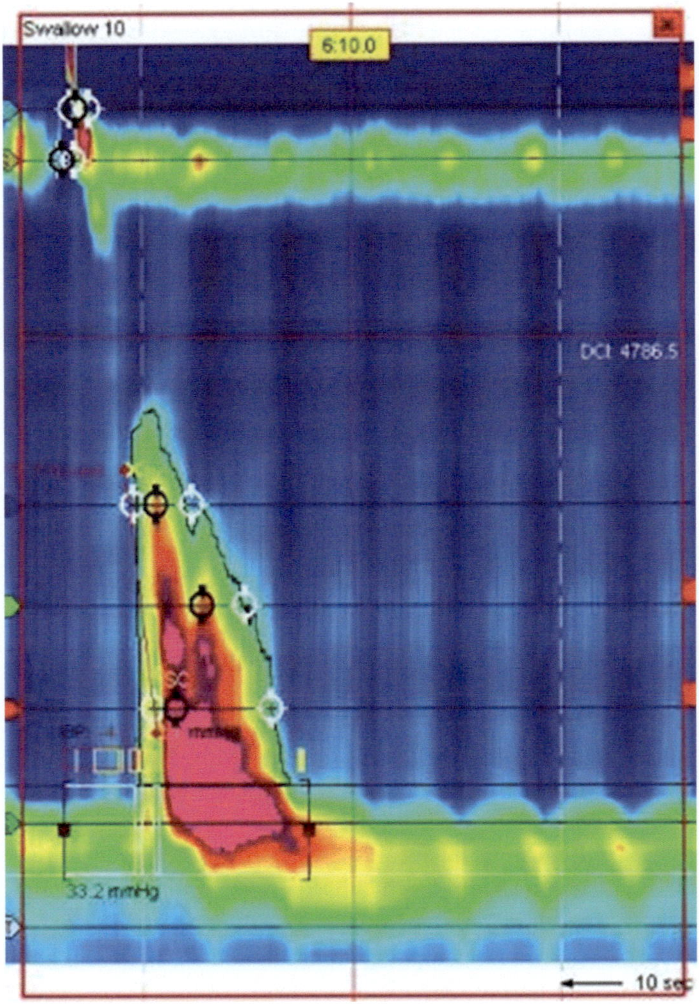

Fig. 11.15 Diffuse esophageal spasm (DES) is defined as normal median IRP and ≥20% premature contractions (DL < 4.5 s) with DCI > 450 mmHg-s-cm*. Some normal peristalsis may be present. This disorder may be attributable not only to a primary esophageal dysmotility but also secondary to reflux disease. Further workup of the patient's symptoms is warranted

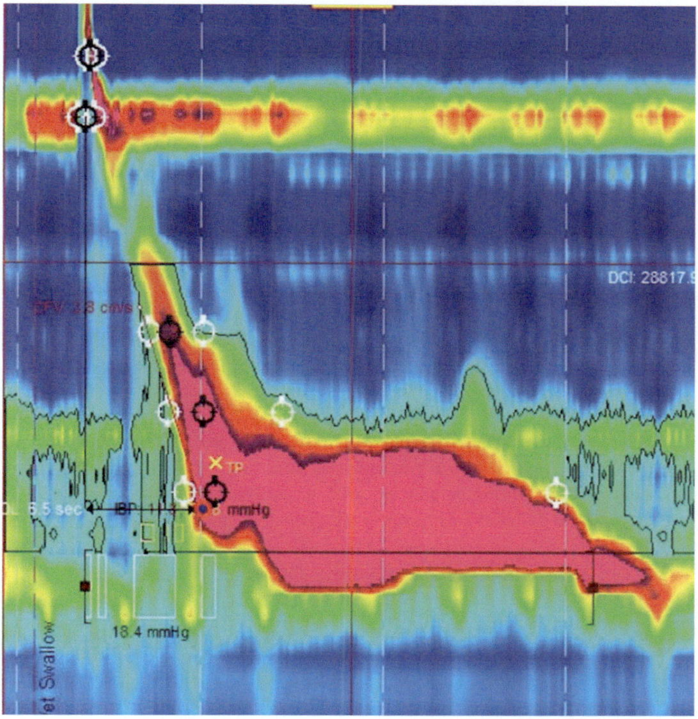

Fig. 11.16 Hypercontractile esophagus (Jackhammer esophagus): at least 20% of propagated swallow-induced contraction with a DCI of >8000 mmHg-s-cm, as that value is extremely rare in asymptomatic subjects. This patient's study was characterized by contraction amplitudes of >200 mmHg in the distal esophagus, and average DCI (contraction vigor) of 14,919. Patients with these disorders may present with dysphagia and/or noncardiac chest pain

least 20% of swallows and normal DL. Hypercontractility may be involved, or even be localized to the LES. DCI > 8000 is never seen in asymptomatic controls. The occurrence of a multipeaked contraction seems to be of limited relevance (Fig. 11.16).

Absent Contractility: It is characterized by aperistalsis (100% failed swallows) in the setting of normal LES relaxation (IRP <15 mmHg). This motility pattern is

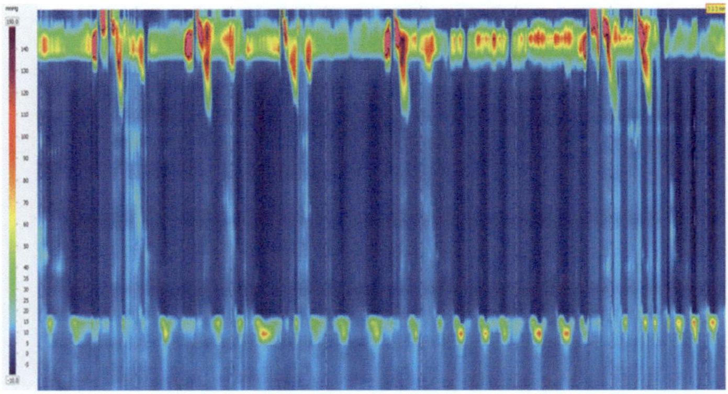

Fig. 11.17 Aperistaltic esophagus and low LES resting pressure. This type of HRM may be seen in patients with connective tissue disorders such as scleroderma. It is a common finding in absent contractility (major motility disorder) and occasionally can be seen in ineffective esophageal motility (minor motility disorder). Hypomotility disorders carry an increased risk of GERD due to delayed esophageal clearance. In addition, unexplained dysphagia can be seen in patients with normal GE junction relaxation

classically seen in patients with systemic scleroderma (Fig. 11.17).

(d) **Esophageal Motility Disorders with Normal IRP**—Minor Disorders of Peristalsis.

Ineffective esophageal motility: It is diagnosed when >50% of swallows are ineffective, determined as either failed (DCI < 100 mmHg cm s) or weak (DCI 100–450 mmHg cm s) (Fig. 11.18).

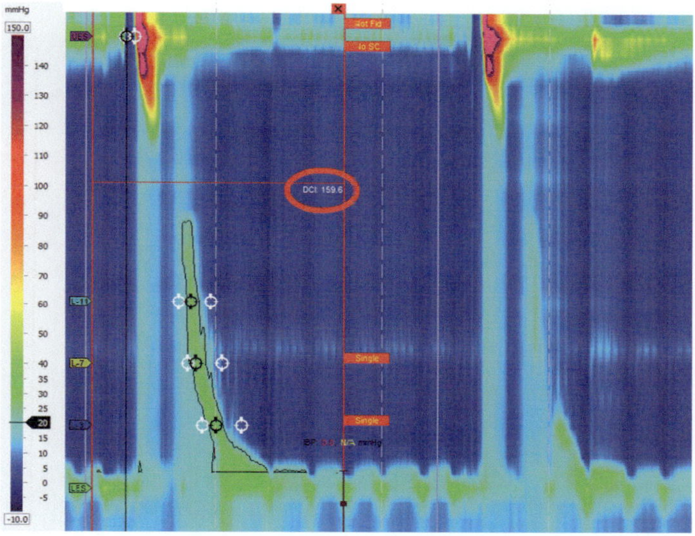

Fig. 11.18 Ineffective esophageal motility is defined by ≥50% ineffective swallows (failed or weak—DCI < 450 mmHg-s-cm). Manometry in a patient with severe GERD

Multiple repetitive swallow (MRS) assessments may be helpful in determining peristaltic reserve (Fig. 11.29).

Fragmented peristalsis: is defined as >50% of swallows with a large break (>5 cm) and not meeting criteria for ineffective esophageal motility (DCI > 450) (Fig. 11.19).

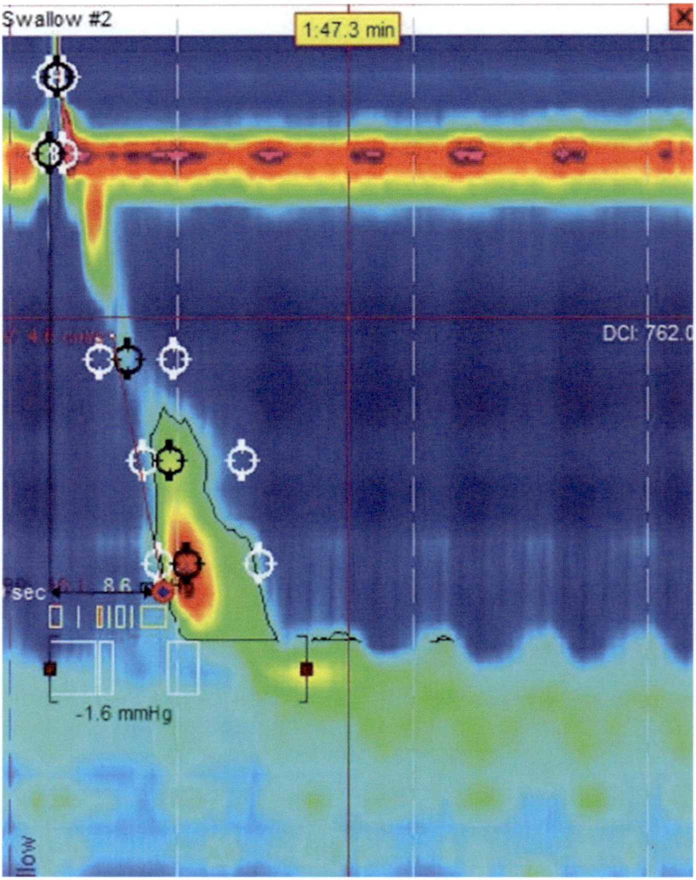

Fig. 11.19 Fragmented peristalsis: ≥50% fragmented contractions with DCI > 450 mmHgs cm. Large breaks (>5 cm in length) in the 20 mmHg isobaric contour. In this HRM, there is a 6-cm break in the 20 mmg isobaric contour (consistent with a large break (>5 cm)). Large peristaltic breaks could be associated with delayed bolus clearance and higher acid exposure time

High-Resolution Manometry with Impedance (HRIM)

High-resolution impedance manometry (HRIM) has been introduced as a technique that combines the benefits of HRM and impedance-based bolus transit assessment. The combination of HRM and multichannel intraluminal impedance (MII) provides information regarding esophageal motility, bolus transit, and esophageal clearance. This technology has demonstrated a good correlation with video fluoroscopy but does not have associated radiation exposure [10]. HRIM was accomplished by adding multiple impedance electrodes on HRM catheters to facilitate the measurement and display of impedance. The basic principles of impedance are based on the measurement of resistance to the electrical flow of the intraluminal contents. Impedance decreases temporarily during the passage of a bolus due to its increased conductivity but returns to baseline when the bolus moves past each pair of electrodes [11] (Figs. 11.20, 11.21, and 11.22).

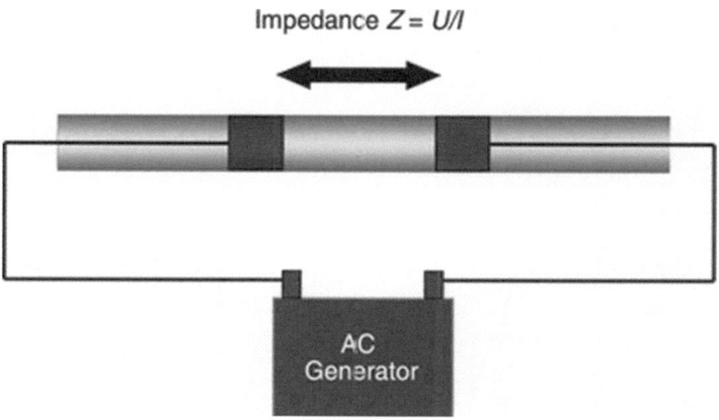

Fig. 11.20 Principles of intraluminal impedance monitoring: An alternating current (AC) circuit is generated between two ring electrodes mounted on a nonconductive catheter placed in a hollow organ such as the esophagus. Electrical impedance (*Z*) of the electric field between two electrodes is the ratio between applied voltage (*U*) and resulting current (*I*)

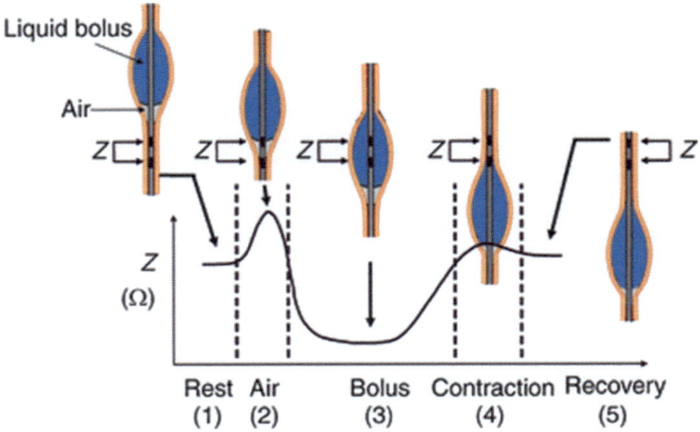

Fig. 11.21 Bolus passage along a neighboring pair of electrodes yields a typical impedance tracing, including five phases: baseline impedance during resting stage of the esophagus (phase 1); impedance rise caused by arrival and passage of an air volume ahead of the bolus (phase 2); impedance drop and recovery caused by arrival and passage of the bolus (phase 3); impedance rise caused by wall contraction associated with lumen occlusion (phase 4) and recovery of impedance signal to baseline levels during transition to resting stage (phase 5)

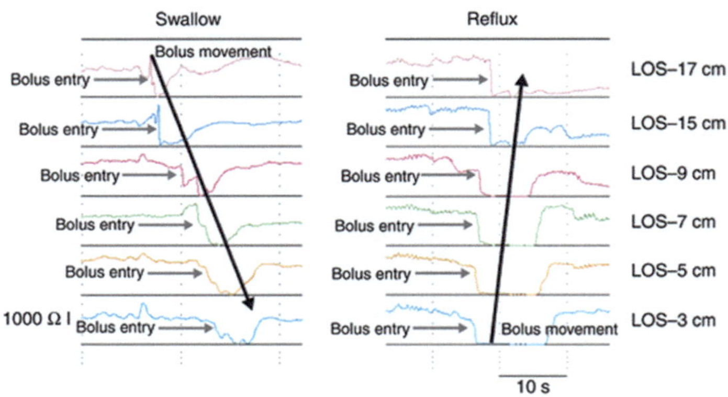

Fig. 11.22 Impedance changes during swallowing and reflux of a bolus, detected by multichannel impedance monitoring. Proximal to distal progression of changes in impedance indicates antegrade bolus movement as seen during swallowing, whereas distal to proximal progression indicates retrograde bolus movement, as seen during reflux. LOS, lower esophageal sphincter

HRIM could distinguish the intraluminal air, which exhibits high impedance from liquid, which exhibits low impedance. Impedance data from several pairs of electrodes can be integrated using dedicated software and displayed superimposed on pressure topography plots, thereby allowing visualization of the bolus as it travels down the esophagus in conjunction with esophageal peristalsis (Fig. 11.22).

HRIM has contributed significantly to current metrics utilized in the Chicago Classification. Measurements such as peristaltic integrity at 20 mmHg being adequate for bolus transit were determined with the use of HRIM. Peristaltic breaks (<2 cm) in the 20 mmHg isobaric contour were associated with complete bolus clearance by impedance criteria using HRIM; therefore, these small breaks were demonstrated not to be pathognomonic for abnormal bolus transit in subsequent studies [12]. Likewise, large breaks (>5 cm) in the 20 mmHg isobaric contour demonstrated incomplete bolus transit on HRIM. Therefore, HRIM data contributed to the criteria developed for the diagnosis of fragmented peristalsis and ineffective esophageal motility (IEM) in the newest Chicago Classification (version 3.0). Of note, the assessment of impedance is not covered by the Chicago Classification of esophageal motility disorders.

Indications for HRIM

HRIM can be valuable in the differential diagnosis of disorders resembling GERD. This includes behavioral disorders such as rumination syndrome (unconscious postprandial abdominal musculature contractions that can return food back into the mouth), by distinguishing rumination episodes from regurgitation or because impedance sensors can detect gas movement. HRIM can detect supragastric belching (where air rapidly enters and subsequently exits the esophagus without reaching the stomach) from gastric belching (diaphragmatic contractions forcing air into the esophagus, which can then be expelled) [13]. Furthermore, the combination of HRM with intraluminal impedance has been shown to discriminate reflux episodes associated with TLESRs better than those after swallow-induced LES relaxations [14].

HRIM has been used to characterize bolus transit in patients with esophageal motor disorders and nonobstructive dysphagia. This testing can diagnose whether a functional defect truly exists in patients with dysphagia and other symptoms such as noncardiac chest pain, especially in patients with manometric diagnoses of ineffective esophageal motility and diffuse esophageal spasm, since it may identify a functional defect in approximately half of these patients [15].

Studies suggest that, in patients with nonobstructive dysphagia and normal manometry, impedance testing will identify a subset of patients with impaired bolus transit [16]. In patients with achalasia, HRIM can be utilized to assess bolus retention in the esophagus and after therapy it can assess the adequacy of LES disruption. However, in achalasia patients, low-baseline impedance levels and air entrapment in the proximal esophagus limit the value of intraluminal impedance monitoring as a test of esophageal emptying [17]. HRIM has also been used to evaluate post-fundoplication dysphagia [18].

Technique

As previously described, the HRIM catheter is a solid state with 36 circumferential pressure sensors at 1-cm intervals and impedance measuring segments including 18 segments at 2-cm intervals (Medtronic Inc., Shoreview, MN). The catheter is also placed transnasally and positioned to record from the hypopharynx to the stomach with approximately 2–3 intragastric sensors, with the most distal impedance measuring segment at 5 cm above the LES.

The HRIM protocol includes a five-minute baseline recording and then ten 5 ml swallows of normal saline (better conductivity) in a supine position for test swallows at 20- to 30-s intervals.

After placement, the supine patient is asked to take 10 liquid (normal saline solution) and 10 viscous swallows.

HRIM Interpretation

- Esophageal bolus clearance can be assessed by the measurement of *bolus presence time* (BPT) and *total bolus transit time* (TBTT).
- BPT represents the time for the bolus to transverse completely an individual recording segment and is measured at each recording segment from the time the bolus enters the segment, as indicated by a drop-in impedance to 50% of the baseline value, until the bolus has cleared the segment, as evidenced by the recovery of the impedance level to 50% of the baseline value for ≥5 s.
- TBTT represents the time for the bolus to transverse the whole esophagus and is measured from the time the bolus enters the proximal esophageal recording segment (Z1) until it has cleared the most distal recording segment (Z4).
- Complete bolus transit if bolus entry occurs at the most proximal site and bolus exit points are recorded in all distal recording segments.
- Incomplete bolus transit if bolus exit is not identified at any of the three distal recording segments.
- Based on the above definitions, normal individuals have a complete bolus transit in at least 80% of liquid and at least 70% of viscous swallows [19]. Conversely, patients with more than 20% of swallows with incomplete bolus transit for liquid and more than 30% of swallows with incomplete bolus transit for viscous are considered to have abnormal bolus transit for liquid and viscous, respectively.

High-Resolution Manometry: Esophageal Disorders Not Addressed by the "Chicago Classification"

In clinical practice, there are a number of patients that have findings in HRM, which are not described by the Chicago classification. The CC is a work in progress, and it is likely that future versions will incorporate new categories of manometric abnormalities.

1. **Upper Esophageal Sphincter:** Oropharyngeal dysphagia and globus sensation could result from disorders of the upper esophageal sphincter (UES). These symptoms demonstrate impaired bolus transit from the hypopharynx into the esophagus. HRM evaluates mainly baseline pressures and relaxation of the UES. Increased intrabolus pressure during swallows may suggest either a cricopharyngeal bar (Fig. 11.23) or Zenker's diverticulum. In patients with cricopharyngeal bar, the UES does not fully relax with a wet swallow because of a thickening of the cricopharyngeal muscle. Of course, barium esophagogram offers more sensitivity for the diagnosis of cricopharyngeal bar. There are no manometric criteria that could help identify a Zenker's diverticulum unless the diverticulum is associated with a cricopharyngeal bar. HRM does not change the management of patients with oropharyngeal dysphagia.
2. **Hiatal Hernia:** A hiatal hernia is the sliding of the stomach into the chest cavity and is demonstrated in HRM as the separation between the diaphragmatic crura and the LES (Fig. 11.24). The measurement of the distance between the crura and the LES represents the size of the hiatal hernia.

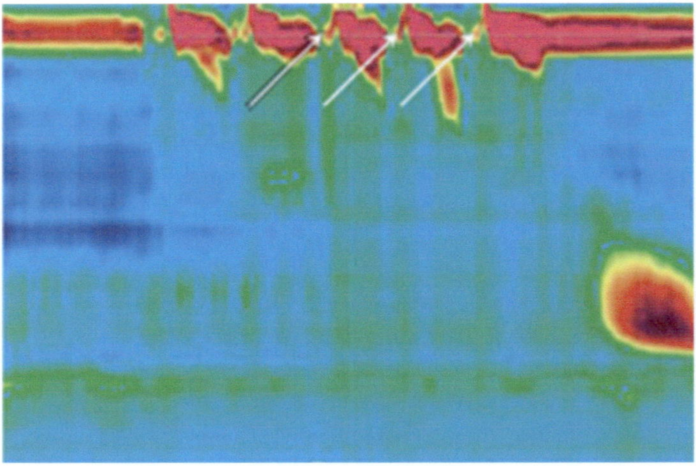

Fig. 11.23 HRM demonstrating a cricopharyngeal bar. The white arrows show raised intrabolus pressure

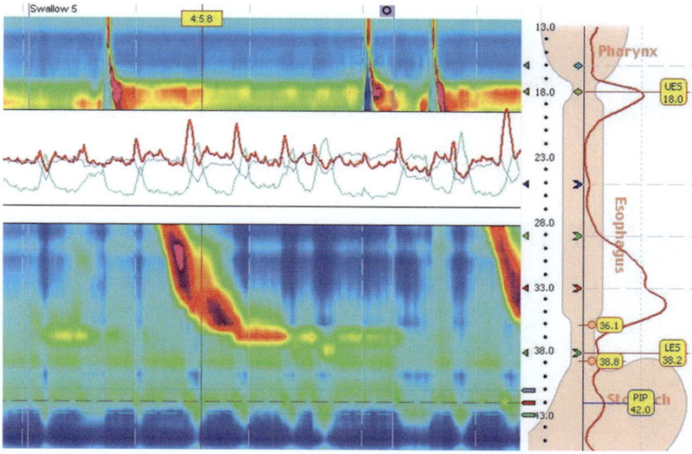

Fig. 11.24 Hiatul hernia. Identification of a hiatul hernia. A 4-cm hiatus hernia is identified in this HRM color contour. There are two zones of high pressure in proximity to the gastroesophageal junction. One appears as a horizontal band of green color about 43 cm from the nares. This band of color coincides with the pressure inversion point (PIP) (red line) that defines the location of the diaphragm. The second zone of high pressure arises as a horizontal band of green color at the distal extent of the peristaltic pressure wave, roughly at 38 cm from the nares. A software tool that aids in identifying the diaphragm (PIP) is shown. At the bottom of the figure, there are three horizontal, colored lines that are 1 cm apart: blue at 41 cm, red at 42 cm, and green at 43 cm from the nares. The white box near the middle of the contour also displays three colored lines. These lines show the pressures recorded at the positions of their corresponding colored lines at 41, 42, and 43 cm from the nares. The three colored lines at the bottom can be moved up and down as a unit. They are positioned here to identify the location of the diaphragm (PIP). Notice that with inspiration the blue line indicates a drop-in pressure and the green line indicates a rise in pressure

3. **Hypotensive LES and Transient LES Relaxations (TLESRs):** Patients with hypotensive LES pressures are at higher risk of developing GERD. However, the majority of patients with GERD have normal LES pressure. In these patients, relaxation of the LES not associated with swallowing (TLESRs) (Fig. 11.25) is the most common mechanism of GERD.

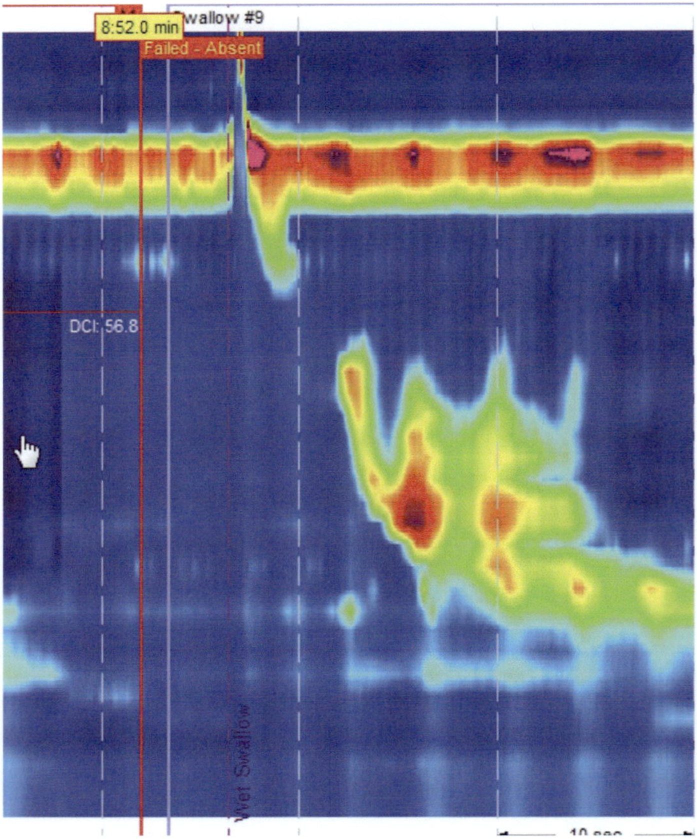

Fig. 11.25 Transient lower esophageal sphincter relaxation (TLESR). This study demonstrated the relaxation of the LES not associated with a wet swallow (WS) before the subject takes the WS

4. **Rumination Syndrome and Belching:** The diagnosis of rumination is facilitated with the use of HRIM, which demonstrates an increase in intragastric pressure that eventually overcomes the LES pressure and results in retrograde movement of gastric contents. The use of impedance helps differentiate between gas and liquid gastric contents. In patients with intragastric belching, there is a similar increase in the intragastric

pressure, but in this case, there is no retrograde movement of gastric fluid but only retrograde movement of gas. Patients with supraesophageal belching show a decrease in UES pressure not associated with swallow, demonstrating esophageal venting.

5. **Post-Fundoplication HRM:** HRM is useful in the evaluation of post-fundoplication patients not only for the accurate placement of the pH probe, but also to assess patients that have persistent, recurrent, or newly developed symptoms after surgery. HRM analyzes the efficacy of the antireflux barrier (LES—Crura), LES pressure and position, and IRP. In general, if there is normal LES pressure and relaxation and the LES and the crura generate a single distal high-pressure zone, it is assumed that the fundoplication is intact and in an intraabdominal position. If there is a hypotensive LES pressure with normal relaxation and the LES and the crura generate a single distal high-pressure zone, it is possible that the fundoplication is disrupted. On the other hand, if there is hypertensive LES pressure and incomplete relaxation, it is assumed that the fundoplication is too tight, twisted, or misconstructed (Fig. 11.26). A dual distal high-pressure zone suggests that a slipped fundoplication is intact and in an intraabdominal position [20] (Fig. 11.27).
6. **Post-Myotomy HRM:** HRM is very useful for the preoperative and postoperative evaluation of patients with esophageal motility disorders with elevated IRP such as achalasia, DES, and in some patients with EGJ outflow obstruction (Fig. 11.28).

   In such patients, HRM can be useful for the assessment of patients with recurrent symptoms after either surgical or endoscopic treatment. This can be caused by an incomplete myotomy, scarring at the myotomy site, a tight partial fundoplication, or megaesophagus. The presence of a persistent LES pressure of >10 mmHg, elevated IRP, and failure to achieve at least 50% reduction in LES pressure from baseline have been associated with poor outcomes [21].

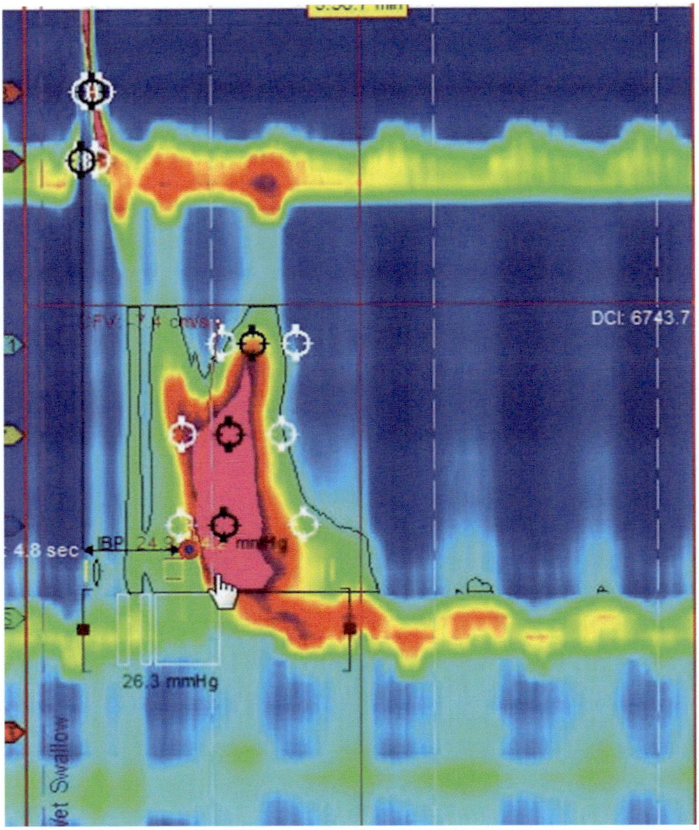

Fig. 11.26 Twisted fundoplication

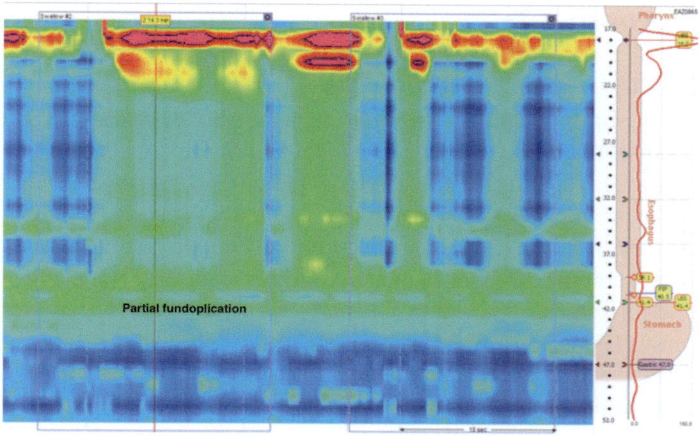

Fig. 11.27 Achalasia post-fundoplication

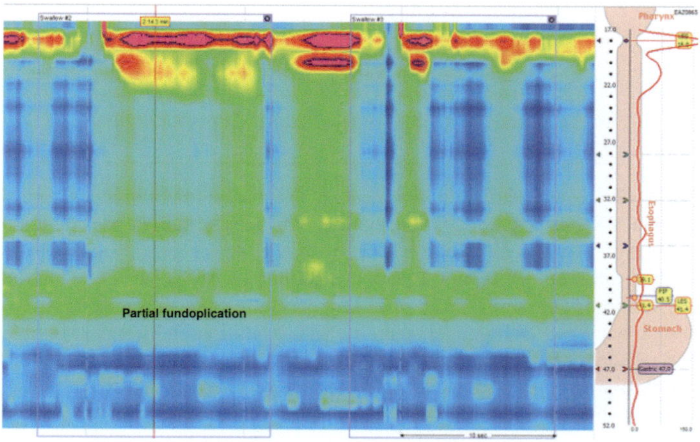

Fig. 11.28 High-resolution esophageal manometry after a failed Heller's myotomy with Dor fundoplication in a patient with achalasia Type II. The patient had ongoing dysphagia. The LES does not relax appropriately (IRP 31) and suggests a persistently elevated LES pressure along with a relatively tight wrap. There is a horizontal band of high pressure from 38 to 42 cm

Provocative Tests

1. **Multiple Rapid Swallows (MRS)**

   Multiple rapid swallows assess the ability of the esophageal smooth muscle to withhold contraction during repetitive swallowing (deglutitive inhibition) and to produce a strong esophageal body peristaltic contraction following the last swallow (peristaltic reserve). The absence of peristaltic reserve is associated with a higher likelihood of dysphagia following antireflux surgery. The MRS consists of at least four 2-ml water swallows performed in rapid succession, with ≤4-s interval between swallows and the LES [22] (Fig. 11.29).
2. **Rapid Drink Challenge**

   The patient drinks 100 to 200 mL of water through a straw as quickly as possible. The rapid drink challenge assesses for esophageal outflow obstruction, and the increased volume of fluid can create a visible obstructive pattern with the compart-

Fig. 11.29 Multiple rapid swallow (MRS) responses. (**a**) Normal and reproducible MRS response showing profound inhibition of the esophageal body and lower esophageal sphincter (LES) during the swallows and rebound esophageal body contraction with the regaining of LES tone following the last swallow of the series. Both MRS sequences are alike and concordant. (**b**) Discordant MRS response, showing normal inhibition and normal contraction response with the first MRS sequence, and normal inhibition but absent contraction response with the second sequence. (**c**) Discordant MRS response, showing abnormal inhibition with both sequences, intact contraction with the first sequence and absent contraction with the second. The esophageal body and lower esophageal sphincter (LES) during the swallows and rebound esophageal body contraction with regaining of LES tone following the last swallow of the series. Both MRS sequences are alike and concordant. (B) Discordant MRS response, showing normal inhibition and normal contraction response with the first MRS sequence, and normal inhibition but absent contraction response with the second sequence. (C) Discordant MRS response, showing abnormal inhibition with both sequences, intact contraction with the first sequence and absent contraction with the second

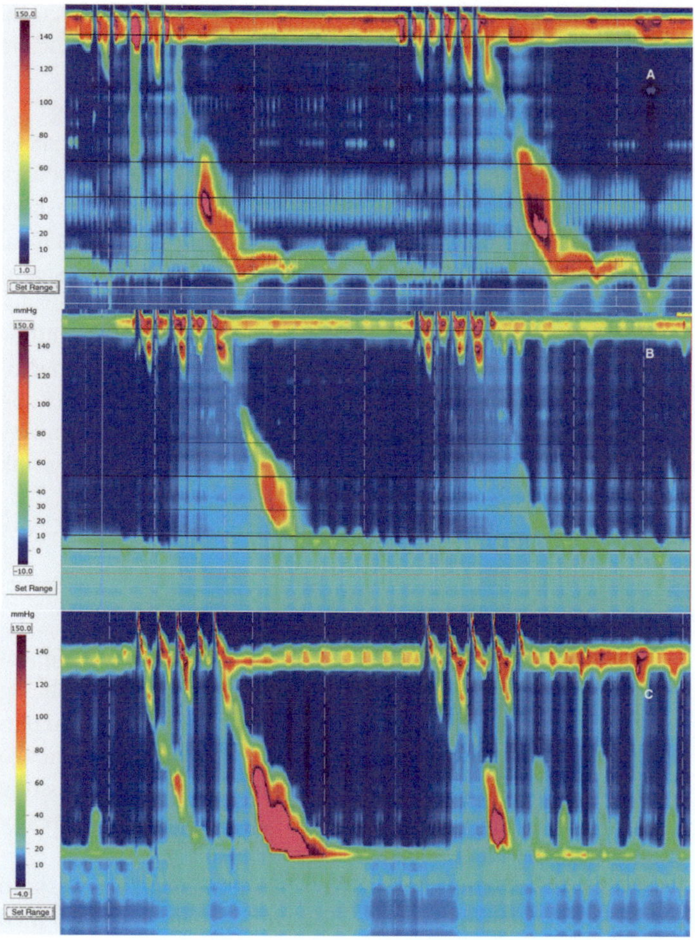
150.0
140
120
100
80
60
40
30
20
10
1.0
Set Range
A
mmHg
150.0
140
120
100
80
60
40
30
20
10
0
-10.0
Set Range
B
mmHg
150.0
140
120
100
80
60
40
30
20
10
-4.0
Set Range
C

mentalization of intrabolus pressure or panesophageal pressurization in the esophageal body if there is an obstructive process at the EGJ.

3. **Standardized Test Meal and Postprandial Monitoring**

   Administration of a meal during the HRM procedure can be useful in demonstrating an obstructive pattern in patients with dysphagia when standard water swallows do not demonstrate abnormality. Monitoring for 30 to 60 min following a test meal can be helpful in diagnosing rumination syndrome and supragastric belching. Upright swallows can be beneficial in evaluating the reliability of the identification of esophageal outflow obstruction. Viscous swallows, bread swallows, and marshmallow swallows have been used as part of provocative testing during HRM with stationary impedance but are not as universally utilized as multiple rapid swallows and the rapid drink challenge.

Updates with Chicago Classification v4.0

In the 5 years since the publication of CCv3.0, both the clinical and research applications of HRM have expanded, introducing novel metrics and the widespread adoption of new therapies, particularly endoscopic myotomy. In order to update the Chicago Classification, an International HRM Working Group consisting of 52 diverse experts worked for 2 years and utilized formally validated methodologies [23].

CC4 has sought to address issues regarding the patient position that were a criticism of CC3. However, that protocol is often insufficient to establish a definitive motility diagnosis that explains symptoms and guides therapy. The new protocol described suggests that clinicians start with the patient in whichever position they usually start and regard this as the "primary position." The study should proceed for the ten wet swallows as usual. An additional set of five wet swallows should then be performed with the patient in the alternate or "secondary position." The differences in normative values for catheter design and patient position should be considered with some example references. Clinicians should

Table 11.2 Supportive manometric measures which may increase confidence for a disorder. Adapted from CC41

Supportive measure	Protocol	Normal response
Multiple Rapid Swallows (MRS)	Five swallows of 2-mL liquid at 2-3 s intervals	Absense of esophageal body contractility (DCI <100 mmHg*s*cm) with complete degulatitive inhibition of the LES during MRS and presense of post-MRS contraction augmentation (DCI post-MRS greater than single swallow mean DCI)
Rapid Drink Challenge (RDC)	Rapid drink of 200 ml of liquid	Absense of esophageal body contractility (DCI <100 mmHg*s*cm) with complete degulatitive inhibition of the LES during RDC and no evidence of major motility disorder post-RDC.
Solid Test Swallows	Ten swallows of ~1-cm³ soft solid (eg bread, soft boiled rice, marshmallow)	Presence of >20% pharyngeal swallows being followed by an effective esophageal contraction defined by DCI >1000 mmHg*s*cm and without a large break (>5 cm) in the contractile front.
Solid Test Meal (STM)	200 g of soft solid meal (eg soft boiled) rice, bread) ingested at normal rate for patient. Study stopped if STM not completed in 8-min.	Presence of >20% pharyngeal swallows being followed by an effective esophageal contraction defined by DCI >1000 mmHg-s-cm and without a large break (>5 cm) in the contractile front. No Symptoms during STM (any symptoms should be recorded in electronic record to assess association with abnormal motility or function). Show eating with <200 g ingested during 8 minuted also considered abnormal.
Post-Prandial Meal (High-resolution impedance manometry)	Administration of a STM or self-identified symptom inducing meal followed by extended monitoring (minimum of 10 min and occurrence of abnormal activity)	Absense of symptoms and abnormal motility or function during post-prandial period. Maximum 4 transient LES relaxations (TLESRs) with belching during initial 10-min post-prandial, no volume regurgitation, no remination or supra-gastric belching episodes.

also consider performing two provocation tests as standard. The Multiple Rapid Swallow 2 (MRS or 5 × 2 ml challenge) is now well established and can indicate the peristaltic reserve [24]. The Rapid Drink Challenge 3 (RDC or 200 ml challenge) can further assess esophagogastric junction (EGJ) outflow [25]. Both are defined in terms of execution and normative parameters within the classification. Parameters are given for solid swallows (e.g., bread, rice, and marshmallow) with the suggestion given for a solid test meal (Table 11.1). However, it is stressed that any abnormal findings should correspond to the patient's symptoms (e.g., dysphagia or chest pain), the absence of which may render the findings clinically insignificant (Table 11.2).

Motility Disorders

The use of a hierarchy of disorders is maintained in CC4 with a note that the classification applies to normal anatomy (i.e., an absence of previous significant intervention/surgery or large Hiatal hernia). The need for initial endoscopy or a Barium study is also emphasized. A scheme for applying the classification can be found in Fig. 11.1. Achalasia and absent contractility have

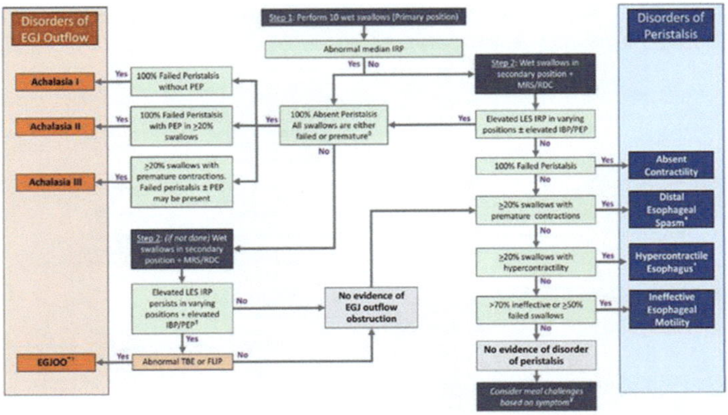

Fig. 11.30 Chicago Classification 4.0 Hierarchical Classification Scheme

stood the test of time and remain essentially unchanged. EGJOO and IEM underwent a complete redefinition. Changes to DES and hypercontractile esophagus were considered, but there were insufficient data to merit major revision; however, both require further investigation and future updates (Fig. 11.30).

Conclusions

High-resolution manometry (HRM) has become the gold standard for the diagnosis of esophageal motility disorders. This technique has not only made esophageal manometry more comfortable and tolerable for the patient since pull-through is not required, but also easier and faster for the operator. The combination of HRM and multichannel intraluminal impedance (MII) provides information regarding esophageal motility, bolus transit, and esophageal clearance and can be valuable in the differential diagnosis of disorders resembling GERD.

Using HRM metrics and utilizing an algorithmic scheme, the Chicago Classification (CC) has significantly improved the recognition and management of esophageal motor disorders. However, the CC is a work in progress. While the manometry software provides a computer-generated analysis of the study, the computerized analysis is imperfect. For that reason, an experienced clinician must review each swallow and provide a final interpretation since an inadequate diagnosis can adversely affect patient outcomes.

The combination of HRM and multichannel intraluminal impedance (MII) provides information regarding esophageal motility, bolus transit, and esophageal clearance. For those reasons, HRIM can be valuable in the differential diagnosis of disorders resembling GERD, in patients with nonobstructive dysphagia, post-fundoplication dysphagia, and discriminate reflux episodes associated with TLESRs.

Lastly, HRM should ideally be performed in a practice environment with therapeutic expertise in treating motility disorders.

References

1. Clouse RE, Staiano A. Topography of the esophageal peristaltic pressure wave. Am J Physiol. 1991;261(4 Pt 1):677–84.
2. Schlottmann F, Herbella FA, Patti MG. Understanding the Chicago classification: from tracings to patients. J Neurogastroenterol Motil. 2017;23(4):487–94.
3. Conklin JL. Evaluation of esophageal motor function with high-resolution manometry. J Neurogastroenterol Motil. 2013;19:281.
4. Kahrilas PJ, Bredenoord AJ, Fox M, Gyawali CP, Roman S, Smout AJPM, et al. The Chicago classification of esophageal motility disorders, v3.0. Neurogastroenterol Motil [Internet]. 2015;27(2):160–74. Available from: http://web.a.ebscohost.com.libproxy.tulane.edu:2048/ehost/detail/detail?vid=0&sid=0b86f1de-375c-4480-85c4-1925e20d34d3%40sdc-v-sessmgr03&bdata=JkF1dGhUeXBlPWlwLHNzbyZzaXRlPWVob3N0LWxpdmUmc2NvcGU9c2l0ZQ%3D%3D#AN=100631580&db=a9h.
5. Kahrilas PJ, Ghosh SK, Pandolfino JE. Esophageal motility disorders in terms of pressure topography: the Chicago classification. J Clin Gastroenterol. 2008;42:627.
6. Bredenoord AJ, Fox M, Kahrilas PJ, Pandolfino JE, Schwizer W, Smout AJPM. Chicago classification criteria of esophageal motility disorders defined in high resolution esophageal pressure topography. Neurogastroenterol Motil. 2012;24:57.

7. Carlson DA, Kahrilas PJ. How to effectively use high-resolution esophageal manometry. Gastroenterology [Internet]. 2016;151(5):789–92. https://doi.org/10.1053/j.gastro.2016.09.024.
8. Herregods TVK, Roman S, Kahrilas PJ, Smout AJPM, Bredenoord AJ. Normative values in esophageal high-resolution manometry. Neurogastroenterol Motil. 2015;27:175.
9. Xiao Y, Read A, Nicodème F, Roman S, Kahrilas PJ, Pandolfino JE. The effect of a sitting vs supine posture on normative esophageal pressure topography metrics and Chicago Classification diagnosis of esophageal motility disorders. Neurogastroenterol Motil. 2012;24:e509.
10. Patel A, Gyawali CP. How to optimally apply impedance in the evaluation of esophageal dysmotility. Curr Gastroenterol Rep. 2016;18:60.
11. Conchillo JM, Smout AJ. Review article: intra-oesophageal impedance monitoring for the assessment of bolus transit and gastro-oesophageal reflux. Aliment Pharmacol Ther. 2009;29:3.
12. Roman S, Lin Z, Kwiatek MA, Pandolfino JE, Kahrilas PJ. Weak peristalsis in esophageal pressure topography: classification and association with dysphagia. Am J Gastroenterol. 2011;106:349.
13. Dhawan I, O'Connell B, Patel A, Schey R, Parkman HP, Friedenberg F. Utility of esophageal high-resolution manometry in clinical practice: first, do HRM. Dig Dis Sci. 2018;63:3178.
14. Roman S, Zerbib F, Belhocine K, Bruley Des Varannes S, Mion F. High resolution manometry to detect transient lower oesophageal sphincter relaxations: diagnostic accuracy compared with perfused-sleeve manometry, and the definition of new detection criteria. Aliment Pharmacol Ther. 2011;34:384.
15. Tutuian R, Castell DO. Combined multichannel intraluminal impedance and manometry clarifies esophageal function abnormalities: study in 350 patients. Am J Gastroenterol. 2004;99:1011.
16. Koya DL, Agrawal A, Freeman JE, Castell DO. Impedance detected abnormal bolus transit in patients with normal esophageal manometry. Sensitive indicator of esophageal functional abnormality? Dis Esophagus. 2008;21(6):563–9.
17. Conchillo JM, Selimah M, Bredenoord AJ, Samsom M, Smout AJPM. Assessment of oesophageal emptying in achalasia patients by intraluminal impedance monitoring. Neurogastroenterol Motil. 2006;18:971.
18. Yigit T, Quiroga E, Oelschlager B. Multichannel intraluminal impedance for the assessment of post-fundoplication dysphagia. Dis Esophagus. 2006;19:382.
19. Tutuian R, Vela MF, Balaji NS, Wise JL, Murray JA, Peters JH, et al. Esophageal function testing with combined multichannel intraluminal impedance and manometry: multicenter study in healthy volunteers. Clin Gastroenterol Hepatol. 2003;1:174.

20. Wang YT, Yazaki E, Sifrim D. High-resolution manometry: esophageal disorders not addressed by the "Chicago classification". J Neurogastroenterol Motil. 2012;18:365.
21. Ghoshal UC, Kumar S, Saraswat VA, Aggarwal R, Misra A, Choudhuri G. Long-term follow-up after pneumatic dilation for achalasia cardia: factors associated with treatment failure and recurrence. Am J Gastroenterol. 2004;99:2304.
22. Stoikes N, Drapekin J, Kushnir V, Shaker A, Brunt LM, Gyawali CP. The value of multiple rapid swallows during preoperative esophageal manometry before laparoscopic antireflux surgery. Surg Endosc. 2012;26:3401.
23. Yadlapati R, Kahrilas PJ, Fox MR, et al. Esophageal motility disorders on high-resolution manometry: Chicago classification version 4.0©. Neurogastroenterol Motil. 2021;33(1):e14058. https://doi.org/10.1111/nmo.14058.
24. Shaker A, Stoikes N, Drapekin J, et al. Multiple rapid swallow responses during esophageal high-resolution manometry reflect esophageal body peristaltic reserve. Am J Gastroenterol. 2013;108(11):1706–12. https://doi.org/10.1038/ajg.2013.289.
25. Ang D, Hollenstein M, Misselwitz B, et al. Rapid drink challenge in high-resolution manometry: an adjunctive test for detection of esophageal motility disorders. Neurogastroenterol Motil. 2017;29(1):e12902. https://doi.org/10.1111/nmo.12902.

Impedance Planimetry: EndoFLIP

12

Michelle Campbell and Michael Ujiki

Background

Impedance planimetry has been used since the late 1980s to measure compliance and cross-sectional area (CSA) of luminal organs and sphincters [1]. Over the next 20 years, it was refined for use in all hollow organs but found particular utility in the lumen of the esophagus [2, 3]. In 2004, a new probe was developed allowing simultaneous measurement of multiple luminal CSAs [4] and was quickly adopted for use at the esophagogastric junction (EGJ) [5]. The new method, known as functional lumen imaging probe (FLIP), was validated in 2005 as a quantitative method for assessing the EGJ in diseases such as achalasia and GERD [6].

M. Campbell
University of Chicago Medical Center, Chicago, IL, USA

M. Ujiki (✉)
NorthShore University HealthSystem, Evanston, IL, USA
e-mail: mujiki@northshore.org

A. D. Patel et al. (eds.), *The SAGES Manual of Physiologic Evaluation of Foregut Diseases*,
https://doi.org/10.1007/978-3-031-39199-6_12

Definition

FLIP is an endoscopic catheter-based device that utilizes high-resolution impedance planimetry to measure luminal CSA and pressure allowing for calculation of distensibility, compliance, and depiction of luminal geometry [7]. The distal end of the 72-cm flexible catheter carries impedance electrodes within a distensible polyester urethane balloon, impermeable to body fluids and electrical current [6]. The FDA has approved FLIP in two available configurations: 8-cm balloon with 16 paired sensors spaced 0.5 cm apart (EF-325) utilized for evaluation of esophagogastric junction (EGJ) or 16-cm balloon with 16 paired sensors spaced 1 cm apart (EF-322) utilized for esophageal body in addition to EGJ. The catheter is most often placed transorally into the esophagus with the most distal few sensors in the stomach, thereby spanning the EGJ (Fig. 12.1). Transnasal placement is also possible; however, most existing data is based on transoral placement.

Using a mechanical pump within the attached FLIP machine, the balloon is distended at controlled speed to a target fill volume with proprietary electrolyte solution of known conductance [7]. A continuous low electric current is emitted by electrodes at either end of the balloon and the voltage across paired electrodes measured. Making use of Ohm's law (*voltage = current x resistance*), the electrical resistance (impedance) of the fluid is proportional to CSA. The original FLIP 1.0 module, available for use with either catheter, displays the calculated CSA measurements in a 3D depiction of the lumen (Fig. 12.1). More recently, the FLIP 2.0 panometry module was released for use with the 16 cm balloon catheter which topographically depicts diameter-pressure changes across space-time continuum representing contraction and distension of the esophageal lumen.

Clinical Role The FLIP system's primary utility is in evaluating the biophysical and motor properties of the esophagus and lower esophageal sphincter (LES), although theoretically its use can be expanded to any gastrointestinal sphincter, including the anal

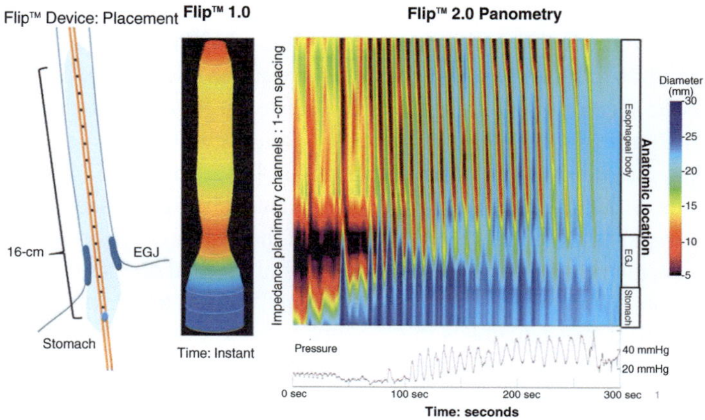

Fig. 12.1 Left: FLIP device position at the EGJ. Center: correlating FLIP 1.0 images. Right: FLIP 2.0 panometry topography representing diameter changes that represent contraction and distention of the esophageal lumen. *EGJ* esophagogastric junction, *FLIP* functional lumen imaging probe

canal [8–11]. Reported metrics obtained during FLIP evaluation include minimum diameter (mm), CSA (mm^2), intra-balloon pressure (mmHg), distensibility index (mm^2/mmHg), and compliance. Of these, distensibility index (DI), defined as the narrowest CSA divided by the corresponding pressure, is the most widely studied with the greatest clinical utility. Normal values for DI at the EGJ range from 3.1 to 9.0 mm^2/mmHg [12].

Achalasia and Motility Disorders

FLIP may be considered as a diagnostic adjunct to endoscopy, manometry, and cross-sectional imaging in the evaluation of suspected mechanical or motor obstruction at the EGJ. High-resolution manometry (HRM) is considered the gold standard in diagnosis of motility disorders, including achalasia in which integrated relaxation pressure (IRP) of the LES is >15 mmHg and peristalsis is absent. FLIP analysis reliably detects major esophageal motility disorders and achalasia when compared to HRM

[13]. In treatment-naïve achalasia patients, the EGJ demonstrates impaired distensibility with DI <1.0 mm^2/mmHg [14–17]. Moreover, FLIP may show a slight advantage over HRM, having been shown to detect impaired EGJ distensibility despite normal IRP on manometry in a subgroup of patients with typical achalasia symptoms and abnormal peristalsis [18]. Volumetric distension within the esophagus during FLIP analysis triggers secondary peristalsis [19]. The second iteration of the FLIP system, FLIP 2.0 panometry, allows serial measurements of luminal diameters plotted as a function of time in topographic fashion using interpolation to depict peristalsis in the esophagus akin to high-resolution manometry. This has led to an expanded role for FLIP 2.0 panometry in accurately identifying achalasia subtypes or other motility disorders using distension-induced contractility mapping [20]. FLIP panometry which is discordant from HRM may be useful in clarifying equivocal or undetected abnormalities on manometry.

The esophagus responds to distention by a bolus with contractions. Similar to a food bolus, FLIP distends the esophagus and induces contractions that are repetitive and antegrade in patients with normal motility. In patients with achalasia, FILP panometry or topography can be used to identify the different achalasia classes. All three classes present with a low distensibility index at the lower esophageal sphincter, but vary in the contractile response. A patient with type I achalasia will have an absent contractile response. Those with type II achalasia will have decreased and disordered contractions. A patient with type III achalasia will have a topography pattern with abnormal retrograde and often, rapid contractions (Fig. 12.2). (ref: Donnan EN, Pandolfino JE. EndoFLIP in the esophagus: assessing sphincter function, wall stiffness, and motility to guide treatment. Gastroenterol Clin North Am. 2020 Sep;49 [3]:427–435.)

In addition to diagnostic utility, FLIP has shown excellent advantage in the assessment of treatment efficacy for achalasia. FLIP measurements obtained following pneumodilation, laparoscopic Heller myotomy, or per oral endoscopic myotomy (POEM)

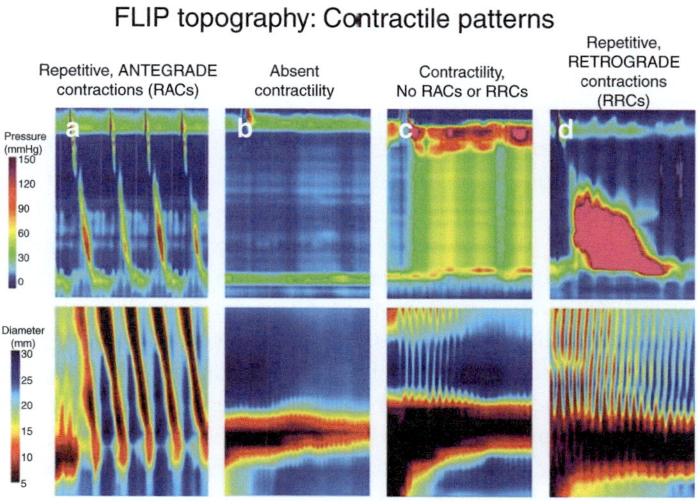

Fig. 12.2 Motility patterns in response to volumetric distention. The top panel is the high-resolution manometry image, and the bottom panel is the FLIP topography image of the representative patient. Panel (**a**) is a normal subject with a RAC pattern. Panel (**b**) is a patient with type I achalasia, and the FLIP depicts an absent contractile response and a poorly relaxing sphincter. Panel (**c**) is type II achalasia, and the FLIP suggests that there are disordered non-occluding contractions in the body of the esophagus and the sphincter does not open. Panel (**d**) is a patient with type III achalasia, and the FLIP topography reveals an abnormal pattern where the contractions are retrograde and rapid in terms of the rate of contractions. Courtesy of the Esophageal Center at Northwestern, Chicago, IL

have been shown to have significant association with treatment success as reported by Eckardt scores [17, 21] and in fact show greater association when compared to manometric measurement of LES pressure [14]. Achieving an optimal DI range (4.5–8.5 mm^2/mmHg) can successfully alleviate achalasia symptoms while minimizing risk of GERD [22]. Therefore, FLIP is now used with increasing frequency intraoperatively to assess extent and completeness of myotomy during laparoscopic Heller myotomy or per oral endoscopic myotomy (POEM) [15, 23, 24].

GERD

Although there was initially early excitement at the prospect of utilizing FLIP technology to diagnose and stratify GERD patients for management planning [25], FLIP has since proven to be a poor diagnostic study for GERD with distensibility and CSA showing poor correlation to clinical symptoms or pH testing [26, 27]. However, FLIP does have an important role in the intraoperative setting in guiding adequacy of fundoplication during reflux procedures. Hiatus repair and fundoplication result in a significant reduction in distensibility of the EGJ during reflux surgery [28–30]. These distensibility changes can be measured by FLIP in real time in the operating room at intervals throughout the procedure (e.g., initial, following hiatal dissection and hernia reduction, following crural closure, and following fundoplication) [28]. Toupet fundoplication results in a more distensible EGJ than Nissen fundoplication [29]. FLIP can be used to provide objective measurement of distensibility when performing fundoplication with early evidence suggesting that maintaining a DI between 2.0 and 3.5 $mm^2/mmHg$ alleviates reflux symptoms while limiting risk of gas bloat from an overly tight wrap [30]. Similarly, using additional metrics provided by FLIP, a decrease in minimum EGJ diameter of 0.15 mm or less, or a decrease in CSA of 1.5 mm^2 or less from initial to post-fundoplication results in greater association with severe heartburn in the postoperative period [31].

Gastroparesis

FLIP has also found utility in evaluating the pylorus in the setting of gastroparesis. Patients with diabetic and idiopathic gastroparesis show decreased sphincter diameter and CSA which correlate inversely with presence of symptoms of early satiety and postprandial fullness [32]. Similar to achalasia and GERD treatments, FLIP can be used in evaluating the efficacy of interventions including gastric peroral endoscopic myotomy (G-POEM). Following G-POEM, FLIP has shown higher CSA and DI in those who achieve clinical relief of symptoms and improvement on gastric emptying scan [33]. Further studies are yet to be performed to better characterize the predictive value of FLIP in gastroparesis, as well as the potential role for tailoring intervention such as with POEM in the achalasia population.

Summary

EndoFLIP is a novel technique with rapidly expanding clinical use in diagnostics and treatment guidance in achalasia, GERD, gastroparesis, and other motility disorders of the foregut and beyond. It is an excellent diagnostic tool in esophageal motility disorders including achalasia, serving currently as an adjunct to manometry with potential to replace HRM as further refinement is made to diagnostic parameters. While not as useful in the diagnosis of GERD, FLIP serves as a valuable tool in the intervention of both achalasia and GERD by allowing the foregut surgeon or interventional endoscopist to guide the POEM or fundoplication procedure in real time for greater treatment efficacy. Application of FLIP to other foregut disorders such as gastroparesis diagnosis and management shows similar promise. As FLIP analysis is more widely adopted, we anticipate a corresponding increase in the availability of both normative data and in-depth applications to the study of foregut pathophysiology and beyond.

References

1. Gregersen H, Stodkilde-Jorgensen H, Djurhuus JC, Mortensen SO. The four-electrode impedance technique: a method for investigation of compliance in luminal organs. Clin Phys Physiol Meas. 1988;9(Suppl A):61–4.
2. Drewes AM, Pedersen J, Liu W, Arendt-Nielsen L, Gregersen H. Controlled mechanical distension of the human oesophagus: sensory and biomechanical findings. Scand J Gastroenterol. 2003;38(1):27–35.
3. Rao SSC, Gregersen H, Hayek B, Summers RW, Christensen J. Unexplained chest pain: the hypersensitive, hyperreactive, and poorly compliant esophagus. Ann Intern Med. 1996;124(11):950–8.

4. Andersen IS, Gregersen H, Buntzen S, Djurhuus JC, Laurberg S. New probe for the measurement of dynamic changes in the rectum. Neurogastroenterol Motil. 2004;16(1):99–105.
5. McMahon BP, Frøkjaer JB, Drewes AM, Gregersen H. A new measurement of oesophago-gastric junction competence. Neurogastroenterol Motil. 2004;16(5):543–6.
6. McMahon BP, Frøkjaer JB, Liao D, Kunwald P, Drewes AM, Gregersen H. A new technique for evaluating sphincter function in visceral organs: application of the functional lumen imaging probe (FLIP) for the evaluation of the oesophago-gastric junction. Physiol Meas. 2005;26(5):823–36.
7. Savarino E, di Pietro M, Bredenoord AJ, Carlson DA, Clarke JO, Khan A, et al. Use of the functional lumen imaging probe in clinical esophagology. Am J Gastroenterol. 2020;115:1786.
8. Alqudah MM, Gregersen H, Drewes AM, McMahon BP. Evaluation of anal sphincter resistance and distensibility in healthy controls using EndoFLIP ©. Neurogastroenterol Motil. 2012;24(12):e591–9.
9. Sørensen G, Liao D, Lundby L, Fynne L, Buntzen S, Gregersen H, et al. Distensibility of the anal canal in patients with idiopathic fecal incontinence: a study with the functional lumen imaging probe. Neurogastroenterol Motil. 2014;26(2):255–63.
10. Gourcerol G, Granier S, Bridoux V, Menard JF, Ducrotté P, Leroi AM. Do endoflip assessments of anal sphincter distensibility provide more information on patients with fecal incontinence than high-resolution anal manometry? Neurogastroenterol Motil. 2016;28(3):399–409.
11. Leroi AM, Melchior C, Charpentier C, Bridoux V, Savoye-Collet C, Houivet E, et al. The diagnostic value of the functional lumen imaging probe versus high-resolution anorectal manometry in patients with fecal incontinence. Neurogastroenterol Motil. 2018;30(6):e13291.
12. Carlson DA, Kou W, Lin Z, Hinchcliff M, Thakrar A, Falmagne S, et al. Normal values of esophageal Distensibility and distension-induced contractility measured by functional luminal imaging probe panometry. Clin Gastroenterol Hepatol. 2019;17(4):674–681.e1.
13. Carlson DA, Kahrilas PJ, Lin Z, Hirano I, Gonsalves N, Listernick Z, et al. Evaluation of esophageal motility utilizing the functional lumen imaging probe. Am J Gastroenterol. 2016;111(12):1726–35.
14. Rohof WO, Hirsch DP, Kessing BF, Boeckxstaens GE. Efficacy of treatment for patients with achalasia depends on the distensibility of the esophagogastric junction. Gastroenterology. 2012 Aug;143(2):328–35.
15. Rieder E, Swanström LL, Perretta S, Lenglinger J, Riegler M, Dunst CM. Intraoperative assessment of esophagogastric junction distensibility during per oral endoscopic myotomy (POEM) for esophageal motility disorders. Surg Endosc. 2013;27(2):400–5.
16. Carlson DA, Lin Z, Kahrilas PJ, Sternbach J, Donnan EN, Friesen L, et al. The functional lumen imaging probe detects esophageal contractil-

ity not observed with manometry in patients with achalasia. Gastroenterology. 2015;149(7):1742–51.

17. Pandolfino JE, de Ruigh A, Nicodème F, Xiao Y, Boris L, Kahrilas PJ. Distensibility of the esophagogastric junction assessed with the functional lumen imaging probe (FLIP™) in achalasia patients. Neurogastroenterol Motil. 2013;25(6):496–501.
18. Ponds FA, Bredenoord AJ, Kessing BF, Smout AJPM. Esophagogastric junction distensibility identifies achalasia subgroup with manometrically normal esophagogastric junction relaxation. Neurogastroenterol Motil. 2017;29(1).
19. Carlson DA, Lin Z, Rogers MC, Lin CY, Kahrilas PJ, Pandolfino JE. Utilizing functional lumen imaging probe topography to evaluate esophageal contractility during volumetric distention: a pilot study. Neurogastroenterol Motil. 2015;27(7):981–9.
20. Carlson DA, Kou W, Rooney KP, Baumann AJ, Donnan E, Triggs JR, et al. Achalasia subtypes can be identified with functional luminal imaging probe (FLIP) panometry using a supervised machine learning process. Neurogastroenterol Motil. 2020;33(3):e13932.
21. Ngamruengphong S, von Rahden BHA, Filser J, Tyberg A, Desai A, Sharaiha RZ, et al. Intraoperative measurement of esophagogastric junction cross-sectional area by impedance planimetry correlates with clinical outcomes of peroral endoscopic myotomy for achalasia: a multicenter study. Surg Endosc. 2016;30(7):2886–94.
22. Teitelbaum EN, Soper NJ, Pandolfino JE, Kahrilas PJ, Hirano I, Boris L, et al. Esophagogastric junction distensibility measurements during Heller myotomy and POEM for achalasia predict postoperative symptomatic outcomes. Surg Endosc. 2015;29(3):522–8.
23. Su B, Callahan ZM, Novak S, Kuchta K, Ujiki MB. Using impedance planimetry (EndoFLIP) to evaluate myotomy and predict outcomes after surgery for achalasia. J Gastrointest Surg. 2020;24(4):964–71.
24. Holmstrom AL, Campagna RAJ, Cirera A, Carlson DA, Pandolfino JE, Teitelbaum EN, et al. Intraoperative use of FLIP is associated with clinical success following POEM for achalasia. Surg Endosc. 2020;35:3090.
25. Kwiatek MA, Pandolfino JE, Hirano I, Kahrilas PJ. Esophagogastric junction distensibility assessed with an endoscopic functional luminal imaging probe (EndoFLIP). Gastrointest Endosc. 2010;72(2):272–8.
26. Tucker E, Sweis R, Anggiansah A, Wong T, Telakis E, Knowles K, et al. Measurement of esophago-gastric junction cross-sectional area and distensibility by an endoluminal functional lumen imaging probe for the diagnosis of gastro-esophageal reflux disease. Neurogastroenterol Motil. 2013;25(11):904–10.
27. Carlson DA, Kathpalia P, Craft J, Tye M, Lin Z, Kahrilas PJ, et al. The relationship between esophageal acid exposure and the esophageal response to volumetric distention. Neurogastroenterol Motil. 2018;30(3).

28. Ilczyszyn A, Botha AJ. Feasibility of esophagogastric junction distensibility measurement during Nissen fundoplication. Dis Esophagus. 2014;27(7):637–44.
29. DeHaan RK, Davila D, Frelich MJ, Gould JC. Esophagogastric junction distensibility is greater following Toupet compared to Nissen fundoplication. Surg Endosc. 2017;31(1):193–8.
30. Su B, Novak S, Callahan ZM, Kuchta K, Carbray J, Ujiki MB. Using impedance planimetry (EndoFLIP™) in the operating room to assess gastroesophageal junction distensibility and predict patient outcomes following fundoplication. Surg Endosc. 2020 Apr;34(4):1761–8.
31. Turner B, Helm M, Hetzel E, Gould JC. Is that "floppy" fundoplication tight enough? Surg Endosc. 2020;34(4):1823–8.
32. Malik Z, Sankineni A, Parkman HP. Assessing pyloric sphincter pathophysiology using EndoFLIP in patients with gastroparesis. Neurogastroenterol Motil. 2015;27(4):524–31.
33. Vosoughi K, Ichkhanian Y, Jacques J, Aadam AA, Benias PC, Law R, et al. Role of endoscopic functional luminal imaging probe in predicting the outcome of gastric peroral endoscopic pyloromyotomy (with video). Gastrointest Endosc. 2020;91(6):1289–99.

Catheter-Based pH Testing 13

Fermin Fontan, Oscar Talledo,
and Peter Nau

Introduction

Catheter-based pH testing dates to 1969 when Spencer J. published in the British Journal of Surgery the first report on prolonged intraesophageal pH monitoring in patients with gastroesophageal reflux [1]. He documented up to 18 h of esophageal pH monitoring in the inpatient setting and showed that prolonged monitoring was feasible and well tolerated by patients. Later in the 1970s, Johnson and DeMeester reported full 24-h pH testing. It was during this initial work that they developed their composite scoring system that would later evolve into a validated scoring system for the identification of pathologic gastroesophageal reflux [2, 3].

With the advent of proton pump inhibitors (PPI) in 1989, the management of acid-related pathologies such as peptic ulcer disease and gastroesophageal reflux disease (GERD) underwent a dramatic change. At present, antisecretory therapy has become the mainstay in the treatment of GERD [4]. Low-risk patients pre-

F. Fontan · O. Talledo · P. Nau (✉)
University of Iowa Carver College of Medicine, Iowa City, IA, USA
e-mail: oscar-talledozevallos@uicwa.edu; peter-nau@iowa.edu

A. D. Patel et al. (eds.), *The SAGES Manual of Physiologic Evaluation of Foregut Diseases*,
https://doi.org/10.1007/978-3-031-39199-6_13

senting with uncomplicated GERD symptoms are offered 4–8 weeks of empiric PPI treatment as the initial approach. The preponderance of trials assessing for resolution of esophagitis 4 and 8 weeks after medical management showed a higher proportion of patients with all grades healed at week 8 compared with week 4 [5, 6].

Response to medical therapy can have a high sensitivity in the diagnosis of GERD but a low and variable specificity [7]. In up to 40% of these subjects, there is no response to therapy. Following confirmation of compliance of the dosing and appropriate timing, most providers will switch to a second-generation PPI or increase the dose to twice daily [8]. In cases where symptoms persist despite optimal medical therapy and lifestyle modifications, a diagnostic workup including pH testing becomes fundamental [9]. A special subset of patients including those with underlying risk factors (Caucasians, male, 50 years of age or older, obese, smokers, heavy alcohol user), and/or alarms symptoms, should be offered endoscopy early on in their workup in order to exclude esophageal metaplasia and potential esophageal malignancies [10].

Defining GERD

Another critical evolution that has paralleled the advent of PPIs has been the significant improvement in the general understanding of the full spectrum of GERD. This disease is defined by the presence of gastric acid reflux into the esophagus which is associated with mild or moderate/severe symptoms occurring two or more times per week and at least once per week, respectively. Heartburn, regurgitation, and dysphagia are classically known as typical symptoms, whereas belching, nausea, wheezing, globus sensation, chest pain, hoarseness, and cough are considered atypical symptoms [11].

Classic GERD is characterized by reflux symptoms in association with various degrees of esophageal erosive findings. The Los Angeles (LA) classification system for esophagitis grading was published in 1999 and is currently implemented as a stan-

Table 13.1 Los Angeles classification

Grade A	At least one mucosal break no longer than 5 mm that does not extend between the tops of two mucosal folds
Grade B	At least one mucosal break more than 5 mm long that does not extend between the tops of two mucosal folds
Grade C	At least one mucosal break that is continuous between the tops of two or more mucosal folds but which involve less than 75% of the circumference
Grade D	At least one mucosal break which involves at least 75% of the esophageal circumference

dardized tool to categorize the degree of erosive esophagitis (Table 13.1) [12].

Interestingly, up to 70% of patients with classic GERD symptoms have no evidence of erosive changes on endoscopy. Of this group, 50% have abnormal pH test results and thus belong to the non-erosive reflux disease (NERD) category [13, 14]. The remaining 50% belong to a subset of patients with esophageal hypersensitivity and functional heartburn. These patients have chronic typical heartburn symptoms attributed to the esophagus without evidencing any other underlying etiology. Together, these presentations account for 90% of the heartburn patients who fail optimal antisecretory therapy.

The importance in distinguishing this subset of patients with physiologic acid levels in the setting of subjective reflux disease is the disparate responses to available therapeutic modalities. Not every patient will require conventional antireflux medication, and not every patient would benefit from surgery.

Catheter-Based pH Testing Device

The general components of catheter-based pH monitoring systems are a flexible catheter with pH sensors and a data logger (Fig. 13.1).

The reference electrodes can be placed either outside the esophagus or internally, built into the catheter. The probes measure approximately 2 mm in diameter which facilitates transnasal

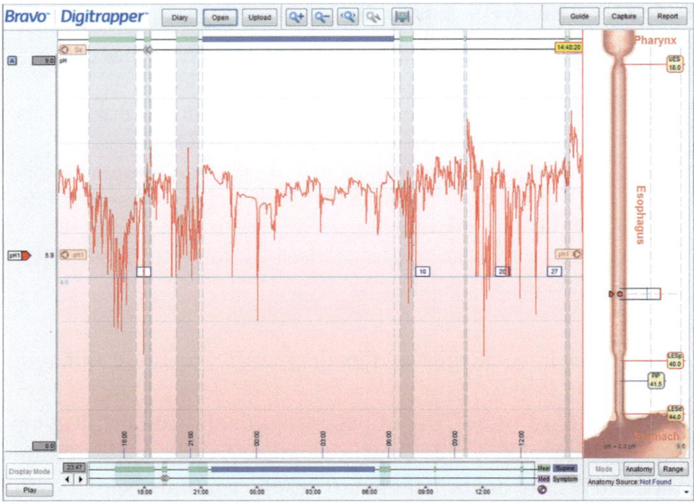

Fig. 13.1 Catheter-based pH testing system. (Courtesy of Diversatek Healthcare Milwaukee, WI)

placement. Most commercially available devices sample data every 4–10 s, and pH testing is usually carried out for approximately 24 h or more, depending on patient tolerance. The data logger varies across the different brands, but in general it is available to be worn on a shoulder strap or a waist belt. Patients are instructed to select the "ingestion" setting at the beginning of their meals and to leave this option selected for the duration of the meal. If ingestion is not occurring, the default "no ingestion" setting is selected. There are other buttons to indicate presence of symptoms and to indicate when the patient is laying supine or sleeping.

If patients are inaccurate, study results may be reported as falsely positive or negative. In addition to the artifacts generated by meal periods, isolated pH drops can be seen and are referred to as "pseudo-reflux" and originating from the monitoring circuit itself [15]. On the other hand, gradual acidification can be seen in patients who have esophageal retention, due to inefficient emptying such as in achalasia.

Different studies have demonstrated that the sensitivity of catheter-based pH monitoring is not as high as previously thought. The percentage of false-negative results in patients with typical symptoms has been shown to be greater than 20%, and in the case of atypical symptomatology, outcomes have shown to be even less accurate. This is in part due to proximal probes, which sensitivity has been reported to be as low as 50% [16, 17]. Hence, patient compliance to test instructions and detail to their recordings are a critical component for test accuracy.

Technique

Esophageal pH testing is considered a safe procedure usually performed in the ambulatory setting. For safety reasons, patients are typically requested to fast for 6 h, depending on the institutional protocol. After calibration of the sensors, patient education, and consent, local aerosol/topical anesthetics is applied to the nasopharynx to decrease patient discomfort and to facilitate transnasal catheter introduction. The placement of the probe takes approximately 10 min. The sensors are typically positioned 5 cm above the upper level of the lower esophageal sphincter (LES) as determined by esophageal manometry. Depending on the manufacturer, there may be additional sensors that can be placed 10 cm below the stomach or 15 cm proximal to the LES. These extra sensors can better define the proximal extent of reflux in the setting of atypical manifestations of GERD [18]. After confirming an adequate location, and securely taping the catheter in place, patients are instructed to resume daily activities and attempt to reproduce normal scenarios that would usually precipitate their symptoms [19]. No clear guidelines on dietary restrictions exist, and recommendations vary across different providers and specialties. Patients are discharged home and provided with diaries for them to document time of symptom occurrence, time of their meals and content, time of upright and recumbent positions, and time of administration of any acid-suppressing medication if taken during the study.

Indications

When considering the utility of objective pH analysis, the ultimate trajectory of the patient's care must be considered. For those patients who do not desire or would not be candidates for operative intervention, the value of pH testing differs from an individual being considered for a surgery. Indications for testing in those who are on a medical management pathway are those with classic GERD symptoms who fail 4 weeks of PPI therapy or have an incomplete response. This is also the management algorithm for those with atypical symptoms of GERD who do not see symptom resolution after a trial of PPIs. In contrast, patients with complications of reflux such as erosive esophagitis (LA grade C or D esophagitis), peptic stricture, or Barrett's esophagus, pH testing to confirm the diagnosis is of low utility [20].

The preponderance of patients being evaluated for an endoscopic or surgical antireflux procedure should be tested prior to proceeding with any interventions. This is secondary to the fact that up to 25% of patients with LA grade B esophagitis will have normal acid exposure on objective testing [21]. It is critical to identify those individuals with esophageal hypersensitivity and functional heartburn as they will not improve with an antireflux procedure. In the case of patients who have undergone previous endoscopic or surgical antireflux therapy and who continue to have GERD symptoms, pH testing is also recommended [22]. Another common indication for testing is obese patients with subjective GERD symptoms that are being evaluated for bariatric surgery. In a recent study, preoperative GERD evaluation including intraesophageal pH testing detected pathology which altered procedure selection from sleeve gastrectomy to Roux-en-Y gastric bypass in 24.8% [23].

An important aspect when considering pH monitoring is the decision to test the patient while on PPI therapy or to request full cessation of antireflux medications. A retrospective study including 250 patients tested while on PPI showed normal pH monitoring data, demonstrating that the clinical yield for pH testing while on PPI therapy could be low [24]. The Lyon Consensus proposes that testing should always be performed off therapy to demonstrate baseline acid exposure time (AET) in "unproven GERD," meaning no (or low-grade) esophagitis at endoscopy, and no prior positive pH testing. In contrast, the Lyon Consensus proposes that patients with "proven GERD" be evaluated on double-dose PPI therapy to establish correlation between refractory symptoms and reflux episodes and/or to exclude inadequate acid suppression or poor compliance as the mechanism of persisting symptoms. This assessment requires pH-impedance (vs. pH) monitoring since most reflux episodes on PPI therapy are weakly acidic (pH 4–7) [25]. It is also reasonable to consider pH monitoring on PPIs in a revisional setting where there are only minor anatomic issues and the underlying goal may be to defer a reoperation. When electing to test off medication, the classic recommendation is to discontinue PPI medications at least 7 days before the study. Other antiacids are typically discontinued 2 days prior to the study, and these include Zantac (ranitidine), Tagamet (cimetidine), Axid (nizatidine), Pepcid (famotidine).

Interpretations

The key interrogans that should be answered by pH testing are as follows: Is the distal esophageal acid exposure in excess of that noted in normal individuals? And are the symptoms reported by the subject, during pH monitoring, associated or not with reflux?

Software packages generally provide a standard readout of pH levels, which is later analyzed by providers for a more accurate result (Fig. 13.2). Time is displayed along the *x*-axis, and the pH levels ranging from 0 to 8 are represented along the *y*-axis. The data recorded by the catheter sensor in conjunction with patient documentation allow providers to obtain the symptom index for reflux (SI), symptom association probability (SAP), and the DeMeester score. The SAP determines the statistical validity of symptom-reflux association, while the SI provides data on the strength of the association [26, 27]. The DeMeester score is a composite calculation of severity characteristics of reflux. It contemplates six different parameters [2, 28].

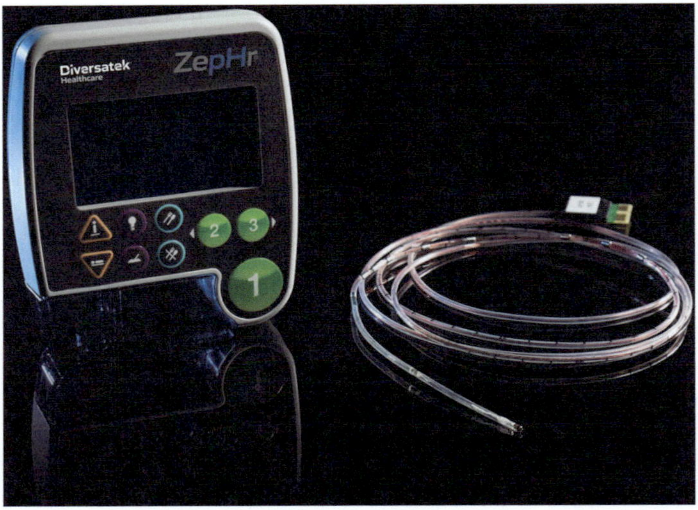

Fig. 13.2 Screenshot of reflux analysis software Digitrapper by Medtronic (Covidien LP, a Medtronic company)

DeMeester score
Total number of reflux episodes
Total time esophageal pH < 4
Upright time esophageal pH < 4
Supine time esophageal pH < 4
Number of reflux episodes lasting >5 min
Longest reflux episode

Among the pH monitoring metrics, AET (esophageal pH < 4) is the most reproducible, is reliably extracted from automated analysis, and is predictive of response from medical and surgical reflux therapy. Acid exposure time < 4% is considered definitively normal (physiological) and >6%, considered definitively abnormal [2, 28]. The physiologic significance of a pH < 4 lies in the fact that mucosal damage and symptoms occur when the esophageal lining is exposed to pH levels lower than 4 [20]. By analyzing these parameters, providers can have a better understanding of the patient's reflux pattern, time of the day, esophageal clearance, and triggers. DeMeester score serves as an objective tool that, in conjunction with endoscopic evaluation and clinical assessment, allows for a more accurate diagnosis.

Conclusion

Catheter-based pH testing is, although less sensitive than other available testing options, still a cost-effective and safe technology, readily available in the armamentarium to diagnose GERD in symptomatic patients.

References

1. Spencer J. Prolonged pH recording in the study of gastroesophageal reflux. Br J Surg. 1969;56:912–4.
2. Johnson LF, DeMeester TR. Twenty-four-hour pH monitoring of the distal esophagus. A quantitative measure of gastroesophageal reflux. Am J Gastroenterol. 1974;62:325–32.
3. Johnson LF, DeMeester TR. Development of the 24-hour intraesophageal pH monitoring composite scoring system. J Clin Gastroenterol. 1986;8:52–8.
4. Vakil N, van Zanten SV, Kahrilas P, et al. The Montreal definition and classification of gastroesophageal reflux disease: a global evidence-based consensus. Am J Gastroenterol. 2006;101:1900–20.
5. Castell DO, Kahrilas PJ, Richter JE, et al. Esomeprazole (40 mg) compared with lansoprazole (30 mg) in the treatment of erosive esophagitis. Am J Gastroenterol. 2002;97:575–83.
6. Richter JE, Kahrilas PJ, Sontog SJ, et al. Comparing lansoprazole and omeprazole in onset of heartburn relief: results of a randomized, controlled trial in erosive esophagitis patients. Am J Gastroenterol. 2001;96:3089–98.
7. Numans ME, et al. Short-term treatment with proton-pump inhibitors as a test for gastroesophageal reflux disease: a meta-analysis of diagnostic test characteristics. Ann Intern Med. 2004;140:518–27.
8. Inadomi JM, McIntyre L, Bernard L, et al. Step-down from multiple- to single-dose proton pump inhibitors (PPIs): a prospective study of patients with heartburn or acid regurgitation completely relieved with PPIs. Am J Gastroenterol. 2003;98:1940–4.

9. Banks M. The modern investigation and management of gastro-oesophageal reflux disease (GORD). Clin Med. 2009;9(6):600–4. Epub 2010/01/26.
10. Shaheen NJ, Weinberg DS, Denberg TD, Chou R, Qaseem A, et al.; Clinical guidelines Committee of the American College of Physicians. Upper endoscopy for gastroesophageal reflux disease: best practice advice from the clinical guidelines committee of the American College of Physicians. Ann Intern Med. 2012;157:808–16.
11. Martinez SD, Malagon IB, Garewal HS, Cui H, Fass R. Non-erosive reflux disease (NERD)--acid reflux and symptom patterns. Aliment Pharmacol Ther. 2003;17:537–45.
12. Lundell LR, Dent J, Bennett JR, et al. Endoscopic assessment of oesophagitis: clinical and functional correlates and further validation of the Los Angeles Classification. Gut. 1999;45:172–80.
13. Hartono JL, Qua CS, Goh KL. Non-erosive reflux disease (NERD), symptomatic and asymptomatic erosive reflux disease (ERD): from hypersensitive to hyposensitive esophagus. Dig Dis Sci. 2011;56(1):90–6. Epub 2010/05/15.
14. Dean BB, Gano AD Jr, Knight K, et al. Effectiveness of proton pump inhibitors in nonerosive reflux disease. Clin Gastroenterol Hepatol. 2004;2:656–64.
15. Vaezi MF. Laryngeal manifestations of gastroesophageal reflux disease. Curr Gastroenterol Rep. 2008;10(3):271–7. Epub 2008/07/16.
16. Mathus-Vliegen EMH, Smit CF, Devriese PP. Artifacts in 24-h pharyngeal and oesophageal pH monitoring: is simplification of pH data analysis feasible? Scand J Gastroenterol. 2004;39(1):14–9.
17. Adhami T, Goldblum JR, Richter JE, Vaezi MF. The role of gastric and duodenal agents in laryngeal injury: an experimental canine model. Am J Gastroenterol. 2004;99(11):2098–106. Epub 2004/11/24.
18. Ahmed T, Vaezi MF. The role of pH monitoring in extraesophageal gastroesophageal reflux disease. Gastrointest Endosc Clin N Am. 2005;15:319–31.
19. Lim PL, Gibbons MJ, Crawford EJ, Watson RGP, Johnston BT. The effect of lifestyle changes on results of 24-h ambulatory oesophageal pH monitoring. Eur J Gastroenterol Hepatol. 2000;12(6):655–6.
20. Jamieson JR, Stein HJ, DeMeester TR, et al. Ambulatory 24-h esophageal pH monitoring: normal values, optimal thresholds, specificity, sensitivity, and reproducibility. Am J Gastroenterol. 1992;87:1102–11.
21. Schwameis K, Lin B, Roman J, Olengue K, Siegal S, DeMeester SR. Is pH testing necessary before Antireflux surgery in patients with endoscopic erosive esophagitis? J Gastrointest Surg. 2018;22(1):8–12.
22. Hong S-KS, Vaezi MF. Gastroesophageal reflux monitoring: pH (catheter and capsule) and impedance. Gastrointest Endosc Clin N Am. 2009;19(1):1–22.

23. Kavanagh R, Smith J, Bashir U, et al. Optimizing bariatric surgery outcomes: a novel preoperative protocol in a bariatric population with gastroesophageal reflux disease. Surg Endosc. 2020;34:1812–8.
24. Charbel S, Khandwala F, Vaezi MF. The role of esophageal pH monitoring in symptomatic patients on PPI therapy. Am J Gastroenterol. 2005;100:283–9.
25. Gyawali CP, Kahrilas PJ, Savarino E, et al. Modern diagnosis of GERD: the Lyon consensus. Gut. 2018;67:1351–62. https://doi.org/10.1136/gutjnl-2017-314722.
26. Wiener GJ, Richter JE, Copper JB, Wu WC, Castell DO. The symptom index: a clinically important parameter of ambulatory 24-hour esophageal pH monitoring. Am J Gastroenterol. 1988;83:358–61.
27. Weusten BL, Roelofs JM, Akkermans LM, Van Berge-Henegouwen GP, Smout AJ. The symptom-association probability: an improved method for symptom analysis of 24-hour esophageal pH data. Gastroenterology. 1994;107:1741–5.
28. Richter JE, et al. Normal 24-hr ambulatory esophageal pH values. Influence of study center, pH electrode, age, and gender. Dig Dis Sci. 1992;37:849–56.

Wireless pH Testing 14

Jennwood Chen and Kyle A. Perry

While gastroesophageal reflux disease (GERD) is a common disorder, making the diagnosis can be challenging because symptoms are often vague. Symptom presentations can be variable between patients, and manifestations of GERD overlap with other foregut pathologies including functional dyspepsia, esophagitis, and gastroparesis [1–4]. Consequently, identifying GERD based on symptoms alone leads to the wrong diagnosis in 30–50% of patients [5–7]. Similarly, esophageal acid exposure alone is insufficient to predict the presence of GERD symptoms or their severity; however, it can help predict response to anti-reflux surgery [8, 9]. Therefore, it is imperative to document objective pathologic reflux in GERD patients, especially for those being considered for anti-reflux surgery (ARS) [6, 10].

J. Chen
Division of Gastroesophageal and Bariatric Surgery, University of Utah, Salt Lake City, UT, USA
e-mail: Jennwood.Chen@hsc.utah.edu

K. A. Perry (✉)
Division of General and Gastrointestinal Surgery, Ohio State University, Columbus, OH, USA
e-mail: Kyle.Perry@osumc.edu

A. D. Patel et al. (eds.), *The SAGES Manual of Physiologic Evaluation of Foregut Diseases*,
https://doi.org/10.1007/978-3-031-39199-6_14

In the absence of clear endoscopic evidence, the current gold standard test to diagnose GERD is the 24-h ambulatory esophageal pH metry or alternatively, the wireless esophageal pH monitoring probe (Bravo™, Medtronic, Shoreview, MN) which most consider an equivalent option [11]. In fact, the recent GERD consensus panel in Lyon recommends that the optimal diagnostic for initial proton pump inhibitor (PPI) non-responders without prior endoscopic demonstration of GERD is pH monitoring done while withholding anti-secretory therapy [12]. In this chapter, we will discuss the evolution, interpretation, and utility of wireless pH monitoring.

A Brief History of pH Monitoring

The diagnosis of gastroesophageal reflux has been evolving for over a century since 1884, when Reichmann lowered a sponge in the esophagus of patient with heartburn and showed that it contained acid [13]. In 1958, using a modified manometry probe, Tuttle and Grossman measured the in situ pH of the esophagus 2 cm above the "respiratory inflection point" [14]. Based on their work, pH would eventually become the standard metric to quantify gastroesophageal reflux.

Designed to measure the hydrogen-ion concentration throughout the gastrointestinal tract, the first wireless pH capsule was created by Jacobson and Mackay in 1957 [15]. Although not specifically geared toward detecting esophageal reflux, its creation provided the fundamentals for what would later become the ambulatory wireless pH monitoring device [16]. In 1974, DeMeester and Johnson studied gastroesophageal reflux in normal individuals and patients with GERD symptoms. Their landmark study established the modern parameters of pH monitoring to diagnose GERD. In particular, they established the location at which the pH sensor is to be placed (5 cm above the lower esophageal sphincter), defined the threshold pH ($\leq$4) for acid reflux, and created a composite score (Johnson-DeMeester Score) to categorize patients as having pathologic acid reflux [17–19].

Catheter-Based pH Monitoring

Until the early 2000s, the primary options for ambulatory esophageal pH monitoring were catheter-based systems. First introduced in the 1970s, these require passage of a nasopharyngeal catheter placed 5 cm above the endoscopically or manometrically identified lower esophageal sphincter (LES) [20]. The catheter runs over and behind the ear and is taped securely to the nose. The catheter connects to a portable digital data recorder that the patient wears around the waist or over the shoulder. The patient is instructed to refrain from changing their daily routine, abstain from bathing, and remain upright until bedtime. Using the digital data recorder, a virtual diary of events is kept which includes symptom events (e.g., heartburn, regurgitation, cough, and sore throat), beginning and end of mealtimes, each time the patient lays down and gets up, and duration of events.

Interpreting the output of the digital recorder involves analyzing both graphical and numerical data. The graphical output comprises a pH tracing that shows acid reflux episodes (drops in pH to a level below pH of 4) over time. The recording system is calibrated to a sampling rate (usually 4 s) at which the pH data are recorded [21]. The numerical data include the percent time of reflux over the monitoring period, percent time of reflux in the upright and supine positions, total number of reflux episodes, number of episodes that last longer than 5 min, duration of the longest episode, and a composite score [22]. The composite score, commonly referred to as the DeMeester score, is based on the standard deviation of the mean of each of the six components measured in normal subjects [23]. Finally, the data also include three measures of symptom correlation: symptom index (SI) defined as the percentage of reflux-related symptom episodes, symptom-sensitivity index (SSI), defined as the percentage of symptom-associated reflux episodes, and symptom association probability (SAP) which is a measure of correlation between symptoms and reflux episodes [21]. Of the three symptom correlation schemes, the SAP and the SI, interpreted in conjunction, are the most statistically valid for symptom-reflux association [24].

The normative thresholds for diagnosing pathologic reflux, as agreed upon by professional consensus groups, are as follows: (1)

24-h total % time pH < 4 greater than 4–5.5% (2) DeMeester score ≥ 14.7 (3) SAP > 95% for primary symptom, SI > 50% for primary symptom [25].

The total duration of the catheter-based ambulatory pH study is typically 24 h. This allows for measurements to be characterized over a complete circadian cycle and captures the effect of physical activity and body position on esophageal acid exposure [26].

It should be apparent from the above description that the ability of ambulatory pH monitors to accurately detect abnormal reflux is largely dependent on patient's tolerance of the test, adherence to a "normal routine," and adequate duration of monitoring. It is these areas which catheter-based systems tend to be most problematic.

Patient discomfort and social embarrassment from the passage and fixation of the nasoesophageal pH catheter are ubiquitous [27, 28]. In fact, up to 10% of patients fail to complete the 24-h monitoring period due to intolerance [29, 30]. For those that are able to endure the duration of the test, studies have shown that patients do significantly alter their daily routine [31, 32]. In particular, patients are more sedentary and spend less time eating, drinking, and being physically active [33]. Unfortunately, these compensatory behaviors may alter the reliability of the test [27, 32]. Finally, it has been suggested that limiting the test to 24 h decreases the diagnostic yield due to the high day-to-day variability in acid exposure and symptom reporting [29, 34, 35]. Studies comparing repeated 24-h monitoring estimated the reproducibility to be 77–83% which may explain why a significant portion of patients with erosive reflux have a normal ambulatory 24-h pH study [28, 36, 37]. Furthermore, studies reporting on the detection performance of catheter-based systems vary widely with reported sensitivities ranging between 73 and 96% [28, 38, 39].

Wireless pH Monitoring

In response to these limitations, the Bravo™ wireless pH monitoring device was developed in 2001 and approved by the US Food and Drug Administration in 2005 for the evaluation of patients with GERD [40].

The Bravo™ wireless pH monitoring system utilizes a radio-telemetry pH sensing capsule that is attached to the mucosa of the distal esophagus. The capsule measures 6 mm × 5.5 mm × 25 mm and contains an antimony pH electrode, a reference electrode, a battery, and a radio-transmitter [40]. The capsule is mounted onto the end of a delivery catheter for oral or nasal insertion, with the former being the preferred method [41].

Prior to insertion, an upper endoscopy is generally performed and the squamocolumnar junction (SCJ) is identified and measured from the incisors. Ideally, the capsule is deployed 6 cm proximal to the SCJ [42]. This is due to the fact that the SCJ is approximately 1 cm distal to the proximal border of the LES [43]. Therefore, endoscopic placement of the Bravo™ capsule 6 cm proximal to the SCJ corresponds to manometric placement of the traditional pH catheter 5 cm proximal to the LES. Transoral placement of the capsule based on manometric landmarks is an alternative option. However, the positioning requires a correction factor to account for the longer pathway of the transnasal manometry catheter [44].

Once the device is activated and calibrated, the delivery catheter is inserted with or without direct endoscopic guidance. With the catheter in its desired location, a vacuum pump is used to apply suction to the wall of the capsule. A pressure between 510 and 700 mmHg is applied for approximately 10–30 s, after which time an activation button is pressed to deploy a spring-loaded pin that attaches the Bravo™ capsule to the mucosa [40, 45, 46]. If placed without direct endoscopic guidance, a repeat endoscopy may be performed to confirm placement. The capsule measures pH and transmits data to a pager-sized receiver that can be worn on the patient's belt [47]. As long patients stay within signal detection range of the receiver (approximately 1 m or 3 ft.), patients are encouraged to follow their daily routine, including bathing. Patients keep a virtual diary of their reflux-related symptoms and events.

The parameters measured during wireless pH monitoring are similar to catheter-based systems [19, 48]. However, in contrast to the 4 s sampling rate of catheter-based systems, the Bravo™ capsule samples esophageal pH every 6 s [27]. Another important difference is that the duration of wireless pH monitoring can be extended to 96 h.

Wireless Versus Catheter-Based pH Monitoring

The clear advantage of wireless pH monitoring over traditional catheter-based systems is patient comfort and ability to adhere to routine activities. In a randomized cross-over trial, Wenner et al. showed that 87% of patients undergoing esophageal pH monitoring preferred the wireless pH capsule over the catheter-based technique, citing less interference with normal activities and social embarrassment [32]. In a study of 133 patients who underwent pH monitoring (78 catheter-based; 55 wireless), Grigolon et al. found that the wireless technique was far better tolerated than the catheter-based, with minor impact on daily activities including food intake [31]. Sweis et al. showed that 96% of patients, who were previously unable to tolerate 24-h catheter-based monitoring, successfully completed 48 h of wireless testing and due to less restriction in activities of daily living, nasopharyngeal discomfort, dysphagia, and chest pain [30]. Finally, in a meta-analysis of randomized control trials that included 167 patients, authors concluded that the Bravo™ wireless pH monitor interfered less with daily activities compared to the catheter-system system [49].

Second, proponents of wireless pH monitoring often discuss the potential increased sensitivity for detecting reflux events due to the prolonged monitoring capability. While catheter-based monitoring is carried out over a 24-h cycle, which typically provides 20–22 h of interpretable data, the Bravo™ capsule captures pH levels for up to 96 h [25]. In a study of 186 patients undergoing wireless pH monitoring, extended monitoring for 48 h identified 22% more patients with abnormal esophageal acid exposure [50]. Sweis et al. found that 96-h monitoring using the Bravo™ capsule diagnosed GERD in 76% of patients with typical reflux symptoms but with previously negative 24-h catheter-based pH studies [51]. Authors comparing 48 to 96-h wireless pH monitoring reported a 23.5% increase in GERD diagnosis when the test was extended by 2 days [52]. Similarly, in a study of 99 patients undergoing 96-h wireless pH testing, Capovilla et al. found an increase in diagnostic yield of 12% when the wireless testing interval was extended to 96 h. However, at long-term follow-up, only 25% of these patients, who would have otherwise had negative tests at 48 h, reported good outcomes post-fundoplication. The authors concluded that while prolonged testing does increase diagnostic yield, it comes at the expense of potentially recruiting complex patients who may not respond to surgical therapy [53]. Currently, the most widely adopted duration for wireless testing is 48 h.

Head-to-head studies comparing performance of wireless versus catheter-based pH monitoring are intriguing. Pandolfino et al. subjected 25 asymptomatic patients to simultaneous 24-h catheter-based and 48-h wireless pH monitoring [54]. Digitized fluoroscopic images were employed to ensure proper and equivalent positioning of the pH electrodes. A pH reference was established using swallows of orange juice (pH = 3.88). The result of the study showed that the catheter-based system over-reported the number of acid exposure events by nearly three times (117.0 vs. 41.8). Forty percent of this discrepancy was attributable to flawed software calibration while the majority of the remainder were brief events with poor reproducibility between systems. In an almost identical study, Pandolfino et al. again noted a significant discrepancy between the two systems [55]. In terms of percent time, the pH was less than 4; Pandolfino found that the catheter-based system reported acid exposure values twice those reported by the Bravo™ capsule. The tendency of catheter-based systems to over-report esophageal acid exposure has been a consistent finding in additional studies [48, 56]. Further examination reveals that the majority of the reflux episodes missed by the Bravo™ capsule are short-duration events that are attributable to the longer sampling rate of the wireless system (6 vs. 4 s), the significance of which, is questionable [20]. Moreover, unlike the Bravo™ capsule which moves with the esophageal mucosa, catheter-based probes can "dip down" toward the stomach with each swallow [26]. Therefore, what is perceived to be an increase in reflux events is simply artifact [57].

Wireless pH monitoring does have limitations. Despite the overall comfort of the Bravo™ capsule, chest pain can be significant and is reported much more often when compared to catheter-based systems [49, 58]. Unintended and early detachment of the capsule can be as high as 10% [59]. Furthermore, when positioned endoscopically, misplacement is common. In a retrospective study of 161 patients, investigators reported that nearly 30% of Bravo™ capsules placed were mal-positioned. The majority of which were >3 cm proximal to the ideal location [42]. Interestingly, upon reanalysis, the authors concluded that even misplacement of 5 cm did not affect the frequency of positive pH studies. Finally, compared to catheter-based systems, the Bravo™ wireless capsule is considerably more expensive [40, 45].

Conclusion

Ambulatory pH monitoring is an invaluable tool in the diagnosis of GERD. The primary end points of pH monitoring are esophageal acid exposure time, number of reflux events, and, to a lesser extent, the association between symptoms and episodes. Wireless pH monitoring is particularly useful for those patients who are unable to tolerate catheter-based testing. Extending the duration of monitoring time to 48 or 96 h may increase diagnostic yield and reproducibility. However, wireless pH monitoring is considerably more expensive and thus may be cost-prohibitive in some instances.

References

1. Johnson LF, DeMeester TR. Development of the 24-hour intraesophageal pH monitoring composite scoring system. J Clin Gastroenterol. 1986;8:S52–8.
2. Penagini R, Sweis R, Mauro A, et al. Inconsistency in the diagnosis of functional heartburn: usefulness of prolonged wireless pH monitoring in patients with proton pump inhibitor refractory gastroesophageal reflux disease. J Neurogastroenterol Motil. 2015;21:265–72.
3. Clayton S, Emerson JF. Eosinophilic esophagitis: a mimic of gastroesophageal reflux disease. Am Fam Physician. 2018;97:628–9.
4. Savarino E, de Bortoli N, De Cassan C, et al. The natural history of gastro-esophageal reflux disease: a comprehensive review. Dis Esophagus. 2016;22:331–9.

5. Patti MG, Diener U, Tamburini A, et al. Role of esophageal function tests in diagnosis of gastroesophageal reflux disease. Dig Dis Sci. 2001;46:597–602.
6. Bello B, Zoccali M, Gullo R, et al. Gastroesophageal reflux disease and antireflux surgery: what is the proper preoperative work-up? J Gastrointest Surg. 2012;17:14–20.
7. Chan K, Liu G, Miller L, et al. Lack of correlation between a self-administered subjective GERD questionnaire and pathologic GERD diagnosed by 24-h esophageal pH monitoring. J Gastrointest Surg. 2010;14:427–36.
8. Campos GM, Peters JH, DeMeester TR, et al. Multivariate analysis of factors predicting outcome after laparoscopic Nissen fundoplication. J Gastrointest Surg. 1999;3:292–300.
9. Khajanchee YS, Hong D, Hansen PD, Swanstrom LL. Outcomes of anti-reflux surgery in patients with normal preoperative 24-hour pH test results. Am J Surg. 2004;187:599–603.
10. Jobe BA, Richter JE, Hoppo T, et al. Preoperative diagnostic workup before antireflux surgery: an evidence and experience-based consensus of the esophageal diagnostic advisory panel. J Am Coll Surg. 2013;217:586–97.
11. Stefanidis D, Hope WW, Kohn GP, et al. Guidelines for surgical treatment of gastroesophageal reflux disease. Surg Endosc. 2010;24:2647–69.
12. Gyawali CP, Kahrilas PJ, Savarino E, et al. Modern diagnosis of GERD: the Lyon consensus. Gut. 2018;67:1351–62.
13. Bennett JR. pH measurement in the oesophagus. Baillieres Clin Gastroenterol. 1987;1:747–67.
14. Tuttle SG, Grossman MI. Detection of gastro-esophageal reflux by simultaneous measurement of intraluminal pressure and pH. Proc Soc Exp Biol Med. 1958;98:225–7.
15. Jacobson B, Mackay RS. A pH-endoradiosonde. Lancet. 1957;272:1224.
16. Herbella FAM, Nipominick I, Patti MG. From sponges to capsules: the history of esophageal pH monitoring. Dis Esophagus. 2009;22:99–103.
17. Johnson LF, DeMeester TR. Twenty-four-hour pH monitoring of the distal esophagus: a quantitative measure of gastroesophageal reflux. Am J Gastroenterol. 1974;62:325–32.
18. Jamieson JR, Stein HJ, DeMeester TR, et al. Ambulatory 24-h esophageal pH monitoring: normal values, optimal thresholds, specificity, sensitivity, and reproducibility. Am J Gastroenterol. 1992;87:1102–11.
19. Neto RML, Herbella FAM, Schlottmann F, Patti MG. Does DeMeester score still define GERD? Dis Esophagus. 2019;32:1900.
20. Vaezi MF. Should we bravo? Gastroenterology. 2006;130:2238–9.
21. Kim GH. How to interpret ambulatory 24-hr esophageal pH monitoring. J Neurogastroenterol Motil. 2010;16:207–10.

22. Hong SS, Vaezi MF. Gastroesophageal reflux monitoring: pH (catheter and capsule) and impedance. Gastrointest Endosc Clin N Am. 2009;19:1–22.
23. DeMeester TR, Wang CI, Wernly JA, et al. Technique, indications, and clinical use of 24 hour esophageal pH monitoring. J Thorac Cardiovasc Surg. 1980;79:656–70.
24. Weusten BL, Roelofs JM, Akkermans LM, et al. The symptom-association probability: an improved method for symptom analysis of 24-hour esophageal pH data. Gastroenterology. 1994;107:1741–5.
25. Richter JE, Pandolfino JE, Vela MF, et al. Utilization of wireless pH monitoring technologies: a summary of the proceedings from the Esophageal Diagnostic Working Group. Dis Esophagus. 2012;26:755–65.
26. Streets CG, DeMeester TR. Ambulatory 24-hour esophageal pH monitoring: why, when, and what to do. J Clin Gastroenterol. 2003;37:14–22.
27. Ayazi S, Lipham JC, Portale G, et al. Bravo catheter-free pH monitoring: normal values, concordance, optimal diagnostic thresholds, and accuracy. Clin Gastroenterol Hepatol. 2009;7:60–7.
28. Lee JS. Is wireless capsule pH monitoring better than catheter systems? J Neurogastroenterol Motil. 2012;18:117–9.
29. Gillies RS, Stratford JM, Booth MI, Dehn TCB. Oesophageal pH monitoring using the Bravo catheter-free radio capsule. Eur J Gastroenterol Hepatol. 2007;19:57–63.
30. Sweis R, Fox M, Anggiansah R, et al. Patient acceptance and clinical impact of Bravo monitoring in patients with previous failed catheter-based studies. Aliment Pharmacol Ther. 2009;29:669–76.
31. Grigolon A, Bravi I, Cantù P, et al. Wireless pH monitoring: better tolerability and lower impact on daily habits. Dig Liver Dis. 2007;39:720–4.
32. Wenner J, Johnsson F, Johansson J, Öberg S. Wireless esophageal pH monitoring is better tolerated than the catheter-based technique: results from a randomized cross-over trial. Am J Gastroenterol. 2007;102:239–45.
33. Fass R, Hell R, Sampliner RE, et al. Effect of ambulatory 24-hour esophageal pH monitoring on reflux-provoking activities. Dig Dis Sci. 1999;44:2263–9.
34. Prakash C, Clouse R. Value of extended recording time with wireless pH monitoring in evaluating gastroesophageal reflux disease. Clin Gastroenterol Hepatol. 2005;4:329–34.
35. Scarpulla G, Camilleri S, Galante P, et al. The impact of prolonged pH measurements on the diagnosis of gastroesophageal reflux disease: 4-day wireless pH studies. Am J Gastroenterol. 2007;102:2642–7.
36. Johnsson F, Joelsson B. Reproducibility of ambulatory oesophageal pH monitoring. Gut. 1988;29:886–9.
37. Ang D, Teo EK, Ang TL, et al. To Bravo or not? A comparison of wireless esophageal pH monitoring and conventional pH catheter to evaluate non-

erosive gastroesophageal reflux disease in a multiracial Asian cohort. J Dig Dis. 2010;11:19–27.
38. Johnsson F, Joelsson B, Isberg PE. Ambulatory 24 hour intraesophageal pH-monitoring in the diagnosis of gastroesophageal reflux disease. Gut. 1987;28:1145–50.
39. Schindlbeck NE, Heinrich C, König A, et al. Optimal thresholds, sensitivity, and specificity of long-term pH-metry for the detection of gastroesophageal reflux disease. Gastroenterology. 1987;93:85–90.
40. Chotiprashidi P, Liu J, Carpenter S, et al. ASGE technology status evaluation report: wireless esophageal pH monitoring system. Gastrointest Endosc. 2005;62:485–7.
41. Pandolfino JE, Kwiatek MA. Use and utility of the Bravo pH capsule. J Clin Gastroenterol. 2008;42:571–3.
42. Doma S, Paladugu S, Parkman HP, Friedenberg FK. Wireless capsules for esophageal pH monitoring: are we placing them correctly? Digestion. 2010;82:54–9.
43. Csendes A, Maluenda F, Braghetto I, et al. Location of the lower oesophageal sphincter and the squamous columnar mucosal junction in 109 healthy controls and 778 patients with different degrees of endoscopic oesophagitis. Gut. 1993;34:21–7.
44. Lacy BE, O'Shana T, Hynes M, et al. Safety and tolerability of transoral Bravo capsule placement after transnasal manometry using a validated conversion factor. Am J Gastroenterol. 2007;102:24–32.
45. Lawenko RMA, Lee YY. Evaluation of gastroesophageal reflux disease using the Bravo capsule pH system. J Neurogastroenterol Motil. 2015;22:25–30.
46. Wood RK. Endoscopic aspects in diagnosis of gastroesophageal reflux disease and motility disorders: Bravo, capsule, and functional lumen imaging probe. Tech Gastrointest Endosc. 2014;16:2–9.
47. Ang D, Xu Y, Ang TL, et al. Wireless oesophageal pH monitoring: establishing values in a multiracial cohort of asymptomatic Asian subjects. Dig Liver Dis. 2013;45:371–6.
48. Varannes des SB, Mion F, Ducrotté P, et al. Simultaneous recordings of oesophageal acid exposure with conventional pH monitoring and a wireless system (Bravo). Gut. 2005;54:1682–6.
49. Iluyomade A, Olowoyeye A, Fadahunsi O, et al. Interference with daily activities and major adverse events during esophageal pH monitoring with bravo wireless capsule versus conventional intranasal catheter: a systematic review of randomized controlled trials. Dis Esophagus. 2017;30:1–9.
50. Tseng D, Rizvi AZ, Fennerty MB, et al. Forty-eight-hour pH monitoring increases sensitivity in detecting abnormal esophageal acid exposure. J Gastrointest Surg. 2005;9:1043–51.
51. Sweis R, Fox M, Anggiansah A, Wong T. Prolonged, wireless pH-studies have a high diagnostic yield in patients with reflux symptoms and nega-

tive 24-h catheter-based pH-studies. Neurogastroenterol Motil. 2011;23:419–26.

52. Grigolon A, Bravi I, Duca P, et al. Prolonged wireless pH monitoring: importance of how to analyse oesophageal acid exposure. Scand J Gastroenterol. 2010;45:1133–4.
53. Capovilla G, Salvador R, Spadotto L, et al. Long-term wireless pH monitoring of the distal esophagus: prolonging the test beyond 48 hours is unnecessary and may be misleading. Dis Esophagus. 2017;30:1–8.
54. Pandolfino JE, Zhang Q, Schreiner MA, et al. Acid reflux event detection using the Bravo wireless versus the Slimline catheter pH systems: why are the numbers so different? Gut. 2005;54:1687–92.
55. Pandolfino JE, Schreiner MA, Lee TJ, et al. Comparison of the Bravo wireless and Digitrapper catheter-based pH monitoring systems for measuring esophageal acid exposure. Am J Gastroenterol. 2005;100:1466–76.
56. Håkanson BS, Berggren P, Granqvist S, et al. Comparison of wireless 48-h (Bravo) versus traditional ambulatory 24-h esophageal pH monitoring. Scand J Gastroenterol. 2009;44:276–83.
57. Fox M. Bravo wireless versus catheter pH monitoring systems. Gut. 2006;55:434–5.
58. Kessels SJ, Newton SS, Morona JK, Merlin TL. Safety and efficacy of wireless pH monitoring in patients suspected of gastroesophageal reflux disease: a systematic review. J Clin Gastroenterol. 2017;51:777–88.
59. Pandolfino JE, Richter JE, Ours T, et al. Ambulatory esophageal pH monitoring using a wireless system. Am J Gastroenterol. 2003;98:740–9.

15 Proximal pH Testing for Laryngopharyngeal Reflux

Umashankkar Kannan,
Krzystof M. Nowak, and Subhash Kini

Laryngopharyngeal Reflux

Laryngopharyngeal reflux (LPR) is an inflammatory condition of the upper aerodigestive tract secondary to reflux of gastroduodenal contents and characterized by morphologic changes in the upper aerodigestive tract [1]. There is currently no agreed gold standard diagnostic criteria. Consequently, many patients may not be diagnosed with LPR and incidence is therefore underreported. J. Koufman reported the prevalence of LPR to be 10% in patients who presented to laryngology clinics and 50% in patients with voice disorders [2, 3].

The common symptoms of LPR include globus sensation, hoarseness, sensation of excess throat mucus, dry cough, nonpro-

U. Kannan · S. Kini (✉)
Institute for Bariatric and Minimally Invasive Surgery, Mount Sinai Morningside Medical Center, New York, NY, USA
e-mail: umashankkar.kannan@mountsinai.org; subhash.kini@mountsinai.org

K. M. Nowak
ENT and Allergy Associates, Yonkers, NY, USA
e-mail: knowak@entandllaergy.com

A. D. Patel et al. (eds.), *The SAGES Manual of Physiologic Evaluation of Foregut Diseases*,
https://doi.org/10.1007/978-3-031-39199-6_15

ductive throat clearing, dryness or itching of the throat, difficulties breathing (especially inspiratory dyspnea), and dysphagia. Complaints of heartburn and regurgitations are reported inconsistently. Major physical findings include posterior commissure hypertrophy, laryngeal/arytenoid erythema and edema, subglottic edema, and excess endolaryngeal mucus [1]. Laryngopharyngeal reflux is associated with laryngeal granuloma, leukoplakia, laryngeal carcinoma, contact ulcers, vocal nodules, and subglottic stenosis [4]. The abovementioned symptoms and signs are nonspecific and overlap with other diagnoses such as postnasal drip due to allergic rhinitis and infection, vocal abuse, effects of smoking, and alcohol abuse. Further, these findings are also noticed in some healthy individuals. Hence, making the diagnosis of LPR can be very challenging. LPR can also be associated with nonacid and bile reflux. Therapeutic trial of a proton pump inhibitor (PPI) may often not be diagnostic. Hence, performing objective testing to support the clinical diagnosis of LPR is always necessary.

The objective tests currently in use to make a diagnosis of LPR include the following:

1. Oropharyngeal pH monitoring.
2. Pepsin detection.
3. Multichannel intraluminal impedance (MII)—pH monitoring.

Presently available diagnostic tests are considered to be suboptimal since their sensitivity and specificity remain uncertain, and further research is required. Many studies evaluating the diagnostic efficacy of these tests are based on reflux symptom index (RSI) and reflux findings score (RFS) which by themselves are nonspecific and nondiagnostic. The lack of gold standard diagnostic criteria for LPR emphasizes that the interpretation of the results must be made with caution and in the context of clinical presentation and consideration of overlapping diagnoses.

Oropharyngeal pH Monitoring

The Dx-pH measurement system (Restech, Respiratory Technology Corp, Houston, TX, United States) is a transnasal device to monitor the oropharyngeal pH [5]. The Restech probe has a sensor made of antimony that records changes in voltage potentials relative to pH in the surrounding environment in the pharynx. The sensor located at the tip of the probe includes reference electrodes and antimony within a 1 mm miniature package. The location of the sensor at the tip rather than side as in traditional probes and the antimony element in the sensor ensures accuracy by preventing artifacts from dryness of pharynx [6].

The nasal passage is anesthetized with 2% lidocaine, and the probe is inserted until the light-emitting diode (LED) flashlight is 5–10 mm below the uvula (Fig. 15.1). The LED light at the tip of

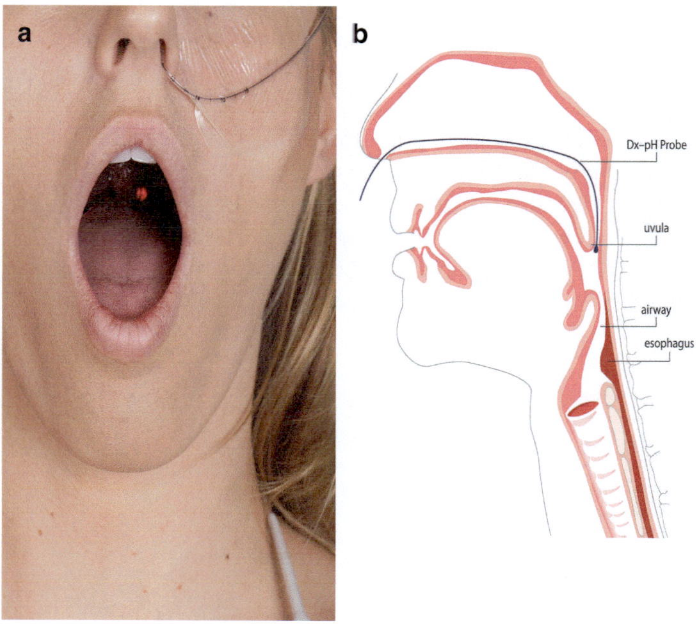

Fig. 15.1 (**a**) LED light at the tip of the catheter is positioned below the uvula; (**b**) transnasal passage of the pH catheter

the probe helps in positioning the catheter. The catheter is secured to the patient's face, and the transmitter at the end of the catheter is fixed to the patient's clothing. Patient carries the data recorder during testing. The pH is measured at the frequency of two times per second and transmitted to the data recorder.

Patients are requested to keep a diary of symptoms and mealtimes along with the duration of time spent in supine and upright positions. Patient's recorded events are then added to the proprietary software (Dataview v4) to calculate data for threshold pH from 6.5 to 5.

At each pH level (<6.5, <6, <5.5, and <5), the following are calculated along with other data (Fig. 15.2):

- The total %time with pH below baseline.
- The total %time with pH below baseline in upright position.
- The total %time with pH below baseline in supine position.

The values are then plotted in a bar graph in relation to the 75th and 95th percentile of the normative data in upright and supine positions at each pH levels (<6.5, <6, <5.5 and <5).

The acid exposure is termed mild, moderate, and severe depending on the % time exposure at each pH levels (Fig. 15.3). The software also provides the number of episodes of reflux and allows for symptom correlation at each pH level.

The RYAN score was created to identify severe reflux patients with high specificity. A positive RYAN score denotes severe

EVENT CALCULATIONS	pH < 6.5	pH < 6.0	pH < 5.5	pH < 5.0
Total time of all pH events	17:15	7:02	1:05	0:00
Total % pH below baseline	72.9%	29.7%	4.6%	0.0%
Total time below baseline pH, upright	9:17	1:40	0:02	0:00
Total % pH below baseline, upright	67.1%	12.1%	0.3%	0.0%
Total time below baseline pH, supine	7:58	5:22	1:02	0:00
Total % pH below baseline, supine	80.9%	54.5%	10.6%	0.0%
Longest time of a pH Event	7:27	1:26	0:10	0:00
Number of events > 5 minutes	27	15	6	0
Total Number of Events	132	105	16	0

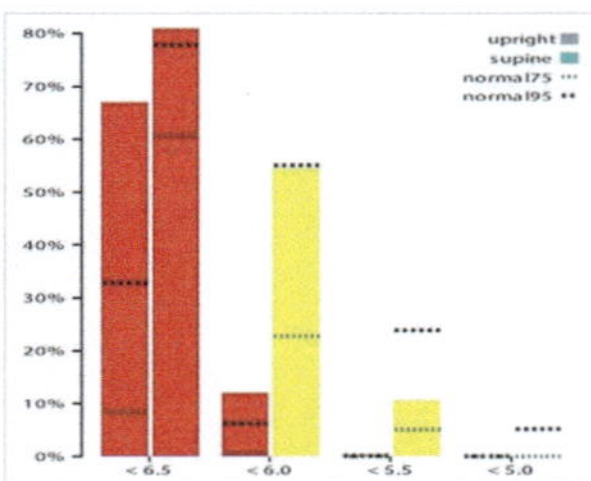

Fig. 15.2 pH event calculations in upright and supine position and its relation to 75th and 95th percentile of normative data

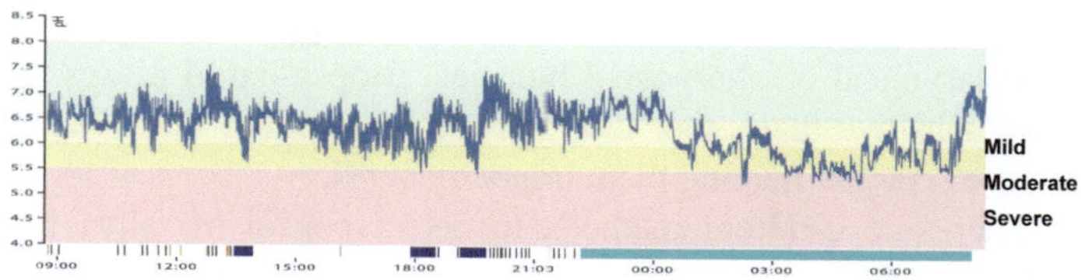

Fig. 15.3 Acidic reflux graph

reflux, while a negative score does not rule out mild or moderate disease.

The RYAN score is calculated based on the following three values:

1. The number of pH episodes falling below the established threshold.
2. The duration of the longest episode with pH below the threshold.
3. The total duration of time below the threshold.

A composite score is calculated from the three components. The score is pathological if the software-generated RYAN score is >9.41 in upright position (pH 5.5) or >6.81 in supine position (pH > 5.0). If a patient with a positive RYAN score does not show response to medical treatment, the patient can be considered for surgical intervention [5].

Pepsin

Pepsin, a proteolytic enzyme secreted in the stomach, is one of the most deleterious constituents of gastric juice. In addition to being directly destructive to the laryngeal epithelium, pepsin can also be endocytosed and activated at low pH inside the cell to cause intracellular injury. Trace amounts of pepsin can be detected in the saliva of normal individuals, but higher concentrations are seen in patients with LPR. At this time, there are no clearly established cutoff values for pepsin assays.

Pepsin assays are performed in saliva, sputum samples, or from laryngeal or pharyngeal biopsies. Biopsy-based assays are more sensitive than other tests but are much more invasive and require sedation making them impractical [7].

There are different methods to detect pepsin in saliva like Peptest (RD Biomed, Hull, UK, distributed as “Pepsincheck” in USA) or more complex immunohistochemical techniques such as Western blot or enzyme-linked immunosorbent assay (ELISA). The techniques based on western blot or ELISA are expensive and are not available easily. Salivary pepsin assay is a noninvasive, cost-effective, and convenient way to diagnose LPR and can be performed on any individual suspected of LPR. Peptest (Pepsincheck) is an easily available and FDA-approved immunological in vitro method to detect the presence of pepsin in saliva at a concentration equal to or greater than 16 ng/mL [8]. Peptest (Pepsincheck) requires three samples collected over 24 h. It is recommended that the first sample be obtained upon waking up, before eating and cleaning teeth. The second and third samples should be collected after 60 min of lunch and dinner, respectively. If the patient has symptoms during the 24 h testing period, the sample can be collected within 15 min of symptoms. The three samples are mailed for analysis. Proton pump inhibitors or H2 blockers do not interfere with pepsin detection and need not be held prior to testing. Antacids and alginate suspensions are stopped for 48 h prior to testing. Patients can eat and drink as they would normally do during 24 h of sample collection. A meta-analysis has shown a pooled sensitivity and specificity of salivary pepsin in diagnosing LPR to be 64% and 68%, respectively [9]. For diagnosing GERD, salivary pepsin has higher efficacy with sensitivity and specificity are 73% and 88%. Repeated saliva testing and timing the collection upon waking or after refluxes have shown to increase the sensitivity of the test. Pepsin testing on other samples like tracheal aspirates, bronchoalveolar lavage fluid, nasal lavage, and middle ear fluid needs further research to be clinically validated. Further research is still needed to find the optimal cutoff value, number of samples, and timing of samples to diagnose LPR.

Multichannel Intraluminal Impedance (MII): pH Testing

In addition to upper and lower esophageal pH measurements, MII-pH testing allows for detection of esophageal bolus (liquid and air) movements by sensing changes in electrical impedance along the catheter. Classical pH monitoring measures only pH and does not detect nonacid reflux or some aerosolized molecules. A detailed discussion is outside the scope of this chapter.

Conclusion

The techniques mentioned above can be very helpful in making the diagnosis of LPR. It is important to emphasize that still a gold standard to identify LPR patients is lacking. Currently, the diagnosis of LPR requires careful review of symptoms, physical findings, and objective testing, ruling out other competing etiologies.

References

1. Lechien JR, Akst LM, Hamdan AL, Schindler A, Karkos PD, Barillari MR, et al. Evaluation and management of laryngopharyngeal reflux disease: state of the art review. Otolaryngol Head Neck Surg. 2019;160(5):762–82.
2. Koufman JA. The otolaryngologic manifestations of gastroesophageal reflux disease (GERD): a clinical investigation of 225 patients using ambulatory 24-hour pH monitoring and an experimental investigation of the role of acid and pepsin in the development of laryngeal injury. Laryngoscope. 1991;101(4 Pt 2 Suppl 53):1–78.
3. Koufman JA, Aviv JE, Casiano RR, Shaw GY. Laryngopharyngeal reflux: position statement of the committee on speech, voice, and swallowing disorders of the American Academy of Otolaryngology-Head and Neck Surgery. Otolaryngol Head Neck Surg. 2002;127(1):32–5.
4. Campagnolo AM, Priston J, Thoen RH, Medeiros T, Assunção AR. Laryngopharyngeal reflux: diagnosis, treatment, and latest research. Int Arch Otorhinolaryngol. 2014;18(2):184–91.

5. Ayazi S, Lipham JC, Hagen JA, Tang AL, Zehetner J, Leers JM, et al. A new technique for measurement of pharyngeal pH: normal values and discriminating pH threshold. J Gastrointest Surg. 2009;13(8):1422–9.
6. Vailati C, Mazzoleni G, Bondi S, Bussi M, Testoni PA, Passaretti S. Oropharyngeal pH monitoring for laryngopharyngeal reflux: is it a reliable test before therapy? J Voice. 2013;27(1):84–9.
7. Johnston N, Dettmar PW, Ondrey FG, Nanchal R, Lee SH, Bock JM. Pepsin: biomarker, mediator, and therapeutic target for reflux and aspiration. Ann N Y Acad Sci. 2018;1434(1):282–9.
8. Barona-Lleo L, Barona-De Guzman R, Krstulovic C. The diagnostic usefullness of the salivary pepsin test in symptomatic laryngopharyngeal reflux. J Voice. 2019;33(6):923–8.
9. Wang J, Zhao Y, Ren J, Xu Y. Pepsin in saliva as a diagnostic biomarker in laryngopharyngeal reflux: a meta-analysis. Eur Arch Otorhinolaryngol. 2018;275(3):671–8.

16 Endoscopic Evaluation of the Bariatric Surgery Patient

Sofiane El Djouzi

Introduction

A frequently discussed advantage of upper endoscopy is its diagnostic and therapeutic potential compared to gastrointestinal imaging studies (i.e., contrast upper gastrointestinal series). An upper endoscopy allows for direct visualization of the foregut mucosa, enables practitioners to obtain biopsy samples, and performs endoluminal interventions. Endoscopists must remain vigilant when concern exists for postoperative complications. As an example, when a gastrointestinal staple line leak is suspected, a water-soluble upper GI study should be performed as the initial diagnostic test [1]. Air insufflation of the foregut may be deleterious in patients that are less than 4 weeks postsurgery, as it could convert a small contained leak into a free perforation or disrupt a healing anastomosis. In this setting, carbon dioxide, as opposed to air insufflation, should be used as its rapid absorption will prevent persistent dilation of the GI tract.

S. El Djouzi (✉)
Barijuve Surgical, Darien, IL, USA
e-mail: sofiane.eldjouzi@barijuve.com

A. D. Patel et al. (eds.), *The SAGES Manual of Physiologic Evaluation of Foregut Diseases*,
https://doi.org/10.1007/978-3-031-39199-6_16

Periprocedural Recommendations

It is recommended that no food is taken 8 hours before the upper endoscopy. Clear liquids can be taken up to 2 hours before endoscopy [2]. Antibiotic prophylaxis is not recommended due to the low risk of infection from this procedure [3]. Pre-endoscopy laboratory and imaging studies should be performed based on individual patient risk factors. The risk of discontinuing antiplatelet therapy and systemic anticoagulation must require a case-by-case review [4].

Technical Considerations

To safely and successfully perform an upper endoscopy in a bariatric surgery patient, it is imperative to be familiar with the patient's operative reports, postoperative imaging, and select the appropriate equipment required to complete the procedure [5]. Proper equipment, including the choice of the endoscope, will depend on the patient's surgical history. In patients that previously underwent restrictive procedures, a standard adult gastroscope is sufficient. A balloon-assisted enteroscope or pediatric colonoscope may become handy in those requiring evaluation of jejunojejunal anastomosis, retrograde evaluation of the biliopancreatic limb, or bypassed stomach [6]. Balloon-assisted enteroscopy uses a balloon attached to an over the tube to allow for a more distal assessment of the gastrointestinal tract in patients who have undergone Roux-en-Y gastric bypass (RYGB) with long (150 cm) Roux limb [7]. Regardless of the endoscopic technique, the endoscopist must be familiar with the prior operative reports to appreciate the possible variation in postsurgical anatomy.

Sedation

In most instances, periprocedural sedation requires conscious sedation or monitored anesthesia care (MAC). That being said, a patient with high body mass index (BMI) and obstructive sleep apnea (OSA) might require endotracheal intubation under general anesthesia as it becomes much more challenging to proceed with the procedure otherwise. In a study of patients undergoing advanced endoscopic procedures, higher BMI patients had an increased frequency of sedation-related complications, including apnea, oxygen desaturations, and airway obstructions [8–10]. Such a statement should be taken into consideration when selecting office versus hospital-based endoscopy to minimize any peri-procedural risks.

Conscious sedation is frequently performed using a combination of narcotic analgesia and benzodiazepine sedatives under the surgeon or gastroenterologist's direction performing the procedure. In a study comparing obese patients that have undergone RYGB and those who have not, postsurgical patients required more sedation, possibly from improved liver function post-op [11]. The involvement of the anesthesia team might become vital in the context of complex cases. A major advantage of conscious sedation is that patients are sedated yet still able to follow commands during the procedure. Alternatively, MAC anesthesia is performed under the direct care of an anesthesiologist or Certified Registered Nurse Anesthetist (CRNA) supervised by an anesthesiologist.

The patient's sedation is titrated to a level that preserves spontaneous breathing and airway reflexes [10]. Patients undergoing MAC anesthesia are unconscious but still breathing without the assistance of a ventilator. The safety of conscious sedation in bariatric surgery patients with metabolic syndrome has been challenged before. Nonetheless, one study of 1385 patients reported a cardiopulmonary event rate during conscious sedation of 0.6% in Roux-en-Y gastric bypass patients [11], which is similar to 0.9% described in the general population [11, 12].

Procedural Technique

Pre- or postbariatric surgery upper endoscopy is frequently performed in the outpatient setting. The choice of anesthesia is dictated by the patient's clinical characteristics and the operator's experience level.

Upper endoscopy begins with passage of the endoscope through the mouth into the oropharynx to evaluate for upper esophageal abnormalities. Next the endoscope is advanced down the esophagus to the esophagogastric junction to evaluate the squamocolumnar junction or Z-line. Biopsies may be taken through cold or hot forceps to evaluate for any mucosal abnormalities (i.e., Barrett's esophagus and distal esophagitis). Next, the scope is passed into the stomach and retroflexed to look for a hiatal hernia. From this point, it all depends on whether the patient has or has not had weight loss surgery yet. It also depends on the layout of the Foregut anatomy. The rest of the stomach is examined as well as the gastrojejunal anastomosis or the duodenum depending on the patient's surgery. Biopsies, mucosal brushings, and cultures may be taken throughout the procedure. Any adjunct to the procedure depends on the indication(s) of the intervention and the goals yet to be achieved. More details on those technical aspects are detailed along the subsequent sections of the chapter.

Timing of Endoscopy Evaluation in the Bariatric Patient

The Preoperative Period

It is well accepted and endorsed that patients with symptomatic gastroesophageal reflux disease (GERD) or a history of chronic upper gastrointestinal complaints should have an upper GI endoscopy before undertaking the planned bariatric procedure [13, 14]. However, routine preoperative endoscopic evaluation of all bariatric patients remains controversial [15, 16]. Multiple studies have reported the routine use of preoperative esophagogastroduodenoscopy (EGD) with variable incidence of findings of clinically relevant abnormalities such as hiatal hernia, esophagitis, Barrett's esophagus, esophageal dysplasia, duodenitis, ulcers, and tumors [15, 17, 18]. On the other hand, a large study reported that over half of the patients were found to be harboring endoscopically significant findings while remaining clinically asymptomatic [17]. Such results delayed or altered the planned surgical procedure in 1.7–7.6% of the patients [15, 17, 18].

Evidence of reflux esophagitis and hiatal hernia is more concerning if a vertical sleeve gastrectomy (VSG) is planned as these findings are relative contraindications due to the increased risk of developing de novo GERD. Several studies have shown incidence variability in the development of de novo GERD, Barrett's esophagus, erosive esophagitis, as well as the increased use of proton pump inhibitors (PPIs) after VSG [19, 20]. If a hiatal hernia is discovered at the time of the endoscopy, the repair is highly recommended at the time of the weight loss surgery [21].

The most recent recommendations by the Standards of Practice Committee of the American Society for Gastrointestinal Endoscopy (ASGE) along with the Society of Gastrointestinal and Endoscopic Surgeons (SAGES) and the American Society for Metabolic and Bariatric Surgery (ASMBS) were published in 2015. The recommendation to perform preoperative screening endoscopy should be individualized based on patient need, symptomatology, discussion with the surgeon, and type of procedure to be performed [22].

The Intraoperative Period

The intraoperative use of endoscopy remains controversial, with some surgeons making it mandatory. It is used primarily to test for intraoperative gastrointestinal staple line leak, evaluate the anatomy outlook during revisional procedures, identify and control bleeding, and access surgical lumen and anastomosis diameter [23]. Upon researching the surgical literature, two studies assessing the value of the routine application of intraoperative endoscopy at the time of bariatric surgery identified abnormalities such as staple and suture line leaks and other technical errors that were promptly corrected. Luckily, the incidence of such findings was very low [24, 25].

The Postoperative Period

Endoscopy is not the first line of assessment in the postoperative period. It remains indicated when other non-invasive testings have remained inconclusive in the evaluation of persistent nausea, vomiting, intolerance to oral intake, and new epigastric pain [1]. There are a number of etiologies behind such symptoms. While some could be managed expectantly along with counseling and behavioral modifications, others might require surgical or endoscopic intervention.

GERD

Postoperative GERD is not uncommon after certain bariatric procedures. As related earlier, reflux symptoms and the development of de novo GERD are more prevalent after VSG. On the other hand, the RYGB has proven to be an excellent surgical indication for GERD treatment in patients who also suffer from obesity [26, 27]. Postoperative GERD symptoms should first be managed medically for an extended period of time [28]. Weight loss alone could potentially reduce or ablate the complaints [29]. If medical management fails, endoscopy could be considered to investigate for any anatomical abnormalities such as severe gastrojejunal anastomotic stricture or gastrogastric fistula after RYGB, and twisted gastric tube after VSG [22].

Adjustable Gastric Band (AGB) Slippage and Erosion

AGB slippage and erosion into the gastric lumen can be assessed endoscopically (it could also be suspected through contrast imaging studies). A meta-analysis of 19 studies and 500 patients recently estimated the rates of slippage and erosion to be 5% and 1%, respectively [30]. Band erosion may cause an array of symptoms (abdominal pain, nausea, vomiting, port site infection, increased food intake with weight gain, and GI bleeding), or it may remain asymptomatic [31]. If any portion of the band is seen on endoscopy, the surgeon needs to be consulted for further management [22]. Similarly, band slippage can cause abdominal pain, weight gain, reflux symptoms, or dysphagia. Acute band slippage can lead to life-threatening gastric necrosis and require a prompt surgical correction [32, 33].

Marginal Ulcers

Marginal ulcers typically occur after RYGB surgery with an incidence of 0.6–36% [34–36]. Patients may present with abdominal pain, bleeding, and nausea or could potentially be asymptomatic. The ulcers are usually on the intestinal side and believed to be due to many possible mechanisms (i.e., local ischemia, acidic effects on the intestinal mucosa, staple line disruption, and exposed staple or suture material on the intraluminal side) [37]. Other factors include the presence of a gastrogastric fistula, H pylori infection, smoking, uncontrolled diabetes, excessive gastric pouch length, and chronic use of NSAIDs or corticosteroids [34, 36, 37]. Marginal ulcers are first treated medically with acid reduction and cytoprotective agents. Refractory ulceration will require revisional surgery [38].

Gastric Leak and Fistulae

Gastric leaks and gastric fistulae have an incidence of 1–6% in weight loss surgery patients and can result in enterocutaneous fistula, peritonitis, abscess, sepsis, organ failure, and death [39–43]. Leaks after RYGB most commonly occur at the gastrojejunal anastomosis. Jejunojejunal leaks, though exceedingly rare, can occur and may require reoperation [44]. After VSG, leaks typically occur along the very proximal staple line and most commonly at the proximal one-third of the greater curvature of the staple line [45]. Diagnosis is usually made with an upper GI contrast study or CT. However, early endoscopy can be performed if there is diagnostic uncertainty or for endoscopic intervention [46, 47]. The injection of fibrin glue, application of clips, placement of self-expandable metal stents (SEMS), or insertion of the pigtail catheter are all handy tools to manage such leaks [48, 49]. Gastric fistulae can also be treated endoscopically using fibrin glue [50, 51] or SEMS [52–54]. These patients may eventually need surgical closure of the fistula as endoscopic interventions typically serve as a bridge to definitive management [55].

Anastomotic Strictures

Gastrojejunal anastomotic strictures, defined as anastomoses less than 10 mm in diameter (accepted normal diameter is 14–16 mm), are not uncommon complications of the RYGB. Such complication triggers nausea, vomiting, and or dysphagia. A stricture can be diagnosed with an upper GI contrast study but endoscopy is preferred as it is both diagnostic and therapeutic [56].

Anastomotic strictures can be dilated endoscopically with either through-the-balloon dilators or wire-guided bougie dilators [57, 58]. These should be serially dilated over multiple sessions to prevent perforation [59]. There is debate over dilating the stoma to >15 mm due to concern of weight regain. However, one study noted the reduced need for repeat dilation and no association with weight regain [58].

One important consideration in RYGB patients is whether the Roux limb was delivered in antecolic or retrocolic fashion. A tight tunnel created through the transverse colon mesentery can cause narrowing of the Roux limb and subsequent obstruction [60]. On endoscopy, there will be a normal gastrojejunal anastomosis with dilated jejunum distally until the point where the Roux limb traverses the mesocolon. Dilation at this point is not advised given a high risk for perforation [61].

Short-segment gastric lumen stenosis after VSG can be treated endoscopically. However, long-segment stenosis may require surgical intervention, such as seromyotomy or revision to gastric bypass [62].

Foreign Body and Bezoars

Lodged foreign material and bezoars can be diagnosed and retrieved endoscopically. Foreign material includes staple and suture material that can contribute to marginal ulcers, stomal stenosis, abdominal pain, and dysphagia [63, 64]. These should be removed once the gastrojejunal anastomosis has matured. Food bezoars usually occur after AGB [65, 66], but can occur after RYGB within the gastric pouch or at the jejunojejunal anastomosis [67–69]. These can be removed endoscopically after fragmentation [70].

Anemia and GI Bleed

Anemia in the postbariatric patient can be from iron or vitamin B12 deficiency. GI bleeding can also contribute to anemia and should be evaluated with endoscopy. Bleeding from the staple tines occurs in 1–4% of patients undergoing any stapled bariatric surgery [71]. The excluded stomach and the Roux limb lumens should also be visually inspected, although access to both may be challenging. Endoscopy or enteroscopy may need to be used [72]. A surgical gastrostomy may be needed for unsuccessful attempts at accessing the excluded stomach [73].

Endoscopic Retrograde Cholangiopancreatography (ERCP) After RYGB

Performing an ERCP in a post-RYGB patient presents a unique set of challenges. A standard endoscope cannot traverse the entire length of a Roux limb and thus cannot reach the duodenal papillae [74]. Choledocholithiasis can be diagnosed through non-endoscopic modalities such as MRCP or percutaneous transhepatic cholangiography. There have been case reports of successful ERCPs using colonoscopes, double-balloon enteroscopy, single balloon enteroscopy, and spiral-assisted enteroscopy [75–77]. Minimally invasive laparoscopic transgastric ERCP can be performed as well, with success rates greater than with enteroscopy alone [78–80]. Retrograde ERCP can also be performed through an enterotomy in the Roux limb [81].

Conclusion

Upper gastrointestinal endoscopy is an essential tool in the diagnosis and treatment of bariatric surgery patients. Preoperatively endoscopy is used to evaluate pathology that may alter the surgical planning, yet routine and liberal use remains a subject of debate. Intraoperatively, endoscopy could be used with the proper indication and concerns to address any technical matters or complications promptly. Endoscopy might require expert skills when it comes to managing postoperative complications. As technology evolves, gastrointestinal endoscopy will likely gain an even more prominent role in the care of the bariatric patient.

Editors' Note

See Figs. 16.1, 16.2, 16.3, and 16.4.

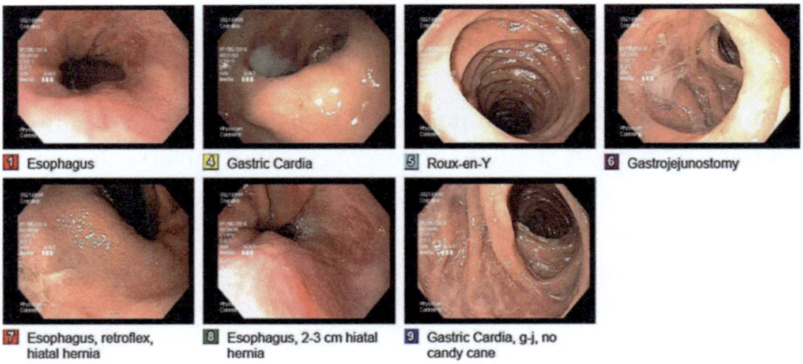

Fig. 16.1 Endoscopic views in a patient after Roux-en-Y gastric bypass. Important factors to note include the length of the pouch, the size of the outlet of the pouch (in scope diameters), and the presence/absence of a hiatal hernia. The LES can also be examined to subjectively determine whether it is patulous. Finally, the scope should be passed as distally as possible in the roux limb to determine length (if the jejunojejunostomy can be reached) and there should be no bile in the roux limb

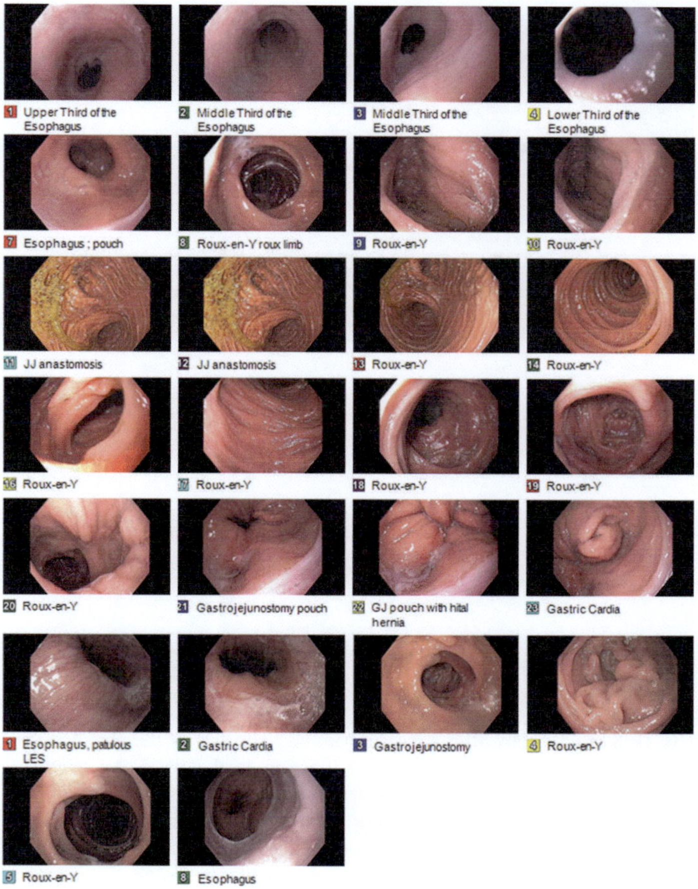

Fig. 16.2 Another patient's upper endoscopy after a gastric bypass. This patient had a hiatal hernia, a normal outlet size at the gastrojejunostomy. However, the roux limb was noted to be short at 50 cm and bile seen at the jejunojejunostomy as expected

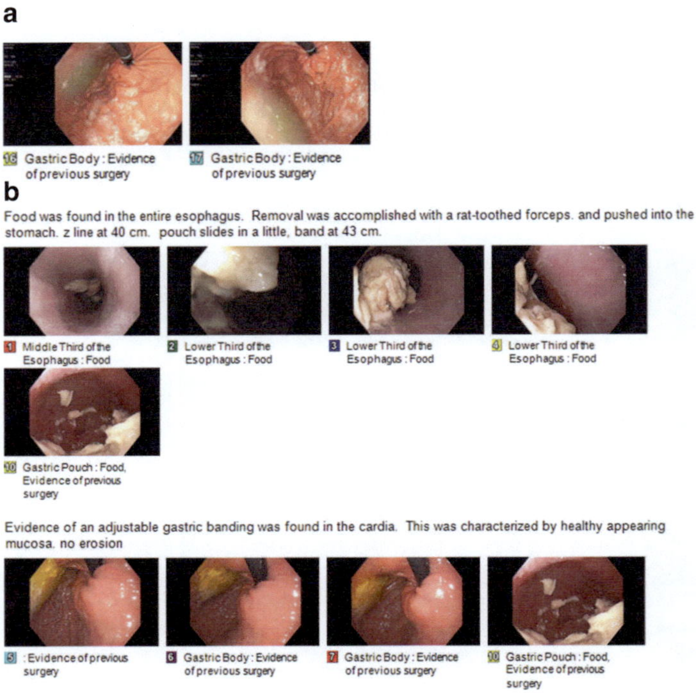

Fig. 16.3 Endoscopy after a gastric banding. The size of the pouch is very important from the gastroesophageal junction to the band. An excessive amount of stomach above the band is considered a slip. Also, a retroflexed view beyond the band can be helpful to identify erosions. (**a**) Retroflexed view showing band in place with no erosion. (**b**) Food in esophagus after band placed suggesting band to tight. Band in place with no erosion

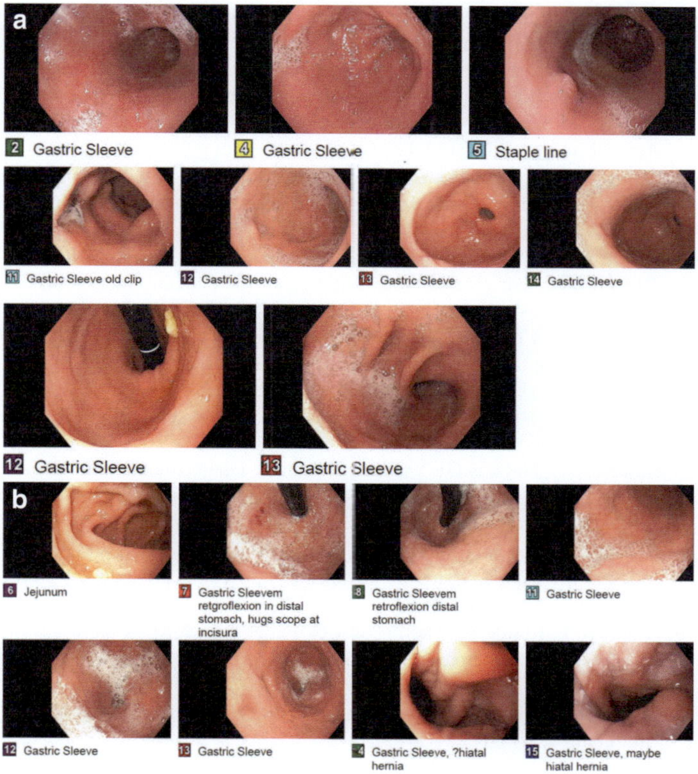

Fig. 16.4 Endoscopy after vertical sleeve gastrectomy. (**a**) The sleeve should be tubular proximally and have a reasonable view through the incisura into the distal stomach where the staple line ends 5–7 cm proximal to the pylorus. Retroflexion in the distal stomach shows an open incisura as in panel 12. Retroflexion in the proximal stomach can be difficult in tighter sleeves. (**b**). In panel 7, the incisura tightly holds the scope on retroflexion. This is an undesirable finding on endoscopy in a sleeve. In panels 14 and 15, one can see a hiatal hernia and patulous LES, which can contribute to reflux after a sleeve

References

1. Lee JK, Van Dam J, Morton JM, et al. Endoscopy is accurate, safe, effective in the assessment and management of complications following gastric bypass surgery. Am J Gastroenterol. 2009;104:575–82.

2. American Society of Anesthesiologists Committee. Practice guidelines for preoperative fasting and the use of pharmacologic agents to reduce the risk of pulmonary aspiration: application to healthy patients undergoing elective procedures: an updated report by the American Society of Anesthesiologists Committee on Standards and Practice Parameters. Anesthesiology. 2011;114:495.
3. ASGE Standards of Practice Committee, Khashab MA, Chithadi KV, et al. Antibiotic prophylaxis for GI endoscopy. Gastrointest Endosc. 2015;81:81.
4. ASGE Standards of Practice Committee, Acosta RD, Abraham NS, et al. The management of antithrombotic agents for patients undergoing GI endoscopy. Gastrointest Endosc. 2016;83:3.
5. Stellato TA, Crouse C, Hallowell PT. Bariatric surgery: creating new challenges for the endoscopist. Gastrointest Endosc. 2003;57:86.
6. Sinar DR, Flickinger EG, Park HK, Sloss RR. Retrograde endoscopy of the bypassed stomach segment after gastric bypass surgery: unexpected lesions. South Med J. 1985;78:255.
7. Moreels TG, Hubens GJ, Ysebaert DK, et al. Diagnostic and therapeutic double-balloon enteroscopy after small bowel Roux-en-Y reconstructive surgery. Digestion. 2009;80:141.
8. Kilic ET, Sayar S, Kahraman R, Ozdil K. The effects of obesity on sedation-related outcomes of advanced endoscopic procedures. North Clin Istanb. 2019;6(4):321–6.
9. Jirapinyo P, Kumar N, Thompson CC. Patients with Roux-en-Y gastric bypass require increased sedation during upper endoscopy. Clin Gastroenterol Hepatol. 2015;13(8):1432–6.
10. Das S, Ghosh S. Monitored anesthesia care: an overview. J Anaesthesiol Clin Pharmacol. 2015;31:27–9.
11. Jirapinyo P, Abu Dayyeh BK, Thompson CC. Conscious sedation for upper endoscopy in the gastric bypass patient: prevalence of cardiopulmonary adverse events and predictors of sedation requirement. Dig Dis Sci. 2014;59(9):2173–7.
12. Sharma VK, Nguyen CC, Crowell MD, et al. Cardiopulmonary unplanned events after GI endoscopy. Gastrointest Endosc. 2007;66:27–34.
13. Hampel H, Abraham NS, El-Serag HB. Meta-analysis: obesity and the risk for gastroesophageal reflux disease and its complications. Ann Intern Med. 2005;143:199–211.
14. Abd Ellatif ME, Alfalah H, Asker WA, et al. Place of upper endoscopy before and after bariatric surgery: a multicenter experience with 3219 patients. World J Gastrointest Endosc. 2016;8(10):409–17.
15. Parikh M, Liu J, Vieira D, et al. Preoperative endoscopy prior to bariatric surgery: a systematic review and meta-analysis of the literature. Obes Surg. 2016;26:2961–6.

16. Lee J, Wong SK, Liu SY, Ng EK. Is preoperative upper gastrointestinal endoscopy in obese patients undergoing bariatric surgery mandatory? An Asian perspective. Obes Surg. 2017 Jan;27(1):44–50.
17. Saarinen T, Kettunen U, Pietiläinen KH, et al. Is preoperative gastroscopy necessary before sleeve gastrectomy and Roux-en-Y gastric bypass? Surg Obes Relat Dis. 2018;14:757–62.
18. Salama A, Saafan T, El Ansari W, et al. Is routine preoperative esophagogastroduodenoscopy screening necessary prior to laparoscopic sleeve gastrectomy? Review of 1555 cases and comparison with current literature. Obes Surg. 2018;28:52–60.
19. Genco A, Soricelli E, Casella G, et al. Gastroesophageal reflux disease and Barrett's esophagus after laparoscopic sleeve gastrectomy: a possible, underestimated long-term complication. Surg Obes Relat Dis. 2017;13:568–74.
20. Sebastianelli L, Benois M, Vanbiervliet G, et al. Systematic endoscopy 5 years after sleeve gastrectomy results in a high rate of Barrett's esophagus: results of a multicenter study. Obes Surg. 2019;29:1462–9.
21. Dolan K, Finch R, Fielding G. Laparoscopic gastric banding and crural repair in the obese patient with a hiatal hernia. Obes Surg. 2003;13:772–5.
22. ASGE Standards of Practice Committee, Evans JA, Muthusamy VR, et al. The role of endoscopy in the bariatric surgery patient. Surg Obes Relat Dis. 2015;11:507–17.
23. Haddad A, Tapazoglou N, Singh K, et al. Role of intraoperative esophagogastroenteroscopy in minimizing gastrojejunostomy-related morbidity: experience with 2,311 laparoscopic gastric bypasses with linear stapler anastomosis. Obes Surg. 2012;22:1928–33.
24. Champion JK, Hunt T, DeLisle N. Role of routine intraoperative endoscopy in laparoscopic bariatric surgery. Surg Endosc. 2002;16:1663–5.
25. Nimeri A, Maasher A, Salim E, et al. The use of intraoperative endoscopy may decrease postoperative stenosis in laparoscopic sleeve gastrectomy. Obes Surg. 2016;26:1398–401.
26. Stefanidis D, Navarro F, Augenstein VA, et al. Laparoscopic fundoplication takedown with conversion to Roux-en-Y gastric bypass leads to excellent reflux control and quality of life after fundoplication failure. Surg Endosc. 2012;26:3521–7.
27. Kim M, Navarro F, Eruchalu CN, Augenstein VA, Heniford BT, Stefanidis D. Minimally invasive Roux-en-Y gastric bypass for fundoplication failure offers excellent gastroesophageal reflux control. Am Surg. 2014;80(7):696–703.
28. Soricelli E, Iossa A, Casella G, et al. Sleeve gastrectomy and crural repair in obese patients with gastroesophageal reflux disease and/or hiatal hernia. Surg Obes Relat Dis. 2013;9:356–61.
29. Singh M, Lee J, Gupta N, et al. Weight loss can lead to resolution of gastroesophageal reflux disease symptoms: a prospective intervention trial.

Obesity (Silver Spring). 2013;21(2):284–90. https://doi.org/10.1002/oby.20279.
30. Singhal R, Bryant C, Kitchen M, et al. Band slippage and erosion after laparoscopic gastric banding: a meta-analysis. Surg Endosc. 2010;24:2980–6.
31. El Djouzi S. Role of endoscopy in managing foreign body erosions after bariatric surgery. In: Chand B, editor. Endoscopy in obesity management. Cham: Springer; 2018. https://doi.org/10.1007/978-3-319-63528-6_10.
32. Foletto M, De Marchi F, Bernante P, et al. Late gastric pouch necrosis after Lap-Band, treated by an individualized conservative approach. Obes Surg. 2005;15:1487–90.
33. Iannelli A, Facchiano E, Sejor E, et al. Gastric necrosis: a rare complication of gastric banding. Obes Surg. 2005;15:1211–4.
34. Azagury DE, Abu Dayyeh BK, Greenwalt IT, et al. Marginal ulceration after Roux-en-Y gastric bypass surgery: characteristics, risk factors, treatment, and outcomes. Endoscopy. 2011;43:950–4.
35. El-Hayek K, Timratana P, Shimizu H, et al. Marginal ulcer after Roux-en-Y gastric bypass: what have we really learned? Surg Endosc. 2012;26:2789–96.
36. Wilson JA, Romagnuolo J, Byrne TK, et al. Predictors of endoscopic findings after Roux-en-Y gastric bypass. Am J Gastroenterol. 2006;101:2194–9.
37. MacLean LD, Rhode BM, Nohr C, et al. Stomal ulcer after gastric bypass. J Am Coll Surg. 1997;185:1–7.
38. Marcotte E. Treatment of marginal ulcers after gastric bypass. In: Chand B, editor. Endoscopy in obesity management. Cham: Springer; 2018.
39. Carrodeguas L, Szomstein S, Soto F, et al. Management of gastrogastric fistulas after divided Roux-en-Y gastric bypass surgery for morbid obesity: analysis of 1,292 consecutive patients and review of literature. Surg Obes Relat Dis. 2005;1:467–74.
40. Filho AJ, Kondo W, Nassif LS, et al. Gastrogastric fistula: a possible complication of Roux-en-Y gastric bypass. JSLS. 2006;10:326–31.
41. Gould JC, Garren MJ, Starling JR. Lessons learned from the first 100 cases in a new minimally invasive bariatric surgery program. Obes Surg. 2004;14:618–25.
42. Gumbs AA, Duffy AJ, Bell RL. Management of gastrogastric fistula after laparoscopic Roux-en-Y gastric bypass. Surg Obes Relat Dis. 2006;2:117–21.
43. Carucci LR, Turner MA, Conklin RC, et al. Roux-en-Y gastric bypass surgery for morbid obesity: evaluation of postoperative extraluminal leaks with upper gastrointestinal series. Radiology. 2006;238:119–27.
44. Ballesta C, Berindoague R, Cabrera M, Palau M, Gonzales M. Management of anastomotic leaks after laparoscopic Roux-en-Y gastric bypass. Obes Surg. 2008 Jun;18(6):623–30.

45. Aurora AR, Khaitan L, Saber AA. Sleeve gastrectomy and the risk of leak: a systematic analysis of 4,888 patients. Surg Endosc. 2012;26:1509–15.
46. Eisendrath P, Cremer M, Himpens J, et al. Endotherapy including temporary stenting of fistulas of the upper gastrointestinal tract after laparoscopic bariatric surgery. Endoscopy. 2007;39:625–30.
47. Merrifield BF, Lautz D, Thompson CC. Endoscopic repair of gastric leaks after Roux-en-Y gastric bypass: a less invasive approach. Gastrointest Endosc. 2006;63:710–4.
48. Brolin RE, Lin JM. Treatment of gastric leaks after Roux-en-Y gastric bypass: a paradigm shift. Surg Obes Relat Dis. 2013;9:229–33.
49. Spyropoulos C, Argentou MI, Petsas T, et al. Management of gastrointestinal leaks after surgery for clinically severe obesity. Surg Obes Relat Dis. 2012;8:609–15.
50. Evans JA, Branch MS, Pryor AD, et al. Endoscopic closure of a gastrojejunal anastomotic leak (with video). Gastrointest Endosc. 2007;66:1225–6.
51. Papavramidis ST, Eleftheriadis EE, Papavramidis TS, et al. Endoscopic management of gastrocutaneous fistula after bariatric surgery by using a fibrin sealant. Gastrointest Endosc. 2004;59:296–300.
52. Fukumoto R, Orlina J, McGinty J, et al. Use of Polyflex stents in treatment of acute esophageal and gastric leaks after bariatric surgery. Surg Obes Relat Dis. 2007;3:68–71; discussion 71–2.
53. Kriwanek S, Ott N, Ali-Abdullah S, et al. Treatment of gastro-jejunal leakage and fistulization after gastric bypass with coated self expanding stents. Obes Surg. 2006;16:1669–74.
54. Salinas A, Baptista A, Santiago E, et al. Self-expandable metal stents to treat gastric leaks. Surg Obes Relat Dis. 2006;2:570–2.
55. Tsai C, Kessler U, Steffen R, Merki H, Zehetner J. Endoscopic closure of gastro-gastric fistula after gastric bypass: a technically feasible procedure but associated with low success rate. Obes Surg. 2019;29(1):23–7.
56. Messmer JM, Wolper JC, Sugerman HJ. Stomal disruption in gastric partition in morbid obesity (comparison of radiographic and endoscopic diagnosis). Am J Gastroenterol. 1984;79:603–5.
57. Escalona A, Devaud N, Boza C, Pérez G, Fernández J, Ibáñez L, Guzmán S. Gastrojejunal anastomotic stricture after Roux-en-Y gastric bypass: ambulatory management with the Savary-Gilliard dilator. Surg Endosc. 2007 May;21(5):765–8.
58. Peife KJ, Shiels AJ, Azar R, et al. Successful endoscopic management of gastrojejunal anastomotic strictures after Roux-en-Y gastric bypass. Gastrointest Endosc. 2007;66:248–52.
59. Go MR, Muscarella P 2nd, Needleman BJ, et al. Endoscopic management of stomal stenosis after Roux-en-Y gastric bypass. Surg Endosc. 2004;18:56–9.

60. Hwang RF, Swartz DE, Felix EL. Causes of small bowel obstruction after laparoscopic gastric bypass. Surg Endosc. 2004;18:1631–5.
61. Wetter A. Role of endoscopy after Roux-en-Y gastric bypass surgery. Gastrointest Endosc. 2007;66:253–5.
62. Parikh A, Alley JB, Peterson RM, et al. Management options for symptomatic stenosis after laparoscopic vertical sleeve gastrectomy in the morbidly obese. Surg Endosc. 2012;26:738–46.
63. Ryou M, Mogabgab O, Lautz DB, et al. Endoscopic foreign body removal for treatment of chronic abdominal pain in patients after Roux-en-Y gastric bypass. Surg Obes Relat Dis. 2010;6:526–31.
64. Yu S, Jastrow K, Clapp B, et al. Foreign material erosion after laparoscopic Roux-en-Y gastric bypass: findings and treatment. Surg Endosc. 2007;21:1216–20.
65. Parameswaran R, Ferrando J, Sigurdsson A. Gastric bezoar complicating laparoscopic adjustable gastric banding with band slippage. Obes Surg. 2006;16:1683–4.
66. Veronelli A, Ranieri R, Laneri M, et al. Gastric bezoars after adjustable gastric banding. Obes Surg. 2004;14:796–7.
67. Powers WF, Miles DR. Phytobezoar causing small bowel obstruction seven years after laparoscopic Roux-en-Y gastric bypass. Surg Obes Relat Dis. 2011;7:e3–5.
68. Roy M, Fendrich I, Li J, et al. Treatment option in patient presenting with small bowel obstruction from phytobezoar at the jejunojejunal anastomosis after Roux-en-Y gastric bypass. Surg Laparosc Endosc Percutan Tech. 2012;22:e243–5.
69. Sarhan M, Shyamali B, Fakulujo A, et al. Jejunal bezoar causing obstruction after laparoscopic Roux-en-Y gastric bypass. JSLS. 2010;14:592–5.
70. Pinto D, Carrodeguas L, Soto F, et al. Gastric bezoar after laparoscopic Roux-en-Y gastric bypass. Obes Surg. 2006;16:365–8.
71. Nguyen NT, Longoria M, Chalifoux S, et al. Gastrointestinal hemorrhage after laparoscopic gastric bypass. Obes Surg. 2004;14:1308–12.
72. Sakai P, Kuga R, Safatle-Ribeiro AV, et al. Is it feasible to reach the bypassed stomach after Roux-en-Y gastric bypass for morbid obesity? The use of the double-balloon enteroscope. Endoscopy. 2005;37:566–9.
73. Sundbom M, Nyman R, Hedenstrom H, et al. Investigation of the excluded stomach after Roux-en-Y gastric bypass. Obes Surg. 2001;11:25–7.
74. Baron TH, Chahal P, Ferreira LE. ERCP via mature feeding jejunostomy tube tract in a patient with Roux-en-Y anatomy (with video). Gastrointest Endosc. 2008;68:189.
75. Wright BE, Cass OW, Freeman ML. ERCP in patients with long-limb Roux-en-Y gastrojejunostomy and intact papilla. Gastrointest Endosc. 2002;56:225–32.

76. Lennon AM, Kapoor S, Khashab M, et al. Spiral assisted ERCP is equivalent to single balloon assisted ERCP in patients with Roux-en-Y anatomy. Dig Dis Sci. 2012;57:1391–8.
77. Shah RJ, Smolkin M, Yen R, et al. A multicenter, U.S. experience of single-balloon, double-balloon, and rotational overtube assisted enteroscopy ERCP in patients with surgically altered pancreaticobiliary anatomy (with video). Gastrointest Endosc. 2013;77:593–600.
78. Ceppa FA, Gagne DJ, Papasavas PK, et al. Laparoscopic transgastric endoscopy after Roux-en-Y gastric bypass. Surg Obes Relat Dis. 2007;3:21–4.
79. Martinez J, Guerrero L, Byers P, et al. Endoscopic retrograde cholangiopancreatography and gastroduodenoscopy after Roux-en-Y gastric bypass. Surg Endosc. 2006;20:1548–50.
80. Schreiner MA, Chang L, Gluck M, et al. Laparoscopy-assisted versus balloon enteroscopy-assisted ERCP in bariatric post-Roux-en-Y gastric bypass patients. Gastrointest Endosc. 2012;75:748–56.
81. Baron TH. Approaches to ERCP in patients with Roux-en-Y gastric bypass anatomy. Gastroenterol Hepatol (N Y). 2019;15(11):622–4.

Part IV

Foregut Motility Disorders

17 Achalasia

Luis Serrano, Joel Richter,
Christopher DuCoin,
and Abdul-Rahman Fadi Diab

Case Presentation

A 30-year-old female presents to the office with progressive dysphagia to solids and liquids for the past 6 months. She describes food "sticking" in her mid-chest area and complains of heartburn and food regurgitation after eating. She reports a 28-pound weight loss over the last 6 months and has been seeing a psychologist for an "eating disorder" for the past year. She recently saw a gastroenterologist who performed an upper endoscopy and noted a

L. Serrano
HCA Florida Osceola Surgical Care Specialists, Kissimmee, FL, USA
e-mail: luis.serrano@hcahealthcare.com

J. Richter · C. DuCoin (✉) · A.-R. F. Diab
Division of Gastrointestinal Surgery, Department of Surgery, University of South Florida Morsani College of Medicine, Tampa, FL, USA
e-mail: jrichte1@usf.edu; cducoin@usf.edu; abduldiab@usf.edu

A. D. Patel et al. (eds.), *The SAGES Manual of Physiologic Evaluation of Foregut Diseases*,
https://doi.org/10.1007/978-3-031-39199-6_17

mildly dilated esophagus and difficulty traversing the esophagogastric junction. The gastroenterologist has now ordered a timed barium swallow (TBS) and a high-resolution manometry (HRM). What do we expect to see on TBS and HRM? What are our treatment options?

Introduction

Achalasia is an esophageal motility disorder characterized by failure of the lower esophageal sphincter (LES) mechanism to relax and by disruption of the peristaltic mechanism of the body of the esophagus. Both conditions need to be present to confirm the diagnosis of achalasia. In addition, these symptoms must not be related to other structural or mechanical causes [1]. Achalasia is an uncommon disease that can often be challenging to diagnose and can pose a long and at times frustrating diagnostic process for both the physician and the patient. The reported annual incidence is 1 in 100,000, and the disease has a prevalence of 10 per 100,000 [2, 3]. Achalasia is equally distributed between men and women. It has a bimodal distribution with most patients diagnosed between the ages of 20–40 and 60–70; however, it can also be seen in children [4].

Pathophysiology

Several theories exist that attempt to explain the origin of achalasia; however, no clear explanation has yet to be proven. The fact that it is uncommon in siblings and that it manifests later in life suggests external sources as a possible triggering agent for the development of achalasia. Concepts of viral infections and autoimmune causes have been studied with no consistent evidence to explain the origins of achalasia. As of now, achalasia remains as an idiopathic condition [5].

The normal anatomic function of the esophagus is to allow a food bolus to pass from the oropharynx to the stomach. The bolus moves through the esophagus which transitions from proximal skeletal to distal smooth muscle and traverses both the upper (UES) and the lower esophageal sphincters (LES). These sphincters act as toned muscle that functions to prevent gastric contents from refluxing back into the esophagus and thus preventing aspiration. The muscular function of the esophagus is controlled by the myenteric plexus which contains inhibitory and excitatory neurons. In patients with achalasia, there is a functional loss of the nitric oxide (NO) secreting inhibitory neurons in the myenteric plexus. This loss results in the inability of the LES to relax and failure of peristalsis in the esophageal body [6].

Clinical Presentation

Achalasia presents with a variety of signs and symptoms. The most common clinical complaints are dysphagia, regurgitation, chest pain, and some degree of weight loss. Less common symptoms include epigastric pain, heartburn, and respiratory symptoms secondary to aspiration of regurgitated food and saliva. Patients can present with a single symptom or multiple symptoms. Dysphagia can be for both liquids and solids; however, solids are usually affected first, and then liquids become affected. Dysphagia is caused by failed propulsion of food bolus due to lack of peristalsis and inability of the LES to relax. Heartburn symptoms are related to either retained acidic food in the distal esophagus or to food undergoing the process of fermentation in the esophagus. Physical exam adds little value to the clinical picture; nonetheless, a focused exam can help rule out other conditions that can mimic achalasia as cancer [6].

The Eckardt score is a fast and simple scale (Table 17.1), that aids in making the diagnosis of achalasia and in assessing the

Table 17.1 Eckardt score

Score	Dysphagia	Regurgitation	Chest pain	Weight loss (kg)
0	None	None	None	None
1	Occasional	Occasional	Occasional	<5
2	Daily	Daily	Daily	5–10
3	Every meal	Every meal	Every meal	>10

severity of the disease. It is also a tool that can be used clinically to assess the effectiveness of treatments. It consists of four components addressing degrees of dysphagia, regurgitation, chest pain, and weight loss in kilograms (kg). Each category can receive a score of 0–3 for a maximum of 12 points. If a patient has a score of more than 4 the diagnosis of achalasia should be considered [7].

Diagnostic Workup

If the diagnosis of achalasia is suspected, the workup should start with a barium swallow where the classic "bird's beak" image is seen. We favor the timed barium swallow (TBS) to increase the diagnostic capability of the radiologic evaluation of the esophagus, as this test assesses both esophageal anatomy and upright emptying. To perform a TBS, the patient is given 8 ozs of barium in the upright position and films are obtained at 1- and 5-min intervals (Fig. 17.1). At this point, the esophagus is cleaned of the contrast by drinking water. Lastly, a 13 mm barium pill is swallowed and an additional X-ray is obtained 5 min later. The 13 mm size has been historically used because 13 mm is the size diameter where esophageal strictures are symptomatic [8]. Retention of the barium tablet at 5 min is considered abnormal as well as a liquid barium column greater than 5 cm at the 1-min interval and 2 cm at 5-min interval [9, 10]. A key criteria is liquid retention which shows an 85% accuracy for the diagnosis of achalasia and hold up of the pill which shows a 100% accuracy in achalasia patients [10].

Esophagogastroduodenoscopy (EGD) is a mandatory workup for achalasia to aid with the diagnosis and to rule out pseudoachalasia. Pseudoachalasia is defined as an invasive tumor, usually adenocarcinoma, or an extrinsic compression that mimics the symptoms and the imaging studies of achalasia. In patients with achalasia, there can be a wide variety of findings from normal esophageal anatomy to a markedly dilated esophagus with retained food particles on EGD. In addition, increased resistance can be encountered during passage of the scope through the gas-

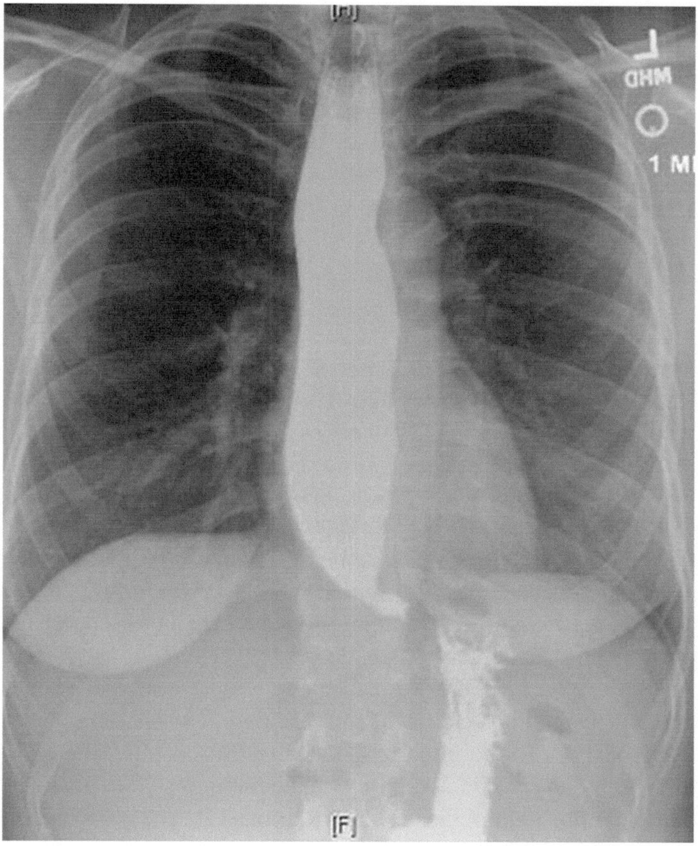

Fig. 17.1 Barium swallow shows a persistently narrowed region at the end of the esophagus (the lower esophageal sphincter) with a positive bird's beak sign and a dilated esophagus above the narrowed region

troesophageal junction, which should alert the endoscopist to the possibility of achalasia. In some cases, puckering of the GE junction can be appreciated by the endoscopist [11].

EGD and TBS aid in the diagnosis of achalasia; however, the final diagnosis is not made until confirmatory high-resolution manometry (HRM) is performed. HRM is considered the gold standard in the diagnosis of achalasia. HRM can distinguish

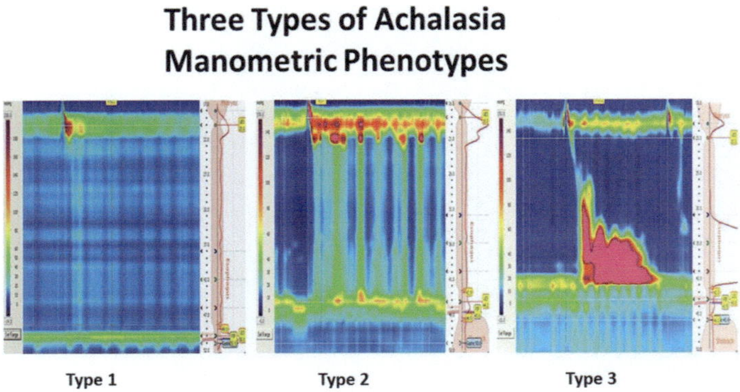

Fig. 17.2 High-resolution manometry (HMR) exemplifying the difference between achalasia types I, II, and III

between three different types of achalasia [12]. HRM evaluates the esophageal motility using a catheter with 36 pressure sensors spaced every 1 cm along its length. The catheter is placed into the nose and advanced into the stomach. Once in place, the patient completes 10 swallows of 5 ml of saline that are then mapped in a pressure and time chart (Fig. 17.2) [13].

During HRM, patients with achalasia will have several characteristics, including failed LES relaxation with swallowing and a hypertensive LES baseline in about 50% of patients. There are three subtypes of achalasia based on the findings of HRM, classified according to the Chicago classification [14]. The combination of TBS and HRM has been studied and together they increase the diagnostic accuracy for achalasia to nearly 100% [10].

Chicago Classification

The Chicago classification is the universal method of interpreting HRM. It was initially published in 2009 and updated in the 2015 consensus to version 3.0 (v3.0). It is important to understand the parameters reported by HRM. These include the UES, the body of the esophagus, the LES, and the intrabolus pressure pattern. The esophageal body is evaluated by both contraction strength and peristalsis. Contraction strength is expressed by the distal contractile index (DCI). A normal DCI is between 450 and 8000 mmHg × cm × s. The DCI can be subclassified as failed if less than 100 mmHg × cm × s, ineffective if 100–450 mmHg × cm × s or hypercontractile when greater than 8000 mmHg × cm × s (Table 17.2). Peristalsis is evaluated by the distal latency (DL), which measures the period from the beginning of the contractile wave to the contractile deceleration point. LES function is expressed by the integrated relaxation pressure (IRP) and basal pressure (BP) of the LES. Lastly, the intrabolus pressure pattern corresponds to areas of the esophagus with a pressure greater than 30 mmHg. Based on the manometric findings, esophageal motility disorders are categorized as either distal disorders with esophagogastric junction outflow obstruction or major disorders and minor disorders of peristalsis [13, 14].

Achalasia falls into the esophagogastric junction outflow obstruction group. In achalasia, there are two issues with the esophagus as follows: (1) incomplete relaxation of the LES expressed as an elevated IRP greater than 15 mmHg and (2) some degree of failed peristalsis. Achalasia is further subdivided into three categories based on the manometry findings, specifically based on the type of peristalsis irregularity. Achalasia type I involves an elevated IRP and 100% failed esophageal contractions. Type II achalasia is the most common type and has an elevated IRP; however, there is panesophageal pressurization in at least 20% of the swallows. Type III achalasia has similar characteristics of IRP and LES, but there are more than 20% spastic contractions on swallows (Fig. 17.2) [15]. Achalasia can evolve into stage IV achalasia, also known as sigmoid type or end-stage achalasia. It consists of a severely enlarged and tortuous esophagus that on imaging resembles a sigmoid colon. There is no mano-

Table 17.2 Distal contractile index (values in mmHg × cm × s)

Failed	Ineffective	Normal	Hypercontractile
<100	100–450	450–8000	>8000

metric equivalent for stage IV achalasia; thus, the diagnosis is made based on descriptive findings on EGD and barium swallow rather than manometry [16].

An additional subtype of the EGJ obstructive condition that is like achalasia but does not meet criteria for achalasia is called esophagogastric junction outlet obstruction (EGJOO). It is characterized by elevated IRP and failed relaxation of the LES. However, normal esophageal contractility is preserved [17].

Treatment

Achalasia cannot be cured. At best treatment is palliative as the disease persists even after all treatment modalities. It is thus vital to discuss with patients the goals and expectations regarding treatment and that interventions are not for cure but rather to improve quality of life and prevent complications such as megaesophagus. As mentioned above, achalasia encompasses two problems, the esophagogastric obstruction and the dysmotility of the esophagus. Currently, there is no treatment for the dysmotility portion of this disease. Treatments efforts are therefore focused toward the obstruction of the distal esophagus [4, 17].

Treatment strategies can be medical, endoscopic, and/or surgical. Medical management with calcium channel blockers like nifedipine or nitrates has shown limited success and is reserved for patients who cannot tolerate a more invasive approach.

Botulinum toxin injection is a temporary treatment modality for achalasia. Typically, 100 units of botulinum toxin are injected into four quadrants of LES. This relaxes the LES by blocking the release of acetylcholine. It is particularly beneficial in older patients that would otherwise not tolerate more invasive procedures [17]. The limitation of botulinum toxin is its short duration of action with only 3–6 months of symptom relief and limited success in subsequent injections [16].

Pneumatic dilatation is the most efficient nonsurgical treatment available. Pneumatic dilators are preferentially performed since they can split the circular fibers of the esophagus which translates into a more effective treatment. Both endoscopic and fluoroscopic guidance can be used to aid in the usage of the dilators. Multiple achalasia balloon sizes exist as 30, 35, and 40 mm [18]. There are variable reports on the success of pneumatic dilation. Overall, pneumatic dilation is 60% effective when using the smallest 30 mm balloon, but using the 35 mm balloon increases the success rate to near 90% [12]. Pneumatic dilation has been shown to be successful in about 60% of patients at 5 years after several treatments; however, symptom relief decreases over time. Some situations like age less than 40 years can predict poor success of dilation [19]. If there is failure of symptom improvement with the first two treatments, pneumatic dilation will unlikely resolve symptoms. In patients with high LES pressure (more than 15–30 mmHg), or if the LES pressure did not drop to more than 50% from the pretreatment numbers, pneumatic dilation will likely fail. Complications associated with pneumatic dilation include perforation (incidence of 1.6%), bleeding, and reflux [16]. The risk of perforation increases with the increase in balloon size. However, dilation to 35 mm and even 40 mm is relatively safe when it is preceded by an initial 30 mm dilation [20].

Surgical myotomy is referred to as a Heller myotomy. It was originally described by Ernest Heller in 1914 and can provide relief of symptoms in approximately 85–100% of patients. Recent minimally invasive approaches to this operation have made it better tolerated by patients. A study reported that the therapeutic success rate of this approach is 93% and 90% after 1 and 2 years, respectively [21]. In the current era, it can be performed either laparoscopically or robotically. The procedure involves the mobilization of the distal esophagus and proximal stomach with a myotomy that must include the inner muscular circular fibers. The external longitudinal fibers and the internal circular fibers can be divided using variable methods as hook cautery, ultrasonic dissection, or blunt dissection. The myotomy should be extended 6 cm onto the esophagus and at least 2 cm onto the gastric muscle [6].

During a Heller myotomy, fundoplication may be performed. It is thought that adding a fundoplication to the myotomy will prevent reflux since the LES mechanism is lost [22]. A systematic review found after a mean follow-up of 26.6 months that the rates of reflux and esophagitis following myotomy with fundoplication are 16.8%

and 7.6%, respectively [23]. However, both the addition of a fundoplication and best type of fundoplication have been debated. Dor fundoplication (anterior 180-degree fundoplication) provides reflux prevention, avoids dissection posterior to the esophagus, and covers the exposed mucosa of the myotomy. Toupet fundoplication (posterior 270-degree fundoplication) is believed to provide a greater antireflux mechanism. The sutures placed on the cut end of the muscle also help keep the myotomy open. Unlike Dor fundoplication, there is no coverage of the myotomy with the Toupet fundoplication [24, 25]. Intraoperative endoscopy is recommended to assess for completion of myotomy and rule out leak.

Peroral endoscopic myotomy (POEM) was first introduced by Dr. Inoue in 2009. POEM is performed entirely endoscopically. The procedures begins with a mucosotomy and accessing the submucosal space. This spaced is used to start the submucosal tunnel, usually begining in the mid to upper esopahgus. This submucosal tunnel will then go roughly 3 cm past the LES. The myotomy is then created roughly from 2 cm distal to the LES on the gastric side, to within 2–3 cm of the origional mucosotomy. Thus the myotomy can be extremely long when performing a POEM, making it an excellent treatment choice for type III achalasia. At the completion of the case the mucosotmy is closed with endoscopic clips. POEM has good efficacy in most patients with achalasia. It is rapidly gaining traction as another gold-standard treatment for achalasia. A systematic review compared the clinical success of POEM against pneumatic dilation (PD). The clinical success with POEM was superior to PD at 12, 24, and 36 months. In addition, POEM was superior to PD in type I, II, and III achalasia, and pooled odds ratio of clinical success at 12 and 24 months were significantly higher with POEM. However, pooled odds ratio of GERD was significantly higher with POEM [26]. Another systematic review compared the risk of GERD and esophagitis after POEM against laparoscopic Heller's myotomy and fundoplication (LHM). The pooled rate of abnormal acid exposure according to pH studies was 39.0% after POEM and 16.8% after LHM, and the rate of esophagitis was 29.4% after POEM and 7.6% after LHM [23].

POEM is particularly useful in patients with type III achalasia, due to long segments of spastic contractions and POEM's ability to create a long myotomy [27]. POEM is well tolerated with good symptomatic improvement. Some potential complications include both pneumothorax and pneumoperitoneum which are decreased by using CO_2 instead of air for insufflation. Another possible complication is bleeding within myotomy tunnel or inadvertent mucosotomy [16, 17, 28]. A study compared rates of serious adverse events following POEM against laparoscopic Heller's myotomy (LHM), and they reported rates of 2.7% and 7.3% for POEM and LHM, respectively. POEM is as safe as LHM if not even safer [29].

Unlike a Heller myotomy, POEM does not include an antireflux procedure such as a Dor or Toupet fundoplication. Due to the lack of an antireflux operation, post-POEM patients can experience gastrointestinal reflux disease up to 50% of the time. Evidence of reflux can even be seen in asymptomatic patients. For this reason, it is good practice to follow POEM patients for reflux using endoscopy. Some advocate treating patients with a proton pump inhibitor (PPI) post-POEM to prevent acid reflux complications such as peptic stricture, Barrett's esophagus, and esophageal cancer [28]. Since its inception, POEM has gained acceptance and been utilized as a treatment modality around the world.

Esophagectomy is reserved as a last resort for end-stage achalasia with megaesophagus. Myotomy, either surgical or endoscopic, will relax the LES, but there is currently no therapy for the aperistalsis seen in achalasia. In these instances, esophagectomy should be considered in patients that have already undergone an appropriate myotomy with resting low LES pressures, a dilated or megaesophagus, and persistent symptoms [6].

Achalasia is a complex disease that requires a combined approach of a primary care physician, a gastroenterologist, and a surgeon for the diagnosis, treatment, and follow-up of such patients. The diagnosis can occasionally be challenging. It is crucial to understand the pathophysiology, the diagnostic algorithm, and the treatment options. At best, the interventions are palliative and not therapeutic, and the risk of disease progression is always present. A key aspect in the treatment of achalasia is having a well-informed and continuous dialog with the patient, so that they are fully informed regarding realistic treatment expectations.

Editors' Note

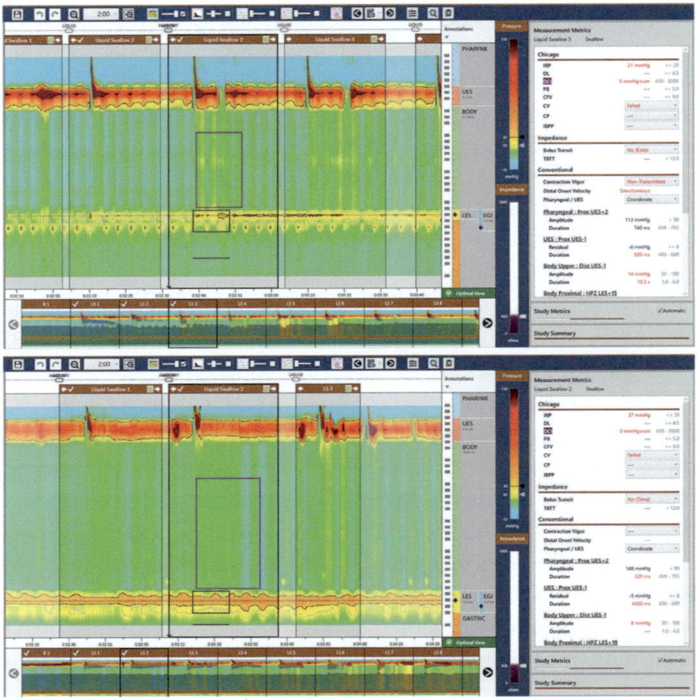

Type 1 achalasia

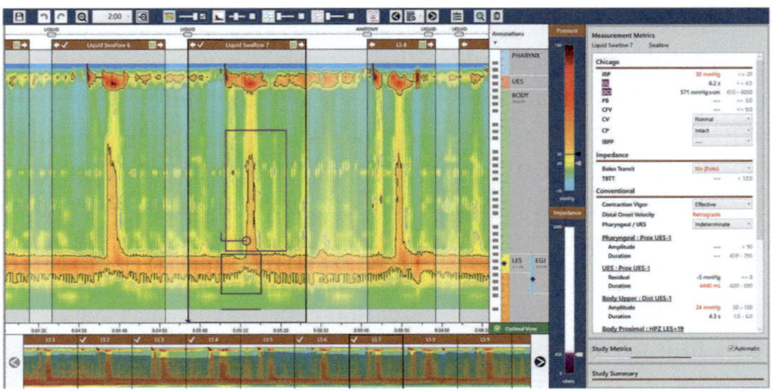

Type 2 achalasia

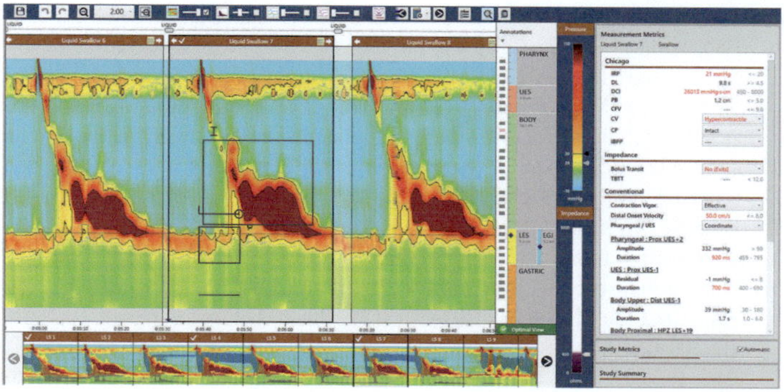

Type 3 achalasia

References

1. Ross D, Richter J, Velanovich V. Health-related quality of life and physiological measurements in achalasia. Dis Esophagus. 2017;30(2):1–5. https://doi.org/10.1111/dote.12494.
2. Niebisch S, Hadzijusufovic E, Mehdorn M, et al. Achalasia-an unnecessary long way to diagnosis. Dis Esophagus. 2017;30(5):1–6. https://doi.org/10.1093/dote/dow004.
3. Kahrilas PJ, Bredenoord AJ, Fox M, et al. Expert consensus document: advances in the management of oesophageal motility disorders in the era of high-resolution manometry: a focus on achalasia syndromes. Nat Rev Gastroenterol Hepatol. 2017;14(11):677–88. https://doi.org/10.1038/nrgastro.2017.132.
4. Swanström LL. Achalasia: treatment, current status and future advances. Korean J Intern Med. 2019;34(6):1173–80. https://doi.org/10.3904/kjim.2018.439.
5. Farrukh A, Mayberry JF. Achalasia: an epidemiology update. Esophagus. 2015;2(12):170–4. https://doi.org/10.1007/s10388-014-0475-z.
6. Schlottmann F, Neto RML, Herbella FAM, Patti MG. Esophageal achalasia: pathophysiology, clinical presentation, and diagnostic evaluation. Am Surg. 2018;84(4):467–72.
7. Slone S, Kumar A, Jacobs J, Velanovich V, Richter JE. Accuracy of achalasia quality of life and Eckardt scores for assessment of clinical improvement post treatment for achalasia. Dis Esophagus. 2021;34(2):doaa080. https://doi.org/10.1093/dote/doaa080.

8. Desai JP, Moustarah F. Esophageal stricture. In: StatPearls. StatPearls Publishing; 2022. http://www.ncbi.nlm.nih.gov/books/NBK542209/. Accessed 31 May 2022.
9. de Oliveira JM, Birgisson S, Doinoff C, et al. Timed barium swallow: a simple technique for evaluating esophageal emptying in patients with achalasia. AJR Am J Roentgenol. 1997;169(2):473–9. https://doi.org/10.2214/ajr.169.2.9242756.
10. Blonski W, Kumar A, Feldman J, Richter JE. Timed barium swallow: diagnostic role and predictive value in untreated achalasia, Esophagogastric junction outflow obstruction, and non-achalasia dysphagia. Am J Gastroenterol. 2018;113(2):196–203. https://doi.org/10.1038/ajg.2017.370.
11. Ates F, Vaezi MF. The pathogenesis and management of achalasia: current status and future directions. Gut Liver. 2015;9(4):449–63. https://doi.org/10.5009/gnl14446.
12. Moonen A, Boeckxstaens G. Current diagnosis and management of achalasia. J Clin Gastroenterol. 2014;48(6):484–90. https://doi.org/10.1097/MCG.0000000000000137.
13. Ju H, Ma Y, Liang K, Zhang C, Tian Z. Function of high-resolution manometry in the analysis of peroral endoscopic myotomy for achalasia. Surg Endosc. 2016;30(3):1094–9. https://doi.org/10.1007/s00464-015-4304-9.
14. Schlottmann F, Herbella FA, Patti MG. Understanding the Chicago classification: from tracings to patients. J Neurogastroenterol Motil. 2017;23(4):487–94. https://doi.org/10.5056/jnm17026.
15. Kahrilas PJ, Bredenoord AJ, Fox M, et al. The Chicago classification of esophageal motility disorders, v3.0. Neurogastroenterol Motil. 2015;27(2):160–74. https://doi.org/10.1111/nmo.12477.
16. Stefanidis D, Richardson W, Farrell TM, et al. SAGES guidelines for the surgical treatment of esophageal achalasia. Surg Endosc. 2012;26(2):296–311. https://doi.org/10.1007/s00464-011-2017-2.
17. Schlottmann F, Herbella F, Allaix ME, Patti MG. Modern management of esophageal achalasia: from pathophysiology to treatment. Curr Probl Surg. 2018;55(1):10–37. https://doi.org/10.1067/j.cpsurg.2018.01.001.
18. Mikaeli J, Bishehsari F, Montazeri G, Yaghoobi M, Malekzadeh R. Pneumatic balloon dilatation in achalasia: a prospective comparison of safety and efficacy with different balloon diameters. Aliment Pharmacol Ther. 2004;20(4):431–6. https://doi.org/10.1111/j.1365-2036.2004.02080.x.
19. Ghoshal UC, Rangan M. A review of factors predicting outcome of pneumatic dilation in patients with achalasia cardia. J Neurogastroenterol Motil. 2011;17(1):9–13. https://doi.org/10.5056/jnm.2011.17.1.9.
20. van Hoeij FB, Prins LI, Smout AJPM, Bredenoord AJ. Efficacy and safety of pneumatic dilation in achalasia: a systematic review and meta-

analysis. Neurogastroenterol Motil. 2019;31(7):e13548. https://doi.org/10.1111/nmo.13548.
21. Boeckxstaens GE, Annese V, des Varannes SB, et al. Pneumatic dilation versus laparoscopic Heller's myotomy for idiopathic achalasia. N Engl J Med. 2011;364(19):1807–16. https://doi.org/10.1056/NEJMoa1010502.
22. Richards WO, Torquati A, Holzman MD, et al. Heller myotomy versus Heller myotomy with dor fundoplication for achalasia. Ann Surg. 2004;240(3):405–15. https://doi.org/10.1097/01.sla.0000136940.32255.51.
23. Repici A, Fuccio L, Maselli R, et al. GERD after per-oral endoscopic myotomy as compared with Heller's myotomy with fundoplication: a systematic review with meta-analysis. Gastrointest Endosc. 2018;87(4):934–943.e18. https://doi.org/10.1016/j.gie.2017.10.022.
24. Patel DA, Lappas BM, Vaezi MF. An overview of achalasia and its subtypes. Gastroenterol Hepatol. 2017;13(7):411–21.
25. Rawlings A, Soper NJ, Oelschlager B, et al. Laparoscopic dor versus Toupet fundoplication following Heller myotomy for achalasia: results of a multicenter, prospective, randomized-controlled trial. Surg Endosc. 2012;26(1):18–26. https://doi.org/10.1007/s00464-011-1822-y.
26. Ofosu A, Mohan BP, Ichkhanian Y, et al. Peroral endoscopic myotomy (POEM) vs pneumatic dilation (PD) in treatment of achalasia: a meta-analysis of studies with ≥ 12-month follow-up. Endosc Int Open. 2021;9(7):E1097–107. https://doi.org/10.1055/a-1483-9406.
27. Hamer PW, Holloway RH, Heddle R, Devitt PG, Thompson SK. Type III achalasia—a clinical description. Dis Esophagus. 2017;30(8):1–6. https://doi.org/10.1093/dote/dox051.
28. Inoue H, Minami H, Kobayashi Y, et al. Peroral endoscopic myotomy (POEM) for esophageal achalasia. Endoscopy. 2010;42(4):265–71. https://doi.org/10.1055/s-0029-1244080.
29. Werner YB, Hakanson B, Martinek J, et al. Endoscopic or surgical myotomy in patients with idiopathic achalasia. N Engl J Med. 2019;381(23):2219–29. https://doi.org/10.1056/NEJMoa1905380.

Minor Disorders of Esophageal Motility

18

Amy Banks-Venegoni, Justin Hsu, and Gregory Fritz

Ineffective Esophageal Motility

Ineffective esophageal motility (IEM) is a manometric diagnosis that is defined as greater than or equal to 50% ineffective swallows that can be combinations of failed or weak (distal contractile integral <450 mmHg·s·cm) swallows with a normal lower esophageal sphincter relaxation pressure of less than 15 mmHg·s·cm [1]. It is associated with impaired bolus transit through the esophagus and nonobstructive dysphagia. This disorder is reportedly found in as high as 30% of patients undergoing high-resolution manometry (HRM) and as many as 17% of asymptomatic patients [2]. IEM has been found to have a higher prevalence in smooth muscle disorders like scleroderma and other diseases that affect neuron function like Parkinson's disease and ALS [3]. The pathophysiology of IEM has therefore been investigated and theorized to arise

A. Banks-Venegoni (✉)
Spectrum Health Medical Group and Corewell Health West-Department of Surgery, Michigan State School of Medicine, East Lansing, MI, USA
e-mail: Amy.banksvenegoni@Corewellhealth.org

J. Hsu · G. Fritz
Corewell Health General Surgery Residency, Michigan State School of Medicine, East Lansing, MI, USA
e-mail: Justin_Hsu@med.unc.edu; Gregory.fritz@Corewellhealth.org

A. D. Patel et al. (eds.), *The SAGES Manual of Physiologic Evaluation of Foregut Diseases*,
https://doi.org/10.1007/978-3-031-39199-6_18

from a combination of neuronal factors that disrupt the circular muscle contraction, esophageal shortening (from longitudinal muscle contraction), and esophageal muscle tone that participate in primary esophageal peristalsis [4]. Impaired secondary peristalsis that is triggered by esophageal distension may also play a significant role in the underlying cause of IEM.

Patients with IEM often have a wide range of symptoms that include cough, heartburn, regurgitation, chest pressure, and dysphagia which makes the diagnosis difficult. The typical workup to distinguish the etiology of these symptoms includes esophagogastroduodenoscopy (EGD), upper GI contrast study (UGI), pH testing, and high-resolution manometry (HRM). IEM impairs esophageal clearance and therefore can participate in the pathophysiology of gastroesophageal reflux disease (GERD) [5]. Patients with IEM and normal pH studies are younger than those with abnormal pH testing, suggesting that IEM could be an early primary event that subsequently leads to abnormal acid burden [6]; however, further studies need to be performed to confirm this. Patients with chronic cough have a higher likelihood of esophageal hypomotility, lower contraction amplitude, and vigor [7]. Identification of severe IEM (>70% ineffective peristalsis) provides supportive evidence for a more severe GERD phenotype marked by supine acid burden [8].

There is no pharmacologic intervention that reliably restores esophageal smooth muscle contractility or improves symptoms. Therefore, unless GERD is identified, symptomatic patients with IEM are challenging to treat. Dietary restriction and lifestyle changes typically recommended to patients with GERD remain the mainstay of clinical IEM management. With the hypothesis that dietary fiber binds nitric oxide (NO) contained in food and could reduce the inhibitory effects of NO in the esophagus, psyllium (15 g/day) was reported to decrease esophageal dysphagia and increase LES resting pressure in patients with GERD [9, 10]. However, effects on esophageal contractility were not reported in this open-label study. Alternative therapies are popular, as they decrease esophageal sensitivity and symptom perception and may benefit esophageal contractility. A pilot study of patients with PPI refractory GERD demonstrated significant increase in esophageal contraction vigor 10 min after an osteopathic intervention on the diaphragm, but long-term effects on esophageal symptoms are unknown [11].

Conventional prokinetic agents (metoclopramide, domperidone) have not been proven to be beneficial in IEM. There are limited data on newer prokinetic agents like mosapride, a 5HT-4 agonist, which may facilitate secondary peristalsis induced by rapid air distension in patients with IEM but had no improvement in primary and secondary esophageal contraction vigor [9, 12]. Buspirone, a mixed partial 5HT-1A agonist and dopamine D2 receptor antagonist, increased esophageal contraction amplitudes and decreased reflux symptoms in scleroderma patients [9, 13, 14], but was not more effective than placebo in patients with IEM and dysphagia [15].

No specific management strategy has been favored over another. Treatment options revolve around management of symptoms for each individual patient. If IEM patients are found to have GERD refractory to pharmacologic management and are pursuing antireflux surgery, then a partial (270-degree) Toupet fundoplication is the surgical treatment of choice so as to not further exacerbate poor esophageal clearance.

Patient Scenarios

1. JV is a 66-year-old female presenting with dysphagia who previously was diagnosed with reflux many years ago. She takes a proton pump inhibitor (PPI) twice daily without symptomatic improvement. Her main complaint is dysphagia to thicker food groups and pills. She endorses early satiety without weight loss and regurgitation of liquids when supine. She denies true heartburn-like symptoms or odynophagia. UGI showed small sliding hiatal hernia without reflux. EGD confirmed hiatal hernia without eosinophilia. pH study had a normal DeMeester score of 0.5 with normal percent time spent in reflux. HRM with normal upper esophageal sphincter (UES) pressures, normal lower esophageal sphincter (LES) pressures, weak distal contractile integral (DCI) with mean of 425 mmHg·s·cm, abnormal peristalsis with 40% weak and 70% ineffective swallows, and 70% incomplete bolus clearance (Figs. 18.1, 18.2, and 18.3). The patient was treated with lifestyle modification only with moderate improvement in symptoms.
2. SB is a 65-year-old male presenting with burning sensation and chest pressure after eating. He endorses liquid regurgita-

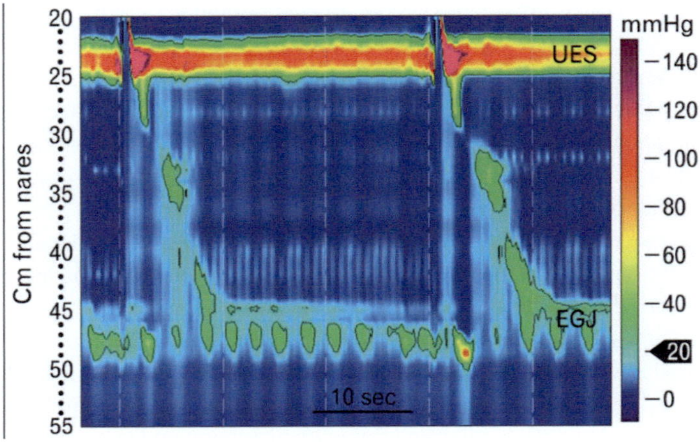

Fig. 18.1 Weak esophageal contractile force with normal peristalsis

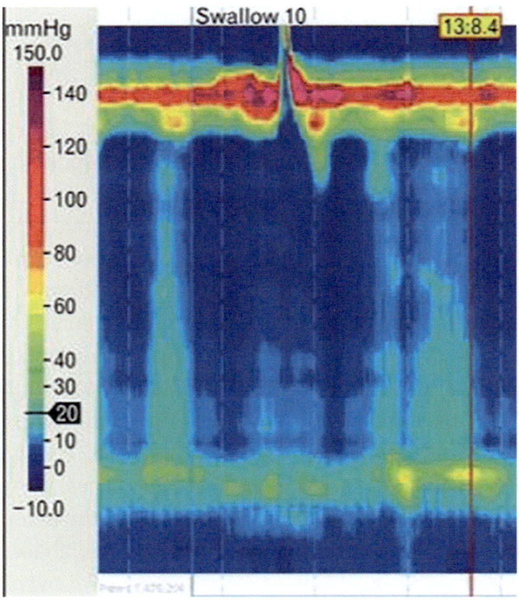

Fig. 18.2 Failed swallow

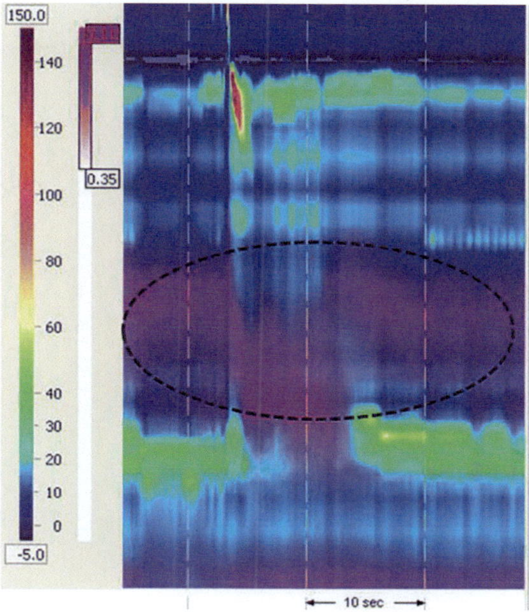

Fig. 18.3 Delayed esophageal bolus clearance by impedance data

tion into his throat mostly at night while supine. He denies dysphagia or shortness of breath. Diet modification and antacid therapy have not provided symptomatic improvement. UGI suggested slightly dilated distal esophagus without delay in passage of contrast or tablet into the stomach and small sliding hiatal hernia. EGD demonstrated normal appearing esophagus with small hiatal hernia and without eosinophilia. pH study confirms GERD by elevated DeMeester score of 21 and high percent time spent in reflux at 6.8%. Heartburn and cough were associated with reflux events by symptom association probability (SAP) of 98% and 99%. HRM demonstrates normal UES resting and relaxation pressures, normal LES resting and relaxation pressures, weak DCI with mean of 398 mmHg·s·cm, abnormal peristalsis with 50% weak and 60% failed swallows, and 40% incomplete bolus clearance (Figs. 18.4 and 18.5). The patient was treated for his GERD with laparoscopic hiatal hernia repair and Toupet fundoplication with resolution in preoperative symptoms.

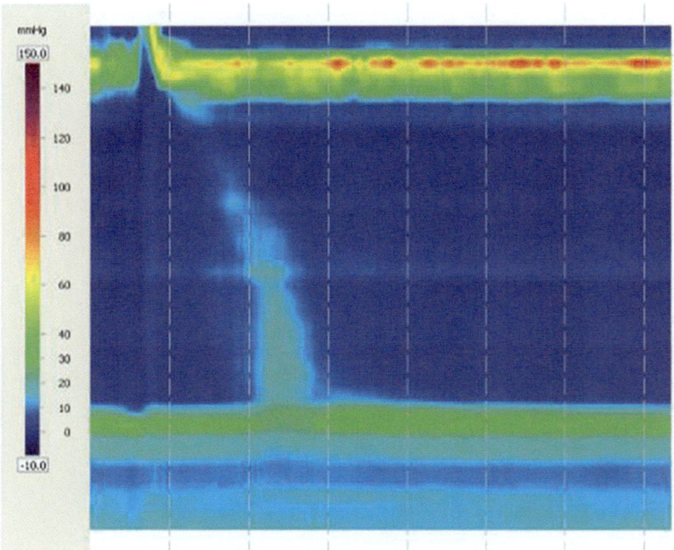

Fig. 18.4 Weak and ineffective esophageal contraction

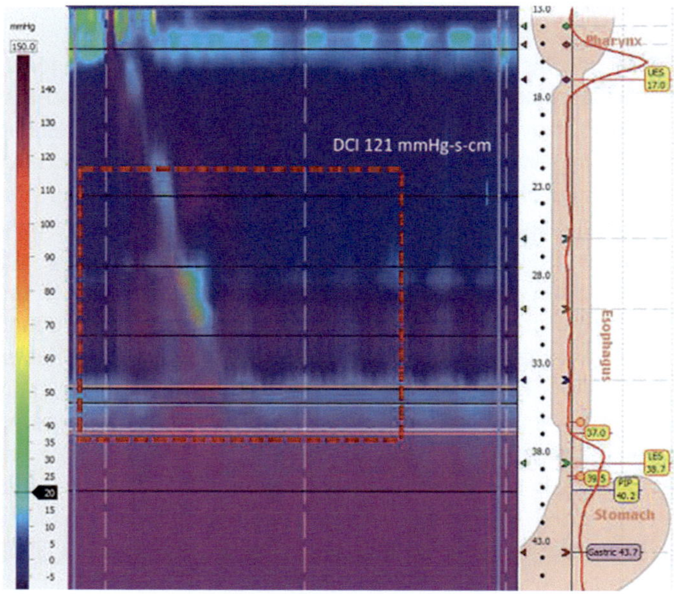

Fig. 18.5 Delayed esophageal bolus clearance by impedance data

Fragmented Peristalsis

Fragmented peristalsis (FP) is defined by the Chicago Classification v3.0 (CC3.0) in 2014 by HRM demonstrating greater than or equal to 50% of fragmented contractions (each with >5 cm break in the 20 mmHg isobaric contour) with a normal distal contractile integral (DCI) and normal lower esophageal sphincter (LES) relaxation pressure [2]. The CC3.0 simplified the descriptions of peristaltic function and retired the terms defined in the 2012 Chicago Classification (CC2.0), namely "weak peristalsis with small breaks" and "weak peristalsis with large breaks," by making contractile vigor (based solely on DCI) independent of contraction pattern (based on latency and breaks). The new classification clarifying diagnostic criteria subsequently not only reduced the number of diagnoses classified as minor motility disorders, but also reduced the number of patients diagnosed with a minor motility disorder [2, 16].

The pathophysiology of FP is unknown but thought to be due to an abnormality of esophageal peristalsis at the transition zone between the proximal and distal contractile segments. This results in a break of the contractile contour that causes incomplete bolus transit [1, 17]. Of note, a normal esophageal peristalsis topography already consists of three natural troughs: one dividing proximal skeletal muscle from distal smooth muscle, one dividing the distal smooth muscle into two contraction segments, and one between the distal smooth muscle segment and LES [18]. The first trough of the esophagus is also the most distinctive on topography as it signifies the transition zone (also termed intersegmental trough) between the proximal and distal contractile segments, which corresponds to the interface between different muscle fiber types and neural control mechanism [1, 19, 20]. A transition zone with a measurement of 2 cm or 1 s in size was identified as the 95th percentile in asymptomatic patients [19]. To correlate these measurements with actual bolus clearance, a high-resolution impedance manometry study revealed that incomplete bolus transit was only found in 16% of the patients with breaks <5 cm, as opposed to 100% of the patients with breaks exceeding 5 cm in length, which became the basis for the definition of FP [17].

Since the new classification, there have been no studies that examined the prevalence of FP in asymptomatic patients. One study that specifically looked at the difference in prevalence between CC3.0 and CC2.0 examined minor disorders of peristalsis and noted a prevalence of 15% in healthy volunteers (down from 25.2% of CC2.0) and 33.3% in symptomatic patients (up from 24.5% in CC2.0) [16]. The study suggested an increase in the prevalence of minor disorders of peristalsis with abnormal results as the diagnostic criteria became more stringent and less asymptomatic patients were diagnosed. A study by Dan Wang et al. from China, assessed patients presenting with a predominant symptom of dysphagia and a normal EGD and found fragmented peristalsis had a prevalence of 16.1% [21].

Like IEM, patients with FP often have a wide range of symptoms that can include cough, heartburn, dysphagia, or regurgitation. Retrospectively, FP has been associated with GERD and Barrett's esophagus [1, 22, 23]. Using HRM, recent studies show that failed peristalsis and fragmented peristalsis had a higher significant correlation with reflux burden as opposed to weak peristalsis, which further supports the new metrics found in CC3.0 [24].

There is no pharmacologic intervention that will restore the break in esophageal peristalsis or improve symptoms. Therefore, unless GERD is identified, symptomatic patients with FP are challenging to treat. In GERD patients undergoing fundoplication without dysphagia symptoms but had a preoperative diagnosis of fragmented peristalsis, current evidence showed no correlation from these diagnoses with post-fundoplication dysphagia in short-term follow-up [25, 26]. However, the question regarding whether to perform a total versus partial fundoplication in GERD patients with dysphagia from FP remains controversial. Newer provocative maneuvers such as multiple rapid swallows (MRS) demonstrate contraction reserve, which detects abnormalities in inhibitory and excitatory esophageal motor function. When the contraction following the last swallow is weak in an MRS maneuver, an impaired integrity of neural excitation and muscle is predicted. Patients with abnormal MRS contraction have increased risk of prolonged bolus transit and poor bolus clearance. MRS evaluation can help identify patients who are at higher risk for post-fundoplication dysphagia [27–29].

Patient Scenario

1. HG is a 76-year-old male presenting with reflux symptoms for 20 years that have worsened over the past 6 months. Symptoms consist of bloating, chest pain, chronic cough, regurgitation of saliva and mucus when supine, and spicy food intolerance. He denies abdominal pain, dysphagia, emesis, food impaction, heartburn, hematemesis, nausea, or odynophagia. Lifestyle modifications including decreased meal size, avoiding spicy foods, not eating 5 h prior to bedtime, and elevating the head of the bed have provided minimal symptomatic relief. The patient has taken a PPI for years with some relief. UGI demonstrated delayed distention in the distal esophagus secondary to multiple, persistent tertiary contractions, and insufficient primary peristaltic waves with moderate esophageal dysmotility. EGD identified mild esophagitis confirmed on biopsy and grade II flap valve. pH study revealed a normal DeMeester score of 0.6 and normal % time spent in reflux at 0.1%. Heartburn was not correlated to reflux events. HRM demonstrated normal UES resting and relaxation pressures, normal LES resting and relaxation pressures, normal LES length, normal DCI, 70% fragmented peristaltic waves, and 100% incomplete bolus clearance (Figs. 18.6 and 18.7). The patient was counseled that his symptoms were due to esophageal stasis and was instructed to continue lifestyle modifications that help with esophageal emptying.

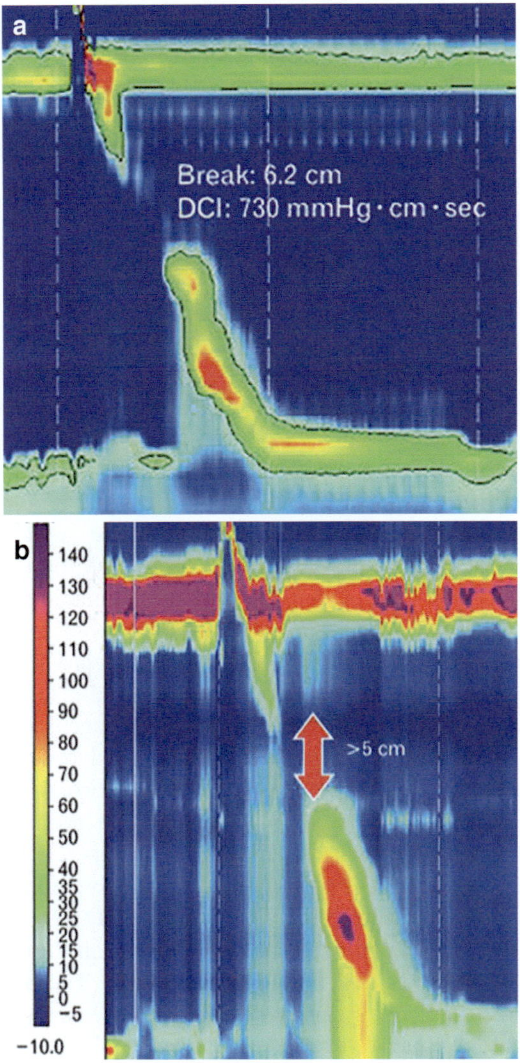

Fig. 18.6 Fragmented swallows

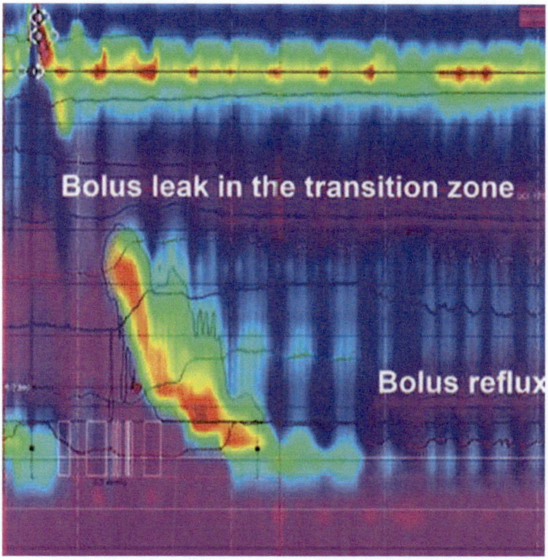

Fig. 18.7 Esophageal stasis and delayed clearance by impedance data

Editors' Note

IEM

IEM in a patient with longstanding GERD and a hiatal hernia.

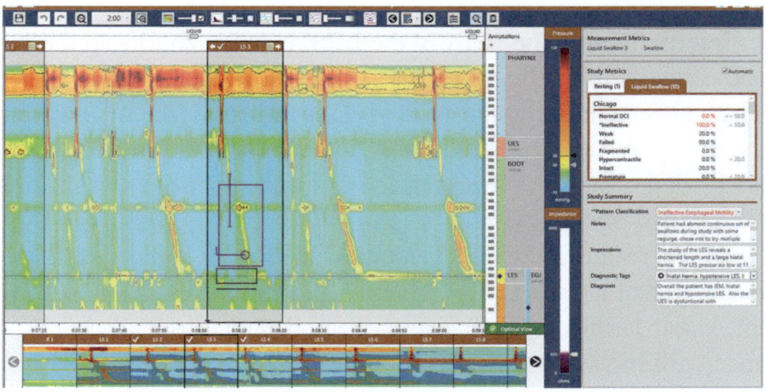

The study of the LES reveals a shortened length and a large hiatal hernia. The LES pressure is low at 11 mmHg and relaxes

completely. The esophageal body study demonstrates normal peristalsis and low contraction amplitudes (DEA 16 mmHg, DCI of 56). Bolus transit is fair at 50%. Overall, the patient has IEM, hiatal hernia, and hypotensive LES. Also, the UES is dysfunctional with non-coordinated contractions and does not relax.

IEM with dysphagia/heartburn: dysphagia of solid food only sticking to the mid-lower chest for the past 2–3 years occurring about once a week that improves with smaller bites; heartburn presenting as a burning sensation for the past 10–12 years occurring 3–4 times a week with certain foods late at night that goes away with Tums; also complains of a raspy voice and cough. Stopped taking Protonix almost 2 months ago.

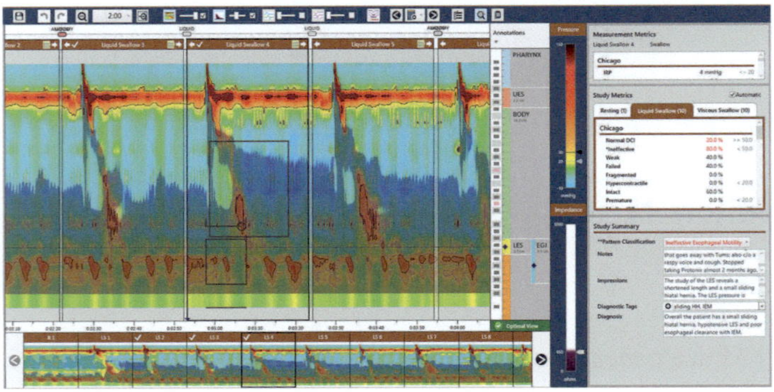

Interpretation: The study of the LES reveals a shortened length and a small sliding hiatal hernia. The LES pressure is negligible. The hiatus appears tighter. With viscous materials, the LES was in the hiatus and showed minimal relaxation. The esophageal body study demonstrates 80% ineffective swallows (40% weak and 40% failed swallows) and amplitudes of only 35 mmHg (DCI 225). There are increased velocities seen with some swallows. Bolus transit is poor (10%). Overall, the patient has a small sliding hiatal hernia, hypotensive LES, and poor esophageal clearance with IEM.

References

1. Porter RF, Kumar N, Drapekin JE, Gyawali CP. Fragmented esophageal smooth muscle contraction segments on high resolution manometry: a marker of esophageal hypomotility. Neurogastroenterol Motil. 2012;24:763–e353.
2. Kahrilas PJ, Bredenoord AJ, Fox M, Gyawali CP, Roman S, Smout AJ, Pandolfino JE. The Chicago classification of esophageal motility disorders, v3.0. Neurogastroenterol Motil. 2015;27:160–74.
3. Carlson DA, Crowell MD, Kimmel JN, et al. Loss of peristaltic reserve, determined by multiple rapid swallows, is the most frequent esophageal motility abnormality in patients with systemic sclerosis. Clin Gastroenterol Hepatol. 2016;14:1502–6.
4. Mittal RK. Regulation and dysregulation of esophageal peristalsis by the integrated function of circular and longitudinal muscle layers in health and disease. Am J Physiol Gastrointest Liver Physiol. 2016;311:G431–43.
5. Triadafilopoulos G, Tandon A, Shetler KP, et al. Clinical and pH study characteristics in reflux patients with and without ineffective oesophageal motility (IEM). BMJ Open Gastroenterol. 2016;3:e000126.
6. Shetler KP, Bikhtii S, Triadafilopoulos G. Ineffective esophageal motility: clinical, manometric, and outcome characteristics in patients with and without abnormal esophageal acid exposure. Dis Esophagus. 2017;30:1–8.
7. Bennett MC, Patel A, Sainani N, Wang D, Sayuk GS, Gyawali CP. Chronic cough is associated with long breaks in esophageal peristaltic integrity on high-resolution manometry. J Neurogastroenterol Motil. 2018;24:387–94.
8. Rengarajan A, Bolkhir A, Gor P, et al. Esophagogastric junction and esophageal body contraction metrics on high resolution manometry predict esophageal acid burden. Neurogastroenterol Motil. 2018;30(5):1647–54.
9. Gyawali CP, Sifrim D, Carlson DA, et al. Ineffective esophageal motility: concepts, future directions, and conclusions from the Stanford 2018 symposium. Neurogastroenterol Motil. 2019;31(9):e13584.
10. Morozov S, Isakov V, Konovalova M. Fiber-enriched diet helps to control symptoms and improves esophageal motility in patients with non-erosive gastroesophageal reflux disease. World J Gastroenterol. 2018;24:2291–9.
11. Pauwels A, Vandingenen N, Vanuytsel T, et al. The effect of an osteopathic intervention on the respiratory diaphragm on lower esophageal function in healthy volunteers and patients with non-erosive reflux disease. Gastroenterology. 2018;154:S-238.
12. Chen C-L, Yi C-H, Liu T-T, Orr WC. Effects of mosapride on secondary peristalsis in patients with ineffective esophageal motility. Scand J Gastroenterol. 2013;48:1363–70.
13. Scheerens C, Tack J, Rommel N. Buspirone, a new drug for the management of patients with ineffective esophageal motility? United European Gastroenterol J. 2015;3:261–5.
14. The 5-HT1A receptor agonist buspirone improves esophageal motor function and symptoms in systemic sclerosis: a 4-week, open-label trial. Arthritis Res Ther. 2016;18:195.

15. Aggarwal N, Thota PN, Lopez R, et al. A randomized double-blind placebo-controlled crossover-style trial of buspirone in functional dysphagia and ineffective esophageal motility. Neurogastroenterol Motil. 2018;30:13213.
16. Monrroy H, Cisternas D, Bilder C, et al. The Chicago classification 3.0 results in more normal findings and fewer hypotensive findings with no difference in other diagnoses. Am J Gastroenterol. 2017;112(4):606–12.
17. Roman S, Lin Z, Kwiatek MA, et al. Weak peristalsis in esophageal pressure topography: classification and association with dysphagia. Am J Gastroenterol. 2011;106:349–56.
18. Clouse RE, Staiano A. Topography of normal and high-amplitude esophageal peristalsis. Am J Phys. 1993;265:G1098–107.
19. Ghosh SK, Pandolfino JE, Kwiatek MA, Kahrilas PJ. Oesophageal peristaltic transition zone defects: real but few and far between. Neurogastroenterol Motil. 2008;20:1283–90.
20. Kumar N, Porter RF, Chanin JM, Gyawali CP. Analysis of intersegmental trough and proximal latency of smooth muscle contraction using high-resolution esophageal manometry. J Clin Gastroenterol. 2012;46:375–81.
21. Wang D, Wang X, Yao Y, Xiaowen X, Wang J, Jia Y, Hong X. Assessment of esophageal motor disorders using high-resolution manometry in esophageal dysphagia with Normal endoscopy. J Neurogastroenterol Motil. 2019;25(1):61–7.
22. Savarino E, Gemignani L, Pohl D, et al. Oesophageal motility and bolus transit abnormalities increase in parallel with the severity of gastro-oesophageal reflux disease. Aliment Pharmacol Ther. 2011;34:476–86.
23. Bazin C, Benezech A, Alessandrini M, et al. Esophageal motor disorders are a strong and independent associated factor of Barrett's esophagus. J Neurogastroenterol Motil. 2018;24:216–25.
24. Rogers BD, Rengarajan A, Mauro A, et al. Fragmented and failed swallows on esophageal high-resolution manometry associate with abnormal reflux burden better than weak swallows. Neurogastroenterol Motil. 2020;32:e13736.
25. Nikolic M, Schwameis K, Kristo I, et al. Ineffective esophageal motility in patients with GERD is no contraindication for Nissen fundoplication. World J Surg. 2020;44:186–93.
26. Bakhos CT, Petrov RV, Parkman HP, Malik Z, Abbas AE. Role and safety of fundoplication in esophageal disease and dysmotility syndromes. J Thorac Dis. 2019;11(Suppl 12):S1610–7.
27. Zerbib F, Roman S. Current therapeutic options for esophageal motor disorders as defined by the Chicago classification. J Clin Gastroenterol. 2015;49(6):451–60.
28. Shaker A, Stoikes N, Drapekin J, et al. Multiple rapid swallow responses during esophageal high-resolution manometry reflect esophageal body peristaltic reserve. Am J Gastroenterol. 2013;108:1706–12.
29. Min YW, Shin I, et al. Multiple rapid swallow maneuver enhances the clinical utility of high-resolution manometry in patients showing ineffective esophageal motility. Medicine (Baltimore). 2015;94(40):e1669.

Distal Esophageal Spasm 19

Sarah Samreen and Dmitry Oleynikov

Introduction

Distal esophageal spasm (DES) is an idiopathic disorder and is the most frequently studied esophageal motility disorder aside from achalasia. It used to be commonly known as diffuse esophageal spasm, but in 2003, Sperandio et al. [1] concluded that due to the limited nature of the disorder, diffuse esophageal spasm is a misnomer and the name "distal" esophageal spasm is more appropriate. The Chicago classification of esophageal motility disorders has since adopted the new name. Due to the rarity of this disorder, the true prevalence in the general population is unknown; however, prevalence is 3–9% in symptomatic patients [2]. The disorder is most often seen in women and most commonly diag-

S. Samreen
University of Texas Medical Branch, Galveston, TX, USA
e-mail: sasamree@utmb.edu

D. Oleynikov (✉)
Department of Surgery, Monmouth Medical Center, Long Branch, NJ, USA
e-mail: dmitry.oleynikov@rwjbh.org

A. D. Patel et al. (eds.), *The SAGES Manual of Physiologic Evaluation of Foregut Diseases*,
https://doi.org/10.1007/978-3-031-39199-6_19

nosed in the 60s to early 70s age range [3, 4]. This may also be secondary to delay in diagnosis due to a lack of physician and public awareness.

Even though the complete neuromuscular physiology is unclear, it is thought to be caused by an impaired neurologic inhibitory pathway due to muscular hypertrophy and degeneration of the branches of the vagus nerve. This allows for premature, repetitive, and simultaneous esophageal smooth muscle contractions [5] most notably in the lower two-thirds of the esophagus. Another suggested pathway is the impairment of inhibitory innervation secondary to deficiency of tissue nitric oxide (NO) [6] once again leading to simultaneous contractions and possibly abnormal relaxation of the esophagogastric junction. This is supported by the fact that healthy subjects administered NO scavenger demonstrate simultaneous contractions in the distal esophagus, which is reversed by the replacement of NO [7]. Since achalasia has a similar pathophysiologic mechanism, some authors have suggested that even though uncommon DES may progress to or overlap with achalasia [8–11]. Some studies employing intraluminal ultrasound or computed tomography (CT) have demonstrated thicker lower esophageal sphincter (LES) and esophageal smooth muscle layer in patients with DES [12, 13]. It is unclear if these findings are the primary cause or secondary to chronically increased neuronal stimulation.

Symptoms and Diagnosis

DES can present with various esophageal symptoms that range widely in severity and frequency. Tutuian et al. [4] demonstrated the most common symptoms by analyzing 71 patients with a manometric diagnosis of DES. They found dysphagia to be the most common symptom (32%), followed by chest pain (22%), typical GERD symptoms (20%), and atypical GERD symptoms (13%). When correlated with manometry, dysphagia may be associated with impaired bolus transit, whereas chest pain may be associated with strong esophageal contraction amplitudes.

However, patients rarely present with a single symptom and most commonly have a combination of several symptoms. Thirty percent of the patients may have some weight loss [3] due to modification of dietary habits.

Symptoms are often triggered by ingestion of solids or fluids, emotional stress, or even exertion. Chest pain can radiate to the back, jaw, bilateral chest, and shoulders and thus can be confused with cardiac angina. Hence, it is prudent to prioritize cardiac investigation and rule out more-prevalent and life-threatening cardiovascular disease as the cause of chest pain, before attributing symptoms to less dangerous and rare disorder like DES [14].

The workup of DES consists of upper endoscopy, pH monitoring, esophageal manometry, and esophagography. Esophageal manometry is considered the gold standard, especially since the introduction of high-resolution manometry (HRM). It is important to remember that due to the intermittent nature of DES, spasm-attributed motility may not always be observed during esophageal manometry. Hence, a negative study does not always rule out the diagnosis of DES.

According to the Chicago classification v4.0, a conclusive manometric diagnosis of DES is defined by premature contractions in more than 20% of swallows, coupled with a normal lower esophageal sphincter pressure [15]. Premature contractions are indicated on manometry as low distal latency (DL) of <4.5 seconds, in the setting of a DCI greater than 450 mmHg.s.cm. DL is defined as the time between the swallow-induced upper esophageal sphincter relaxation and the contractile deceleration point (CDP) in the distal esophagus where propagation velocity slows down [16].

Barium esophagram may demonstrate a "corkscrew" or "rosary bead" pattern of simultaneous contractions, sometimes also referred to as pseudodiverticulosis. This is caused by tertiary contractions indicating advanced disease. However, these findings are neither specific nor sensitive and are not necessary for diagnosis.

Upper endoscopy performed at the initial evaluation allows the exclusion of mechanical obstruction, esophageal stenosis, or esophagitis [6]. Twenty-four- or 48-h pH monitoring should be considered in patients having regurgitation or heartburn to exclude GERD.

Treatment

There is no standardized treatment algorithm for DES. This is due to the rarity of the diagnosis and a lack of clinical trials as well as a lack of understanding of the underlying pathology of the disease. Symptom control is the main focus of treatment. The first step is to eliminate trigger foods or drinks from the diet. Proton pump inhibitors (PPIs) and histamine receptor blockers are used for patient's complaining of GERD, which has the potential to induce spasm. Peppermint oil has smooth muscle relaxing properties and has emerged as a potential treatment for patients with dysphagia and non-cardiac chest pain [17, 18].

Smooth muscle relaxants may be effective in providing symptomatic relief in some cases. Nitrates cause smooth muscle relaxation through an increase in tissue NO. While not tested in a controlled fashion, nitrates have shown manometrically to prolong the DL without an effect on the distal contraction amplitude [7]. Phosphodiesterase-5 inhibitors work by blocking the breakdown of NO controlled by cyclic guanosine monophosphate, leading to the reduction in the esophageal contractile amplitude [19]. However, the high cost and lack of insurance coverage are a barrier to the use of phosphodiesterase-5 inhibitors. Calcium channel blockers are another drug therapy used in the management of DES, but the use is limited by side effects. Since visceral hypersensitivity can be a major driver of symptoms, tricyclic antidepressants are effective at relieving chest pain in patients with esophageal motility disorders [20–22].

Botox injection is currently the best-studied treatment in patients with DES [23]. Botulinum toxin causes muscle relaxation by inhibiting the release of acetylcholine from cholinergic neurons at the neuromuscular junction. Vanuytsel et al. [24] performed a prospective, double-blind, randomized controlled trial comparing Botox injection vs. saline in patients with DES and nutcracker esophagus. They gave botulinum toxin into the esophageal body above the esophagogastric junction and demonstrated reduced symptoms, as well as stabilized unintentional weight loss in those treated with botulinum toxin. Even though botox injections appear effective, the effect is temporary and there is concern over complications. However, complications occur at a low rate of 7.9% and seem to be mild consisting mainly of chest pain, heartburn, and epigastric pain, except for one patient that had a fatal case of mediastinitis after botox injection [25].

Esophageal dilation has a limited role in the management of DES. Pneumatic dilation has been reported to have some success, but it is unclear if the patients could have been more properly categorized as spastic achalasia [26]. Also, pneumatic dilation has a risk for esophageal perforation.

Peroral endoscopic myotomy (POEM) has emerged and shown promise in the treatment of DES. It is especially effective for achieving a long myotomy that is essential to prevent any spastic remnants. However, the procedure can be technically challenging due to hyperactive spastic contractions during the procedure [27]. Studies also seem to suggest that the success rates for POEM are higher in classic achalasia than in patients with DES [28, 29]. Considering that patients with DES are usually older than patients with achalasia, the fact that POEM is minimally invasive appears attractive. The risks associated with POEM procedure include bleeding, mucosal tears, pneumothorax, pneumo-peritoneum, and worsening GERD [2]. Still, the results are favorable and continued research is needed.

Heller myotomy is a well-established treatment for achalasia. However, its role in the management of DES is debatable at best. Leconte et al. [30] performed long myotomy and anterior fundoplication on 20 patients with a diagnosis of DES. Dysphagia and chest pain were significantly improved in 18 and 20 patients, respectively, after 50 months of median follow-up. All of these procedures were performed via laparotomy. With the current advancement in minimally invasive procedures performed via either laparoscopy or robotically, newer studies, especially controlled trials, are necessary to determine if surgical management is superior to endoscopic or medical treatment of DES.

Conclusion

In conclusion, accurate diagnosis of this condition is the most important first step. Once this is completed, then an escalation of management should be started with medical management as the first step. This is followed by endoscopic management using Botox and dilation, and then progression to myotomy, either endoscopic or laparoscopic if the patient is a good candidate. Because of the chronic nature of DES, these patients require prolonged follow-up in a partnership with gastroenterology and surgery is key in the ultimate symptomatic management of these patients.

References

1. Sperandio M, Tutuian R, Gideon RM, Katz PO, Castell DO. Diffuse esophageal spasm: not diffuse but distal esophageal spasm (DES). Dig Dis Sci. 2003;48(7):1380–4. https://doi.org/10.1023/a:1024131814888.
2. Khalaf M, Chowdhary S, Elias PS, Castell D. Distal esophageal spasm: a review. Am J Med. 2018;131(9):1034–40. https://doi.org/10.1016/j.amjmed.2018.02.031.
3. Almansa C, Heckman MG, DeVault KR, Bouras E, Achem SR. Esophageal spasm: demographic, clinical, radiographic, and manometric features in 108 patients. Dis Esophagus. 2012;25(3):214–21. https://doi.org/10.1111/j.1442-2050.2011.01258.x.
4. Tutuian R, Mainie I, Agrawal A, Gideon RM, Katz PO, Castell DO. Symptom and function heterogenicity among patients with distal esophageal spasm: studies using combined impedance-manometry. Am J Gastroenterol. 2006;101(3):464–9. https://doi.org/10.1111/j.1572-0241.2006.00408.x.
5. Roman S, Kahrilas PJ. Distal esophageal spasm. Curr Opin Gastroenterol. 2015;31(4):328–33. https://doi.org/10.1097/MOG.0000000000000187.
6. Roman S, Kahrilas PJ. Management of spastic disorders of the esophagus. Gastroenterol Clin N Am. 2013;42(1):27–43. https://doi.org/10.1016/j.gtc.2012.11.002.

7. Konturek JW, Gillessen A, Domschke W. Diffuse esophageal spasm: a malfunction that involves nitric oxide? Scand J Gastroenterol. 1995;30(11):1041–5. https://doi.org/10.3109/00365529509101604.
8. Longstreth GF, Foroozan P. Evolution of symptomatic diffuse esophageal spasm to achalasia. South Med J. 1982;75(2):217–20. https://doi.org/10.1097/00007611-198202000-00023.
9. Robson K, Rosenberg S, Lembo T. GERD progressing to diffuse esophageal spasm and then to achalasia. Dig Dis Sci. 2000;45(1):110–3. https://doi.org/10.1023/a:1005469629067.
10. Khatami SS, Khandwala F, Shay SS, Vaezi MF. Does diffuse esophageal spasm progress to achalasia? A prospective cohort study. Dig Dis Sci. 2005;50(9):1605–10. https://doi.org/10.1007/s10620-005-2903-3.
11. Fontes LH, Herbella FA, Rodriguez TN, Trivino T, Farah JF. Progression of diffuse esophageal spasm to achalasia: incidence and predictive factors. Dis Esophagus. 2013;26(5):470–4. https://doi.org/10.1111/j.1442-2050.2012.01377.x.
12. Goldberg MF, Levine MS, Torigian DA. Diffuse esophageal spasm: CT findings in seven patients. AJR Am J Roentgenol. 2008;191(3):758–63. https://doi.org/10.2214/AJR.07.3747.
13. Mittal RK, Kassab G, Puckett JL, Liu J. Hypertrophy of the muscularis propria of the lower esophageal sphincter and the body of the esophagus in patients with primary motility disorders of the esophagus. Am J Gastroenterol. 2003;98(8):1705–12. https://doi.org/10.1111/j.1572-0241.2003.07587.x.
14. Goldin A, Lo WK. Approach to esophageal motility disorders. In: Oleynikov D, Fisichella P, editors. A mastery approach to complex esophageal diseases. Cham: Springer; 2018. https://doi.org/10.1007/978-3-319-75795-7_5.
15. Yadlapati R, Kahrilas PJ, Fox MR, et al. Esophageal motility disorders on high-resolution manometry: Chicago classification version 4.0©. Neurogastroenterol Motil. 2021;33(1):e14058. https://doi.org/10.1111/nmo.14058.
16. Pandolfino JE, Roman S, Carlson D, et al. Distal esophageal spasm in high-resolution esophageal pressure topography: defining clinical phenotypes. Gastroenterology. 2011;141(2):469–75. https://doi.org/10.1053/j.gastro.2011.04.058.
17. Khalaf MHG, Chowdhary S, Elmunzer BJ, Elias PS, Castell D. Impact of peppermint therapy on dysphagia and non-cardiac chest pain: a pilot study. Dig Dis Sci. 2019;64(8):2214–8. https://doi.org/10.1007/s10620-019-05523-8.
18. Parvataneni S, Vemuri-Reddy S. Role of peppermint oil in diffuse esophageal spasm in the geriatric population. Cureus. 2020;12(3):e7192. https://doi.org/10.7759/cureus.7192. Published 6 Mar 2020.
19. Eherer AJ, Schwetz I, Hammer HF, et al. Effect of sildenafil on oesophageal motor function in healthy subjects and patients with oesophageal

motor disorders. Gut. 2002;50(6):758–64. https://doi.org/10.1136/gut.50.6.758.
20. Clouse RE, Lustman PJ, Eckert TC, Ferney DM, Griffith LS. Low-dose trazodone for symptomatic patients with esophageal contraction abnormalities. A double-blind, placebo-controlled trial. Gastroenterology. 1987;92(4):1027–36. https://doi.org/10.1016/0016-5085(87)90979-6.
21. Cannon RO 3rd, Quyyumi AA, Mincemoyer R, et al. Imipramine in patients with chest pain despite normal coronary angiograms. N Engl J Med. 1994;330(20):1411–7. https://doi.org/10.1056/NEJM199405193302003.
22. Hershcovici T, Achem SR, Jha LK, Fass R. Systematic review: the treatment of noncardiac chest pain. Aliment Pharmacol Ther. 2012;35(1):5–14. https://doi.org/10.1111/j.1365-2036.2011.04904.x.
23. Bashashati M, Andrews C, Ghosh S, Storr M. Botulinum toxin in the treatment of diffuse esophageal spasm. Dis Esophagus. 2010;23(7):554–60. https://doi.org/10.1111/j.1442-2050.2010.01065.x.
24. Vanuytsel T, Bisschops R, Farré R, et al. Botulinum toxin reduces dysphagia in patients with nonachalasia primary esophageal motility disorders. Clin Gastroenterol Hepatol. 2013;11(9):1115–1121.e2. https://doi.org/10.1016/j.cgh.2013.03.021.
25. van Hoeij FB, Tack JF, Pandolfino JE, et al. Complications of botulinum toxin injections for treatment of esophageal motility disorders†. Dis Esophagus. 2017;30(3):1–5. https://doi.org/10.1111/dote.12491.
26. Irving JD, Owen WJ, Linsell J, McCullagh M, Keightley A, Anggiansah A. Management of diffuse esophageal spasm with balloon dilatation. Gastrointest Radiol. 1992;17(3):189–92. https://doi.org/10.1007/BF01888544.
27. Ponds FA, Smout AJPM, Fockens P, Bredenoord AJ. Challenges of peroral endoscopic myotomy in the treatment of distal esophageal spasm. Scand J Gastroenterol. 2018;53(3):252–5. https://doi.org/10.1080/00365521.2018.1424933.
28. Sharata AM, Dunst CM, Pescarus R, et al. Peroral endoscopic myotomy (POEM) for esophageal primary motility disorders: analysis of 100 consecutive patients. J Gastrointest Surg. 2015;19(1):161–70. https://doi.org/10.1007/s11605-014-2610-5.
29. Khan MA, Kumbhari V, Ngamruengphong S, et al. Is POEM the answer for management of spastic esophageal disorders? A systematic review and meta-analysis. Dig Dis Sci. 2017;62(1):35–44. https://doi.org/10.1007/s10620-016-4373-1.
30. Leconte M, Douard R, Gaudric M, Dumontier I, Chaussade S, Dousset B. Functional results after extended myotomy for diffuse oesophageal spasm. Br J Surg. 2007;94(9):1113–8. https://doi.org/10.1002/bjs.5761.

Jackhammer Esophagus

20

Stuart A. Abel and Joseph R. Broucek

Introduction

Jackhammer esophagus (JE) is a relatively new diagnosis that has been distinguished from nutcracker esophagus and diffuse esophageal spasm (DES). JE was first described in 2012 when esophageal hypercontractility without multipeaked contractions was noted in association with esophagogastric junction outflow obstruction [1]. The definition of JE was defined more specifically by the Chicago Classification published in 2015 [2].

S. A. Abel (✉)
Division of Upper GI and General Surgery, Department of Surgery, Keck Medical Center of USC, University of Southern California, Los Angeles, CA, USA
e-mail: Stuart.Abel@med.usc.edu

J. R. Broucek
Division of General Surgery, Department of Surgery, Vanderbilt University Medical Center, Nashville, TN, USA
e-mail: Joseph.Broucek@vumc.org

A. D. Patel et al. (eds.), *The SAGES Manual of Physiologic Evaluation of Foregut Diseases*,
https://doi.org/10.1007/978-3-031-39199-6_20

Epidemiology

JE is a rare subset of esophageal motility disorders. Early population studies determined prevalence rates of JE to be on the order of 4–5% of patients with esophageal dysmotility [3, 4]. In 2018, Kristo et al. published a cohort study of 2443 patients undergoing surgical evaluation for gastroesophageal reflux and found the prevalence of JE to be 1.7% in that population [5]. A retrospective cohort study of 1099 patients undergoing high-resolution manometry (HRM) revealed a diagnosis of JE in 3% of study patients, 89% of which were female [6]. A small cohort of 74 patients with either JE or nutcracker esophagus was published in 2017 by Al-Qaisi et al. demonstrating similar demographics between the two patient populations. Roughly two-thirds of patients were female with an average BMI of 28 kg/m^2 and an average age in the seventh decade of life [7]. Given the low prevalence of JE, large epidemiologic studies have not been conducted.

Pathophysiology

The pathophysiology of JE has been theorized, but is poorly understood. In contrast to DES which is thought to occur because of a decrease in inhibitory neuronal signaling that leads to early and rapid contractions in the distal esophagus, JE is thought to occur because of either an increase in excitatory neuronal signaling or an increased response to excitatory signaling. This ultimately results in smooth muscle hypertrophy throughout the esophagus. There have been several studies to demonstrate eosinophilic infiltration of the muscularis propria in JE [8]. Eosinophilic infiltration may have a role in facilitating enhanced neuronal signaling; however, it is not always present on histopathology in patients diagnosed with JE. The underlying mechanism of enhanced signaling remains unknown.

Esophagogastric junction (EGJ) obstruction is frequently seen in conjunction with JE. There is also limited evidence of resolution of symptoms of JE and normalization of HRM after addressing the cause of EGJ obstruction such as in one case report of JE developing in a patient with a laparoscopic gastric band and resolving after deflation of the band. This association suggests a possible role of obstruction at the EGJ in the pathophysiology of JE [9]. This role of EGJ dysfunction in the pathophysiology of JE has been studied, and impaired EGJ relaxation in patients with JE has been found to be a predictor of disease progression and a possible indication for early and aggressive treatment [10]. There are several case reports and prospective studies of JE that demonstrate the potential for progression of JE to type III achalasia, especially in the setting of impaired esophagogastric junction relaxation [10–12]. While EGJ dysfunction and eosinophilia are often seen in the setting of JE, not all patients with JE have these characteristics. Furthermore, there are reports in the literature of JE occurring after radiofrequency catheter ablation or in the setting of opioid-induced esophageal dysfunction, pointing to a more complex pathophysiologic process [13, 14].

Clinical Features

Symptoms

Like other esophageal dysmotility disorders, JE presents with a spectrum of symptoms. The most common symptom of JE is dysphagia to both solids and liquids, which occurs in up to two-thirds of patients. Noncardiac chest pain occurs in roughly half of patients and can be either the principle presenting symptom or can be secondary to dysphagia with the sensation of food getting stuck in the thoracic esophagus. Gastroesophageal reflux has been described in one-third of patients and weight loss in roughly a quarter of patients with JE [15, 16].

Patient-reported symptoms are not closely correlated with the number of hypercontractile swallows and mean distal contractile index (DCI). Dysphagia appears to be most closely correlated to elevated lower esophageal sphincter (LES) pressures [17]. Chest pain is a common reason for presentation to the emergency department. Those presenting with noncardiac chest pain will have normal investigational workups. A thorough diagnostic workup in these patients should include esophageal studies when indicated.

Imaging/Tests

Upper gastrointestinal endoscopy is an integral component of any esophageal dysmotility evaluation. It can differentiate between organic causes of dysphagia and mechanical obstruction. It is also a means to obtaining a full-thickness biopsy of the esophagus. Cap-fitted endoscopic mucosal resection (EMR) with peroral endoscopic myotomy (POEM) has been described as a technique for obtaining full-layer histopathology. One particular study using this technique demonstrated reduced numbers of interstitial cells of Cajal in the muscularis propria, providing a possible explanation for the uncoordinated peristalsis seen in JE [18]. A barium esophagram and a pH study can be useful components of the diagnostic evaluation when conditions other than esophageal dysmotility are suspected.

Diagnosis of JE is confirmed on HRM [19]. While the diagnostic criteria of JE are based on HRM results, the diagnostic accuracy of HRM for major esophageal motility disorders has been subject to some debate. Some studies would suggest that the diagnostic accuracy of HRM is higher for achalasia than JE [20]. As an adjunct to HRM, multiple rapid swallows (MRSs) and rapid drink challenge (RDC) can be performed. These adjuncts can yield information about inhibitory/excitatory neuromuscular function and latent obstruction, respectively. One study evaluating these adjuncts reported the presence of abnormal inhibition during MRS in some patients with JE and increased stimulation after single swallows than after MRS. An obstructive pattern on RDC was correlated to symptoms of dysphagia. These adjuncts during HRM may help guide therapeutic strategies [21].

Differential Diagnosis

The differential diagnosis for the most common presenting symptom of JE, dysphagia to both solids and liquids, includes structural and functional etiologies. Structural conditions include different benign or malignant obstructing masses, esophageal ring or web, or esophageal stricture. Esophageal strictures occur secondary to peptic ulcer disease, caustic injury, radiation, prior surgery, or ischemia. Functional conditions include achalasia, ineffective or absent esophageal motility, scleroderma, infectious or eosinophilic esophagitis, or DES. Patient's presenting with chest pain would need to be evaluated for both cardiac etiologies, as well as noncardiac etiologies including peptic ulcer disease, gastroesophageal reflux disease, esophagitis, and hypercontractile esophageal motility disorders such as DES.

Diagnosis

Evaluation

When a patient presents with symptoms suspicious for esophageal dysmotility, a systematic approach to diagnosis is necessary. First, it is important to identify any strong risk factors for esophageal disease such as a history of relevant radiation therapy, caustic injury, surgery, or cancer. Patients with these risk factors should be evaluated first with an esophagram. This may detect an obstructing lesion, prompting further workup to rule out malignancy. Although rare, midesophageal pulsion diverticula have been described in patients with JE [22, 23]. Such a finding on esophagram should not change the focus of further investigation. Other nonspecific findings on esophagram may include multifocal contraction and delayed esophageal emptying, and in patients with EGJ dysfunction, a narrowed gastroesophageal junction may be evident (Fig. 20.1). The next appropriate step in diagnosis is to perform endoscopy with esophageal biopsies. This may reveal an esophageal web, a stricture, a diverticulum, a mass, or it may reveal infectious or eosinophilic esophagitis. If endoscopy with biopsies reveals no abnormalities and a contrast swallow study has already been performed, the next step in diagnostic workup is to perform HRM, upon which the diagnosis of JE is based. Once the diagnosis of JE is confirmed, a thorough systemic workup should be considered. One study demonstrated that 25% of

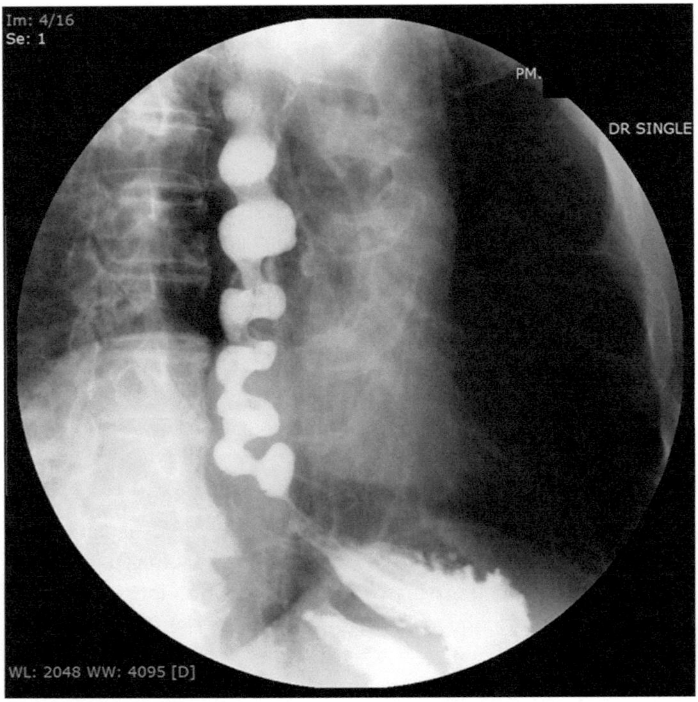

Fig. 20.1 Barium esophagogram showed a constricted and curling of the esophageal lumen resembling a corkscrew. (Sirinawasatien A, Sakulthongthawin P. Manometrically jackhammer esophagus with fluoroscopically/endoscopically distal esophageal spasm: a case report. BMC Gastroenterol. 2021 May 17;21(1):222. doi: 10.1186/s12876-021-01808-3)

patients with JE had systemic inflammatory diseases or synchronous neoplasias at the time of diagnosis [24].

Diagnostic Criteria

The Chicago classification of esophageal motility disorders is an international consensus that has evolved in recent years, first being published in 2009 and later being revised in 2012 and 2014. It relies on high-resolution esophageal pressure topography, derived from the combination of HRM and Clouse plots, to calculate the vigor of each distal esophageal contraction. This calculation accounts for the amplitude, duration, and vertical length of each esophageal contraction and is reported as the DCI.

The Chicago Classification v3.0 is the most updated version of this classification scheme, defining JE as >20% of observed swallows having a DCI >8000 mmHg (Fig. 20.2). JE can occur at any level of the esophagus, including the LES. The diagnosis of nutcracker esophagus, which had been defined by DCI readings between 5000 and 8000 mmHg, was removed due to lack of clinical significance [2].

The integrated relaxation pressure (IRP) is defined as the 4-s mean EGJ pressure measured over 10 s of relaxation following upper esophageal sphincter relaxation with swallowing. The IRP is used to determine the presence or absence of an EGJ outlet obstruction and can help differentiate between different esopha-

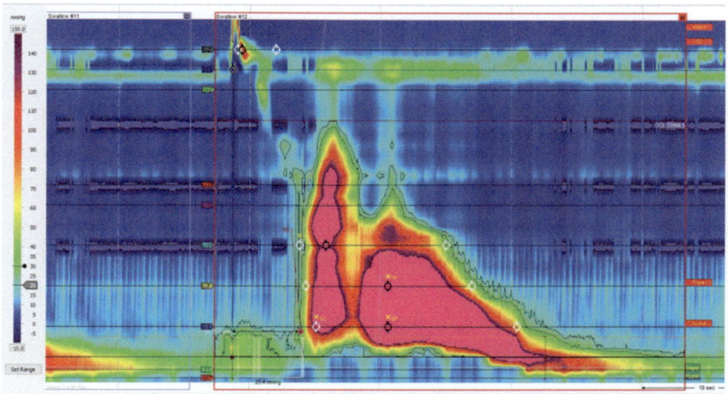

Fig. 20.2 High-resolution esophageal manometry representative of the patient's swallows. The median integrated relaxation pressure (IRP) was borderline high at 15.5 mmHg, a distal latency (DL) was normal at 6.5 s, and the mean distal contractile integral (DCI) was elevated to 14,458 mmHg-s-cm. High-amplitude peristaltic esophageal contraction with a DCI > 8000 mmHg-s-cm represented the hypercontractile (JH) esophagus. (Sirinawasatien A, Sakulthongthawin P. Manometrically jackhammer esophagus with fluoroscopically/endoscopically distal esophageal spasm: a case report. BMC Gastroenterol. 2021 May 17;21(1):222. doi: 10.1186/s12876-021-01808-3)

geal dysmotility disorders. For example, JE is characterized by a markedly elevated DCI with a concomitantly elevated IRP. This differs from spastic achalasia which does not present with an elevated IRP [2].

A key component of the diagnostic evaluation for JE is to distinguish it from DES. Both conditions affect the distal esophagus; however, DES is characterized by premature (distal latency [DL] <4.5 s) but functional (DCI ≥ 450 mmHg·s·cm) contractions. JE is characterized by vigorous contractions with normal latency [2]. One study, however, described two distinct subgroups of JE. Classic JE was characterized by hypercontractility and normal distal latencies, and spastic JE was characterized by hypercontractility and short distal latencies. This study found that classic JE patients responded to anticholinergic agents, while spastic JE patients did not [25].

Management

Initial Management

The initial approach to a patient with a new diagnosis of JE is medical management. JE, however, appears to be heterogeneous, and the nuances of management can be difficult to perfect. The first component of medical management has long been pain control medications. These include conventional medications such as NSAIDS and opioids, as well as anxiolytics, benzodiazepines, and low-dose tricyclic antidepressants [26].

Given that the pathogenesis of JE is thought to involve an imbalance between inhibitory and excitatory signaling; the second component of medical management has long been smooth muscle relaxants such as nitrates, calcium channel blockers, and phosphodiesterase inhibitors. In limited studies, nitrates have demonstrated both clinical and manometric efficacy in patients with esophageal spasm [27]. Studies have demonstrated efficacy of calcium channel blockers in up to nearly 2/3 of patients [28]. Phosphodiesterase inhibitors have been shown to reduce contractile amplitude and velocity in patients with motility disorders

[26]. Anticholinergics are also an option as some studies have demonstrated cholinergic nerve excitation in association with the characteristically strong contractions seen in JE [29].

Systemic steroid administration and antiallergic medications have demonstrated efficacy in the management of JE in patients with eosinophilic esophagitis or eosinophilic infiltration on histopathology [28]. One particular study not only found resolution of symptoms with systemic steroid administration, but also improved esophageal muscularis propria thickening, and normalized manometric findings [30]. Another study found resolution of dysphagia, but not chest pain with high-dose systemic steroid use [31]. Other literature, however, found that while systemic steroids reduced the number of peripheral blood eosinophils and resulted in the disappearance of eosinophils from the epithelium, there was persistent eosinophil infiltration into the muscular layer, ongoing hyperperistaltic contractions on HRM, and no resolution of symptoms [32].

Beyond these mainstays of medical management are some less proven options. Botulinum toxin has been considered as a means of reducing muscle contractility in some patients; however, it has not been well studied in this patient population [33]. There are case reports that demonstrate efficacy of the herbal medication Shakuyakukanzoto in the treatment of JE because of its antispasmodic effect on smooth muscle [28, 34]. It has also been demonstrated to inhibit gastrointestinal motility on endoscopy when sprayed into the lumen of the intestinal tract [35].

Persistent Disease

JE patients who fail to improve with maximal medical therapy may require surgical or endoscopic management. The goal with such management is to decrease the hyperperistaltic contractions and/or EGJ outlet obstruction that drives symptoms. This can be accomplished with a Heller myotomy or with pneumatic dilatation. These techniques have demonstrated variable degrees of success; however, POEM is quickly emerging as an effective alternative.

POEM is a relatively new intervention for which robust data, especially as it pertains to JE, are still emerging. Presently, there is no expert consensus and no official guidelines for the use of POEM in the treatment JE. There are several small prospective studies as well as systematic reviews and meta-analyses that demonstrate the safety and efficacy of this therapeutic modality in the treatment of spastic esophageal disorders, including JE in both the adult and pediatric populations [36–41]. Existing data demonstrate comparable short-term and midterm results when compared to laparoscopic Heller myotomy and superior results when compared to pneumatic dilatation [42].

Some existing literature on the use of POEM in the treatment of JE supports extending the myotomy through the LES to reduce the risk of postprocedural ineffective esophageal motility and the risk of progression to achalasia [38]. This is especially true in patients with JE and impaired esophagogastric junction relaxation [43]. Other studies would suggest that variations in the total myotomy length do not have a significant effect on clinical success, and POEM may cause irreversible fibrotic change, particularly in the LES muscle, which predisposes patients to postprocedural gastroesophageal reflux [44, 45]. There is no consensus for myotomy length; however, consideration of more aggressive management may be prudent for JE patients presenting with dysphagia secondary to EGJ outlet obstruction, and intermittent bolus clearance on impedance exam, as these patients are at risk of further deterioration of esophageal function [43].

Editors' Note

Jackhammer

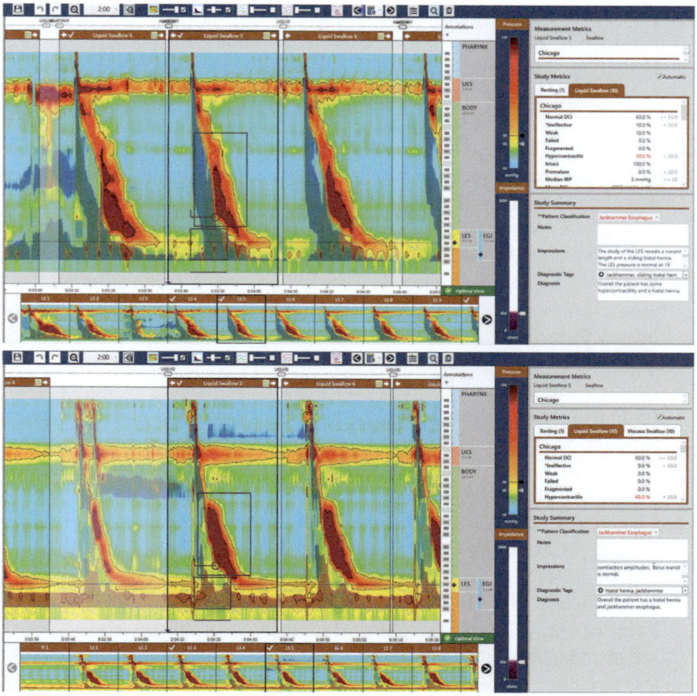

Jackhammer esophagus. 66-year-old female with complaints of chest pain, dysphagia, and GERD. Manometry reading: The study of the LES reveals a shortened length and a hiatal hernia. The LES pressure is normal at 28 mmHg and relaxes completely. The esophageal body study demonstrates normal peristalsis with high contraction amplitudes. Bolus transit is normal. Overall the patient has a hiatal hernia and jackhammer esophagus. *Note the normal bolus transit and normal LES relaxation in the face of hypercontractility in the esophageal body

References

1. Roman S, Pandolfino JE, Chen J, Boris L, Luger D, Kahrilas PJ. Phenotypes and clinical context of hypercontractility in high-resolution esophageal pressure topography (EPT). Am J Gastroenterol. 2012;107(1):37–45. https://doi.org/10.1038/ajg.2011.313. Epub 2011 Sep 20.

2. Kahrilas PJ, Bredenoord AJ, Fox M, Gyawali CP, Roman S, Smout AJ, Pandolfino JE, International High Resolution Manometry Working Group. The Chicago classification of esophageal motility disorders, v3.0. Neurogastroenterol Motil. 2015;27(2):160–74. https://doi.org/10.1111/nmo.12477. Epub 2014 Dec 3.
3. Jia Y, Arenas J, Hejazi RA, Elhanafi S, Saadi M, McCallum RW. Frequency of jackhammer esophagus as the extreme phenotypes of esophageal hypercontractility based on the new Chicago classification. J Clin Gastroenterol. 2016;50(8):615–8. https://doi.org/10.1097/MCG.0000000000000496.
4. Kamal A, Shakya S, Lopez R, Thota PN. Gender, medication use and other factors associated with esophageal motility disorders in non-obstructive dysphagia. Gastroenterol Rep (Oxf). 2018;6(3):177–83. https://doi.org/10.1093/gastro/goy018. Epub 2018 Jun 2.
5. Kristo I, Schwameis K, Maschke S, Kainz A, Rieder E, Paireder M, Jomrich G, Schoppmann SF. Phenotypes of jackhammer esophagus in patients with typical symptoms of gastroesophageal reflux disease responsive to proton pump inhibitors. Sci Rep. 2018;8(1):9949. https://doi.org/10.1038/s41598-018-27756-9.
6. Clément M, et al. Jackhammer esophagus: from manometric diagnosis to clinical presentation. Can J Gastroenterol Hepatol. 2019;2019:5036160. PMID: 30941328.
7. Al-Qaisi MT, Siddiki HA, Crowell MD, Burdick GE, Fleischer DE, Ramirez FC, Vela MF. The clinical significance of hypercontractile peristalsis: comparison of high-resolution manometric features, demographics, symptom presentation, and response to therapy in patients with jackhammer esophagus versus nutcracker esophagus. Dis Esophagus. 2017;30(12):1–7. https://doi.org/10.1093/dote/dox085.
8. Sato H, Takeuchi M, Takahashi K. Eosinophilic infiltration of the muscularis propria in a patient with jackhammer esophagus treated with per-Oral endoscopic myotomy. Clin Gastroenterol Hepatol. 2015;13(4):e33–4. https://doi.org/10.1016/j.cgh.2014.11.005. Epub 2014 Nov 12.
9. Woo M, Andrews CN, Buresi M. Reversible jackhammer esophagus in a patient with a gastric band. Neurogastroenterol Motil. 2019;31(4):e13572. https://doi.org/10.1111/nmo.13572.
10. Huang L, Pimentel M, Rezaie A. Do jackhammer contractions lead to achalasia? A longitudinal study. Neurogastroenterol Motil. 2017;29(3) https://doi.org/10.1111/nmo.12953. Epub 2016 Sep 23.
11. Abdallah J, Fass R. Progression of jackhammer esophagus to type II achalasia. J Neurogastroenterol Motil. 2016;22(1):153–6. https://doi.org/10.5056/jnm15162.
12. Huang L, Rezaie A. Progression of jackhammer esophagus to achalasia. J Neurogastroenterol Motil. 2016;22(2):348–9. https://doi.org/10.5056/jnm16021.

13. Amieva-Balmori M, Cano-Contreras AD, Remes-Troche JM. "Jackhammer esophagus" and eosinophilic esophagitis. Rev Gastroenterol Mex. 2015;80(3):217–9. https://doi.org/10.1016/j.rgmx.2015.03.006. Epub 2015 Aug 12.
14. Snyder DL, Crowell MD, Horsley-Silva J, Ravi K, Lacy BE, Vela MF. Opioid-induced esophageal dysfunction: differential effects of type and dose. Am J Gastroenterol. 2019;114(9):1464–9. https://doi.org/10.14309/ajg.0000000000000369.
15. Herregods TVK, Smout AJPM, Ooi JLS, Sifrim D, Bredenoord AJ. Jackhammer esophagus: observations on a European Cohort. Neurogastroenterol Motil. 2017;29(4) https://doi.org/10.1111/nmo.12975. Epub 2016 Oct 17.
16. Almansa C, Heckman MG, DeVault KR, Bouras E, Achem SR. Esophageal spasm: demographic, clinical, radiographic, and manometric features in 108 patients. Dis Esophagus. 2012;25(3):214–21. https://doi.org/10.1111/j.1442-2050.2011.01258.x. Epub 2011 Sep 23.
17. Csucska M, Masuda T, Bremner RM, Mittal SK. Clinical symptom presentation of hypercontractile peristalsis in the era of high-resolution manometry: a single-center experience. Dig Dis. 2020;38:355–63. https://doi.org/10.1159/000505123.
18. Sato H, Hasegawa G, Takeuchi M, Takahashi K, Sato Y, Hashimoto S, Mizuno K, Kobayashi M. Education and imaging. Gastroenterology: a unique endoscopic technique for full-layer histology of jackhammer esophagus. J Gastroenterol Hepatol. 2015;30(8):1226. https://doi.org/10.1111/jgh.12914.
19. García-Lledó J, Clemente-Sánchez A, Merino-Rodríguez B, Nogales-Rincón Ó, González-Asanza C, Menchén-Fernández-Pacheco P. Hypercontractile "jackhammer esophagus". Rev Esp Enferm Dig. 2015;107(4):234. PMID: 25824925.
20. Kim JH, Kim SE, Cho YK, Lim C-H, In Park M, Hwang JW, Jang J-S, Minkyung O, Motility Study Club of Korean Society of Neurogastroenterology and Motility. Factors determining the inter-observer variability and diagnostic accuracy of high-resolution manometry for esophageal motility disorders. J Neurogastroenterol Motil. 2018;24(1):58–69. https://doi.org/10.5056/jnm17064.
21. Mauro A, Quader F, Tolone S, Savarino E, De Bortoli N, Marianna Franchina C, Gyawali P, Penagini R. Provocative testing in patients with jackhammer esophagus: evidence for altered neural control. Am J Physiol Gastrointest Liver Physiol. 2019;316(3):G397–403. https://doi.org/10.1152/ajpgi.00342.2018. Epub 2018 Dec 13.
22. Goel R, Anggiansah A, Wong T, Wilkinson M. A jackhammer in the gullet: high amplitude oesophageal contractions as a cause of atypical chest pain. BMJ Case Rep. 2015;2015:bcr2015210631. https://doi.org/10.1136/bcr-2015-210631.

23. Carlson DA, Gluskin AB, Mogni B, Koo J, Sood R, Lin Z, Pandolfino JE. Esophageal diverticula are associated with propagating peristalsis: a study utilizing high-resolution manometry. Neurogastroenterol Motil. 2016;28(3):392–8. https://doi.org/10.1111/nmo.12739. Epub 2015 Dec 8.
24. Mallet A-L, Ropert A, Bouguen G, Siproudhis L, Boutroux D, Bretagne J-F, Brochard C. Prevalence and characteristics of acid gastro-oesophageal reflux disease in jackhammer oesophagus. Dig Liver Dis. 2016;48(10):1136–41. https://doi.org/10.1016/j.dld.2016.06.030. Epub 2016 Jul 9.
25. Hong YS, Min YW, Rhee P-L. Two distinct types of hypercontractile esophagus: classic and spastic jackhammer. Gut Liver. 2016;10(5):859–63. https://doi.org/10.5009/gnl15388.
26. Roman S, Kahrilas PJ. Management of spastic disorders of the esophagus. Gastroenterol Clin North Am. 2013;42(1):27–43. https://doi.org/10.1016/j.gtc.2012.11.002. Epub 2013 Jan 4. PMID: 23452629; PMCID: PMC3618975.
27. Swamy N. Esophageal spasm: clinical and manometric response to nitroglycerine and long acting nitrites. Gastroenterology. 1977;72(1):23–7. PMID: 401445.
28. Hosaka H, Kawami N, Manabe N, Kuribayashi S, Sato H, Funaki Y, Ayaki M, Hara K, Ueda C, Matsumura T, Fujiwara Y, Wada M, Kishino M, Yano F, Masaoka T, Ishimura N, Akiyama J, Ochiai Y, Uraoka T, Iwakiri K. Clinical presentation and therapeutic outcome of patients with jackhammer esophagus-a multicenter cohort study in Japan. Esophagus. 2022;19(3):393–400. https://doi.org/10.1007/s10388-022-00916-7. Epub 2022 Mar 6. PMID: 35249162; PMCID: PMC9166863.
29. Babaei A, Shad S, Massey BT. Esophageal hypercontractility is abolished by cholinergic blockade. Neurogastroenterol Motil. 2021;33(8):e14017. https://doi.org/10.1111/nmo.14017. Epub 2020 Nov 13. PMID: 33185322.
30. Funaki Y, Ogasawara N, Kawamura Y, Yoshimine T, Tamura Y, Izawa S, Tsuyuki T, Ebi M, Sasaki M, Kasugai K. Markedly effective steroid treatment of three patients with allergy-related jackhammer esophagus. Intern Med. 2020;59(5):633–9. https://doi.org/10.2169/internalmedicine.3865-19. Epub 2019 Nov 8.
31. Sato H, Takeuchi M, Takahashi K, Sato Y, Hashimoto S, Mizuno K, Suzuki K, Kobayashi M, Honma T, Inoue H, Terai S. Nutcracker and jackhammer esophagus treatment: a three-case survey, including two novel cases of eosinophilic infiltration into the muscularis propria. Endoscopy. 2015;47(9):855–7. https://doi.org/10.1055/s-0034-1391985. Epub 2015 May 11.
32. Tanaka S, Toyonaga T, Kawara F, Watanabe D, Hoshi N, Abe H, Ariyoshi R, Ohara Y, Ishida T, Takao T, Morita Y, Umegaki E. A case of jackhammer esophagus caused by eosinophilic esophagitis in which per-oral

endoscopic myotomy resulted in symptom improvement. Clin J Gastroenterol. 2018;11(5):377–81. https://doi.org/10.1007/s12328-018-0868-y. Epub 2018 May 22.

33. Zerbib F, Roman S. Current therapeutic options for esophageal motor disorders as defined by the Chicago classification. J Clin Gastroenterol. 2015;49(6):451–60. https://doi.org/10.1097/MCG.0000000000000317.
34. Kawami N, Hoshino S, Hoshikawa Y, Takenouchi N, Hanada Y, Tanabe T, Koeda M, Monma E, Goto O, Kaise M, Iwakiri K. Differences in clinical characteristics between conservative-treatment-response group and refractory (surgical-treatment) group in patients with jackhammer esophagus. Esophagus. 2021;18(1):138–43. https://doi.org/10.1007/s10388-020-00748-3. Epub 2020 May 26. PMID: 32458101.
35. Sakai Y, Tsuyuguchi T, Ishihara T, Kato K, Tsuboi M, Ooka Y, Katsuura K, Ohara T, Takayama S, Kimura M, Kasanuki J, Ai M, Yokosuka O. Confirmation of the antispasmodic effect of shakuyaku-kanzo-to (TJ-68), a Chinese herbal medicine, on the duodenal wall by direct spraying during endoscopic retrograde cholangiopancreatography. J Nat Med. 2009;63(2):200–3. https://doi.org/10.1007/s11418-008-0304-6. Epub 2008 Dec 3. PMID: 19050990.
36. Feng J, Ali RW, Hao J-y, Kong G-x, Yang L-h, Huang X-j. Peroral endoscopic myotomy for esophageal motility disorders. Esophagus. 2020;17(1):11–8. https://doi.org/10.1007/s10388-019-00693-w.
37. Khan M, A, Kumbhari V, Ngamruengphong S, Ismail A, Chen Y-I, Chavez YH, Bukhari M, Nollan R, Ismail MK, Onimaru M, Balassone V, Sharata A, Swanstrom L, Inoue H, Repici A, Khashab MA. Is POEM the answer for management of spastic esophageal disorders? A systematic review and meta-analysis. Dig Dis Sci. 2017;62(1):35–44. https://doi.org/10.1007/s10620-016-4373-1. Epub 2016 Nov 17.
38. Bechara R, Ikeda H, Inoue H. Peroral endoscopic myotomy for jackhammer esophagus: to cut or not to cut the lower esophageal sphincter. Endosc Int Open. 2016;4(5):E585–8. https://doi.org/10.1055/s-0042-105204. Epub 2016 Apr 8. PMID: 27274539.
39. Khashab MA, Familiari P, Draganov PV, Aridi HD, Cho JY, Ujiki M, Tinto RR, Louis H, Desai PN, Velanovich V, Albéniz E, Haji A, Marks J, Costamagna G, Devière J, Perbtani Y, Hedberg M, Estremera F, Martin Del Campo LA, Yang D, Bukhari M, Brewer O, Sanaei O, Fayad L, Agarwal A, Kumbhari V, Chen Y-I. Peroral endoscopic myotomy is effective and safe in non-achalasia esophageal motility disorders: an international multicenter study. Endosc Int Open. 2018;6(8):E1031–6. https://doi.org/10.1055/a-0625-6288. Epub 2018 Aug 10.
40. Khashab MA, Messallam AA, Onimaru M, Teitelbaum EN, Ujiki MB, Gitelis ME, Modayil RJ, Hungness ES, Stavropoulos SN, El Zein MH, Shiwaku H, Kunda R, Repici A, Minami H, Chiu PW, Ponsky J, Kumbhari V, Saxena P, Maydeo AP, Inoue H. International multicenter experience with peroral endoscopic myotomy for the treatment of spastic esophageal

disorders refractory to medical therapy (with video). Gastrointest Endosc. 2015;81(5):1170–7. https://doi.org/10.1016/j.gie.2014.10.011. Epub 2015 Jan 26.

41. Ramos RI, Guidi M, Kakisu MH, Rocca AM, Sakai P. Peroral endoscopic myotomy in pediatric jackhammer esophagus. Rev Esp Enferm Dig. 2018;110(7):464–5. https://doi.org/10.17235/reed.2018.5090/2017. PMID: 29667413.
42. Estremera-Arévalo F, Albéniz E, Rullán M, Areste I, Iglesias R, Vila JJ. Efficacy of peroral endoscopic myotomy compared with other invasive treatment options for the different esophageal motor disorders. Rev Esp Enferm Dig. 2017;109(8):578–86. https://doi.org/10.17235/reed.2017.4773/2016.
43. García PV, de Los Ríos CC, Rodríguez-Valcárcel FC, García-Gallardo DH. Progression of jackhammer esophagus to type III achalasia and improvement after extended myotomy. J Neurogastroenterol Motil. 2020;26(1):164–6. https://doi.org/10.5056/jnm19156.
44. Chandan S, Mohan BP, Chandan OC, Jha LK, Mashiana HS, Hewlett AT, Khashab MA. Clinical efficacy of per-oral endoscopic myotomy (POEM) for spastic esophageal disorders: a systematic review and meta-analysis. Surg Endosc. 2020;34(2):707–18. https://doi.org/10.1007/s00464-019-06819-6. Epub 2019 May 9.
45. Sato H, Takahashi K, Mizuno K-I, Hashimoto S, Yokoyama J, Hasegawa G, Terai S. Esophageal motility disorders: new perspectives from high-resolution manometry and histopathology. J Gastroenterol. 2018;53(4):484–93. https://doi.org/10.1007/s00535-017-1413-3. Epub 2017 Nov 13.

21 Secondary Esophageal Motility Disorders: Diagnosis and Management

Meredith A. Harrison, Ronak Modi, Rodrigo Duarte-Chavez, and Andrew M. Brown

Introduction

Disorders of esophageal motility are defined by using high resolution manometry (HRM) with color pressure topography plots and categorized according to version 3.0 of the Chicago Classification of esophageal motility disorders, last updated in 2014 [1]. Using a tiered approach, the Chicago Classification system defines the primary esophageal motility disorders. In addition to those major and minor disorders, there are other systemic and localized pathologies which secondarily lead to disorders of motility. As a result of these secondary esophageal motility disorders being rel-

M. A. Harrison · A. M. Brown (✉)
Department of Surgery, St. Luke's University Hospital, Bethlehem, PA, USA
e-mail: Meredith.harrison@sluhn.org; andrew.brown2@sluhn.org

R. Modi · R. Duarte-Chavez
Department of Gastroenterology, St. Luke's University Hospital, Bethlehem, PA, USA
e-mail: Ronak.Modi@sluhn.org; Rodrigo.Chavez@sluhn.org

A. D. Patel et al. (eds.), *The SAGES Manual of Physiologic Evaluation of Foregut Diseases*,
https://doi.org/10.1007/978-3-031-39199-6_21

atively rare, diagnoses can often be delayed, and management can be challenging. The knowledgeable foregut surgeon should be prepared for the complexities of these conditions and able to treat these patients in conjunction with a multidisciplinary team.

Case #1

Patient Information

A 62-year-old female presents to the outpatient office with atypical chest pain and dysphagia to solids and liquids associated with uncontrollable heartburn despite medical therapy. Physical exam reveals telangiectasia, muscle atrophy with sclerodactyly, and Raynaud phenomenon. On laboratory workup, anti-centromere antibodies were positive.

Manometry

Figure 21.1 shows the HRM for this patient. By Chicago classification, this patient has ineffective esophageal motility with scleroderma pattern. The mean distal contractile integral (DCI) for this patient was 50 mmHg/s/cm, with a median integrated relaxation pressure (IRP) of 1 mmHg.

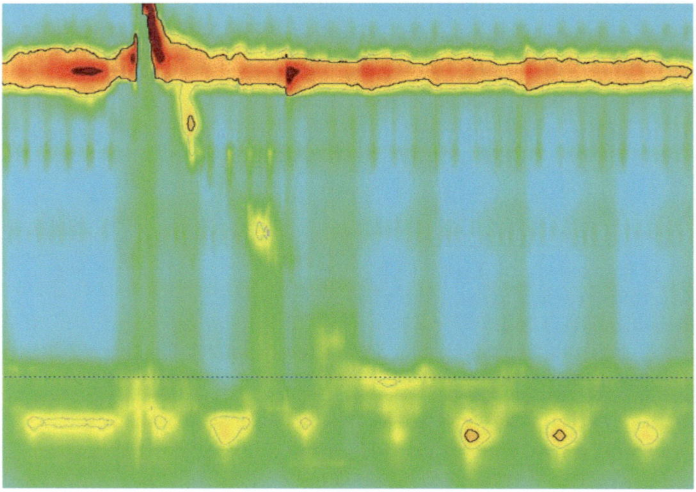

Fig. 21.1 High Resolution Manometry in Scleroderma. Mean DCI: 50 mmHg/s/cm, Median IRP: 1 mmHg

Background

Systemic Sclerosis (SSc) or Scleroderma is a connective tissue disorder with 8:2 female to male predominance and documented histological esophageal involvement in up to 90% of patients [2].

While the percentage of histologic involvement of the esophagus in patients with SSc is quite high, the incidence of esophageal symptoms ranges from 40 to 80%. Patients with esophageal dysfunction have two broad categories of symptoms: heartburn and regurgitation secondary to gastroesophageal reflux disease (GERD), or dysphagia and chest pain secondary to esophageal dysmotility [2].

Workup can include pH testing with or without impedance and upper endoscopy, but manometry is imperative. Classic scleroderma esophagus is characterized by absent or ineffective peristalsis with a hypotensive lower esophageal sphincter (LES). A hypotensive LES is defined as less than 10 mmHg. Upwards of 50% of symptomatic patients will present with this manometric pattern. Additionally, chest CT may reveal a dilated esophagus in >70% of patients who present with the classic scleroderma esophagus pattern on esophageal manometry [3].

Management is aimed at symptom improvement, either managing GERD symptoms or dysmotility symptoms. GERD management is centered on proton pump inhibitor (PPI) therapy, but although there is short term benefit, the long-term efficacy is not sustained, and there is no prevention of progression of esophageal dysfunction [4, 5]. Common practice includes a 2–4× increase in the daily dose of PPI to gain better symptom control [6]. Surgical management for GERD symptoms of SSc should avoid anti-reflux procedures such as Nissen fundoplication, as 38–71% of patients can develop postoperative dysphagia despite improvement of reflux symptoms [7–9]. Some authors advocate Roux-en-y gastric bypass to prevent reflux, which has been shown to have better post-op GER-related quality of life and less dysphagia as compared to Nissen [10]. However, bypass in a scleroderma patient should be pursued with caution given the propensity of small intestinal dysmotility in SSc patients. An esophagectomy can be considered for end-stage scleroderma of the esophagus.

Esophageal dysmotility symptoms can be improved with various prokinetic drugs such as metoclopramide, erythromycin, and cisapride [11–13]. Ciaspride has been shown to increase LES pressure and the amplitude of distal esophageal body peristalsis in SSc patients [11, 14]. Domperidone, a peripheral dopamine antagonist, is commonly used, but the literature questions the effect of symptom and manometric improvement of this drug's administration [15]. An emerging therapy, buspirone a 5-hydroxytryptamine 1A (5-HT1A) agonist, has been shown to increase LES resting pressure and improve the severity of heartburn and regurgitation in SSc patients in small studies [16].

Case #2

Patient Information

A 39-year-old male presents to the office with complaints of significant heartburn and regurgitation. His medical history is significant for chronic GERD on medical therapy and obesity, with a social history significant for smoking.

Manometry

Figure 21.2 shows the HRM for this patient. The manometry pinpoints a specific reflux event.

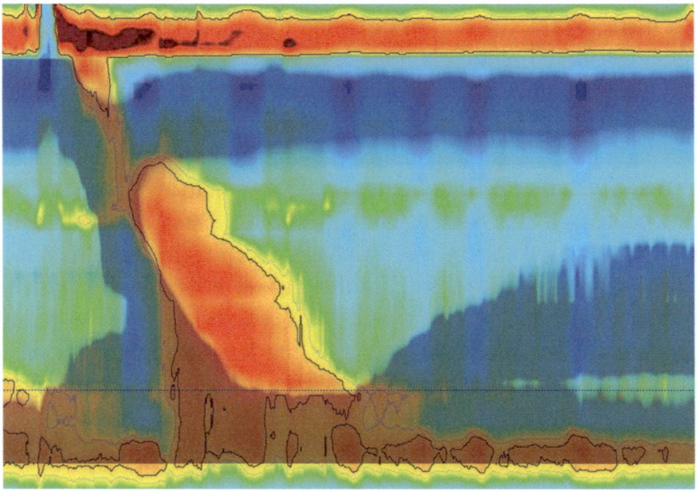

Fig. 21.2 High Resolution Manometry in GERD. Arrow indicates a reflux event during study.

Background

Gastroesophageal reflux disease (GERD), while highly prevalent in Western countries, displays heterogeneity in terms of clinical features, pathophysiologic mechanisms, and response to acid suppression [17]. The pathogenesis is multifactorial, but includes: transient lower esophageal sphincter (LES) relaxations, hypotension of the LES, impairment of the gastroesophageal junction (i.e., hiatal hernia), ineffective esophageal acid and bolus clearance, delayed gastric emptying, and impaired mucosal defensive factors. The major mechanisms for esophageal dysmotility in GERD are due to impairments at the gastroesophageal junction (transient LES relaxation, hypotensive LES, or hiatal hernia) and ineffective esophageal motility [17–19]. Furthermore, persistent injury to the esophageal mucosa is associated with dysmotility.

Transient LES relaxations are 10–60 s periods of LES relaxation that are not preceded by a swallow and are deemed spontaneous [20]. These episodes make up the majority of the periods of reflux in patients with moderate GERD. As the severity of GERD increases, a hypotensive LES becomes the prevalent pathophysiological mechanism. Defined as an LES basal pressure less than 10 mmHg, a hypotensive LES is found with increasing prevalence as the severity of GERD increases, such as in patients with Barrett's esophagus, erosive esophagitis, and nonerosive reflux disease [21, 22].

Ineffective esophageal motility, defined as hypocontractility in greater than 30% of swallows, is the most prevalent esophageal motor disorder in GERD [23, 24]. Furthermore, worsening peristaltic dysfunction is increasingly prevalent with more severe GERD [21, 23, 25, 26]. When contractility is preserved, major peristaltic breaks can be observed resulting in fragmented peristalsis [27].

Diagnosis of esophageal dysmotility in the setting of GERD is done with high resolution manometry, often combined with impedance, which can help identify abnormal bolus transport and clearance during swallows and investigate the relationships between bolus transit and LES relaxation [28]. Treatment with a proton pump inhibitor will decrease acid exposure, but does not improve esophageal dysmotility. Additionally, weight loss will improve the symptomatology of GERD, but it is unknown whether it will improve motor abnormalities. Prokinetic agents (metoclopramide, bethanecol, domperidone) have proven to increase the rate of gastric emptying, increase the LES pressure, and esophageal clearance of reflux [29]. Endoscopic thermal ablation has been shown to decrease esophageal acid exposure and decreases the frequency of transient LES relaxation, but its impact on dysmotility is unclear [30]. Fundoplication, either the laparoscopic gold standard or transoral incisionless fundoplication (TIF), can be effective in improving esophageal acid exposure, but should be viewed with caution in the setting of significant dysmotility [31, 32]. A partial fundoplication, such as a Toupet, is a more appropriate choice than Nissen fundoplication (360°) with esophageal dysmotility.

Case #3

Patient Information

A 42-year-old male presents to the emergency department with chest pain and intermittent dysphagia to solid foods. His medical history is significant for asthma and multiple episodes of food impactions in the past. Endoscopy during his hospitalization with proximal esophageal biopsies reveals 40 eosinophils/high powered field on microscopic evaluation.

Manometry

Figure 21.3 shows the HRM for this patient. Manometry reveals esophagogastric junction outflow obstruction (EGJOO) secondary to distal esophageal eosinophilic esophagitis (EoE) stricture. There is evidence of increased intrabolus pressures; mean DCI of 5200 mmHg/s/cm and median IRP of 16 mmHg.

Manometry normalized with treatment of EoE and esophageal balloon dilation.

Background

Eosinophilic esophagitis (EoE) is one of the most common conditions diagnosed during the assessment of feeding problems in children and during the evaluation of dysphagia and food impaction in adults [33]. Estimated prevalence of EoE is between 1 and 5 per 10,000 persons in the United States and Europe, with

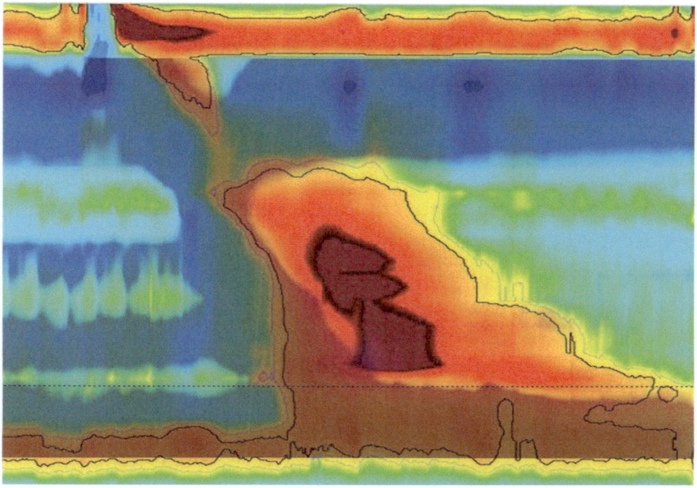

Fig. 21.3 High Resolution Manometry in Eosinophilic Esophagitis. Mean DCI: 5200 mmHg/s/cm, and Median IRP: 16 mmHg

an increasing prevalence in Asia and a 3:1 male:female predominance [34–38].

EoE is currently defined as a chronic, immune-mediated or antigen-mediated esophageal disease characterized by symptoms related to esophageal dysfunction and eosinophil predominant inflammation, with the most dominant antigens being food-based [33]. Additionally, esophageal mucosal eosinophilia of at least 15 eosinophils per high power field is present. This is thought to approach a sensitivity of 100% and specificity of 96% for establishing histologic diagnosis [39]. Eosinophils can release cytokines, growth factors, and other proteins resulting in chronic inflammation. This will affect the esophageal motility via the inhibitory or excitatory pathways. This can lead to abnormal esophageal relaxation or contraction. Symptoms include: feeding problems, vomiting and abdominal pain in children, dysphagia, chronic reflux, and food impaction in adolescents and adults.

Esophageal dysfunction is most often related to stricturing and fibrosis. While this is not always detectable endoscopically, this can be seen using an intraluminal balloon device [40]. Contrast esophagography in patients with abnormal esophageal-wall compliance often reveals that the esophageal caliber is decreased and the esophagus is diffusely less distensible [41]. The most common endoscopic findings are white specks (representative of eosinophilic exudates), mucosal edema, linear furrows, esophageal rings, and strictures [42, 43]. Strictures in patients with EoE may be lengthy, tapered, and commonly escape detection during endoscopy but are evident in contrast esophagram. Two recent studies reported that 71% of adults and 55% of children with eosinophilic esophagitis did not have esophageal narrowing recognized at the time of endoscopy, but did have evidence of narrowing at the time of esophagography [44–46].

Manometry may be used in patients with EoE during the work-up since dysphagia is one of the most common clinical symptoms. EoE can mimic all of the categories of esophageal motility. A recent small study by Hejazi et al. found that one patient had manometric findings including non-peristaltic contractions and incomplete relaxation of the LES, suggesting achalasia. One had total aperistalsis with contraction amplitudes <10 mmHg and a weak LES pressure, criteria suggesting scleroderma. Two had low amplitude (<30 mmHg) non-peristaltic contractions limited to the mid esophagus. Criteria for nutcracker esophagus were met in 2 patients. Isolated low LES pressure was observed in four patients who were also receiving proton pump inhibitors, and the remainder had normal esophageal motility findings [46]. This illustrates the heterogeneity in manometric findings in EoE.

Management of these patients includes alleviation of symptoms, control of inflammation, and restoration of function. Diet, pharmaceutical agents, and dilation can be used to reach these goals [33]. Pharmaceutical agents include the use of proton pump inhibitors and topical glucocorticoids, which specifically decrease fibrosis through the reduction of inflammatory cells [47]. Topical glucocorticoids may also reduce the frequency of subsequent food impactions [48]. Esophageal dilation can alleviate esophageal narrowing particularly in older teenagers and adults. Perforation rates of less than 1% have been seen in several large series [49]. In patients with eosinophilic esophagitis, dilation should be performed gradually over multiple sessions, with an expectation that 75% of patients will have chest pain after the procedure [33].

Case #4

Patient Information

A 42-year-old female presents to the office with complaints of chest pain associated with regurgitation and dysphagia to both solids and liquids. Her medical history is significant for chronic back and knee pain, and she takes chronic opioids for this pain.

Manometry

Figure 21.4 shows the HRM for this patient. Manometry reveals hypercontractile esophagus. Mean DCI is 10,500 mmHg/s/cm and median IRP is 8 mmHg.

Background

Opioids have become the most widely prescribed analgesia in western countries. The effect of opioids on stomach, small intestine, and colon motility has been well characterized, but the effects on esophageal motility are still unclear [50]. Data suggest

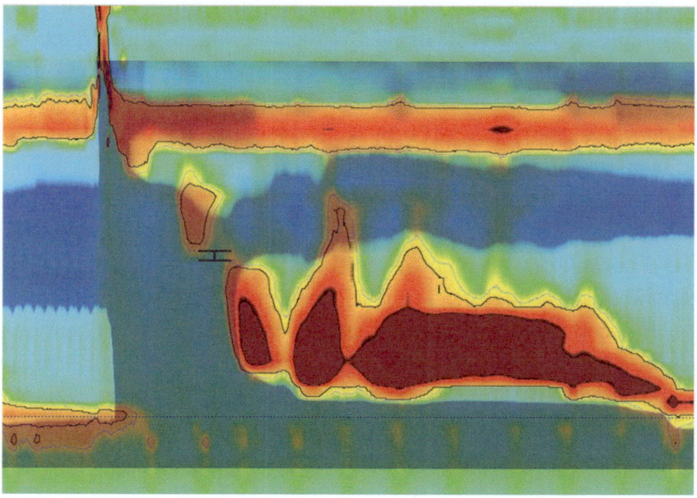

Fig. 21.4 High Resolution Manometry in Opioid-Induced Esophageal Dysmotility. Mean DCI: 10500 mmHg/s/cm, Median IRP: 8 mmHg. This is classified by the Chicago 3.0 classification as hypercontractile esophagus.

that long-term use of opioids can cause esophageal motility dysfunction, reflecting symptoms similar to motility disorders, such as achalasia and functional esophagogastric junction (EGJ) outflow obstruction [51]. This is termed opioid-induced esophageal dysfunction (OIED) [50].

There are multiple theories for how opioids act on the receptors in the esophagus. The μ-opioid receptor stimulation can be associated with symptoms of dysphagia and heartburn. Opioids decrease peristaltic activity and alter the function of the lower esophageal sphincter, mediated mainly by μ-opioid receptors. While the pathophysiologic mechanism is not well understood, one mechanism could be the impairment of the nitric oxide pathway.

While symptoms can vary, the predominant symptom in most patients is dysphagia, especially to liquids, with sudden onset. Other symptoms include weight loss, regurgitation, and chest pain.

According to the Chicago classification and published studies on the use of opioids and esophageal motility, the main opioid-related esophageal disorders are EGJ outflow obstruction and type 3 achalasia, along with distal esophageal spasm and hypercontractile esophagus. Impaired LES relaxation and reduced distal latency in the manometry, observed in EGJ outflow obstruction and type 3 achalasia, can be more frequent in patients undergoing long-term opioid therapy [50].

Limited data exist in the management of OIED. The withdrawal of the opioid is the first line measure, given that studies have observed a reversal of motility dysfunction after the withdrawal of the drug [50]. If the drug cannot be withdrawn, it should be reduced to the minimum effective dosage. Other options include calcium channel blockers, aimed to decrease LES pressure, which have led to little improvement [52]. Other available options include the injection of botulinum toxin. This could be a valid temporary and more rational option for patients who cannot withdraw from opioids. A small number of patients have been treated with pneumatic dilation and per-oral endoscopic myotomy, both with poor results [53, 54].

Case #5

Patient Information

A 55-year-old male from Bolivia, with a history of congestive heart failure secondary to dilated cardiomyopathy presents to clinic complaining of dysphagia to solids, regurgitation, and constipation.

Manometry

Figure 21.5 shows the manometry for this patient. Manometry reveals Achalasia associated with Chagas disease, with elevated IRP and aperistalsis.

Background

Chagas disease is a tropical infectious disease caused by the protozoan *Trypanosoma cruzi*. A large proportion of individuals develop chronic disease many years after the acute phase, often without detectable parasitemia [55]. Gastrointestinal dysfunction occurs in 10–15% of patients with Chagas disease. The

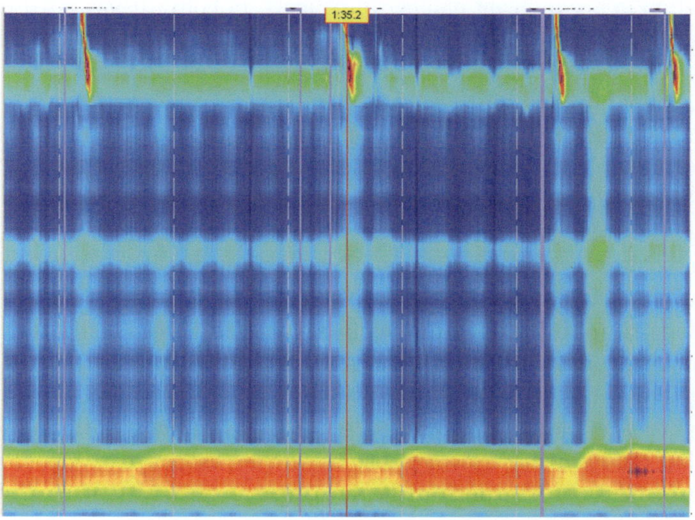

Fig. 21.5 Manometry in Chagas Disease. Mean DCI: 5 mmHg/s/cm, Median IRP: 35 mmHg. This is classified by the Chicago 3.0 classification as Type 1 Achalasia secondary to Chagas disease (Used with permission, courtesy of Dr. Asyia Ahmad)

pathology of the esophageal dysfunction caused by Chagas disease is the loss of the myenteric plexus of the esophagus [55]. The symptoms are characterized by slowly progressive dysphagia, malnutrition, and weight loss. Some patients may also experience regurgitation, heartburn, chest pain, and pulmonary complications due to elementary aspiration [56]. Severity of symptoms is secondary to the degree of denervation that the patient experiences [55].

Manometry shows partial or absent lower esophageal sphincter relaxation and simultaneous contractions in the esophageal body [57–60]. The esophageal manifestations of the disease are very similar, although not completely equal, to those of idiopathic type II achalasia.

Silva et al. observed that the LES was hypotensive or normotensive in the majority of patients with impaired relaxation found in a minority of patients. Aperistalsis was seen in 100% of the patients, and the upper esophageal sphincter had impaired relaxation in a significant number of patients. In both Chagas disease esophagopathy (CDE) and Type II achalasia, the main feature is aperistalsis of the esophageal body. Additionally, the LES shows a failure to relax [56].

Treatment is similar to that of Type II achalasia. The mainstay of treatment is pneumatic dilation and myotomy. However, Meneghelli et al. evaluated the manometric evolution of esophageal involvement and found that worsening of dysphagia was not associated with the longer duration of dysphagia. Patients whose disease did not worsen had dysphagia for a longer time, suggesting that the duration of this symptom may not be associated with changes in the severity of the disease. This is contrary to idiopathic achalasia, where the natural history is progression of dysphagia. While some patients chose to make lifestyle modifications for mild symptom of dysphagia without esophageal dilation, when there is worsening of the dysphagia or an increase in esophageal diameter, patients are more likely to accept invasive treatment, such as myotomy [55].

Summary

The causes and prevalence of secondary esophageal motility disorders range from autoimmune to infectious, and common to very rare. A good clinical understanding of these conditions, and their manometric findings and management, is essential to providing optimal care in these patients.

References

1. Kahrilas PJ, Bredenoord AJ, Fox M, et al. International high resolution manometry working group. The Chicago classification of esophageal motility disorders, v3.0. Neurogastroenterol Motil. 2015;27:160–74.
2. Denaxas K, Ladas SD, Karamanolis GP. Evaluation and management of esophageal manifestation in systemic sclerosis. Ann Gastroenterol. 2018;31(2):165–70.
3. Karamanolis GP, Denaxas K, Panopoulos S, et al. Severe esophageal disease and its associations in systemic sclerosis. Clin Exp Rheumatol. 2017;35((Suppl 106):106):82–5.
4. Hendel L, Hage E, Hendel J, Stentoft P. Omeprazole in the long-term treatment of severe gastrooesophageal reflux disease in patients with systemic sclerosis. Aliment Pharmacol Ther. 1992;6:565–77.
5. Pakozdi A, Wilson H, Black CM, Denton CP. Does long term therapy with lansoprazole slow progression of oesophageal involvement in systemic sclerosis? Clin Exp Rheumatol. 2009;27(3 Suppl 54):5–8.
6. Hansi N, Thoua N, Carulli M, et al. Consensus best practice pathway of the UK scleroderma study group:gastrointestinal manifestations of systemic sclerosis. Clin Exp Rheumatol. 2014;32(6 Suppl 86):S214–21.
7. Poirier NC, Taillefer R, Topart P Duranceau A. Antireflux operations in patients with scleroderma. Ann Thoracic Surg. 1994;58:66–72.
8. Orringer MB, Orringer JS, Dabich L, Zarafonetis CJ. Combined Collis gastroplasty—fundoplication operations for scleroderma reflux esophagitis. Surgery. 1981;90:624–30.
9. Mansour KA, Malone CE. Surgery for scleroderma of the esophagus: a 12-year experience. Ann Thoracic Surg. 1988;46:513–4.
10. Kent MS, Luketich JD, Irshad K, et al. Comparison of surgical approaches to recalcitrant gastroesophageal reflux disease in the patient with scleroderma. Ann Thoracic Surg. 2007;84:1710–5.
11. Sallam H, McNearney TA, Chen JD. Systematic review:pathophysiology and management of gastrointestinal dysmotility in systemic sclerosis (scleroderma). Aliment Pharmacol Ther. 2006;23:691–712.

12. Di Martino N, Ingrosso M, Fei L, Maffettone V, Landolfi V, Del Genio A. Behavior of the pressure of the lower esophageal sphincter after intravenous administration of domperidone in normal subjects. Minerva Med. 1985;76:1411–7.
13. Grande L, Lacima G, Ros E, et al. Lack of effect of metoclopramide and domperidone on esophageal peristalsis and esophageal acid clearance in reflux esophagitis. A randomized, double-blind study. Dig Dis Sci. 1992;37:583–8.
14. Wehrmann T, Caspary WF. Effect of cisapride on esophageal motility in healthy probands and patients with progressive systemic scleroderma. Klin Wochenschr. 1990;68:602–7.
15. Karamanolis GP, Panopoulos S, Karlaftis A, et al. Beneficial effect of the 5-HT1A receptor agonist buspirone on esophageal dysfunction associated with systemic sclerosis: a pilot study. United European Gastroenterol J. 2015;3:266–71.
16. Karamanolis GP, Panopoulos S, Denaxas K, et al. The 5-HT1A receptor agonist buspirone improves esophageal motor function and symptoms in systemic sclerosis:a 4-week, open-label trial. Arthritis Res Ther. 2016;18:195.
17. Martinucci I, de Bortoli N, Giacchino M, et al. Esophageal motility abnormalities in gastroesophageal reflux disease. World J Gastrointest Pharmacol Ther. 2014;5(2):86–96.
18. Castell DO, Murray JA, Tutuian R, Orlando RC, Arnold R. Review article: the pathophysiology of gastro-oesophageal reflux disease - oesophageal manifestations. Aliment Pharmacol Ther. 2004;20(Suppl 9):14–25.
19. Orlando RC. Overview of the mechanisms of gastroesopha- geal reflux. Am J Med. 2001;111(Suppl 8A):174S–7S.
20. Spechler SJ, Castell DO. Classification of oesophageal motility abnormalities. Gut. 2001;49:145–51.
21. Savarino E, Gemignani L, Pohl D, et al. Oesophageal motility and bolus transit abnormalities increase in parallel with the severity of gastro-oesophageal reflux disease. Aliment Pharmacol Ther. 2011;34:476–86.
22. Zentilin P, Conio M, Mele MR, et al. Comparison of the main oesophageal pathophysiological characteristics between short- and long- segment Barrett's oesophagus. Aliment Pharmacol Ther. 2002;16:893–8.
23. Diener U, Patti MG, Molena D, Fisichella PM, Way LW. Esophageal dysmotility and gastroesophageal reflux disease. J Gastrointest Surg. 2001;5:260–5.
24. Lee J, Anggiansah A, Anggiansah R, Young A, Wong T, Fox M. Effects of age on the gastroesophageal junction, esophageal motility, and reflux disease. Clin Gastroenterol Hepatol. 2007;5:1392–8.
25. Kahrilas PJ, Dodds WJ, Hogan WJ, Kern M, Arndorfer RC, Reece A. Esophageal peristaltic dysfunction in peptic esophagitis. Gastroenterology. 1986;91:897–904.

26. Wu JC, Cheung CM, Wong VW, Sung JJ. Distinct clinical characteristics between patients with nonerosive reflux disease and those with reflux esophagitis. Clin Gastroenterol Hepatol. 2007;5:690–5.
27. Gyawali CP, Kahrilas PJ, Savarino E, et al. Modern diagnosis of GERD: the Lyon consensus. Gut. 2018;67(7):1351–62.
28. Savarino E, Tutuian R. Combined multichannel intraluminal impedance and manometry testing. Dig Liver Dis. 2008;40:167–73.
29. Lin S, Li H, Fang X. Esophageal motor dysfunctions in gastroesophageal reflux disease and therapeutic perspectives. J Neurogastroenterol Motil. 2019;25(4):499–507.
30. Franciosa M, Triadafilopoulos G, Mashimo H. Stretta radiofrequency treatment for GERD: a safe and effective modality. Gastroenterol Res Pract. 2013;2013:783815.
31. Broeders JA, Mauritz FA, Ahmed Ali U, et al. Systematic review and meta-analysis of laparoscopic Nissen (posterior total) versus Toupet (posterior partial) fundoplication for gastro-oesophageal reflux disease. Br J Surg. 2010;97:1318–30.
32. Rinsma NF, Smeets FG, Bruls DW, et al. Effect of transoral incisionless fundoplication on reflux mechanisms. Surg Endosc. 2014;28:941–9.
33. Furuta GT, Katzka DA. Eosinophilic esophagitis. N Engl J Med. 2015;373(17):1640–8.
34. Kapel RC, Miller JK, Torres C, Aksoy S, Lash R, Katzka DA. Eosinophilic esophagitis: a prevalent disease in the United States that affects all age groups. Gastroenterology. 2008;134:1316–21.
35. Hruz P, Straumann A, Bussmann C, et al. Escalating incidence of eosinophilic esophagitis: a 20-year prospective, population-based study in Olten County, Switzerland. J Allergy Clin Immunol. 2011;128(6):1349.e5–50.e5.
36. Ronkainen J, Talley NJ, Aro P, et al. Prevalence of oesophageal eosinophils and eosinophilic oesophagitis in adults: the population-based Kalixanda study. Gut. 2007;56:615–20.
37. Dellon ES, Jensen ET, Martin CF, Shaheen NJ, Kappelman MD. Prevalence of eosinophilic esophagitis in the United States. Clin Gastroenterol Hepatol. 2014;12(4):589.e1–96.e1.
38. Ishimura N, Shimura S, Jiao D, et al. Clinical features of eosinophilic esophagitis: differences between Asian and Western populations. J Gastroenterol Hepatol. 2015;30(Suppl 1):71–7.
39. Dellon ES, Speck O, Woodward K, et al. Distribution and variability of esophageal eosinophilia in patients undergoing upper endoscopy. Mod Pathol. 2015;28:383–90.
40. Nicodeme F, Hirano I, Chen J, et al. Esophageal distensibility as a measure of disease severity in patients with eosinophilic esophagitis. Clin Gastroenterol Hepatol. 2013;11(19):101.e1–1107.e1.

41. Lee J, Huprich J, Kujath C, et al. Esophageal diameter is decreased in some patients with eosinophilic esophagitis and might increase with topical corticosteroid therapy. Clin Gastroenterol Hepatol. 2012;10:481–6.
42. Hirano I, Moy N, Heckman MG, Thomas CS, Gonsalves N, Achem SR. Endoscopic assessment of the oesophageal features of eosinophilic oesophagitis: validation of a novel classification and grading system. Gut. 2013;62:489–95.
43. Dellon ES, Gibbs WB, Fritchie KJ, et al. Clinical, endoscopic, and histologic findings distinguish eosinophilic esophagitis from gastroesophageal reflux disease. Clin Gastroenterol Hepatol. 2009;7:1305–13.
44. Gentile N, Katzka D, Ravi K, et al. Oesophageal narrowing is common and frequently under-appreciated at endoscopy in patients with oesophageal eosinophilia. Aliment Pharmacol Ther. 2014;40:1333–40.
45. Menard-Katcher C, Swerdlow MP, Mehta P, Furuta GT, Fenton LZ. Contribution of esophagram to the evaluation of complicated pediatric eosinophilic esophagitis. J Pediatr Gastroenterol Nutr. 2015;61(5):541–6.
46. Hejazi RA, Reddymasu SC, Sostarich S, McCallum RW. Disturbances of esophageal motility in eosinophilic esophagitis: a case series. Dysphagia. 2010;25(3):231–7.
47. Aceves SS, Newbury RO, Chen D, et al. Resolution of remodeling in eosinophilic esophagitis correlates with epithelial response to topical corticosteroids. Allergy. 2010;65:109–16.
48. Kuchen T, Straumann A, Safroneeva E, et al. Swallowed topical corticosteroids reduce the risk for long-lasting bolus impactions in eosinophilic esophagitis. Allergy. 2014;69:1248–54.
49. Moawad FJ, Cheatham JG, DeZee KJ. Meta-analysis: the safety and efficacy of dilation in eosinophilic oesophagitis. Aliment Pharmacol Ther. 2013;38:713–20.
50. Ortiz V, Garcia-Campos M, Saez-Gonzalez E, delPozo P, Garrigues V. A concise review of opioid-induced esophageal dysfunction: is this a new clinical entitiy? Dis Esophagus 2018;31(5).
51. Gonzalez ES, Bellver VO, Jaime FC, et al. Opioid-induced lower esophageal sphincter dysfunction. J Neurogastroenterol Motil. 2015;21:618–20.
52. Wu SD, Zhang ZH, Jin JZ, et al. Effects of narcotic analgesic drugs on human Oddi's sphincter motility. World J Gastroenterol. 2004;10:2901–4.
53. Dorn S, Lembo A, Cremonini F. Opioid-induced bowel dysfunction: epidemiology, pathophysiology, diagnosis, and initial therapeutic approach. Am J Gastroenterol. 2014;2:31–7.
54. Kahrilas PJ, Bredenoord AJ, Fox M, et al. Expert consensus document: advances in the management of oesophageal motility disorders in the era of high-resolution manometry: a focus on achalasia syndromes. Nat Rev Gastroenterol Hepatol. 2017;14:677–88.

55. Meneghelli UG, Peria FM, Darezzo FMR, et al. Clinical, radiographic, and manometric evolution of esophageal involvement by Chagas' disease. Dysphagia. 2005;20(1):40–5.
56. Silva LC, Vicentine FPP, Herbella FAM. High resolution manometric findings in patients with Chagas' disease esophagopathy. Asian Pac J Trop Med. 2012;5(2):110–2.
57. Oliveria RB, Troncon LEA, Dantas RO, Meneghelli UG. Gastrointestinal manifestations of Chagas' disease. Am J Gastroenterol. 1998;93:884–9.
58. Rezende JM. The digestive tract in Chagas' disease. Mem Inst Oswaldo Cruz. 1984;79:97–106.
59. Oliveira RB, Rezende Rilho J, Dantas RO, Lazigi N. The spectrum of esophageal motor disoders in Chagas' disease. Am J Gastroenterol. 1995;90:1119–24.
60. Dantas RO, Deghaide NHS, Donadi EA. Esophageal motility of patients with Chagas' disease and idiopathic achalasia. Dig Dis Sci. 2001;46:1200–6.

Esophagogastric Junction Outflow Obstruction

22

Kelly M. Herremans, J. Christian Brown, and Alexander L. Ayzengart

Case Scenario

67-year-old woman presented with a 3-year history of dysphagia (mostly to solids), associated with occasional regurgitation of undigested food and substernal chest pain. Her workup included a diagnostic upper endoscopy, timed barium esophagram, and high-resolution manometry. Manometry was consistent with esophagogastric junction outflow obstruction and demonstrated elevated lower esophageal sphincter integrated relaxation pressure of 18.8 mmHg (Fig. 22.1). Peristalsis was normal with 100% bolus clearance. No evidence of intraluminal mucosal pathology, strictures, or external compression was noted on endoscopy. Timed barium esophagram showed retention of liquid contrast at 1 min and eventual passage of the barium tablet after 5 min, but no evidence of hiatal hernia, gastric volvulus, or esophageal diverticulum.

K. M. Herremans · J. C. Brown · A. L. Ayzengart (✉)
Department of Surgery, University of Florida Health, Gainesville, FL, USA
e-mail: kelly.herremans@surgery.ufl.edu

A. D. Patel et al. (eds.), *The SAGES Manual of Physiologic Evaluation of Foregut Diseases*,
https://doi.org/10.1007/978-3-031-39199-6_22

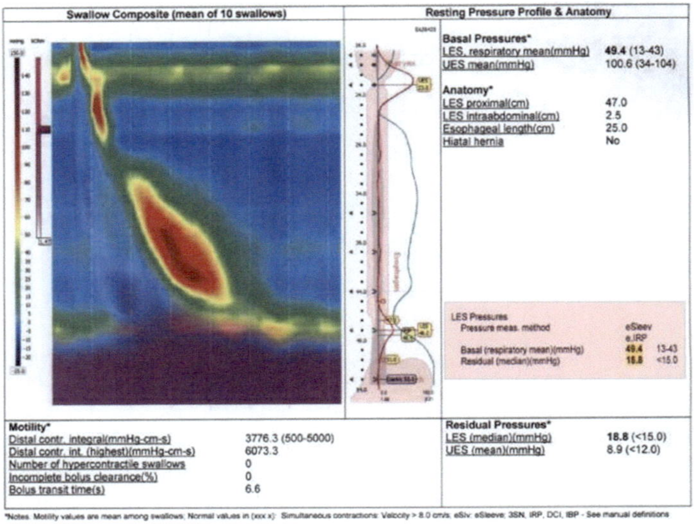

Fig. 22.1 Findings of EGJOO on HRM

Introduction

Esophagogastric junction outflow obstruction (EGJOO) is classified as a major esophageal motility disorder by the Chicago Classification of Esophageal Motility Disorders, version 4.0, and is defined by recently refined findings on high-resolution manometry (HRM) and its associated protocol incorporating patient positioning and provocative swallowing. EGJOO is characterized by an elevated integrated relaxation pressure (IRP) with preserved or weak peristalsis, such that the criteria of achalasia are not met. IRP is considered elevated when above the threshold of 15 mmHg, albeit this is technology-specific.

Etiology

Findings of EGJOO are not uncommon and are reported in up to 14% of HRM studies. It is more commonly found in women (51–88%) and the average age of diagnosis is between 56 and 69 years old. Etiologies of EGJOO vary significantly and include mechanical, inflammatory, medication-related, and functional causes. Secondary causes of EGJOO include a wide range of pathologies (Table 22.1). Functional, or idiopathic, EGJOO is diagnosed once secondary causes have been excluded.

Table 22.1 Secondary Causes

Secondary Causes of EGJOO		
Mechanical	Inflammatory	Medication-related
• Hiatal hernia • Gastric volvulus • Distal esophageal – Stricture – Schatzki ring – Web – Diverticulum • Esophageal varices • Vascular compression • Malignancy • Postsurgical	• Reflux esophagitis • Eosinophilic esophagitis • Systemic sclerosis • Amyloidosis	• Chronic opioid use • Antipsychotics

Clinical Presentation

Patients diagnosed with EGJOO present with a variety of symptoms. The most common symptom prompting HRM evaluation is dysphagia (46%), but other symptoms include chest pain (32%), heartburn (20%), nausea, and vomiting (19%). However, patients typically present with a combination of symptoms. EGJOO may also be found incidentally on routine preoperative evaluation for anti-reflux procedures. Therefore, large volume foregut centers may report higher incidence of EGJOO.

Diagnosis

The diagnosis of EGJOO is made based on HRM findings of an elevated median IRP above 15 mmHg with intact peristalsis. It is differentiated from achalasia based on the presence and degree of peristalsis. IRP measurement is representative of the deglutitive esophagogastric junction relaxation and is recorded as a median pressure (mmHg) of ten test swallows.

Additional information from HRM studies may be utilized to help support the diagnosis of EGJOO and identify patients who would benefit from intervention. Findings of delayed bolus transit combined with patient symptoms of dysphagia and chest pain are highly predictive of clinically relevant EGJOO. Elevated distal contractile integral (DCI) >11,000 mmHg-cm-s in addition to elevated IRP is predictive of symptom persistence after lower esophageal sphincter (LES) directed therapy. Though further research is needed, panesophageal pressurization during rapid drink challenge is found to be related to increased severity of symptoms and likelihood of progression to achalasia.

Additional methods for evaluation of EGJOO include endoscopy, timed barium esophagram (TBE), computed tomography (CT), and endoscopic functional luminal imaging probe (EndoFLIP). If not previously performed, endoscopy should be completed to assess for secondary causes of outlet obstruction. Thorough endoscopic evaluation, including forward and retroflexed views, is necessary to evaluate for secondary causes such as hiatal hernia, postsurgical changes, strictures, rings, gastric and esophageal tumors, and esophagitis. Endoscopic ultrasound may also be used to further elucidate obstructive etiologies if suspicious findings are noted on endoscopy. TBE serves a dual purpose in the evaluation of EGJOO, as it may be used to rule out secondary causes, but may also be used to indicate clinically relevant disease. This test is particularly useful in differentiating EGJOO from untreated achalasia. Addition of a barium tablet may be used to supplement barium esophagram. Delay in passage of barium tablet further indicates functional or anatomical obstruction. CT imaging may be used to evaluate secondary causes of EGJOO. However, CT should be considered on an individual basis as it has been found to yield little additional information. Endoscopic FLIP topography is a relatively new method that has been employed to assess esophageal motility. The EndoFLIP probe uses high-resolution impedance planimetry to measure the relationship between luminal dimensions and distensive pressure during volumetric distension. It may be utilized trans-nasally in an awake patient, but also can be used as a quick 5-min adjunct to endoscopy or in the intraoperative setting. Despite limited adoption in clinical settings, EndoFLIP may be used as a complementary tool to assess EGJ dynamics. It is recommended that data from multiple testing modalities should be evaluated and utilized on a case-by-case basis in order to determine the etiology of patient's EGJOO.

Management

EGJOO is a heterogeneous disorder composed of both mechanical and functional motor abnormalities. As a result, management strategies for the treatment of EGJOO are as diverse as its underlying causes. Appropriate diagnosis, as identified during clinical evaluation, defines the practical treatment modality. However, thorough review of these individual clinical entities and their associated treatment outcomes is beyond the scope of this chapter.

A portion of manometrically identified EGJOO lacks a discrete mechanical obstruction and is classified as functional, or idiopathic, EGJOO (iEGJOO). Some indicate that iEGJOO is a variant phenotype of achalasia; the cardinal feature of impaired lower esophageal sphincter relaxation occurs, but with intact peristalsis. Although tailoring the therapeutic modality to the underlying etiology is likely critical to achieving successful long-term treatment outcomes, a paucity of evidence exists to support an optimal approach.

For patients with incidentally found EGJOO on HRM, watchful waiting is an appropriate option as many resolve without intervention. Differentiating between patients with nil-to-mild symptoms and moderate-to-severe symptoms helps to delineate between further management options. In patients with mild or atypical symptoms, expectant management may be recommended initially, as overall spontaneous resolution rate is approximately 40%.

Patients with significant dysphagia and severe chest pain are less likely to have symptom resolution without intervention. Manometric findings of DCI >11,000 mmHg-cm-s, delayed bolus transit, intrabolus pressure greater than 24 mmHg, and panesophageal pressurization on rapid drink test help to distinguish clinically significant disease. Delayed barium passage as well as retention of barium tablet during further workup may also assist in identifying patients who would benefit from intervention.

Treatment

Clinical evidence regarding the treatment of EGJOO remains sparse as a result of the rarity of this disease. However, due to the overlap with achalasia, multiple therapeutic options have been applied with varying success. If a patient's presentation includes the aforementioned severe symptoms or evaluation findings, targeted lower esophageal sphincter (LES) therapy is warranted and treatment options must be tailored to patient's symptoms, comorbidities, surgical candidacy, and physician expertise.

Pharmaceutical treatments have been explored with mixed outcomes. Medications frequently trialed are calcium channel blockers, PPI's, nitrates, antispasmodics, and prokinetics. Initiation of pharmacologic treatment is a practical starting point given their safety profile and known outcomes in achalasia. However, it has been reported that only 50% of patients with EGJOO exhibit any response to therapy. Acotiamide is a new prokinetic medication that has been heralded for its preliminary results in functional dyspepsia and subsequently EGJOO with up to 83% of patients showing symptomatic improvement. In the United States, it remains in clinical trials at the time of this publication.

Botulinum toxin may also be injected into the LES. The effect is transient and decremental with subsequent injections. Botulinum toxin injections are inferior to myotomy and should be reserved for poor surgical candidates as resultant scarring from injections may obscure esophageal surgical planes if additional interventions need to be carried out.

Bougie dilation may be reserved for EGJOO secondary to inflammatory or peptic strictures, but pneumatic dilation is preferred in functional EGJOO. Pneumatic dilation is a safe, effective option for patients with clinically significant EGJOO. Of note, age less than 40 and male gender were associated with lower rates of sustained symptomatic improvement following pneumatic dilation. However, clinical improvement is typically achieved through repeat dilations. Pneumatic dilation is non-inferior to myotomy in the treatment of EGJOO, though patient characteristics should be considered.

Heller myotomy, performed laparoscopically or robotically, is a successful and sustainable treatment option in EGJOO with 90–100% success in symptom resolution. Classically, a full-thickness myotomy is created at least 5–6 cm proximal and 2–3 cm distal to the esophagogastric junction. At the time of operation, a partial fundoplication is typically performed to reduce postoperative GERD. Heller myotomy remains an excellent option for the treatment of EGJOO in patients who are deemed appropriate surgical candidates.

Peroral endoscopic myotomy (POEM) is a relatively new technique that may be used to perform LES myotomy in EGJOO. In this procedure, a long submucosal tunnel is created using a combination of hydrodissection and electrocautery, followed by an endoscopic myotomy of the circular muscle fibers. The myotomy length can extend beyond 15 cm proximal and 3 cm distal to the esophagogastric junction and can be tailored to the underlying esophageal disease. Short-term data are promising (>90% success rate), but future long-term outcomes require further analysis. Notably, patients undergoing POEM have significant rates of symptomatic reflux and esophagitis following the procedure.

Conclusion

Given the heterogeneity of EGJOO and its unclear clinical significance, a progression of treatment modalities from the least invasive to the most invasive (i.e., surgery) is a reasonable therapeutic approach (Fig. 22.2). An eventual progression to the POEM

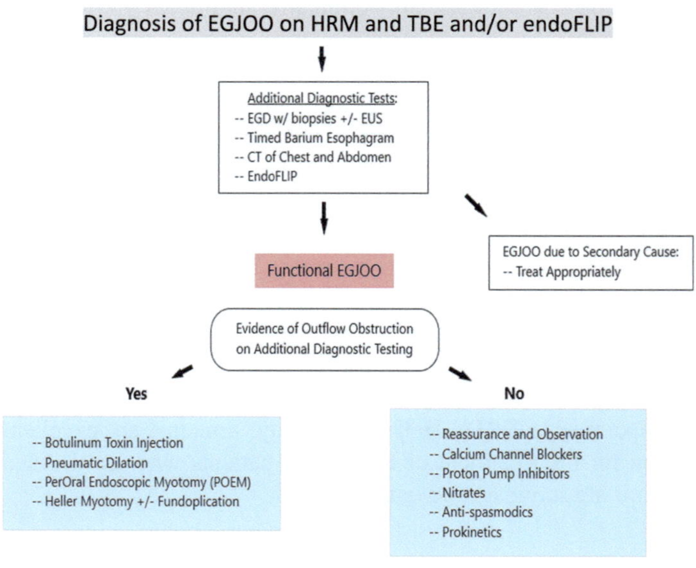

Fig. 22.2 Treatment Algorithm

procedure or to the Heller myotomy with or without a fundoplication may be expected in some of these patients. Treatment decisions ultimately should be tailored to individual patient characteristics, circumstances, and preferences.

Further Reading

Richter JE. Chicago classification version 4.0 and its impact on current clinical practice. Gastroenterol Hepatol. 2021;17(10):468–75.

Clayton SB, Patel R, Richter JE. Functional and anatomic.esophagogastic junction outflow obstruction: manometry, timed barium esophagram findings, and treatment outcomes. Clin Gastroenterol Hepatol. 2016;14(6):907–11.

Khashab MA, et al. Peroral endoscopic myotomy is effective and safe in non-achalasia esophageal motility disorders: an international multicenter study. Endosc int open. 2018;6(8):E1031.

Richter JE, Clayton SB. Diagnosis and management of esophagogastric junction outflow obstruction. Am J Gastroenterol. 2019;114(4):544–7.

Ihara E, et al. Diagnosis and treatment strategy of achalasia subtypes and esophagogastric junction outflow obstruction based on high-resolution manometry. Digestion. 2017;95(1):29–35.

Beveridge C, Lynch K. Diagnosis and Management of Esophagogastric Junction Outflow Obstruction. Gastroenterol Hepatol. 2020;16(3):131.

Porter RF, Gyawali CP. Botulinum toxin injection in dysphagia syndromes with preserved esophageal peristalsis and incomplete lower esophageal sphincter relaxation. Neurogastroenterol Motility. 2011;23(2):139–e28.

Garbarino S, et al. Management of functional esophagogastric junction outflow obstruction: a systematic review. J Clin Gastroenterol. 2020;54(1):35–42.

van Hoeij FB, Smout AJPM, Bredenoord AJ. Characterization of idiopathic esophagogastric junction outflow obstruction. Neurogastroenterol Motil. 2015;27(9):1310–6.

Samo S, Qayad E. Esophagogastric junction outflow obstruction: Where are we now in diagnosis and management? World J Gastroenterol. 2019;25:411–7.

23 Gastric Outlet Obstruction

Michael T. Fastiggi and Mujjahid Abbas

Introduction

Gastric outlet obstruction is a clinical entity that can be defined as a spectrum of disease processes that contribute to a pathophysiologic disruption in gastric emptying due to mechanical obstruction [1]. This obstruction can be intrinsic or extrinsic and can be gastric, duodenal, or extraluminal in nature [2]. Common presenting symptoms include early satiety, bloating, epigastric abdominal pain, and postprandial vomiting.

Historically, the most common cause of gastric outlet obstruction was secondary to benign disease, specifically peptic ulcer disease. However, as proton pump inhibitors, H2 receptor blockers, and eradication of *Helicobacter pylori* became more widespread, malignancy has become the predominant etiology [3, 4]. The most common malignant etiologies include pancreatic adenocarcinoma, distal gastric cancer, duodenal malignancies, and

M. T. Fastiggi · M. Abbas (✉)
New Jersey Bariatric Center, Hackettstown, NJ, USA

University Hospitals Cleveland Medical Center, Cleveland, OH, USA

Case Western University School of Medicine, Cleveland, OH, USA
e-mail: Mujjahid.Abbas@UHhospitals.org

A. D. Patel et al. (eds.), *The SAGES Manual of Physiologic Evaluation of Foregut Diseases*,
https://doi.org/10.1007/978-3-031-39199-6_23

other less common malignancies such as gastric lymphoma or cholangiocarcinoma [5, 6]. Other benign causes include gastric volvulus, inflammatory conditions (ex. caustic injury, acute or chronic pancreatitis, Crohn's disease, tuberculosis), iatrogenic (PEG tube migration, postsurgical narrowing), and other less common causes [2].

In this chapter we will discuss the diagnostic workup and management of gastric outlet obstruction due to varying etiologies.

Diagnostic Workup

History

Like many disease processes, investigation should begin with a thorough history. A detailed investigation into the symptoms, their timing of onset, and chronicity is essential. The most common symptoms include epigastric pain, abdominal bloating, early satiety, weight loss, and postprandial nausea/vomiting, especially of undigested food. Timing of symptoms varies with etiology, from abrupt onset (in rare cases of mechanical obstruction like gallstone impaction in Bouveret syndrome or gastric volvulus) to more insidious in onset (peptic ulcer disease, malignancy).

Physical Examination

Often, there are no specific findings to suggest gastric outlet obstruction. Historically, the presence of a succussion splash was thought to be strongly suggestive of gastric outlet obstruction; however, some reports estimate that a succussion splash is seen in only 50% of patients with gastric outlet obstruction [7, 8]. The technique to assess for succussion splash is as follows: the patient is rocked back and forth at the hips while auscultating in the epigastrium, and if a splashing sound is heard, this is considered positive [2]. The rest of the physical exam may be nonspecific.

Laboratory Values

With severe gastric outlet obstruction, significant nausea/vomiting may be present. This can result in a volume contracted state. Often, metabolic alkalosis is present. This is secondary to both contraction alkalosis with hypokalemia, but can also be compounded by vomiting with a hypochloremic metabolic alkalosis.

Imaging

Imaging is usually via abdominal radiograph, CT scan, or both. Abdominal radiographs are likely to show a distended stomach with retained gastric juices or food particles. Contrast material will often have delayed transit through the pylorus, and the stomach can be large and atonic [3] (Fig. 23.1). CT scan may also show a large distended stomach with retained food particles and can also often better diagnose the etiology of gastric outlet obstruction [9].

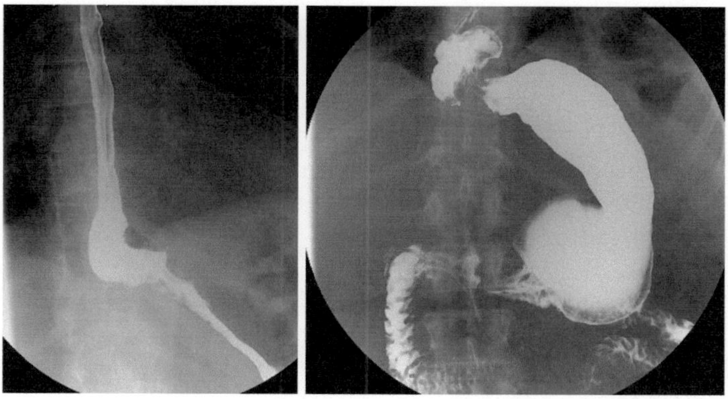

Fig. 23.1 Contrast esophagram of gastric outlet obstruction after sleeve gastrectomy

Endoscopic Evaluation

Endoscopic evaluation of gastric outlet obstruction is an essential step in confirming the diagnosis, and it can also provide therapeutic options.

Preparation

In order to evacuate the stomach and prevent inadequate viewing, it is recommended that patients with gastric outlet obstruction fast for 4 h prior to an endoscopy and have the contents of their stomach suctioned via a nasogastric tube [2].

Technique

Endoscopy should be performed with standard technique, with the patient in the left lateral decubitus position. The entire stomach should be examined to the extent that is possible. If large amounts of retained food remain present, the endoscopy may have to be repeated after another attempt at nasogastric suction and lavage. Care should be taken to examine the pylorus and the site of obstruction with the aim of revealing the etiology, whether intrinsic or extrinsic. Biopsies of suspicious areas should be taken. Depending on the etiology apparent on endoscopy, different endoscopic therapeutic options can be used, and these will be discussed in further detail.

Management

Initial Management

As mentioned previously, patients with gastric outlet obstruction often have long standing nausea/vomiting which can lead to profound electrolyte disturbances, hypovolemia, and malnourishment. Initial management should focus on resuscitation with correction of electrolyte imbalances, as well as nasogastric decompression with replacement. Depending on the degree of malnourishment, the possibility of intervention, and the timing expected to resolution, consideration should be given to the initiation of parenteral or jejunal nutrition [10]. In addition, a proton pump inhibitor should be started regardless of etiology, as proton pump inhibitors can decrease gastric secretions leading to an overall decreased volume of gastric contents [2, 11].

Medical Management

For acute gastric outlet obstruction secondary to peptic ulcer disease, the etiology is often secondary to edema and inflammation adjacent to the area of ulceration. Conservative techniques of gastric decompression through nasogastric suction, acid suppression, and eradication of H. pylori can lead to eventual resolution, with some series reporting up to 90% response rate [11, 12]. In the minority of cases that do not have symptom resolution and are not able to tolerate a liquid diet, further therapy is required.

Management by Etiology

Given that gastric outlet obstruction is a spectrum of diseases, the differences in etiology and thus the variations in treatment are broad, especially when comparing benign and malignant disease. Here the treatment strategies are broken into some subgroups.

Benign Disease

As previously discussed, management of benign gastric outlet obstruction caused by inflammatory states such as peptic ulcer disease begins with medical management. For the minority of cases that fail medical management, the next step is endoscopic therapy.

Endoscopic Dilation

Endoscopic dilation of strictures caused by peptic ulcer disease has been described since 1981 and has essentially become the first line treatment for medically refractory peptic ulcer disease causing gastric outlet obstruction. Long-term outcomes are very favorable, with success and long-term remission rates of 75–100% described for serial dilation [13]. Similarly, endoscopic dilation has been successful in other benign inflammatory conditions, such as anastomotic and caustic strictures, while having variable success with conditions like Crohn's disease and chronic pancreatitis [14–16].

As with the diagnostic upper endoscopy, patients should fast prior to the procedure, and if significant retained gastric contents are present, have these contents suctioned through a nasogastric tube. The procedure can then be done either under conscious sedation in the left lateral decubitus position, or if a difficult procedure is anticipated that will cause significant patient discomfort, under general anesthesia in the supine position.

After identifying the area of stricture, if possible the scope should be passed through in order to fully evaluate the length and diameter of the stricture. If this is not possible with the adult endoscope, a pediatric endoscope may be used. In addition, biopsies of the strictured segment should also be taken to rule out malignancy, if not done already.

After performing this, the endoscopist should attempt to pass a balloon dilator through the stricture. Balloon dilators are available in inflated sizes of 6 mm to 20 mm. Prior to choosing the balloon size, the diameter of the stricture should be measured and the endoscopist should choose the proper diameter balloon [15].

There are two types of balloons - those with a single fixed diameter when inflated, and those that can be dilated to sequential diameters as their pressure increases. The balloon dilators can be filled with water or with diluted water-soluble contrast to aid in confirmation of placement via fluoroscopy [15, 16]. To place the dilator, a through the scope (TTS) balloon is passed. The use of a wire-guided balloon helps aid passage through a narrowed or stenotic pyloric channel compared to non-wire-guided balloon dilators [15]. Fluoroscopy can assist in placement of the wire and balloon dilator, and the center of the balloon dilator should rest at the center of the stricture. The TTS method can allow for limited fluoroscopy, using it to confirm placement and dilation success, rather than performing the entire procedure under fluoroscopy. With a skilled endoscopist and good visualization of the stricture, safety and outcomes are similar to performing the dilation under fluoroscopy, minimizing the need for ionizing radiation [17].

Once the balloon is in place and ready for dilation, the balloon is inflated to the target pressure as specified by the device parameters. The dilation begins when the balloon is inflated and moderate resistance is felt. The general consensus is that for serial dilations, the dilator should not exceed three sequential dilators (3 mm) of increasing size in a single session, also known as the "rule of 3," both for single and multi-diameter balloons [18]. At the completion of the procedure, the strictured area should be inspected for any signs of bleeding or perforation, and the patient should be monitored post-procedure. Any concern for perforation (ex. pain, tenderness) should be immediately investigated with a water-soluble contrast study.

The procedure can be repeated every one to 2 weeks, with a goal endpoint of 15–18 mm stricture diameter. Dilation beyond 12–15 mm increases risk of perforation [15, 19]. After reaching the goal endpoint, the patients should be monitored for recurrence. There is generally a good response in long-term follow-up for serial dilations in peptic ulcer disease with continued acid suppression and avoidance of NSAIDs and smoking/nicotine with long-term remission rates of 80–100% with median follow-up periods of 28–43 months [19, 20].

Endoscopic Steroid Injection

Inflammatory processes can eventually cause fibrosis and strictures from the subsequent narrowing. Intralesional steroid injection can be performed to reduce this by interfering with collagen synthesis and scarring [20, 21]. This can be done as an adjunct to endoscopic balloon dilation for inflammatory strictures related to peptic ulcer disease refractory to balloon dilatation, caustic strictures, and strictures related to Crohn's disease.

The preparation is similar to endoscopic balloon dilation. Triamcinolone acetate (Kenilog) is prepared as a solution of 40 mg/mL. At the narrowest area of the stricture, the triamcinolone can be administered in four quadrant injections of 0.5 mL (20 mg) aliquots [22]. This can be combined with endoscopic balloon dilation for maximal effectiveness. Compared to placebo, intralesional steroid injection was associated with significantly decreased need for repeat dilation, with 10–13% recurrence rates within 1 year, and similarly good long-term response rates up to 5 years [22, 23]. Complications are similar to those in endoscopic balloon dilation. In addition, there is a risk of intramural infection or bleeding [23].

Self-Expanding Metal Stents

In benign disease, self-expanding metal stents are generally reserved for patients with strictures refractory to attempts at dilation who are poor surgical candidates. Most self-expanding metal stents are made from a woven material of wires of nickel and titanium, offering a superior advantage over the historic stainless steel fibers used previously. In addition, the stents can be coated or uncoated, with coats of silicone or PTFE [24].

As mentioned previously, in benign disease patient selection is generally restricted to those with strictures refractory to other endoscopic therapies who are poor surgical candidates. Patient preparation is similar to the previous endoscopic procedures detailed, with most being done under conscious sedation in the left lateral decubitus position. The stent placement is then usually performed under fluoroscopic guidance. A guidewire is passed through the area of stenosis, and the positioning is confirmed on fluoroscopy. The stent can then be carefully deployed with endoscopic and fluoroscopic guidance, with care taken to include one to 2 cm of overlap proximally and distally to ensure that the stricture is fully covered [24, 25]. Injection of water-soluble contrast can then demonstrate that the stent is patent. The stents can then be removed 3–6 months after placement.

Early symptom improvement was demonstrated by Heo et al., with all ten patients reporting success. Ninety percent of the enrolled patients reported being symptom free with long-term follow-up (median 11 months); however, two patients reported worsening symptoms after removal, with one requiring replacement stenting. In addition, one patient's stent was unable to be removed, but was closely observed and had no symptoms over 17 months of follow-up [25]. Thus, major complications include stent migration, stent obstruction, bleeding, or perforation.

Surgical Management

While the majority of patients will respond to conservative management or endoscopic therapy, a subset will require surgical intervention in benign disease. Factors that predict this include duration of treatment >1 year and a need for more than 3 procedures [26].

Surgical management depends on the etiology, but the ultimate goal is to relieve the gastric outlet obstruction. In the case of peptic ulcer disease, this can be accomplished via antrectomy with vagotomy to prevent ulcer recurrence, or with vagotomy and a drainage procedure, either pyloroplasty or gastrojejunostomy. In Csendes et al., there was no significant difference in postoperative course seen between highly selective vagotomy with gastrojejunostomy compared to selective vagotomy with antrectomy, leading the study authors to recommend the highly selective vagotomy with gastrojejunostomy as the recommended choice [27].

Malignant Disease

Malignant disease represents the most common overall cause of gastric outlet obstruction. Palliation of this disease and its symptoms can result in improved quality of life for patients with advanced upper GI malignancies.

Self-Expanding Metal Stents

Similar to benign disease, self-expanding metal stents can be used to stent across malignant obstructions. Differences include that fully covered metal stents are usually used to prevent tumor ingrowth and dysphagia or obstruction [28]. While surgical bypass or gastrojejunostomy provides better long-term resolution of obstructive symptoms from malignant gastric outlet obstruction, endoscopic stent placement is associated with a shorter time to return to food intake and is recommended for patients with a life expectancy <2 months [29].

Surgical Bypass

In severe cases of malignant obstruction, surgical intervention may be necessary. In the setting of metastatic or unresectable locally advanced abdominal malignancies, surgical bypass via gastrojejunostomy may provide better long-term outcomes for reintervention and complications compared to enteral stent placement [29]. Therefore, depending on the specifics related to the patient and his or her preferences, disease staging, and prognosis, a detailed discussion should be held to determine an informed individual decision.

Surgical bypass can be performed laparoscopically unless significant disease burden limits working space. A gastrojejunostomy should be performed distal to the area of obstruction. If the disease burden is locally advanced but has a focal area of obstruction, palliative surgical resection can be considered. A decompressive gastrostomy tube may also be placed to vent proximal secretions if not fully drained via the surgical bypass.

Special Considerations

Esophagogastric Junction Outflow Obstruction

Care must be taken not to confuse gastric outlet obstruction with the disease spectrum of esophagogastric junction outflow obstruction (EGJOO). EGJOO is a motility disorder resulting in obstruction at the esophagogastric junction with preserved peristalsis [30]. While presenting symptoms can mimic some symptoms of gastric outlet obstruction, especially postprandial nausea/vomiting, it is a different disease entirely. Diagnosis can be made via high resolution manometry, with further investigation via endoscopy and contrast esophagrams to help delineate the etiology [30].

Bariatric Surgery Complications

Several complications of bariatric surgical procedures can cause or mimic gastric outlet obstruction. Complications from Roux-en-Y gastric bypass, sleeve gastrectomy, and gastric banding will be discussed.

Roux-En-Y Gastric Bypass

The Roux-en-Y gastric bypass is a malabsorptive and restrictive procedure, during which a small gastric pouch is anastomosed to a limb of jejunum, while the gastric remnant, duodenum, and proximal jejunum are bypassed and anastomosed downstream of the gastrojejunal anastomosis. Rates of stomal stenosis at the gastrojejunostomy range from 4% to 26% and is thought to be secondary to tissue ischemia, marginal ulceration, tension, and the use of 21 mm EEA staplers [31, 32]. Stomal stenosis occurs when luminal diameter falls below 10 mm and clinically presents several weeks after surgery as progressively worsening nausea, vomiting, dysphagia, and inability to tolerate diet [33]. Diagnosis can be made via endoscopy or contrast studies, and manometry may show impaired esophageal motility (Fig. 23.2).

Management is usually successful with endoscopic dilation, usually over the course of several attempts [34]. Strictures refractory to attempts at dilation may ultimately require surgical revision.

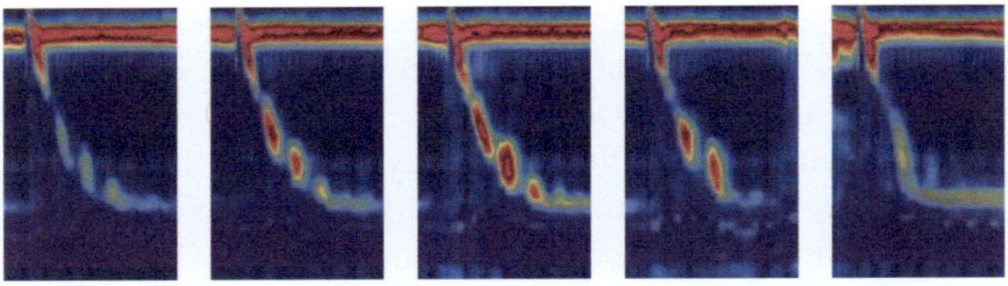

Findings

LES		Normal
LESP (mid resp.)	11 mmHg	10-45
Total Length	2.4 cm	
Median IRP	6 mmHg	<= 20
EGJ Morphology	Type III	
Lower Esophageal Body (Liquid: 10 swallows)		
Chicago Classification Metrics		
Normal DCI (450 - 8000)	80.0 %	>= 50.0
Mean DCI	1650 mmHg·s·cm	
DCI Ratio	0.75	> 0.85
*Ineffective	20.0 %	< 50.0
Hypercontractile (DCI > 8000)	0.0 %	< 20.0
Premature (DL < 4.5)	10.0 %	< 20.0
Panesophageal	0.0 %	<= 0.0
**Pattern Classification	Normal Esophageal Motility	

* Ineffective includes weak, failed, and fragmented swallows.

** Pattern Classification does not constitute a diagnosis. It may be invalid if the patient has had prior related surgeries.

Impedance		
Distal Baseline Impedance	1072 ohms	
Complete Transit (Liquid: 10 swallows)	60.0 %	>= 80.0
Complete Transit (Viscous: 10 swallows)	80.0 %	>= 70.0

Fig. 23.2 Impaired esophageal motility following Roux-en-Y gastric bypass

Sleeve Gastrectomy

The sleeve gastrectomy involves creation of a restrictive "sleeve" of a stomach over a bougie, resecting the greater curvature. Narrowing can occur at the incisura angularis or gastroesophageal junction and is seen in 0.6–1% of sleeve gastrectomy patients [35].

Narrowing at the incisura angularis can mimic a gastric outlet obstruction as there is essentially a mechanical obstruction preventing passage of contents through the pyloric channel (Figs. 23.1 and 23.3). This most commonly occurs either from selection of a bougie that was too small, stapling too close to the pylorus, or narrowing after stapling secondary to oversewing of the staple line. Management can be performed initially with endoscopic dilation or stenting, and if unsuccessful, may require conversion to Roux-en-Y gastric bypass.

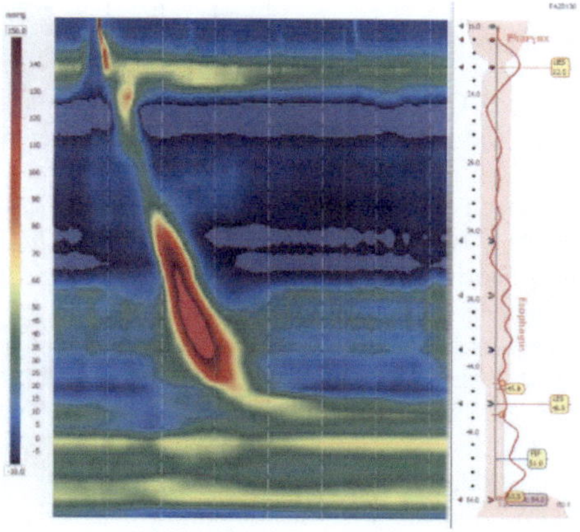

Lower Esophageal Sphincter Region		Normal
Landmarks		
Proximal LES (from nares)(cm)	45.8	
LES length(cm)	**8.0**	2.7-4.8
Esophageal length (LES-UES centers)(cm)	24.9	
Intraabdominal LES length(cm)	2.8	
Hiatal hernia?	No	
LES Pressures		
Pressure meas. method	eSleeve,IRP	
Basal (respiratory mean)(mmHg)	**4.7**	13-43
Residual (mean)(mmHg)	11.2	
Residual (median)(mmHg)	4.4	<15.0

Esophageal Motility		Normal
Number of swallows evaluated	10	
Chicago Classification		
% failed	0	
% weak	0	
% ineffective	0	
% panesophageal pressurization	0	
% premature contraction	10	
% fragmented	0	
% intact	100	
Number of hypercontractile swallows	0	
Additional High Resolution Parameters		
Distal latency	3.3	
Distal contractile integral(mean)(mmHg-cm-s)	3402.8	500-5000
Distal contractile integral(highest)(mmHg-cm-s)	4749.4	
Contractile front velocity(cm/s)	4.4	<9.0
Impedance analysis		
Incomplete bolus clearance(%)	0	
Bolus transit time (sec)	3.7	

Fig. 23.3 Gastric outlet obstruction following sleeve gastrectomy, with two high pressure zones distal to the lower esophageal sphincter

Gastric Banding

Gastric banding is a purely restrictive procedure that involves the placement of a restrictive band around the cardia of the stomach. The procedure has largely fallen out of favor due to disappointing long-term weight loss and relatively high morbidity with high revision rates [36]. Acute stomal obstruction is an early postoperative complication that can mimic gastric outlet obstruction. The etiology can be secondary to edema or due to an error in technique. If due to edema, obstruction may resolve with nasogastric decompression. Obstruction secondary to technical error usually requires band revision or removal [33].

References

1. Appasani S, Kochhar S, Nagi B, Gupta V, Kochhar R. Benign gastric outlet obstruction–spectrum and management. Trop Gastroenterol. 2012;32(4):259–66.
2. Frederickson D, Gan SI, Howell DA, Travis AC. Gastric outlet obstruction in adults. Waltham, MA: UpToDate; 2020. Accessed 14 Aug 2020.
3. Kreel L, Ellis H. Pyloric stenosis in adults: a clinical and radiological study of 100 consecutive patients. Gut. 1965;6(3):253.
4. Shone DN, Nikoomanesh P, Smith-Meek MM, Bender JS. Malignancy is the most common cause of gastric outlet obstruction in the era of H2 blockers. Am J Gastroenterol. 1995;90(10):1769.
5. Tendler DA. Malignant gastric outlet obstruction: bridging another divide. Am J Gastroenterol. 2002;97(1):4.
6. Samad AB, Whanzada TW, Shoukat IM. Gastric outlet obstruction: change in etiology. Pak J Surg. 2007;23(1):29–32.
7. Arabi NA, Musaad AM, Ahmed EE, Ibnouf MM, Abdelaziz MS. Primary gastric tuberculosis presenting as gastric outlet obstruction: a case report and review of the literature. J Med Case Rep. 2015;9(1):265.
8. Lau JY, Chung SS, Sung JJ, Chan AC, Ng EK, Suen RC, Li AK. Through-the-scope balloon dilation for pyloric stenosis: long-term results. Gastrointest Endosc. 1996;43(2):98–101.
9. Awan A, Johnston DE, Jamal MM. Gastric outlet obstruction with benign endoscopic biopsy should be further explored for malignancy. Gastrointest Endosc. 1998;48(5):497–500.
10. Jaka H, Mchembe MD, Rambau PF, Chalya PL. Gastric outlet obstruction at Bugando medical Centre in Northwestern Tanzania: a prospective review of 184 cases. BMC Surg. 2013;13(1):1–8.
11. Taskin V, Gurer I, Ozyilkan E, Sare M, Hilmioglu F. Effect of helicobacter pylori eradication on peptic ulcer disease complicated with outlet obstruction. Helicobacter. 2000;5(1):38–40.
12. Brandimarte G, Tursi A, Gasbarrini G. Antimicrobial treatment for peptic stenosis: a prospective study. Eur J Gastroenterol Hepatol. 1999;11(7):731–4.
13. Storm AC, Ryou M. Advances in the endoscopic management of gastric outflow disorders. Curr Opin Gastroenterol. 2017;33(6):455–60.
14. Kozarek RA, Botoman VA, Patterson DJ. Long-term follow-up in patients who have undergone balloon dilation for gastric outlet obstruction. Gastrointest Endosc. 1990;36(6):558–61.
15. Kochhar R, Kochhar S. Endoscopic balloon dilation for benign gastric outlet obstruction in adults. World J Gastrointest Endosc. 2010;2(1):29.
16. Sonntag CC, Pauli EM. Medical and endoscopic management of gastric outlet obstruction. In: The SAGES manual of foregut surgery. Cham: Springer; 2019. p. 749–78.

17. Rana SS, Bhasin DK, Chandail VS, Gupta R, Nada R, Kang M, Nagi B, Singh R, Singh K. Endoscopic balloon dilatation without fluoroscopy for treating gastric outlet obstruction because of benign etiologies. Surg Endosc. 2011;25(5):1579–84.
18. Siddiqui UD, Banerjee S, Barth B, Chauhan SS, Gottlieb KT, Konda V, Maple JT, Murad FM, Pfau PR, Pleskow DK, Tokar JL. Tools for endoscopic stricture dilation. Gastrointest Endosc. 2013;78(3):391–404.
19. Cherian PT, Cherian S, Singh P. Long-term follow-up of patients with gastric outlet obstruction related to peptic ulcer disease treated with endoscopic balloon dilatation and drug therapy. Gastrointest Endosc. 2007;66(3):491–7.
20. DiSario JA, Fennerty MB, Tietze CC, Hutson WR, Burt RW. Endoscopic balloon dilation for ulcer-induced gastric outlet obstruction. Am J Gastroenterol. 1994;89(6):868.
21. Kim JH, Shin JH, Song HY. Benign strictures of the esophagus and gastric outlet: interventional management. Korean J Radiol. 2010;11(5):497–506.
22. Ramage JI Jr, Rumalla A, Baron TH, Pochron NL, Zinsmeister AR, Murray JA, Norton ID, Diehl N, Romero Y. A prospective, randomized, double-blind, placebo-controlled trial of endoscopic steroid injection therapy for recalcitrant esophageal peptic strictures. Am J Gastroenterol. 2005;100(11):2419–25.
23. Kochhar R, Poornachandra KS. Intralesional steroid injection therapy in the management of resistant gastrointestinal strictures. World J Gastrointest Endosc. 2010;2(2):61.
24. Kim KY, Tsauo J, Song HY, Kim PH, Park JH. Self-expandable metallic stent placement for the palliation of esophageal cancer. J Korean Med Sci. 2017;32(7):1062–71.
25. Heo J, Jung MK. Safety and efficacy of a partially covered self-expandable metal stent in benign pyloric obstruction. World J Gastroenterol: WJG. 2014;20(44):16721.
26. Boylan JJ, Gradzka MI. Long-term results of endoscopic balloon dilatation for gastric outlet obstruction. Dig Dis Sci. 1999;44(9):1883–6.
27. Csendes A, Maluenda F, Braghetto I, Schutte H, Burdiles P, Diaz JC. Prospective randomized study comparing three surgical techniques for the treatment of gastric outlet obstruction secondary to duodenal ulcer. Am J Surg. 1993;166(1):45–9.
28. Wang C, Wei H, Li Y. Comparison of fully-covered vs partially covered self-expanding metallic stents for palliative treatment of inoperable esophageal malignancy: a systematic review and meta-analysis. BMC Cancer. 2020;20(1):73.
29. Jeurnink SM, Steyerberg EW, van Hooft JE, van Eijck CH, Schwartz MP, Vleggaar FP, Kuipers EJ, Siersema PD, Dutch SUSTENT Study Group. Surgical gastrojejunostomy or endoscopic stent placement for the pallia-

tion of malignant gastric outlet obstruction (SUSTENT study): a multicenter randomized trial. Gastrointest Endosc. 2010;71(3):490–9.
30. Samo S, Qayed E. Esophagogastric junction outflow obstruction: where are we now in diagnosis and management? World J Gastroenterol. 2019;25(4):411.
31. Schneider BE, Villegas L, Blackburn GL, Mun EC, Critchlow JF, Jones DB. Laparoscopic gastric bypass surgery: outcomes. J Laparoendosc Adv Surg Tech. 2003;13(4):247–55.
32. Qureshi A, Podolsky D, Cumella L, Abbas M, Choi J, Vemulapalli P, Camacho D. Comparison of stricture rates using three different gastrojejunostomy anastomotic techniques in laparoscopic roux-en-Y gastric bypass. Surg Endosc. 2015;29(7):1737–40.
33. Ellsmere J, Jones D, Chen W. Late complications of bariatric surgical operations. Waltham, MA: UpToDate; 2020. Accessed 14 Aug 2020.
34. Barba CA, Butensky MS, Lorenzo M, Newman R. Endoscopic dilation of gastroesophageal anastomosis stricture after gastric bypass. Surg Endosc Other Interv Tech. 2003;17(3):416–20.
35. Burgos AM, Csendes A, Braghetto I. Gastric stenosis after laparoscopic sleeve gastrectomy in morbidly obese patients. Obes Surg. 2013;23(9):1481–6.
36. DeMaria EJ, Sugerman HJ, Meador JG, Doty JM, Kellum JM, Wolfe L, Szucs RA, Turner MA. High failure rate after laparoscopic adjustable silicone gastric banding for treatment of morbid obesity. Ann Surg. 2001;233(6):809.

Gastroparesis

24

Bora Kahramangil, Emanuele Lo Menzo, Samuel Szomstein, and Raul Rosenthal

Introduction

Gastrointestinal motility is a complex process resulting from an interplay between sympathetic and parasympathetic nervous systems, interstitial cells of Cajal, and intestinal smooth muscle cells. Abnormality in any of these components can lead to delayed gastric emptying [1]. Gastroparesis is a pathology of gastrointestinal motility characterized by objectively delayed gastric emptying, absence of mechanical obstruction, and a combination of clinical symptoms including upper abdominal pain, nausea, vomiting, early satiety, and belching [2].

Epidemiology and Etiology

Gastroparesis is a rare disorder with a prevalence of 38 per 100,000 in females and 9.6 per 100,000 in males [3]. Most cases are idiopathic with up to 1/3 of gastroparesis patients having no

B. Kahramangil · E. Lo Menzo (✉) · S. Szomstein · R. Rosenthal
Cleveland Clinic Florida, Department of General Surgery, Bariatric and Metabolic Institute, Weston, FL, USA
e-mail: lomenze@ccf.org

A. D. Patel et al. (eds.), *The SAGES Manual of Physiologic Evaluation of Foregut Diseases*,
https://doi.org/10.1007/978-3-031-39199-6_24

identifiable underlying cause [4]. The most common form of non-idiopathic gastroparesis is diabetes mellitus [4]. Main hypotheses explaining diabetic gastroparesis include diabetic neuropathy-related changes in gastric emptying [5], decrease in interstitial cells of Cajal [6], and hyperglycemic oxidative stress [7]. Another well-recognized form of gastroparesis is postsurgical. Any abdominal or thoracic surgical procedure causing injury to the vagus nerve can result in delayed gastric emptying [8]. Surgical procedures noted to be commonly associated with gastroparesis include fundoplication, distal gastrectomy, and Roux-en-Y gastric reconstruction. Other rare causes of gastroparesis include viral infections [9], autoimmune gastric dysmotility [10], and Parkinson's disease [11]. Finally, several medications including narcotics [12], anticholinergics, antidopaminergics [13], and tricyclic antidepressants [14] can trigger gastroparesis-like symptoms.

Clinical Presentation

Gastroparesis typically presents with a combination of symptoms including nausea, vomiting, abdominal pain, early satiety, postprandial fullness, and abdominal distension. Severe gastroparesis can cause weight loss [13]. When present, emesis typically occurs several hours after a meal and contains undigested food particles. Gastroparesis-related abdominal pain is typically epigastric and may be exacerbated by eating. Patients may describe a cramping, vague, or burning pain. Physical examination may reveal epigastric tenderness, but rebound or guarding is not typical. In non-idiopathic cases, there may be additional signs and symptoms related to the underlying pathologic condition.

Diagnosis

Gastroparesis should be suspected in patients presenting with a combination of the above symptoms. However, diagnosis can only be made after exclusion of mechanical obstruction and objective demonstration of delayed gastric emptying. Radiologic imaging and/or endoscopy can be used to rule out mechanical obstruction. Delayed gastric emptying is typically demonstrated by gastric scintigraphy.

Clinical Evaluation and Diagnostic Modalities

Clinical evaluation starts with a thorough history and physical exam. In patients with signs and symptoms consistent with gastroparesis, exclusion of mechanical obstruction and objective demonstration of delayed gastric emptying are needed.

- **Exclusion of mechanical obstruction:** The work-up in patients suspected to have gastroparesis should start with an upper endoscopy to rule out other causes. Following a normal upper endoscopy, computed tomography (CT) enterography or magnetic resonance (MR) enterography may be obtained to rule out distal obstruction.
- **Demonstration of delayed gastric emptying:** Gastric emptying scintigraphy is the mainstay for the evaluation of gastric emptying. When possible, a solid meal with radioisotopes should be utilized for optimal test results [13]. In patients too sick to tolerate solids, a liquid meal can also be utilized [15]. All medications that can potentially alter gastric motility need to be stopped 48 h prior to scintigraphy. Adequate glycemic control with glucose <180 mg/dL has to be achieved in diabetic patients. Typically, a meal consisting of (99 m)Tc labeled egg whites or egg white substitutes is used [16, 17]. Scintigraphic imaging is obtained immediately after ingestion as well as at 1-, 2-, and 4- h marks. Normal values with a low-fat meal are 37–90% gastric retention at 1 h, 30–60% retention at 2 h, and < 10% retention at 4 h. Delayed gastric emptying is diagnosed if there is >60% food retention at 2 h or > 10% retention at 4 hours [17]. Based on the degree of retention at 4 h, gastroparesis can be categorized as mild (10–15%), moderate (15–35%), or severe (>35%).

Treatment

Treatment of gastroparesis should be undertaken in a stepwise fashion starting with dietary modification followed by pharmacologic treatment with prokinetics and antiemetics. Surgical treatment is reserved for severe and refractory cases. Glucose control is also important in diabetic gastroparesis.

- **Dietary modification:** Dietary modification is the first line treatment for gastroparesis in all patients. Patients should refrain from fatty, spicy, and acidic foods, and limit the amount of dietary roughage [18]. In all forms of gastroparesis, oral nutrition should be maximized as tolerated. For patients who are unable to meet nutrition goals by oral intake, other enteral or parenteral routes may become necessary.
- **Pharmacologic treatment:** Pharmacologic treatment of gastroparesis starts with avoidance of medications that can delay gastric emptying. Such medications include narcotics, tricyclic antidepressants, anticholinergics, octreotide, and calcium blockers **(REF: Parkman HP. American Gastroenterological Association technical review on the diagnosis and treatment of gastroparesis. Gastroenterology 2004).** For those patients who continue to experience symptoms despite dietary modification and avoidance of exacerbating medications, prokinetic agents are the next step in treatment. These medications are typically administered before every meal and at bedtime. Metoclopramide, a dopamine 2 receptor antagonist, is usually the first line prokinetic drug. A 5 mg dose before meals and at bedtime is appropriate for most patients. In patients who do not tolerate metoclopramide, domperidone 20 mg three times daily can be an alternative [19]. Other pharmacologic options include erythromycin, a motilin receptor agonist, and cisapride, a 5-HT4 agonist. Acute hypoglycemia has been shown to delay gastric emptying [20] and decrease the effect of prokinetic drugs [21]. Good glycemic control is paramount in diabetic patients with gastroparesis. Finally, antiemetic

medications without prokinetic effects can also be useful for symptomatic relief.

- **Endoscopic and surgical treatment options:** Surgical and endoscopic treatments are the last resort for patients who remain severely symptomatic despite dietary modification and pharmacologic treatment. In general, these procedures can be grouped under gastric electrical stimulator (GES) placement, botulinum toxin injection, pyloromyotomy, surgical gastric resection, and enteric access procedures.
  - **GES placement:** Although the precise mechanism of action remains unknown, GES placement can lead to significant symptomatic improvement with good patient selection. The typical stimulator device consists of two leads which are placed in the muscularis layer of the greater curvature of the stomach approximately 10 cm proximal to the pylorus along with a subcutaneous pulse generator [22] (Fig. 24.1). In some patients, a temporary device may be tried to ensure symptomatic improvement prior to placement of a permanent stimulator. These stimulators can be effective in diabetic and idiopathic forms of gastroparesis [23]. Gastroparesis-related nausea, vomiting, and abdominal pain have been reported to decrease after GES placement

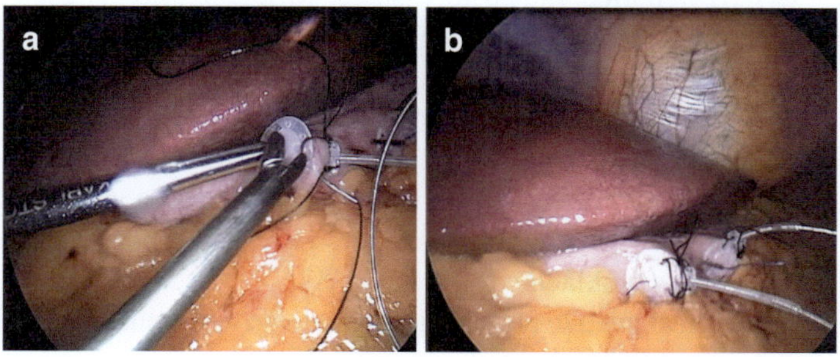

Fig. 24.1 Intraoperative pictures demonstrating the laparoscopic placement of gastric stimulator leads. Leads are placed in the submucosal layer and fixed in place with laparoscopic suturing (**a**). At completion, both leads are located along the greater curvature of the stomach (**b**)

[24]. GES can also improve quality of life [25] and decrease prokinetic drug dose [26] in carefully selected patients.

- **Botulinum toxin injection:** Botulinum toxin injection has been attempted to treat gastroparesis-related symptoms based on the observation that pyloric dysfunction could be seen in a subset of patients with gastroparesis [27]. Patients with gastroparesis and normal gastric body function have been reported to experience significant symptomatic relief with botulinum toxin injection and pyloric balloon dilation [28]. On the other hand, two randomized controlled trials have failed to show efficacy of injections in gastroparesis treatment [29, 30]. Although there is no evidence to support widespread use of botulinum injection, certain subsets of patients with gastroparesis may benefit from this procedure.
- **Pyloromyotomy:** Up to 70% of patients with gastroparesis have been reported to have loss of interstitial cells of Cajal and fibrosis in the pylorus [31]. This finding along with the improvement of symptoms with botulinum injection in selected patients led to the use of pyloromyotomy in gastroparesis treatment. Pyloromyotomy can be performed endoscopically in centers with advanced endoscopic skills (Fig. 24.2). Most studies with endoscopic pyloromyotomy have reported satisfactory short- to medium-term results [22]. Clinical response rate ranged between 70 and 80% and an improvement in gastric emptying was observed in 4–64% of patients [32–34]. Laparoscopic pyloromyotomy can also be performed when endoscopic procedure is not feasible. Both laparoscopic and endoscopic pyloromyotomy have been shown to improve gastroparesis-related symptoms and decrease prokinetic drug needs [35].
- **Surgical gastric resection:** For patients who remain symptomatic despite the less invasive treatment options, surgical gastric resection may be needed. Extensive subtotal or near total gastrectomy with Roux-en-Y gastrojejunostomy can improve vomiting in diabetic gastroparesis [36]. In obese patients with gastroparesis, a Roux-en-Y gastric bypass

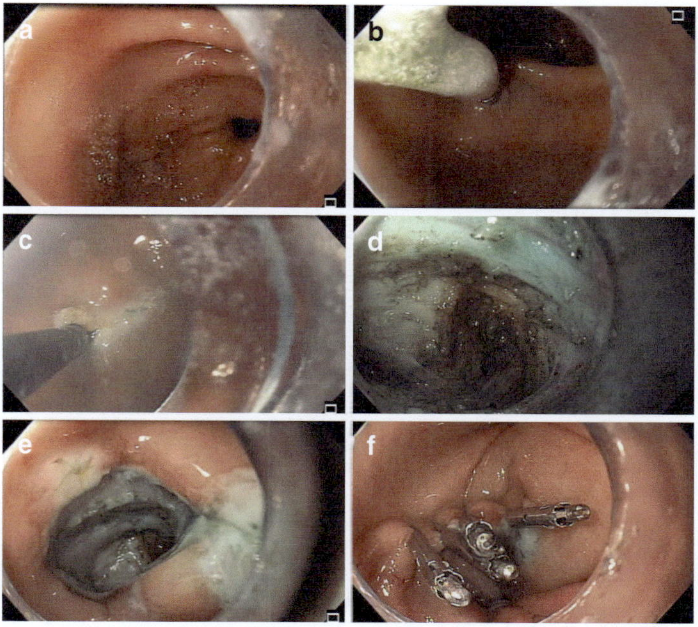

Fig. 24.2 Intraprocedural pictures describing the steps of peroral pyloromyotomy. (**a**) Endoscopic identification of the pylorus, (**b**) Injection of the pyloric mucosa, (**c**) mucosal dissection using endoscopic electrocautery, (**d**) extension of the dissection into the submucosal layers, (**e**) completion of pyloromyotomy, (**f**) closure of the mucosal defect with endoscopic clips

may help decrease nausea in addition to allowing weight loss [24]. For patients who remain severely symptomatic despite all other options including a subtotal gastrectomy, a completion total gastrectomy may be necessary [37].

– **Enteric access procedures:** When patients are unable to meet nutritional goals by oral intake, gastrostomy, jejunostomy, and GJ tubes may become necessary to allow venting and distal enteral access for feeding. These enteral tubes can be placed endoscopically in most cases. When endoscopic placement fails, laparoscopic or open surgical techniques can be utilized.

Conclusion

Gastroparesis is a rare disorder which may cause significant distress when inadequately treated. Diagnosis requires exclusion of mechanical obstruction and demonstration of delayed gastric emptying. Dietary modification is the first line of treatment. Depending on severity of symptoms, pharmacologic treatment with prokinetic agents and surgical interventions may be indicated.

References

1. Lacy BE, Parkman HP, Camilleri M. Chronic nausea and vomiting: evaluation and treatment. Am J Gastroenterol. 2018;113(5):647–59. https://doi.org/10.1038/s41395-018-0039-2.
2. Camilleri M, Parkman HP, Shafi MA, Abell TL, Gerson L. Clinical guideline: management of gastroparesis. Am J Gastroenterol. 2013;108(1):18–37.; quiz 8. https://doi.org/10.1038/ajg.2012.373.
3. Jung HK, Choung RS, Locke GR 3rd, Schleck CD, Zinsmeister AR, Szarka LA, et al. The incidence, prevalence, and outcomes of patients with gastroparesis in Olmsted County, Minnesota, from 1996 to 2006. Gastroenterology. 2009;136(4):1225–33. https://doi.org/10.1053/j.gastro.2008.12.047.
4. Soykan I, Sivri B, Sarosiek I, Kiernan B, McCallum RW. Demography, clinical characteristics, psychological and abuse profiles, treatment, and long-term follow-up of patients with gastroparesis. Dig Dis Sci. 1998;43(11):2398–404. https://doi.org/10.1023/a:1026665728213.
5. Vittal H, Farrugia G, Gomez G, Pasricha PJ. Mechanisms of disease: the pathological basis of gastroparesis—a review of experimental and clinical studies. Nat Clin Pract Gastroenterol Hepatol. 2007;4(6):336–46. https://doi.org/10.1038/ncpgasthep0838.
6. Forster J, Damjanov I, Lin Z, Sarosiek I, Wetzel P, McCallum RW. Absence of the interstitial cells of Cajal in patients with gastroparesis and correlation with clinical findings. J Gastrointest Surg. 2005;9(1):102–8. https://doi.org/10.1016/j.gassur.2004.10.001.
7. Choi KM, Gibbons SJ, Nguyen TV, Stoltz GJ, Lurken MS, Ordog T, et al. Heme oxygenase-1 protects interstitial cells of Cajal from oxidative stress and reverses diabetic gastroparesis. Gastroenterology. 2008;135(6):2055–64, 64.e1–2. https://doi.org/10.1053/j.gastro.2008.09.003.

8. Fich A, Neri M, Camilleri M, Kelly KA, Phillips SF. Stasis syndromes following gastric surgery: clinical and motility features of 60 symptomatic patients. J Clin Gastroenterol. 1990;12(5):505–12.
9. Bityutskiy LP, Soykan I, McCallum RW. Viral gastroparesis: a subgroup of idiopathic gastroparesis—clinical characteristics and long-term outcomes. Am J Gastroenterol. 1997;92(9):1501–4.
10. Dhamija R, Tan KM, Pittock SJ, Foxx-Orenstein A, Benarroch E, Lennon VA. Serologic profiles aiding the diagnosis of autoimmune gastrointestinal dysmotility. Clin Gastroenterol Hepatol. 2008;6(9):988–92. https://doi.org/10.1016/j.cgh.2008.04.009.
11. Jost WH. Gastrointestinal dysfunction in Parkinson's disease. J Neurol Sci. 2010;289(1–2):69–73. https://doi.org/10.1016/j.jns.2009.08.020.
12. Jeong ID, Camilleri M, Shin A, Iturrino J, Boldingh A, Busciglio I, et al. A randomised, placebo-controlled trial comparing the effects of tapentadol and oxycodone on gastrointestinal and colonic transit in healthy humans. Aliment Pharmacol Ther. 2012;35(9):1088–96. https://doi.org/10.1111/j.1365-2036.2012.05040.x.
13. Camilleri M. Gastroparesis: etiology, clinical manifestations, and diagnosis. Accessed 31 Aug 31 2020.
14. Bouras EP, Talley NJ, Camilleri M, Burton DD, Heckman MG, Crook JE, et al. Effects of amitriptyline on gastric sensorimotor function and postprandial symptoms in healthy individuals: a randomized, double-blind, placebo-controlled trial. Am J Gastroenterol. 2008;103(8):2043–50. https://doi.org/10.1111/j.1572-0241.2008.02021.x.
15. Sachdeva P, Kantor S, Knight LC, Maurer AH, Fisher RS, Parkman HP. Use of a high caloric liquid meal as an alternative to a solid meal for gastric emptying scintigraphy. Dig Dis Sci. 2013;58(7):2001–6. https://doi.org/10.1007/s10620-013-2665-2.
16. Abell TL, Camilleri M, Donohoe K, Hasler WL, Lin HC, Maurer AH, et al. Consensus recommendations for gastric emptying scintigraphy: a joint report of the American Neurogastroenterology and motility society and the Society of Nuclear Medicine. J Nucl Med Technol. 2008;36(1):44–54. https://doi.org/10.2967/jnmt.107.048116.
17. Tougas G, Eaker EY, Abell TL, Abrahamsson H, Boivin M, Chen J, et al. Assessment of gastric emptying using a low fat meal: establishment of international control values. Am J Gastroenterol. 2000;95(6):1456–62. https://doi.org/10.1111/j.1572-0241.2000.02076.x.
18. Wytiaz V, Homko C, Duffy F, Schey R, Parkman HP. Foods provoking and alleviating symptoms in gastroparesis: patient experiences. Dig Dis Sci. 2015;60(4):1052–8. https://doi.org/10.1007/s10620-015-3651-7.
19. Camilleri M. Treatment of gastroparesis. Accessed 31 Aug 31 2020.
20. Jebbink RJ, Samsom M, Bruijs PP, Bravenboer B, Akkermans LM, Vanberge-Henegouwen GP, et al. Hyperglycemia induces abnormalities

of gastric myoelectrical activity in patients with type I diabetes mellitus. Gastroenterology. 1994;107(5):1390–7. https://doi.org/10.1016/0016-5085(94)90541-x.
21. Jones KL, Berry M, Kong MF, Kwiatek MA, Samsom M, Horowitz M. Hyperglycemia attenuates the gastrokinetic effect of erythromycin and affects the perception of postprandial hunger in normal subjects. Diabetes Care. 1999;22(2):339–44. https://doi.org/10.2337/diacare.22.2.339.
22. Grover M, Farrugia G, Stanghellini V. Gastroparesis: a turning point in understanding and treatment. Gut. 2019;68(12):2238–50. https://doi.org/10.1136/gutjnl-2019-318712.
23. Shada A, Nielsen A, Marowski S, Helm M, Funk LM, Kastenmeier A, et al. Wisconsin's Enterra therapy experience: a multi-institutional review of gastric electrical stimulation for medically refractory gastroparesis. Surgery. 2018;164(4):760–5. https://doi.org/10.1016/j.surg.2018.04.043.
24. Wakamatsu K, Perez Quirante F, Montorfano L, Lo Menzo E, Seto Y, Rosenthal RJ. Laparoscopic treatment of gastroparesis: a single center experience. Surg Obes Relat Dis. 2018;14(2):200–5. https://doi.org/10.1016/j.soard.2017.07.029.
25. Lin Z, Forster J, Sarosiek I, McCallum RW. Treatment of diabetic gastroparesis by high-frequency gastric electrical stimulation. Diabetes Care. 2004;27(5):1071–6. https://doi.org/10.2337/diacare.27.5.1071.
26. Lin Z, McElhinney C, Sarosiek I, Forster J, McCallum R. Chronic gastric electrical stimulation for gastroparesis reduces the use of prokinetic and/or antiemetic medications and the need for hospitalizations. Dig Dis Sci. 2005;50(7):1328–34. https://doi.org/10.1007/s10620-005-2782-7.
27. Mearin F, Camilleri M, Malagelada JR. Pyloric dysfunction in diabetics with recurrent nausea and vomiting. Gastroenterology. 1986;90(6):1919–25. https://doi.org/10.1016/0016-5085(86)90262-3.
28. Wellington J, Scott B, Kundu S, Stuart P, Koch KL. Effect of endoscopic pyloric therapies for patients with nausea and vomiting and functional obstructive gastroparesis. Auton Neurosci. 2017;202:56–61. https://doi.org/10.1016/j.autneu.2016.07.004.
29. Arts J, Holvoet L, Caenepeel P, Bisschops R, Sifrim D, Verbeke K, et al. Clinical trial: a randomized-controlled crossover study of intrapyloric injection of botulinum toxin in gastroparesis. Aliment Pharmacol Ther. 2007;26(9):1251–8. https://doi.org/10.1111/j.1365-2036.2007.03467.x.
30. Friedenberg FK, Palit A, Parkman HP, Hanlon A, Nelson DB. Botulinum toxin a for the treatment of delayed gastric emptying. Am J Gastroenterol. 2008;103(2):416–23. https://doi.org/10.1111/j.1572-0241.2007.01676.x.
31. Bashashati M, Moraveji S, Torabi A, Sarosiek I, Davis BR, Diaz J, et al. Pathological findings of the antral and pyloric smooth muscle in patients with gastroparesis-like syndrome compared to gastroparesis: similarities and differences. Dig Dis Sci. 2017;62(10):2828–33. https://doi.org/10.1007/s10620-017-4629-4.

32. Davis BR, Sarosiek I, Bashashati M, Alvarado B, McCallum RW. The long-term efficacy and safety of Pyloroplasty combined with gastric electrical stimulation therapy in gastroparesis. J Gastrointest Surg. 2017;21(2):222–7. https://doi.org/10.1007/s11605-016-3327-4.
33. Rodriguez JH, Haskins IN, Strong AT, Plescia RL, Allemang MT, Butler RS, et al. Per oral endoscopic pyloromyotomy for refractory gastroparesis: initial results from a single institution. Surg Endosc. 2017;31(12):5381–8. https://doi.org/10.1007/s00464-017-5619-5.
34. Mekaroonkamol P, Dacha S, Wang L, Li X, Jiang Y, Li L, et al. Gastric Peroral endoscopic Pyloromyotomy reduces symptoms, increases quality of life, and reduces health care use for patients with gastroparesis. Clin Gastroenterol Hepatol. 2019;17(1):82–9. https://doi.org/10.1016/j.cgh.2018.04.016.
35. Hibbard ML, Dunst CM, Swanström LL. Laparoscopic and endoscopic pyloroplasty for gastroparesis results in sustained symptom improvement. J Gastrointest Surg. 2011;15(9):1513–9. https://doi.org/10.1007/s11605-011-1607-6.
36. Watkins PJ, Buxton-Thomas MS, Howard ER. Long-term outcome after gastrectomy for intractable diabetic gastroparesis. Diabet Med. 2003;20(1):58–63. https://doi.org/10.1046/j.1464-5491.2003.00872.x.
37. Forstner-Barthell AW, Murr MM, Nitecki S, Camilleri M, Prather CM, Kelly KA, et al. Near-total completion gastrectomy for severe postvagotomy gastric stasis: analysis of early and long-term results in 62 patients. J Gastrointest Surg. 1999;3(1):15–21, discussion –3. https://doi.org/10.1016/s1091-255x(99)80003-1.

25 Dumping Syndrome

Bora Kahramangil, Emanuele Lo Menzo, Samuel Szomstein, and Raul Rosenthal

Introduction

Dumping syndrome is a gastrointestinal pathology characterized by vasomotor and gastrointestinal symptoms occurring secondary to rapid gastric emptying. The changes in gastric emptying are frequently secondary to postsurgical anatomic alterations following upper gastrointestinal surgery. Although the incidence of dumping syndrome has historically decreased with the discovery of the association of Helicobacter pylori with gastric ulcer and the subsequent decrease in the number of ulcer operations, it is once again on the rise due to the increasing number of bariatric procedures. A good understanding of this pathology remains important for clinical practice.

B. Kahramangil · E. Lo Menzo (✉) · S. Szomstein · R. Rosenthal
Cleveland Clinic Florida, Department of General Surgery, Bariatric and Metabolic Institute, Weston, FL, USA
e-mail: lomenze@ccf.org

A. D. Patel et al. (eds.), *The SAGES Manual of Physiologic Evaluation of Foregut Diseases*,
https://doi.org/10.1007/978-3-031-39199-6_25

Pathophysiology

The main factors in the pathophysiology of dumping syndrome include rapid transit of chyme, pathologic fluid shifts, and the resulting hormonal changes.

1. **Rapid transit of chyme:** Rapid transit of chyme is the major driver of dumping syndrome pathophysiology. The chyme in dumping syndrome is incompletely digested and hyperosmolar [1]. Large volume, hyperosmolar chyme causes duodenal distension, which in turn leads to a reflexive increase in intestinal contractility [2]. This reflex response is mediated by the intestinal smooth muscles and the myenteric neural plexus. It causes abdominal symptoms related to dumping syndrome. Overall, liquid meals are more likely to trigger these symptoms than solids. However, it is worth noting that not every patient with rapid gastric emptying experiences dumping syndrome-related symptoms [1]. Neuroplastic changes in the enteric neural plexus and the resulting adaptation likely underlie the lack of symptoms in some individuals. The patients with dumping syndrome fail to demonstrate adaptive changes to handle rapidly transited chyme.
2. **Fluid shifts:** Distension of the intestine with chyme leads to a fluid shift from the systemic circulation into the intestinal vasculature and lumen. This physiologic response is called splanchnic blood pooling and is mediated by gastrointestinal hormones, as well as the parasympathetic response to the distension of the intestine by chyme [3, 4]. In normal individuals, this is balanced by a compensatory sympathetic discharge. It is hypothesized that in patients with dumping syndrome, the splanchnic blood pooling is potent enough to overcome the compensatory mechanisms [2]. Splanchnic pooling causes symptoms like fatigue, lightheadedness, and in severe cases hypotension. Concurrent sympathetic discharge causes palpitations and sweating. All together, these symptoms constitute the vasomotor symptoms of dumping syndrome.

3. **Hormonal changes:** Alterations in gastrointestinal hormone levels have long been recognized in dumping syndrome. Hyperosmolar, high volume chyme resulting from rapid gastric emptying increases gastrointestinal hormone secretion to supraphysiologic levels [5]. Of the many hormonal abnormalities demonstrated, vasoactive intestinal peptide (VIP) and serotonin appears to have prominent roles in dumping syndrome pathophysiology [6]. VIP increases splanchnic blood flow, intestinal contractions, and secretion of electrolytes and water into the intestinal lumen. Similarly, serotonin causes splanchnic vasodilation. Oversecretion of these hormones may contribute to rapid transit and fluid shifts. Bradykinin has vasodilatory effects and increases vascular permeability [7]. An exaggerated bradykinin response can increase fluid shifts into peripheral vascular tissues, which may contribute to the flushing seen in some patients with dumping syndrome. Norepinephrine levels have also been found to be elevated in dumping syndrome. This may contribute to early sympathetic vasomotor symptoms including tachycardia and sweating [8]. Finally, insulinotropic hormones may be major drivers of late dumping syndrome, which is characterized by delayed hypoglycemia in response to a food bolus. An exaggerated secretion of glucagon-like peptide 1 (GLP-1) and glucose-dependent insulinotropic polypeptide (GIP) in response to hyperosmolar chyme is seen in dumping syndrome [9]. This leads to an increase in insulin secretion and inhibition of glucagon, subsequently causing hypoglycemia.

Epidemiology and Etiology

Dumping syndrome can be caused by surgical and nonsurgical etiologies. Up to 50% of gastric operations can cause rapid gastric emptying, albeit with different rates of symptoms severe enough to warrant work-up and treatment for dumping syndrome [10]. In adults, Roux-en-Y gastric bypass is the most common cause of surgical dumping syndrome [11]. In the pediatric population, dumping syndrome is frequently secondary to Nissen fundoplication [12].

Gastric operations cause dumping syndrome by increasing the rate of chyme transit from the stomach into the intestines [2]. In normal gastric physiology, the antrum and pylorus limit gastric emptying, and the fundus acts as a reservoir for the food bolus. Roux-en-Y gastric bypass can cause dumping syndrome due to a small gastric reservoir and bypassing of the pyloric sphincter. Sleeve gastrectomy, although less frequently, can also cause dumping syndrome due to decreased gastric volume and increased emptying times. Nissen fundoplication can disrupt the reservoir function of the stomach due to decreased fundus volume to accommodate a food bolus. Vagus transections, on the other hand, can have mixed effects on gastric emptying. In patients with an intact pylorus, gastric emptying may be delayed after vagal transection due to a blunted pyloric relaxation. However, vagal reflexes also maintain receptive gastric relaxation following ingestion of a food bolus and inhibition of gastric emptying in response to intestinal stretch. Loss of these arcs can promote rapid gastric emptying.

Nonsurgical causes of dumping syndrome are overall less common. Although early diabetes typically causes gastroparesis, patients with long-standing diabetes sometimes experience dumping syndrome [13]. In a subgroup of patients, the onset of dumping syndrome follows an episode of gastroenteritis. This is likely related to duodenal mucosal damage and the subsequent alteration in duodenal receptors. Finally, there is an idiopathic form of dumping syndrome. In these patients, vagal function may be impaired, resulting in decreased gastric accommodation [5].

Clinical Presentation

Dumping syndrome has two distinct forms based on the constellation of symptoms and timing of their onset after a meal [2] (Table 25.1). Early dumping syndrome occurs within 30 min of a meal and is characterized by systemic and abdominal symptoms. Systemic symptoms include fatigue, lightheadedness, tachycar-

Table 25.1 Clinical presentations of early and late dumping syndrome

Early dumping syndrome	Late dumping syndrome
Onset: Within 30 min of a meal	Onset: 1–3 h after a meal
Driving physiology: Hyperosmolar chyme and fluid shifts	Driving physiology: Reactive hypoglycemia
Systemic symptoms	**Systemic signs**
Palpitations	Sweating
Lightheadedness	Altered level of consciousness
Fatigue	Lightheadedness
Headache	
Hypotension	**Biochemical features**
Abdominal symptoms	Reactive hypoglycemia
Early satiety	
Epigastric pain or fullness	
Diarrhea	
Nausea	
Abdominal cramps	

dia, flushing or pallor, sweating, and in severe cases, syncope. Accompanying gastrointestinal symptoms include early satiety, epigastric pain or fullness sensation, diarrhea, abdominal cramps, and nausea. Early dumping syndrome is the most common presentation. The second form is late dumping syndrome. The symptoms in this form typically manifest 1–3 h after ingestion of a meal and include sweating and lightheadedness in the setting of hypoglycemia, and in severe cases, altered level of consciousness. It is possible to have concurrent early and late dumping syndrome [14]. Severe, long-standing dumping syndrome can lead to protein-energy malnutrition. Other long-term complications include depression, anxiety, and avoidance of social interactions involving eating.

Diagnosis

The diagnosis of dumping syndrome is made with the demonstration of rapid gastric emptying in the presence of appropriate symptoms. Gastric scintigraphy is the gold standard test for gastric emptying, while oral glucose challenge may help demonstrate the maladaptive response to a food bolus. Esophagogastroduodenoscopy, colonoscopy, and stool analysis can be used to rule out other differential diagnoses.

Clinical Evaluation and Diagnostic Modalities

Clinical evaluation for dumping syndrome starts with a thorough history and physical examination. Suggestive signs and symptoms include abdominal fullness, nausea, pallor, palpitations, weakness, and lightheadedness. Severe cases can cause altered mental status and syncope.

- **Demonstration of rapid gastric emptying:** Radionuclide gastric scintigraphy is the gold standard test for demonstration of rapid gastric emptying. Standard meal for the test consists of a 250-calorie egg-substitute labeled with 99mTc, 120 mL of water, and two slices of whole wheat bread [15]. Images are taken immediately after ingestion, at 30 min, and at 1 h, followed by hourly images up to 4 h after meal. In each image, gastric retention is calculated based on the percentage of radioisotopes remaining in the stomach. <35% retention at 1 h is diagnostic for rapid gastric emptying. In late dumping syndrome, <20% retention at 2 h is typical.
- **Oral glucose challenge test:** Oral glucose challenge test can be useful to confirm the diagnosis of dumping syndrome. Patients ingest 50 g of glucose after 10 h of overnight fasting [16]. Pulse and blood pressure are monitored at baseline, during ingestion and after ingestion. Blood glucose and hematocrit can also be measured at these time points and repeated at 30-min intervals. An increase in heart rate of at least 10 beats per minute is considered positive. A 3% increase in hematocrit within the first 30 min after ingestion is compatible with early dumping syndrome. Glucose level < 60 mg/dL at 2–3 h after ingestion indicates late dumping syndrome.

Treatment

Treatment of dumping syndrome starts with lifestyle and dietary modifications. If the symptoms persist despite these changes, pharmacologic treatment is the next step. Surgical procedures are reserved for most severe cases, where symptoms cannot be controlled by any other means (Table 25.2).

- **Dietary modifications:** Dietary modifications are the first line of treatment for dumping syndrome. Patients should ingest smaller but more frequent meals, limit carbohydrate intake, and preferentially eat complex over simple carbohydrates [17]. Lying down after a meal and ingesting solids and liquids separately can also help, as fluids are likely to increase gastric emptying. Increasing dietary fiber may slow down gastric emptying, helping avoid hypoglycemia in late dumping syndrome, and proteins can provide additional calories without worsening symptoms. Despite low patient compliance due to poor taste, guar gum and pectin are useful dietary adjuncts [18]. Both supplements work by increasing the viscosity of food bolus and subsequently help delay gastric emptying.

Table 25.2 Treatment options for dumping syndrome

Dietary modifications	Pharmacologic modifications	Surgical treatment
Ingestion of smaller but more frequent meals	Loperamide	Roux-en-Y gastric bypass reversal
Limited carbohydrate intake	Tincture of opium	Roux-en-Y gastric bypass revision
Preferential ingestion of complex carbohydrates	Acarbose	Continuous enteral feeding
Separation of liquid and solid meals	Octreotide	
Increased dietary fiber	GLP-1 agonists	
Increased protein intake		
Guar gum and pectin		

- **Pharmacologic treatment:** Antimotility drugs can be useful to treat diarrhea associated with dumping syndrome. Loperamide, a gut opioid receptor agonist, and tincture of opium can be used to decrease stool liquidity [19]. Anticholinergic agents can also improve dumping syndrome-related symptoms. They have antidiarrheal effects, slow gastric emptying, and decreased gastrointestinal cramps. Acarbose can be used to prevent hypoglycemia in late dumping syndrome. It is an alpha glycosidase inhibitor, which inhibits the digestion of polysaccharides into monosaccharides [20]. Decreasing carbohydrate absorption can help mitigate the maladaptive insulin and glucagon-like peptide 1 secretion seen in late dumping syndrome. When all other pharmaceutical options fail, octreotide can be tried. Octreotide is a somatostatin analog, which slows gastric emptying and decreases splanchnic blood flow [21]. Furthermore, it inhibits the secretion of intestinal hormones including vasoactive intestinal peptide, insulin, and serotonin. Octreotide improves the symptoms of both early and late dumping syndrome. More recently, GLP-1 agonists have been successfully utilized in the management of late dumping syndrome and hypoglycemia after gastric bypass surgery.
- **Surgical treatment:** Surgery is the last resort for patients who continue to be severely symptomatic despite dietary modifications and maximal pharmacologic treatment. When undertaken, surgical treatment is usually directed at the underlying anatomic abnormality causing dumping syndrome.
  - **Roux-en-Y gastric bypass reversal:** In most cases, dumping syndrome following Roux-en-Y gastric bypass can be adequately controlled with dietary modifications and pharmacologic treatment. However, refractory dumping syndrome, especially in the setting of hypoglycemia, may require surgical revision. Gastric bypass reversal to normal anatomy has been proposed to help control symptoms of dumping syndrome. In 2013, Villalonga et al. reported successful laparoscopic gastric bypass reversal in a series of patients with different pathologies including refractory dumping syndrome [22]. In the six patients who underwent

surgery for dumping syndrome, a leak was observed in one patient, which was managed with laparoscopic drainage. Despite the possibility of a successful conversion to a normal anatomy, weight regain remains a major concern in patients with history of obesity. To overcome this issue, Roux-en-Y gastric bypass reversal with concomitant sleeve gastrectomy has been proposed. Carter et al. analyzed the outcomes of 12 patients who underwent conversion of gastric bypass to sleeve gastrectomy due to various complications including refractory dumping syndrome [23]. Seven major complications were observed in 4 patients including a portal vein thrombosis, postoperative bleed, pancreatic leak, pulmonary embolism, seroma, anastomotic leak, and stricture. Although effective, this is a morbid procedure and requires very careful patient selection.

- **Gastric pouch restriction:** In some patients with Roux-en-Y gastric bypass, refractory hypoglycemia may develop with concurrent loss of gastric restriction due to gastric pouch dilation. In this highly selected group of patients, reconstitution of gastric restriction may help improve hypoglycemia. Different techniques described to restrict gastric pouch volume include the surgical downsizing of the pouch, silastic ring placement, and placement of an adjustable band [17]. Z'graggen et al. analyzed the outcomes of restoration of gastric restriction in 12 patients with refractory hypoglycemia utilizing silastic ring (n = 8) and adjustable gastric band (n = 4) [24]. In this series, perioperative complication rate was 8% with resolution of hypoglycemic episodes in 11 out of 12 patients.
- **Continuous enteral feeding:** Continuous enteral feeding through a feeding jejunostomy can be used in select patients with refractory late dumping syndrome. This eliminates the need for food ingestion and helps prevent hypoglycemia. Enteral access can be obtained by endoscopic or surgical procedures.

References

1. Gulsrud PO, Taylor IL, Watts HD, Cohen MB, Elashoff J, Meyer JH. How gastric emptying of carbohydrate affects glucose tolerance and symptoms after truncal vagotomy with pyloroplasty. Gastroenterology. 1980;78(6):1463–71.
2. Berg P, McCallum R. Dumping syndrome: a review of the current concepts of pathophysiology, diagnosis, and treatment. Dig Dis Sci. 2016;61(1):11–8. https://doi.org/10.1007/s10620-015-3839-x.
3. Aldoori MI, Qamar MI, Read AE, Williamson RC. Increased flow in the superior mesenteric artery in dumping syndrome. Br J Surg. 1985;72(5):389–90. https://doi.org/10.1002/bjs.1800720518.
4. Lipsitz LA, Ryan SM, Parker JA, Freeman R, Wei JY, Goldberger AL. Hemodynamic and autonomic nervous system responses to mixed meal ingestion in healthy young and old subjects and dysautonomic patients with postprandial hypotension. Circulation. 1993;87(2):391–400. https://doi.org/10.1161/01.cir.87.2.391.
5. Lawaetz O, Blackburn AM, Bloom SR, Aritas Y, Ralphs DN. Gut hormone profile and gastric emptying in the dumping syndrome. A hypothesis concerning the pathogenesis. Scand J Gastroenterol. 1983;18(1):73–80. https://doi.org/10.3109/00365528309181562.
6. Sagor GR, Bryant MG, Ghatei MA, Kirk RM, Bloom SR. Release of vasoactive intestinal peptide in the dumping syndrome. Br Med J (Clin Res Ed). 1981;282(6263):507–10. https://doi.org/10.1136/bmj.282.6263.507.
7. Macdonald JM, Webster MM Jr, Tennyson CH, Drapanas T. Serotonin and bradykinin in the dumping syndrome. Am J Surg. 1969;117(2):204–13. https://doi.org/10.1016/0002-9610(69)90305-5.
8. Gebhard B, Holst JJ, Biegelmayer C, Miholic J. Postprandial GLP-1, norepinephrine, and reactive hypoglycemia in dumping syndrome. Dig Dis Sci. 2001;46(9):1915–23. https://doi.org/10.1023/a:1010635131228.
9. Lin HC, Neevel C, Chen PS, Suh G, Chen JH. Slowing of intestinal transit by fat or peptide YY depends on beta-adrenergic pathway. Am J Physiol Gastrointest Liver Physiol. 2003;285(6):G1310–6. https://doi.org/10.1152/ajpgi.00230.2003.
10. Davis JL, Ripley RT. Postgastrectomy syndromes and nutritional considerations following gastric surgery. Surg Clin North Am. 2017;97(2):277–93. https://doi.org/10.1016/j.suc.2016.11.005.
11. Abell TL, Minocha A. Gastrointestinal complications of bariatric surgery: diagnosis and therapy. Am J Med Sci. 2006;331(4):214–8. https://doi.org/10.1097/00000441-200604000-00008.
12. Samuk I, Afriat R, Horne T, Bistritzer T, Barr J, Vinograd I. Dumping syndrome following Nissen fundoplication, diagnosis, and treatment. J

Pediatr Gastroenterol Nutr. 1996;23(3):235–40. https://doi.org/10.1097/00005176-199610000-00006.
13. Hejazi RA, Patil H, McCallum RW. Dumping syndrome: establishing criteria for diagnosis and identifying new etiologies. Dig Dis Sci. 2010;55(1):117–23. https://doi.org/10.1007/s10620-009-0939-5.
14. Eagon JC, Miedema BW, Kelly KA. Postgastrectomy syndromes. Surg Clin North Am. 1992;72(2):445–65. https://doi.org/10.1016/s0039-6109(16)45689-6.
15. Tougas G, Eaker EY, Abell TL, Abrahamsson H, Boivin M, Chen J, et al. Assessment of gastric emptying using a low fat meal: establishment of international control values. Am J Gastroenterol. 2000;95(6):1456–62. https://doi.org/10.1111/j.1572-0241.2000.02076.x.
16. van der Kleij FG, Vecht J, Lamers CB, Masclee AA. Diagnostic value of dumping provocation in patients after gastric surgery. Scand J Gastroenterol. 1996;31(12):1162–6. https://doi.org/10.3109/00365529609036905.
17. van Beek AP, Emous M, Laville M, Tack J. Dumping syndrome after esophageal, gastric or bariatric surgery: pathophysiology, diagnosis, and management. Obes Rev. 2017;18(1):68–85. https://doi.org/10.1111/obr.12467.
18. Leeds AR, Ralphs DN, Ebied F, Metz G, Dilawari JB. Pectin in the dumping syndrome: reduction of symptoms and plasma volume changes. Lancet. 1981;1(8229):1075–8. https://doi.org/10.1016/s0140-6736(81)92242-x.
19. Schiller LR. Chronic diarrhea. Curr Treat Options Gastroenterol. 2005;8(3):259–66. https://doi.org/10.1007/s11938-005-0018-8.
20. De Cunto A, Barbi E, Minen F, Ventura A. Safety and efficacy of high-dose acarbose treatment for dumping syndrome. J Pediatr Gastroenterol Nutr. 2011;53(1):113–4. https://doi.org/10.1097/MPG.0b013e31820ae6d1.
21. Hasler WL, Soudah HC, Owyang C. Mechanisms by which octreotide ameliorates symptoms in the dumping syndrome. J Pharmacol Exp Ther. 1996;277(3):1359–65.
22. Vilallonga R, van de Vrande S, Himpens J. Laparoscopic reversal of roux-en-Y gastric bypass into normal anatomy with or without sleeve gastrectomy. Surg Endosc. 2013;27(12):4640–8. https://doi.org/10.1007/s00464-013-3087-0.
23. Carter CO, Fernandez AZ, McNatt SS, Powell MS. Conversion from gastric bypass to sleeve gastrectomy for complications of gastric bypass. Surg Obes Relat Dis. 2016;12(3):572–6. https://doi.org/10.1016/j.soard.2015.07.001.
24. Z'Graggen K, Guweidhi A, Steffen R, Potoczna N, Biral R, Walther F, et al. Severe recurrent hypoglycemia after gastric bypass surgery. Obes Surg. 2008;18(8):981–8. https://doi.org/10.1007/s11695-008-9480-4.

Normal Physiology Findings After Hiatal Hernia Repair and Fundoplication

26

Ramses A. Saavedra and Edward Auyang

Introduction

Hiatal hernia repair and fundoplication are performed in symptomatic patients to help provide relief from the symptoms produced by the abnormal hiatal anatomy. The goal of surgical repair is restoration of "normal" anatomy. This is achieved by reduction of the hernia and recreation of a functional gastroesophageal junction (GEJ) below the level of the diaphragm. Various techniques can be used to achieve this, including Nissen, Toupet, and Dor fundoplications. Upon recreation of the normal anatomy, restoration of physiologic function is expected. There are several common studies used to assess postoperative anatomy and physiology. The studies discussed here include contrasted upper gastrointestinal esophagram (UGI), computed tomography (CT) scan, esophageal manometry, pH testing, endoscopy, gastric emptying studies, and endoluminal functional imaging. Through analysis of these studies, we will clarify what findings can be considered as normal and address some common variations seen after different operative techniques.

R. A. Saavedra · E. Auyang (✉)
Department of Surgery, University of New Mexico School of Medicine, Albuquerque, NM, USA
e-mail: rasaavedra@salud.unm.edu; eauyang@salud.unm.edu

A. D. Patel et al. (eds.), *The SAGES Manual of Physiologic Evaluation of Foregut Diseases*,
https://doi.org/10.1007/978-3-031-39199-6_26

Upper GI/Esophagram

UGI is a powerful tool in assessing esophageal and gastric anatomy. Images can be obtained in upright, oblique, and supine positions and can also dynamically evaluate function by observing contrast flow in real-time and passage of a radiolucent tablet during a swallow. While the anatomic and functional information that these studies provide in the preoperative evaluation of a hiatal hernia is valuable, routine use in the postoperative evaluation of asymptomatic patients is not required [1]. However, postoperative contrast studies are still obtained by some providers to evaluate for leak immediately post-procedure or to evaluate the anatomic results [2, 3].

After hiatal hernia repair and fundoplication, contrast imaging should show a smooth, tapered narrowing of the distal esophagus and GEJ with a 2–3 cm wrap seen below the level of the diaphragm (Fig. 26.1) [2, 4, 5]. There should not be any evidence of hernia recurrence or reflux. Immediately postoperatively, there may be evidence of swelling near the fundoplication due to tissue edema. However, this swelling should not interfere with passage of radio-opaque material or cause any significant esophageal dilation proximally (Fig. 26.2). When visualized, the leaves of the fundoplication will appear as blind ends surrounding the esophagus. The anterior leaf of the fundoplication may not be visualized as it is challenging to reflux contrast into this area [4]. Patient positioning should be verified as the fundal wrap defect may form an acute angle created by the plication and the nonsurgical gastric wall when the patient is supine [5]. It is important to know the surgical procedure performed as the type of fundoplication performed may alter interpretation of imaged results. For example, a Toupet or Dor fundoplication may be misinterpreted as a disrupted fundoplication. If an esophageal lengthening procedure was necessary, the presence of gastric folds within the wrap is expected.

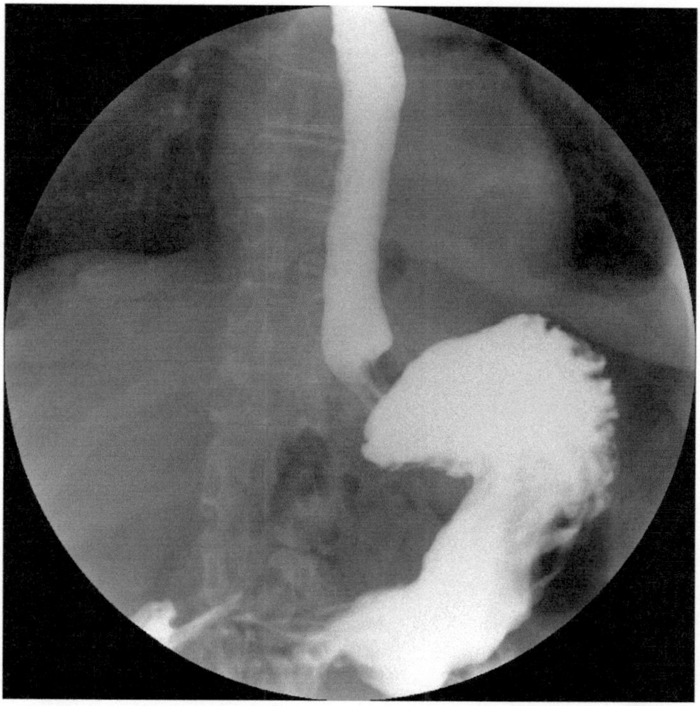

Fig. 26.1 Normal UGI showing contrast easily passing through an intact fundoplication into stomach

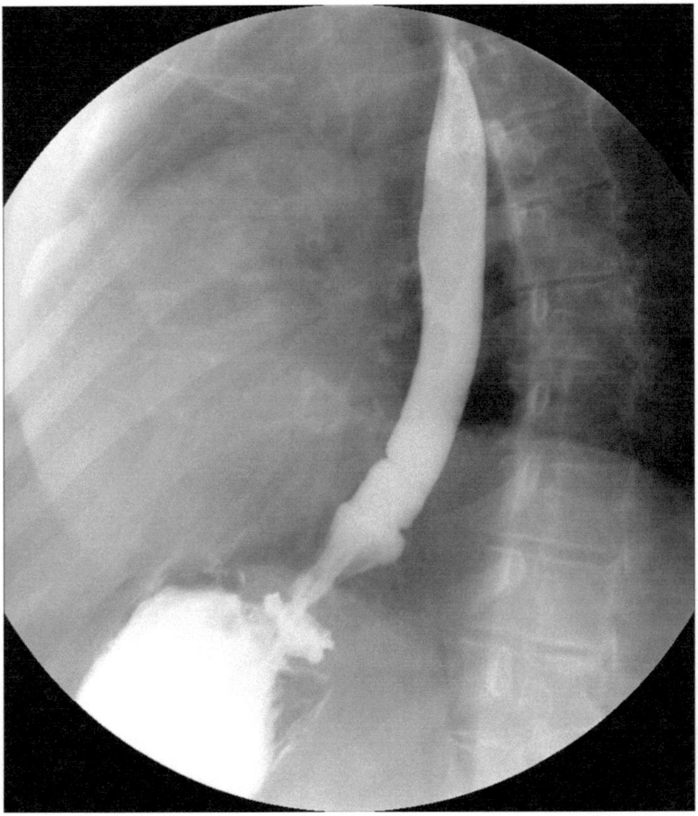

Fig. 26.2 Normal UGI from a lateral perspective showing an intact wrap with contrast entering the leaflets of the fundoplication

Computed Tomography

CT imaging may be obtained for various reasons in patients post-fundoplication. The patient may be symptomatic from the wrap itself, or the wrap may be incidentally seen during evaluation of another anatomical pathology. Similar to the discussion of UGI, understanding the performed surgical procedure and subsequent expected anatomy is critical to proper interpretation of CT imaging.

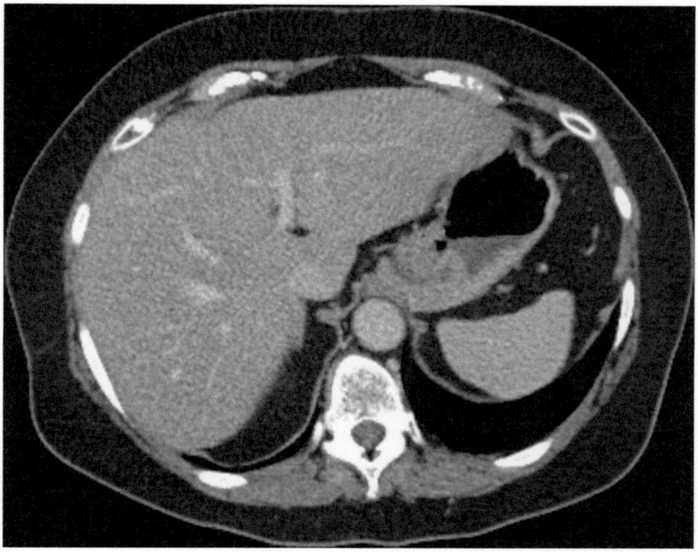

Fig. 26.3 CT scan showing leaflets of the fundoplication wrapping around the distal esophagus

Imaging should clearly show the gastric fundus wrapped around the distal esophagus. Again, the GEJ will lie below the diaphragm with a 2–3 cm wrap surrounding it (Fig. 26.3). No evidence of hernia recurrence should be present. Gaseous distension of the body and fundus of the stomach do not suggest underlying pathology and should still permit for proper fundoplication evaluation [6]. In the first several weeks postoperatively, thickening of the gastric mucosa at the fundoplication secondary to edema is expected [6]. If contrast is used, it ought to pass through the fundoplication easily and there should not be significant esophageal dilation. A slight "whirled" appearance of the fundoplication is within normal limits [5]. As discussed above, Toupet or Dor fundoplication may again appear as a disrupted fundoplication on CT and so reference to the original procedure should be made when possible.

Manometry and Motility

There is extensive literature regarding evaluation of the physiology of the esophagus in the preoperative and postoperative settings. Esophageal manometry allows for assessment of global motility as well as the subcomponents of the esophagus. It is not typically conducted on a routine basis after fundoplication as its association with symptomatology has been controversial. The normal pressures produced by the esophagus in the asymptomatic patient can vary widely [7]. Hiatal hernia repair and fundoplication do not affect the physiologic function of the esophagus and are not associated with motility changes in the esophageal body [8]. Therefore, peristaltic function is expected to be unchanged due to a repair and fundoplication. The lower esophageal sphincter (LES) may see some change in pressures. Patients' LES resting pressures tend to be lower preoperatively, with mean pressure ranging from 6 to 16 mmHg [8–10]. Postoperatively, there is a statistically significant increase in mean pressures, with a range of 17–24 mmHg [8–10]. These changes are expected and are not associated with symptomatology such as dysphagia.

pH Testing

pH testing is typically performed using catheter-based pH monitoring or the portable BRAVO system. This testing evaluates for reflux and can be clinically correlated to the patient's symptoms. Similar to manometry, pH testing is not routinely done in asymptomatic patients postoperatively. However, pH testing has been used for objective confirmation of surgical success in postoperative patients via examination of time with pH <4.0 and DeMeester score. Preoperatively, patients have an increased time with a pH <4.0 in the esophagus compared to normal and a DeMeester score > 14.7 which indicates abnormally high amount of reflux [9, 10]. The anatomical restoration of the LES provided by fundoplication improves both of these metrics. Postoperatively, patients should experience a normalization of DeMeester score to <14.7 and the time of pH <4.0 decreases to ≤5.5% of the time on 24-hr evaluation [9, 10]. These results have also been seen in BRAVO pH analysis. This analysis reiterates decreased reflux episodes, decreased percentage time with pH < 4.0, and significant improvements in DeMeester score to as low as 1.25 in postoperative patients [11]. Those who undergo giant hiatal hernia repair in addition to fundoplication will show the same normalization of DeMeester score and percentage time pH < 4.0, though the objective data may show slightly more episodes of reflux compared to fundoplication alone [12]. These data do not correlate with any clinically significant change in patient symptomatology and is still within normal limits of objective findings. If patients have recurrent or atypical symptoms postoperative, the pH study can be used as a test to rule out GERD as an etiology especially when symptoms do not correlate with objective episodes of reflux.

Endoscopy

Endoscopy is standard in the evaluation of upper gastrointestinal tract pathology, including hiatal hernia evaluation in the preoperative setting. It can also be utilized postoperatively to evaluate the integrity of hiatal hernia repair and fundoplication. It is important to understand endoscopic findings in both settings. The Hill classification is a grading system that has been utilized for evaluation of hiatal hernias. Its principles can be used in both pre- and postoperative settings to evaluate the gastroesophageal flap [13]. Hill classification grades the valve integrity from I-IV. Grade I shows a prominent fold of gastric tissue directly against the endoscope. As the grades increase, the evidence of the gastroesophageal flap is less apparent and the tissue no longer approximates the scope. Grade IV will show an open esophageal lumen and an obvious hiatal hernia. Appropriate surgical repair should reapproximate

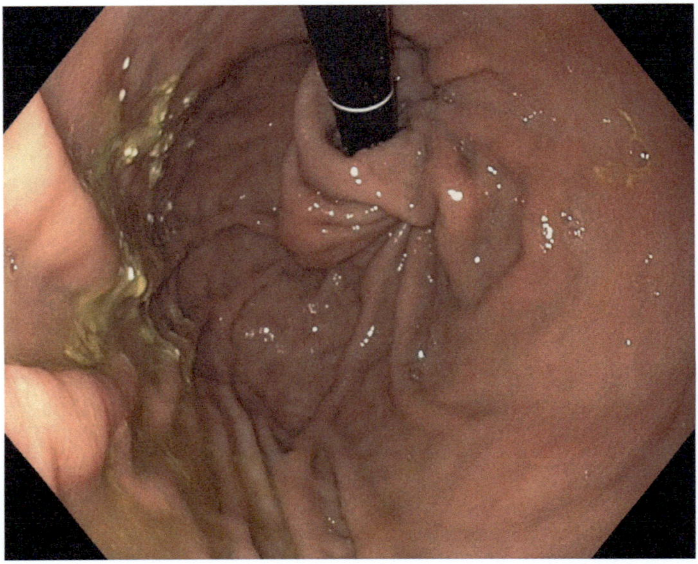

Fig. 26.4 Endoscopy showing an intact Nissen fundoplication

the normal anatomy; however, it is important to reiterate that anatomy visualized on endoscopic evaluation is dependent on the specific repair used.

For example, Nissen fundoplication will lead to creation of a nipple valve on endoscopy with a deep posterior and shallow anterior groove (Fig. 26.4) [14]. The valve will have an "omega" shape to it and should closely approximate the endoscope. Similarly, a Toupet fundoplication will have a flap valve in an "omega" shape and may look identical to that of a Nissen fundoplication (Fig. 26.5) [14]. Lastly, a Dor fundoplication will have a flap valve that is wide and "S"-shaped and should moderately approximate the scope [14]. Regardless of the operative technique used, the gastroesophageal flap should closely approximate the scope, thus resembling a Hill grade I without evidence of a recurrent hiatal hernia.

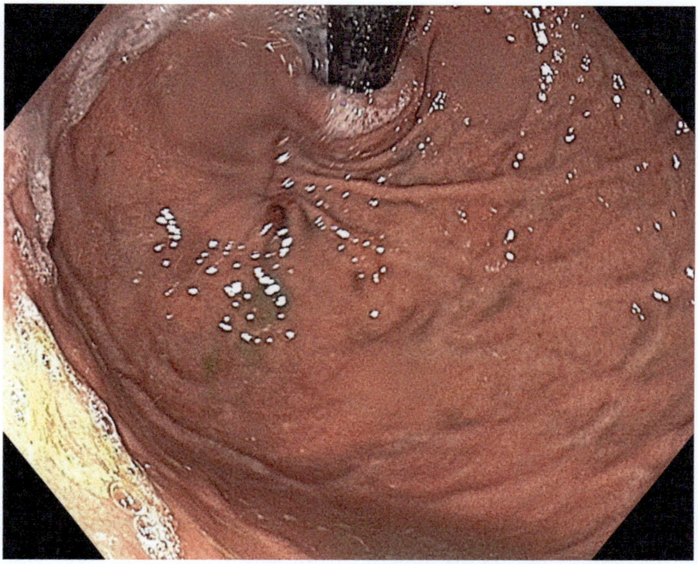

Fig. 26.5 Endoscopy showing an intact Toupet fundoplication

Gastric Emptying

Gastric emptying is usually measured over 2–4 h using Tc-99 sulfur colloid foods. Normal values are 10% emptying at 1 hr., 65% at 2 h, and 90% at 4 h [15]. Delayed gastric emptying is uncommon after surgery; however, it is more commonly reported in cases after very large hiatal hernia repairs or redo paraesophageal hernia repairs [16, 17], likely from gastric atony and not true gastroparesis. Hiatal hernia repair with fundoplication should not result in worsened gastric emptying. The vagus nerve should be left intact during the operation. Thus, vagal nerve function and gastric emptying should be preserved. The restoration of a more normal anatomy can potentially even improve gastric emptying in those with preoperative delayed gastric emptying [18, 19]. Overall, gastric emptying should be expected to have normal results postoperatively in the absence of preexisting gastroparesis.

EndoFLIP

Endoluminal functional luminal-imaging probe (EndoFLIP) is a newer technology that can be used to assess GEJ function, measuring its diameter, area, pressure, and distensibility. EndoFLIP has been used intraoperatively to tailor fundoplications, and its use has shown that a drop in the distensibility index (DI) is associated with nonrecurrence of symptoms in short-term follow-up [20]. Fundoplication will generally reduce the DI as the intervention is decreasing the cross-sectional area of the GEJ. The type of fundoplication used may vary the degree of DI reduction [21]. Exact numeric values identifying a functional fundoplication are still lacking due to the recent introduction of this device. One study has suggested that minimal diameter changes of <0.15 mm and cross-sectional area changes of <1.5 mm^2 may lead to recurrence of symptoms [22]. EndoFLIP may prove a valuable tool in determining the adequacy of fundoplication and tailoring repairs for patients. However, further data are needed to clarify what measurements or changes can be verified as normal for the patient.

Discussion

Hiatal hernia repair with fundoplication should recreate normal anatomy, and thus restore the physiologic function of the GEJ. When performing postoperative testing, reference to the original operation helps delineate what findings are expected, especially with image-directed studies looking at the anatomy. With physiologic testing, such as manometry, pH testing, and gastric emptying, findings should be similar to those of an asymptomatic patient. Normal physiologic findings suggest that reoperation will not benefit the patient. Significant deviation from findings discussed here should be viewed as abnormal. However, abnormal findings alone do not necessarily indicate a need for operative repair. Correlation to symptoms needs to be established.

Editors' Note

Reflux/Dysphagia After a Sleeve

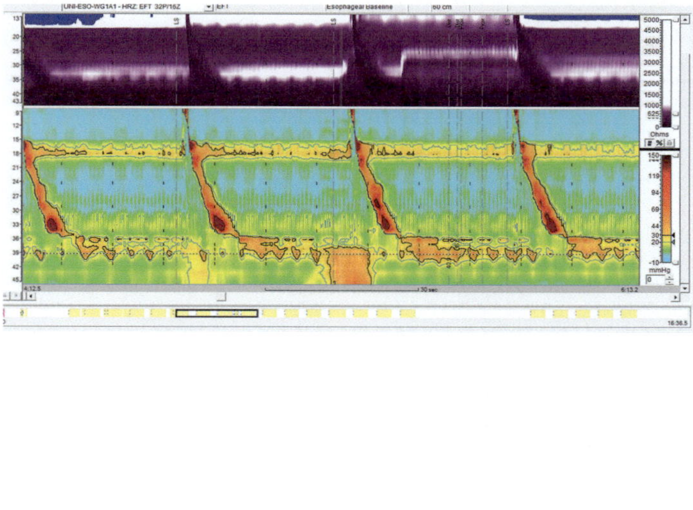

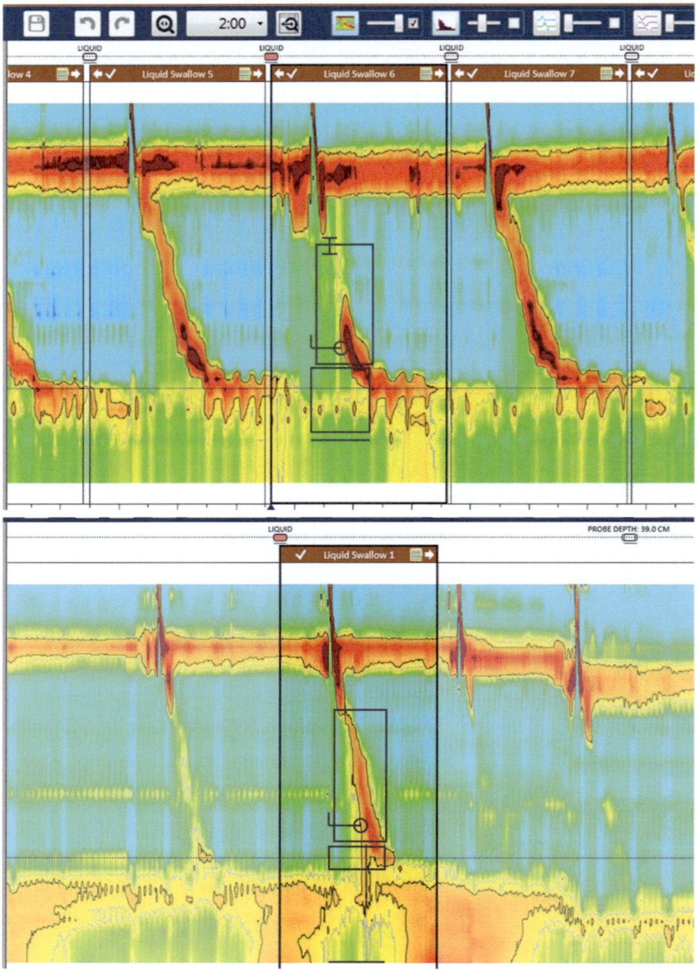

After a sleeve gastrectomy, high pressure is often discussed within the gastric lumen. HRM with impedance is a way to evaluate the pressure within the sleeve. In the figures above, high pressure is noted distal to the LES and hiatus (within the gastric lumen). This may be helpful in determining whether conversion to RYGBP (a decompressive procedure) will help in improving reflux.

Dysphagia or Cough After Sleeve

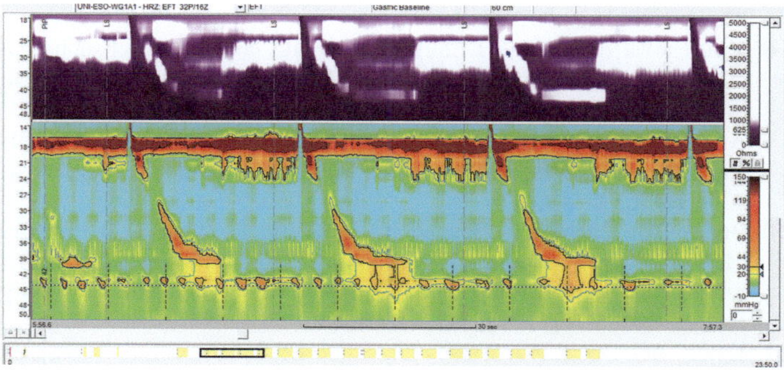

In this study, the patient had a sleeve gastrectomy and did well with weight loss. However, she presented 2 years post-sleeve with globus and cough. She was noted to have a hypotensive LES and hiatal hernia. High pressure was noted between the LES and the hiatus. The patient underwent hiatal hernia repair and LES augmentation with magnetic beads with relief of symptoms. Note there is no high pressure seen within the gastric lumen.

References

1. SAGES Guidelines Committee, Kohn GP, Price RR, DeMeester SR, Zehetner J, Muensterer OJ, et al. Guidelines for the management of hiatal hernia. Surg Endosc. 2013;27(12):4409–28.
2. Carbo AI, Kim RH, Gates T, D'Agostino HR. Imaging findings of successful and failed fundoplication. Radiographics. 2014;34(7):1873–84.
3. Dempsey DT. Barium upper GI series in adults: a surgeon's perspective. Abdom Radiol. 2018;43(6):1323–8.
4. Baker ME, Einstein DM, Herts BR, Remer EM, Motta-Ramirez GA, Ehrenwald E, et al. Gastroesophageal reflux disease: integrating the barium esophagram before and after antireflux surgery. Radiology. 2007;243(2):329–39.
5. Canon CL, Morgan DE, Einstein DM, Herts BR, Hawn MT, Johnson LF. Surgical approach to gastroesophageal reflux disease: what the radiologist needs to know. Radiographics. 2005;25(6):1485–99.
6. Pavone P, Laghi A, Catalano C, Cardone G, Messina A, Neri T, et al. CT of Nissen's fundoplication. Abdom Imaging. 1997;22(5):457–60.

7. Bogte A, Bredenoord AJ, Oors J, Siersema PD, Smout AJPM. Normal values for esophageal high-resolution manometry. Neurogastroenterol Motil. 2013;25(9):762–e579.
8. Yang H, Watson DI, Kelly J, Lally CJ, Myers JC, Jamieson GG. Esophageal manometry and clinical outcome after laparoscopic Nissen fundoplication. J Gastrointest Surg. 2007;11(9):1126–33.
9. Arca MJ, Gagner M, Garcia-Ruiz A, Todd HB. The significance of pH and manometric testing after laparoscopic fundoplication. Surg Endosc. 2002;16(3):395–400.
10. Boddy AP, Mehta S, Bennett J, Lowndes R, Mahon D, Rhodes M. Postoperative esophageal physiology studies may help to predict long-term symptoms following laparoscopic Nissen fundoplication. Surg Endosc. 2008;22(5):1298–302.
11. Knight BC, Devitt PG, Watson DI, Smith LT, Jamieson GG, Thompson SK. Long-term efficacy of laparoscopic anti-reflux surgery on regression of Barrett's esophagus using BRAVO wireless pH monitoring. J Am Coll Surg. 2015;221(4):e1–2.
12. Arnold BN, Dunst CM, Gill AB, Goers TA, Swanström LL. Postoperative impedance–pH testing is unreliable after Nissen fundoplication with or without Giant hiatal hernia repair. J Gastrointest Surg. 2011;15(9):1506–12.
13. Hansdotter I, Björ O, Andreasson A, Agreus L, Hellström P, Forsberg A, et al. Hill classification is superior to the axial length of a hiatal hernia for assessment of the mechanical anti-reflux barrier at the gastroesophageal junction. Endosc Int Open. 2016;04(03):E311–7.
14. Yadlapati R, Hungness ES, Pandolfino JE. Complications of antireflux surgery. Am J Gastroenterol. 2018;113(8):1137–47.
15. Seok JW. How to interpret gastric emptying scintigraphy. J Neurogastroenterol Motil. 2011;17(2):189–91.
16. Tog C, Liu DS, Lim HK, Stiven P, Thompson SK, Watson DI, et al. Risk factors for delayed gastric emptying following laparoscopic repair of very large hiatus hernias: gastroparesis following hiatal hernia repair. BJS Open. 2017;1(3):75–83.
17. Hamrick MC, Davis SS, Chiruvella A, Coefield RL, Waring JP, Sweeney JF, et al. Incidence of delayed gastric emptying associated with revisional laparoscopic paraesophageal hernia repair. J Gastrointest Surg. 2013;17(2):213–7.
18. Farrell TM, Richardson WS, Halkar R, Lyon CP, Galloway KD, Waring JP, et al. Nissen fundoplication improves gastric motility in patients with delayed gastric emptying. Surg Endosc. 2001;15(3):271–4.
19. Lindeboom MYA, Ringers J, van Rijn PJJ, Neijenhuis P, Stokkel MPM, Masclee AAM. Gastric emptying and vagus nerve function after laparoscopic partial fundoplication. Ann Surg. 2004;240(5):785–90.

20. Kim MP, Meisenbach LM, Chan EY. Tailored fundoplication with endoluminal functional lumen imaging probe allows for successful minimally invasive hiatal hernia repair. Surg Laparosc Endosc Percutan Tech. 2018;28:178.
21. DeHaan RK, Davila D, Frelich MJ, Gould JC. Esophagogastric junction distensibility is greater following Toupet compared to Nissen fundoplication. Surg Endosc. 2017;31(1):193–8.
22. Turner B, Helm M, Hetzel E, Gould JC. Is that 'floppy' fundoplication tight enough? Surg Endosc. 2020;34(4):1823–8.

K. Normal Foregut Function After Bariatric Surgery 27

Megan Lundgren and Talar Tatarian

Introduction

Bariatric surgery has proven to be the most effective solution for sustained long-term weight loss in patients with morbid obesity. These procedures, while successful, have unintended consequences on the esophagus, esophageal motility, and GERD by causing mechanical and functional changes of the upper gastrointestinal tract [1]. Postoperative alterations in gastric volume and intraluminal pressure contribute to functional motility changes [1]. Each bariatric procedure uniquely alters intragastric volume, pressure, gastroesophageal pressure gradients, and gastric emptying [2]. As such, each procedure will be discussed separately. Herein, we review the impact of obesity and bariatric surgery on esophageal health, specifically esophageal motility. Reflux following bariatric surgery, the most notable outcome of functional motility postoperatively, will be discussed in detail in a later chapter.

M. Lundgren
Department of Surgery, Penn Highlands Healthcare, Dubois, PA, USA

T. Tatarian (✉)
Department of Surgery, Thomas Jefferson University Hospital, Philadelphia, PA, USA
e-mail: talar.tatarian@jefferson.edu

A. D. Patel et al. (eds.), *The SAGES Manual of Physiologic Evaluation of Foregut Diseases*,
https://doi.org/10.1007/978-3-031-39199-6_27

The Lower Esophageal Sphincter and Esophageal Function in Patients with Obesity

The natural anti-reflux barrier is comprised of the lower esophageal sphincter (LES), diaphragmatic hiatus, phrenoesophageal ligament, and angle of His [3]. This barrier relies predominantly on a competent LES, which can be compromised by decreased intrinsic pressure, overall length, intra-abdominal length, esophageal peristalsis, and gastric motility [4]. Obesity can contribute to the breakdown of several of these components. Increased intra-abdominal girth and pressure are thought to cause increased rates of hiatal hernia, transient LES relaxation, and slower esophageal clearance, all of which lead to the development of GERD [5]. Increased estrogen levels as a result of increased adipose tissue in obesity may contribute to increased transient relaxation of the LES [6]. Not surprisingly, patients with obesity have been shown to have a 2.5-fold increase in the risk of hiatal hernia and a 50% increase in the risk of GERD symptoms [7, 8].

High-resolution impedance manometry allows for detailed evaluation of the crural diaphragm and LES, including their anatomic position and relationship during contraction. Preoperative manometry in the bariatric population has identified disruption of the natural anti-reflux barrier with high rates of separation of the crural diaphragm from the LES mechanism [9]. Manometric studies have also shown subclinical, asymptomatic findings of esophageal dysmotility at higher rates than in the nonobese population [10]. This includes hypertensive LES, nutcracker esophagus, diffuse esophageal spasm, and nonspecific esophageal disorders [10]. These changes in the natural antireflux barrier and the potential for higher rates of esophageal motility disorders need to be taken into account in the planning stages of bariatric surgery. Furthermore, procedure choice needs to be made with the knowledge of normal physiologic findings postoperatively, which are discussed below.

Normal Physiologic Findings After Bariatric Surgery

In this next section, we discuss the functional upper gastrointestinal motility changes that occur "normally" following the most commonly performed bariatric procedures. Each procedure will be discussed separately as the various anatomic configurations contribute to differing effects.

Adjustable Gastric Banding

Adjustable gastric banding (AGB) involves the placement of an inflatable silicone band around the upper stomach to provide restriction and affect satiety. Luminal distension of the cardia above the gastric band causes gastric peristalsis until the lumen above the band is emptied [11]. In an optimally filled gastric band, passage of semisolids into the infraband compartment is briefly delayed without limiting total meal size. If the compartment above the band is not fully cleared, residual bolus may reflux back into the esophagus until additional peristalsis allows for passage.

Following AGB, symptoms such as dysphagia and regurgitation are commonly reported. Recent studies using high-resolution impedance manometry (HRM) have provided some insight into the physiologic causes for these symptoms. Cruziat et al. used HRM to evaluate esophageal motility and clearance in symptomatic patients a median of 6.3 years after surgery [12]. Twenty of 22 patients were found to have abnormal manometric findings including pseudo-achalasia, functional EGJ obstruction, and weak peristalsis. In this study, the most frequent disorder was a functional esophageal gastric junction obstruction defined by increased intra-bolus pressure. Band deflation or removal resulted in improvement of symptoms for the majority of patients. HRM has also identified secondary contractions of the esophagus in banded patients, which increase in frequency with higher filling of the band. These excessive contractions against a high-pressure zone are hypothesized to lead to the trans-hiatal dilation of the esophagus [12]. Due to the significant resistance presented by the band, esophageal peristalsis is required to mediate episodes of liquid or semisolid flow across the gastric band [11]. Band slippage, a known complication of AGB, can augment these physiologic changes and worsen dysphagia, esophageal dysmotility, and trans-hiatal dilation.

Sleeve Gastrectomy

Sleeve gastrectomy (SG) is currently the most commonly performed weight loss procedure in the United States. It involves resection of the greater curvature of the stomach, leaving a long tubular stomach comprised of the lesser curvature and antrum. By removing approximately two thirds of the stomach, there are direct effects on both volume and distensibility as well as neurohormonal effects on receptive relaxation and the gastric pacemaker [13]. These changes not only directly affect the esophagus and stomach, but also cause global alterations in gastrointestinal motility. A recent systematic review of three studies found an increase in small bowel transit time following SG [13]. However, the most studied alterations in motility are in the stomach and esophagus.

The anatomic and mechanical changes following SG have secondary effects on esophageal function. Gastric volume and compliance are decreased causing increased intragastric pressure [1]. Mion et al. found that on HRM, increased intragastric pressure was present only after completion of the swallows, during the LES after-contraction, and not during the relaxation period of the esophagogastric junction [1]. The authors concluded that these findings are manometric markers for SG. Increased intragastric pressure, however, has not been shown to decrease esophagogastric junction bolus transit. The reduced compliance of the gastric sleeve may have an effect on esophageal bolus clearance and transit in certain cases, particularly in those with evidence of reflux on impedance [1].

Gastric emptying after SG has been studied extensively. There has been debate regarding the emptying of the so called "tight-sleeve" versus "antral-sparing" sleeve gastrectomy. Initial studies using gastric emptying found antral preservation to have no effect on gastric emptying [14]. More recently, Baumann et al. used dynamic MRI to better evaluate gastric motility before and after SG. The authors found that following SG, movement of a food bolus through the sleeve segment was passive with no propulsive motility, whereas the antrum maintained its motility with active acceleration during bolus transit [15]. There is some indication that the amount of antrum remaining, in other words, the number of centimeters from the pylorus at which the first staple line is taken, does affect emptying time – however no randomized controlled trials have studied this specifically.

Roux-En-Y Gastric Bypass

The Roux-en-Y gastric bypass (RYGB) is both a restrictive and malabsorptive procedure. It includes the creation of a small proximal gastric pouch which is then connected to a distal segment of jejunum (Roux or alimentary-limb). Individual surgeon practice varies with regard to the lengths of the Roux and biliopancreatic limbs, but these function to decrease intestinal absorption whereas the gastric pouch serves to restrict the volume of oral intake. These subsequently induce weight loss.

More recently, alterations in motility and neurohormonal changes after RYGB have been studied as drivers of weight loss. Björklund et al. used manometry to better define esophago-gastro-Roux limb motor activity following RYGB [16]. The authors performed manometric measurements on eight patients with stable weight loss at least 2 years postoperatively. A manometric catheter was advanced across the GEJ, gastric pouch, and into the Roux limb and intraluminal pressure differences and migrating motor complexes of the Roux limb were measured. The authors found significant pressure differences between the gastric pouch and the LES, as well as no pressure difference between the pouch and the Roux limb at rest. After ingestion, food intake caused a moderate and gradual pressure increase in the gastric pouch as well as in the Roux segment, which reached a peak pressure in the Roux limb around 8 min and then decreased from then on,– independent of further food intake. So, unlike previously proposed, there is no hypertension of the gastric pouch after RYGB. The authors also found interdigestive migrating motor complexes that started beyond the gastrojejunal anastomosis and occurred aborally along the Roux limb at regular intervals [16].

There have been several studies of esophageal motility in the obese population as well as in postoperative patients after RYGB. Studies have had conflicting results. Early studies called for preoperative evaluation of esophageal motility prior to bypass [17] due to a high frequency of lower esophageal sphincter motor dysfunction, motility disorders, and preoperative reflux in patients with obesity. More recent studies have suggested this preoperative evaluation is unnecessary especially in asymptomatic patients [18]. A recent study combining impedance pH and high-resolution manometry found no change in esophageal peristalsis after RYGB [19]. However, patients who report dysphagia to solid foods after RYGB are more likely to have abnormal findings on high-resolution manometry, including incomplete lower esophageal sphincter relaxation and hypertensive lower esophageal sphincter. The causes, however, and direct relationship to the RYGB have not been mapped, although effects on vagal innervation have been suggested [20].

Duodenal Switch and Single Anastomosis Duodenoileal Bypass with Sleeve Gastrectomy

Duodenal Switch (DS) combines a longitudinal sleeve gastrectomy with a small bowel bypass. The duodenum is transected proximal to the ampulla and an anastomosis is created between the proximal duodenum and the distal small bowel, usually 250–300 cm proximal to the terminal ileum. The distal end of the biliopancreatic limb is then anastomosed to the Roux limb approximately 100–150 cm proximal to ileocecal valve. More recently, Single Anastomosis Duodenoileal Bypass with Sleeve Gastrectomy (SADI-S) has gained popularity, during which a single loop anastomosis is created between the proximal duodenum and the small bowel, 250–300 cm proximal to the ileocecal valve.

Both procedures reduce caloric intake and induce fat malabsorption by diverting bile and pancreatic secretions. The changes in esophageal motility are similar to those seen with sleeve gastrectomy, as described in the section above. Studies of gastrointestinal motility following DS or SADI-S are limited. In the Ellias et al. studies using a wireless motility capsule, gastric emptying was found to be rapid in about 30% of patients 1 year after DS. This is in keeping with earlier studies of SG alone. The maximum pressures in the antrum and stomach increased slightly, while small bowel pressures declined significantly postsurgery [21].

In a quality of life study after DS, patients reported more flatus, number of loose bowel movements, urgency, and fecal incontinence compared to patients who had undergone RYGB [22]. This would suggest faster transit, but may also be related to the length of the common channel which is shorter in DS.

Abnormal Physiologic Findings After Bariatric Surgery

While some degree of physiologic and manometric changes are expected after bariatric surgery, occasionally pathologic changes can contribute to worsening reflux, dysphagia, and regurgitation. When this occurs, a thorough workup should commence consisting of upper endoscopy, upper gastrointestinal series with small bowel follow through, pH studies, and manometry. Depending on the findings, a patient should be referred to a bariatric surgeon for consideration of revision surgery. For more detailed review of abnormal findings after bariatric surgery and subsequent management, please refer to the chapter "Reflux After Bariatric Surgery".

Conclusion

Bariatric surgery, while highly effective for weight loss and management of obesity related comorbidities, has unintended consequences on foregut physiology. Advances in high-resolution manometry have led to a better understanding of esophageal motility and the anti-reflux barrier in patients with obesity, both pre- and postoperatively. Preoperative workup is paramount to ensuring that the appropriate procedure is selected for each patient. Procedure choice should be made with thorough understanding of the anticipated physiologic and manometric effects as well as each patient's baseline esophageal health and symptoms.

Editors' Note

Reflux/Dysphagia After a Sleeve Gastrectomy

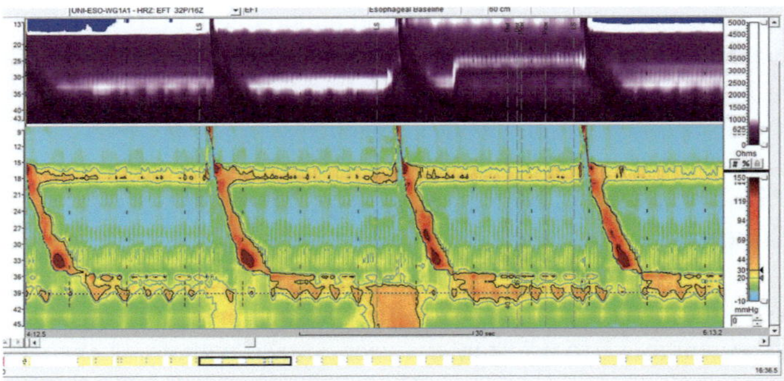

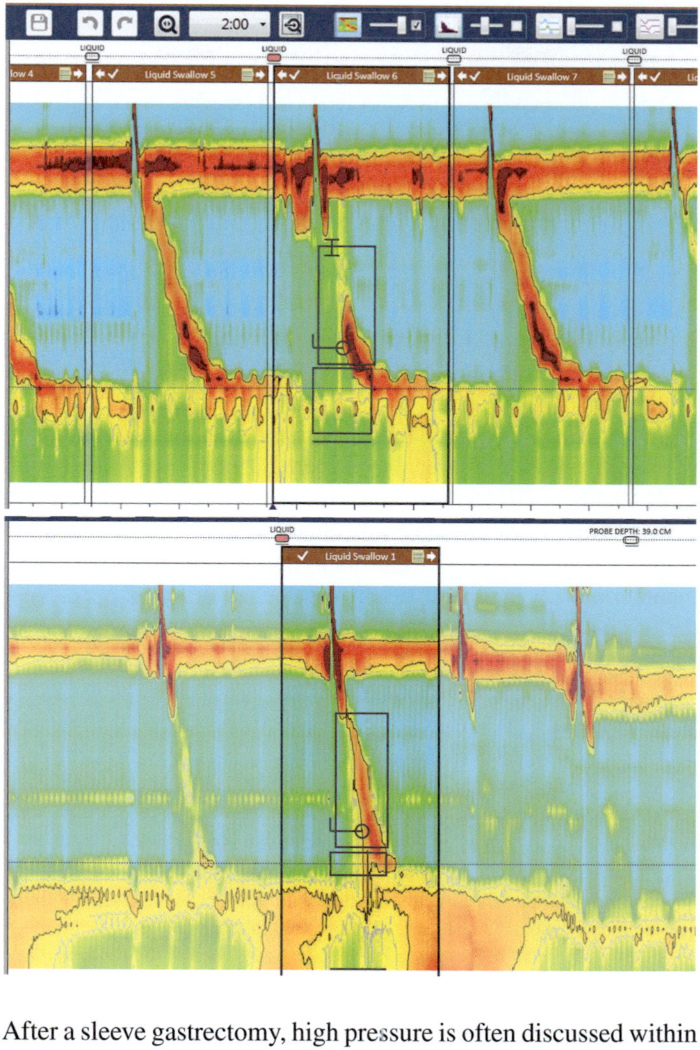

After a sleeve gastrectomy, high pressure is often discussed within the gastric lumen. HRM with impedance is a way to evaluate the pressure within the sleeve. In the figures above, high pressure is noted distal to the LES and hiatus (within the gastric lumen). This may be helpful in determining whether conversion to Roux-en-Y gastric bypass (a decompressive procedure) will help in improving reflux.

Dysphagia or Cough After Sleeve

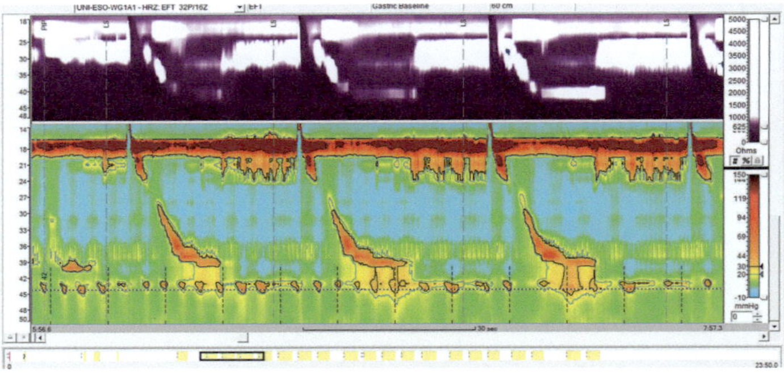

In this study, the patient had a sleeve gastrectomy and did well with weight loss. However, she presented 2 years post-sleeve with globus and cough. She was noted to have a hypotensive LES and hiatal hernia. High pressure was noted between the LES and the hiatus. The patient underwent hiatal hernia repair and LES augmentation with magnetic beads with relief of symptoms. Note there is no high pressure seen within the gastric lumen.

References

1. Mion F, Tolone S, Garros A, et al. High-resolution impedance manometry after sleeve gastrectomy: increased Intragastric pressure and reflux are frequent events. Obes Surg. 2016;26(10):2449–56.
2. Salvatore T. Esophageal high-resolution manometry can unravel the mechanisms by which different bariatric techniques produce different reflux exposures. J Gastrointest Surg. 2020;24(1):1–7.
3. Tatarian T, Pucci MJ, Palazzo F. A modern approach to the surgical treatment of gastroesophageal reflux disease. J Laparoendosc Adv Surg Tech A. 2016;26(3):174–9.
4. Peters JH, DeMeester TR. The gastroesophageal barrier. In: Yeo CJ, editor. Shackelford's surgery of the alimentary tract. Philadelphia, PA: Elsevier Saunders; 2013. p. 194–200.
5. Naik RD, Choksi YA, Vaezi MF. Impact of weight loss on esophageal physiology. Gastroenterol Hepatol. 2015;11(12):801–9.

6. Nilsson M, Johnsen R, Ye W, Hveem K, Lagergren J. Obesity and estrogen as risk factors for gastroesophageal reflux symptoms. JAMA. 2003;290(1):66–72.
7. Hampel H, Abraham NS, El-Serag HB. Meta-analysis: obesity and the risk for gastroesophageal reflux disease and its complications. Ann Intern Med. 2005;143(3):199–211.
8. Wilson LJ, Ma W, Hirschowitz BI. Association of obesity with hiatal hernia and esophagitis. Am J Gastroenterol. 1999;94(10):2840–4.
9. Tolone S, Savarino E, de Bortoli N, et al. Esophagogastric junction morphology assessment by high resolution manometry in obese patients' candidate to bariatric surgery. Int J Surg. 2016;28:S109–13.
10. Hong D, Khajanchee Y, Pereira N, Lockhart B, Patterson E, Swanstrom L. Manometric abnormalities and gastroesophageal reflux disease in the morbidly obese. Obes Surg. 2004;14(6):744–9. https://doi.org/10.1381/0960892041590854.
11. Burton PR, Yap K, Brown WA, et al. Effects of adjustable gastric bands on gastric emptying, supra- and infraband transit and satiety: a randomized double-blind crossover trial using a new technique of band visualization. Obes Surg. 2010;20(12):1690–7.
12. Cruiziat C, Roman S, Robert M, et al. High-resolution esophageal manometry evaluation in symptomatic patients after gastric banding for morbid obesity. Dig Liver Dis. 2011;43(2):116–20.
13. Sioka E, Tzovaras G, Perivoliotis K, et al. Impact of laparoscopic sleeve gastrectomy on gastrointestinal motility. Gastroenterol Res Pract. 2018;2018:4135813.
14. Bernstine H, Tzioni-Yehoshua R, Groshar D, et al. Gastric emptying is not affected by sleeve gastrectomy-scintigraphic evaluation of gastric emptying after sleeve gastrectomy without removal of the gastric antrum. Obes Surg. 2009;19:293–8.
15. Baumann T, Kuesters S, Grueneberger J, et al. Time-resolved MRI after ingestion of liquids reveals motility changes after laparoscopic sleeve gastrectomy—preliminary results. Obes Surg. 2011;21(1):95–101.
16. Björklund P, Lönroth H, Fändriks L. Manometry of the upper gut following roux-en-Y gastric bypass indicates that the gastric pouch and roux limb act as a common cavity. Obes Surg. 2015;25(10):1833–41.
17. Merrouche M, Sabaté J-M, Jouet P, et al. Gastro-esophageal reflux and esophageal motility disorders in morbidly obese patients before and after bariatric surgery. Obes Surg. 2007;17(7):894–900.
18. Valezi A, Herbella F, Junior J, Almeida MM. Esophageal motility after laparoscopic roux-en-Y gastric bypass: the manometry should be preoperative examination routine? Obes Surg. 2012;22(7):1050–4.
19. Pohl D, Mueller MK, Wildi S, et al. 81 gastroesophageal reflux and esophageal peristalsis before and after gastric bypass surgery—an interim

analysis of combined impedance-pH and high-resolution manometry data. Gastroenterology. 2008;134(4):A-13.
20. Mangla S, Tuyama AC, Burakoff R, Lautz DB, Thompson CC, Chan WW. Mo1731 incomplete lower esophageal sphincter relaxation on high-resolution manometry is an independent predictor of solid diet failure in post-roux-en-Y gastric bypass patients. Gastroenterology. 2013;144(5):S-1102. https://doi.org/10.1016/S0016-5085(13)64106-2.
21. Elias K, Semler JR, Webb D-L, Sundbom M, Hellström PM. Gastric sleeve surgery with duodenal switch has minor effects on gastric emptying times and intestinal transit times. Luminal pressures and motility indices as evaluated with wireless motility capsules (SMARTPILL). Gastroenterology. 2020;158(6):S-208.
22. Elias K, Bekhali Z, Hedberg J, Graf W, Sundbom M, Elias K. Changes in bowel habits and patient-scored symptoms after roux-en-Y gastric bypass and biliopancreatic diversion with duodenal switch. Surg Obes Relat Dis. 2018;14(2):144–9.

Normal Physiologic Findings After Esophageal Myotomy

28

Abdulaziz Ali Karam
and Mohammed Al Mahroos

Introduction

Gastrointestinal motility disorders are considered rare conditions worldwide, and this may lead to a lack of full understanding of multiple aspects related to these disorders. Achalasia is by far the best understood foregut motility disorder. It is estimated to have an annual incidence rate of 0.5–1.5 per 100,000 population with a predilection to affect young women [1–3]. The main diagnostic feature of achalasia is incomplete lower esophageal sphincter (LES) relaxation with associated varying degrees of esophageal aperistalsis [4]. The consequence is failure of food to transit smoothly through the esophagus into the stomach, leading patients to experience dysphagia, regurgitation, and chest pain due to food stasis. Even though the understanding of most motility disorders

A. A. Karam
Department of Surgery, St Mary's Hospital, McGill University, Montreal, QC, Canada

M. Al Mahroos (✉)
Department of Surgery, McGill University, Montreal, QC, Canada

Department of Surgery, St Mary's Hospital, McGill University, Montreal, QC, Canada
e-mail: Mohammed.Almahroos@mail.mcgill.ca

A. D. Patel et al. (eds.), *The SAGES Manual of Physiologic Evaluation of Foregut Diseases*,
https://doi.org/10.1007/978-3-031-39199-6_28

is poor, the pathogenesis for achalasia is thought to be loss of inhibitory neurons in Auerbach's plexus. Theories suggesting the cause to be idiopathic or infectious were both proposed. The diagnosis of achalasia requires an esophagram and endoscopic examination. However, esophageal manometry studies are the gold standard modality to confirm the diagnosis. The findings in these studies may vary based on the type and severity of achalasia. Unfortunately, there is no definitive treatment that can restore LES function and esophageal peristalsis. Most available successful therapeutic options are targeted to disrupt the lower esophageal sphincter to help relieve the symptoms yielded from the functional obstruction. The conventional way to treat achalasia is through a surgical myotomy, a method called Heller myotomy. However, in 2010, Inoue et al. described the first per oral endoscopic myotomy (POEM) as a new approach to treating achalasia. Since then, the utilization of POEM has only grown and we have learned more about the physiological changes after per oral myotomy.

Post-myotomy normal physiological findings are widely arguable, because of the lack of fixed post-op normal standardized thresholds [5]. To simplify the process of postoperative follow-up and to achieve better understanding for post-myotomy physiologic findings, we will categorize the findings based on the type of diagnostic study.

Normal Physiologic Findings in Diagnostic Tests Post-Myotomy

Radiological Findings after Myotomy

Most experienced foregut surgeons who treat achalasia on a regular basis investigate the response to treatment at 6–12 months after myotomy. This can serve as the new baseline for future follow-ups. Multiple studies have looked at the radiological findings post-myotomy including Stephen et al. and Yoo et al. in 1988 and 2004, respectively. Both stated that 50–65% of patients will show normal esophageal caliber in early post-op course, as radiological studies were performed within 7 days of myotomy [6]. However, about one third of the patients will show mild dilatation of the esophagus and a smaller group of patients will show moderate dilation. The size of the esophagus in imaging does not always correlate with the presence of symptoms. Expected findings post successful myotomy include free passage of contrast through the lower esophageal sphincter into the stomach, usually without the previous bird's beak-like appearance. In some instances, the body of the esophagus will increase in caliber, which is called ballooning of the esophagus, and the lower gastroesophageal junction will be larger, within first month post-myotomy [7].

Stephen et al. examined esophageal focal outpouching along the myotomy. In their study published in 1988, they noted postoperative outpouching when they examined their patients using upper GI studies. They reported it as a normal postoperative finding [7]. The reported incidence of this finding varies between 33% and 95% in post-myotomy; however, it also did not correlate with the presence of symptoms or lack thereof [8]. Although the study reported no consequences of this finding, in theory it can act as a potential site for stasis of food or rarely food impaction.

It is important for upper GI surgeons and radiologists not to confuse post-myotomy esophageal ballooning with epiphrenic diverticulum which is a saccular protrusion that has a discrete neck. It should also not be mistaken for residual dilatation of the aperistaltic esophagus. The outpouching has an eccentric and focal characteristic.

After POEM, one would still expect a small amount of pneumoperitoneum immediately after the procedure with no clinical significance. This could be attributed to the lack of a serosal layer on the esophagus. Some centers prefer to do a close follow-up X-ray on the first or second day after the procedure [9]. However, it is unlikely to change management if the patient is not showing any worrisome symptoms or signs.

During POEM, the mucosotomy site is usually closed with endoscopic clips. These might be seen if radiological examination is performed during the first few weeks after the procedure. These clips loosen and fall off spontaneously at a later stage. It is worth noting that mucosal edema surrounding the clips can be seen as a rounded small focal lucency and this image can remain even after the clips loosen and disappear [10].

Similar findings were observed in a number of studies using CT-scan on the first day after undergoing POEM. In these instances, the common radiological finding on CT scan was pneumomediastinum (87%), pneumoperitoneum (66%), subcutaneous emphysema (52%), and pleural effusion (46%) [11].

As discussed earlier, most radiological findings which are considered expected post-POEM do not require any intervention. Upper GI surgeons and radiologists should be aware of these findings and their significance or lack thereof. However, these findings might not represent an expected outcome if patients are experiencing unexpected symptoms such as worsening dysphagia, severe pain, or high-grade fever. In cases where symptoms recur, previous findings seen in preoperative imaging might reappear. An esophagogram is an important modality in patients with new onset dysphagia. A patient suffering from recurrent dysphagia might show delayed emptying of esophageal content or esophageal dilatation.

Manometric Findings Post-Myotomy

Manometry is the gold standard test for diagnosing achalasia. It not only helps differentiate it from other esophageal motility disorders, but also helps determine the type of achalasia [12]. There are no specific guidelines for surveillance after a patient undergoes myotomy for achalasia. In most instances, manometry is an important tool to evaluate patients with persistent or recurrence of symptoms.

Attempts have been made to quantify normal values in both manometry and pH studies at 6 months after myotomy. While there is still no consensus regarding specific values, new manometric readings were considered the new baselines after surgery [8]. In part, the new findings may depend on the type of antireflux repair post-laparoscopic myotomy or the lack of an antireflux component post-POEM. In 2018, Torres-Villalobos et al., in their study "Dor vs Toupet Fundoplication After Laparoscopic Heller Myotomy: Long-Term Randomized Controlled Trial Evaluated by High-Resolution Manometry", compared the findings of esophageal manometry for two groups of patients post-myotomy. Group A had Dor fundoplication while group B had Toupet fundoplication. Their findings showed that the "integrated relaxation pressure" (IRP) and basal lower esophageal sphincter (LES) pressure were within normal parameters in both groups at 6 and 24 months. Early on, specifically at the very first month, the IRP was significantly higher ($p < 0.001$) in Dor (9.78 ± 4.20 mmHg) compared to that Toupet (5.91 ± 3.04 mmHg). At 6–24 months, however, there was no statistically significant difference between the two groups. A similar pattern was found for the basal LES pressure at 1 month and at 6–24 months [13]. In none of these scenarios, patients showed symptoms of concern. On the other hand, POEM was reported to have significant improvement of LES relaxation pressure and enhanced esophageal bolus clearance as measured by HRM over 1–12 month period post-myotomy [14].

Recurrence of dysphagia might be a sign of stricture, incomplete myotomy, or recurrence. Manometry would differentiate among all three by indicating an increase in IRP and failure of LES to relax. In cases of an incomplete myotomy, the patients might experience short-term symptomatic relief or no relief. This will be accompanied with an unsatisfactory postoperative IRP results, classically >10 mmHg.

Esophageal pH Study and Endoscopic Findings Post-Myotomy

It was shown in different studies that in short-term follow-up, POEM is non-inferior and, in some case, even potentially more effective than LHM in relieving dysphagia. The downside of POEM is that it was associated with a higher incidence of postoperative gastroesophageal reflux [15].

Using esophageal pH studies, it was found that acid exposure was significantly higher among patients who underwent POEM compared to those who underwent LHM. The percentage of acid reflux reported was up to 48% in POEM vs 14% in LHM. Interestingly, this was reported for all the parameters encountered including total reflux time, upright reflux, supine reflux, postprandial reflux and DeMeester scores [16]. Regardless of the degree of reflux observed in pH studies, in most cases, it was not clinically significant gastroesophageal reflux disease (GERD). The recent Lyon consensus indicates that the diagnosis of GERD requires more objective endoscopic findings such as severe esophagitis, long segment of esophageal mucosa with intestinal metaplasia or stenosis, or the time of esophageal acid exposure is >6% of the time studied through the 24-h pH monitoring [17].

A meta-analysis done by Repici A. et al. found that the average rate of esophagitis post-POEM was found to be 35% during the first 2 years. However, the majority of cases (92%) had mild esophagitis, while only minority of cases were considered moderate to severe [16]. In contrast, esophagitis post-LHM, regardless of severity, was found to be approximately 7.6%, and the majority were classified as mild (48.5%) [18].

The lack of anti-reflux procedure in POEM is thought to be the primary cause of the increase in the incidence of acid exposure to esophageal mucosa. However, the clinical implication of such higher reflux incidence appeared to be less relevant. When performing POEM, the peri-esophageal anti-reflux barriers like suspensory ligaments and angle of His are preserved which can help reduce incidence of clinically significant GERD afterwards.

References

1. Sadowski DC, Ackah F, Jiang B, et al. Achalasia: incidence, prevalence and survival. A population-based study. Neurogastroenterol Motil. 2010;22:e256–61.
2. Zhong C, Tan S, Ren Y, Lü M, Peng Y, Fu X, Tang X. Quality of life following Peroral endoscopic myotomy for esophageal achalasia: a systematic review and meta-analysis. Ann Thorac Cardiovasc Surg. 2020;26:113–24.

3. Townsend CM, Beauchamp RD, Evers BM, Mattox KL. Sabiston textbook of surgery: the biological basis of modern surgical practic. 20th ed. Philadelphia, PA: Elsevier Saunders; 2017. p. 1015–8.
4. Barker JR, Franklin RH. Heller's operation for achalasia of the cardia. A study of the early and late results. Br J Surg. 1971;58(6):466–8.
5. Korean Society of Neurogastroenterology and Motility. 2019 Seoul consensus on esophageal achalasia guidelines. J Neurogastroenterol Motil. 2020;26(2):180–203.
6. Yoo C, Levine MS, Redfern RO, et al. Laparoscopic Heller myotomy and fundoplication: findings and predictive value of early postoperative radiographic studies. Abdom Imaging. 2004;29(6):643–7.
7. Rubesin S, E, Mary Kennedy BA, Levine MS, Rosato EF, Laufer I. Distal esophageal ballooning following Heller myotomy. Radiology. 1988;167(2):345–7.
8. Gockel I, Rabe SM, Niebisch S. Before and after esophageal surgery: which information is needed from the functional laboratory. Visc Med. 2018;34(2):116–2.
9. Rieder E, Dunst CM, Kastenmeier AS, Makris KI, Swanstrom LL. Development and technique of per oral endoscopic myotomy (POEM) for achalasia. Eur Surg. 2011;43(3):140–5.
10. Harmath C, Horowitz J, Berggruen S, et al. Fluoroscopic findings post-peroral esophageal myotomy. Abdom Imaging. 2015;40:237–45.
11. Pannu D, Yang D, Abbitt PL, Draganov PV. Prospective evaluation of CT esophagram findings after peroral endoscopic myotomy. Gastrointest Endosc. 2016;84:408–15. https://doi.org/10.1016/j.gie.2016.02.022.
12. Townsend CM, Beauchamp RD, Evers BM, Mattox KL. Sabiston textbook of surgery: the biological basis of modern surgical practice. 20th ed. Philadelphia, PA: Elsevier Saunders; 2017. p. 1015–8.
13. Torres-Villalobos G, Coss-Adame E, Furuzawa-Carballeda J, et al. Dor vs Toupet fundoplication after laparoscopic Heller myotomy?: long-term randomized controlled trial evaluated by high-resolution manometry. J Gastrointest Surg. 2018;22:13–22.
14. Teitelbaum EN, Soper NJ, Santos BF, et al. Symptomatic and physiologic outcomes one year after peroral esophageal myotomy (POEM) for treatment of achalasia. Surg Endosc. 2014;28:3359–65.
15. Schlottmann F, Luckett DJ, Fine J, Shaheen NJ, Patti MG. Laparoscopic Heller myotomy versus peroral endoscopic myotomy (POEM) for achalasia: a systematic review and meta-analysis. Ann Surg. 2018;267:451–60.
16. Repici A, Fuccio L, Maselli R, et al. GERD after per-oral endoscopic myotomy as compared with Heller's myotomy with fundoplication: a systematic review with meta-analysis. Gastrointest Endosc. 2018;87(4):934.e18–43.e18.

17. Gyawali CP, Kahrilas PJ, Savarino E, et al. Modern diagnosis of GERD: the Lyon consensus. Gut. 2018;67:1351–62.
18. Sanaka MR, Thota PN, Parikh MP, et al. Peroral endoscopic myotomy leads to higher rates of abnormal esophageal acid exposure than laparoscopic Heller myotomy in achalasia. Surg Endosc. 2019;33:2284–92.

Part V

Pathology/Symptom Based

Barrett's Esophagus: A Review of Current Literature

29

Justin Eagleston, Lauren Yoder,
and Kshitij Kakar

Introduction

The definition of Barrett's esophagus (BE) is "the condition in which metaplastic columnar epithelium replaces the stratified squamous epithelium that normally lines the distal esophagus and predisposes to cancer development" [1–5]. The change in epithelium to columnar is a consequence of continued and recurrent esophageal epithelial injury, most commonly from gastroesophageal reflux disease (GERD) (Fig. 29.1).

J. Eagleston
Trihealth Good Samaritan Hospital, Cincinnati, OH, USA

Carolinas Medical Center, Charlotte, NC, USA

L. Yoder
Trihealth Good Samaritan Hospital, Cincinnati, OH, USA
e-mail: lauren_yoder@trihealth.com

K. Kakar (✉)
Trihealth Bethesda North Hospital, Cincinnati, OH, USA

A. D. Patel et al. (eds.), *The SAGES Manual of Physiologic Evaluation of Foregut Diseases*,
https://doi.org/10.1007/978-3-031-39199-6_29

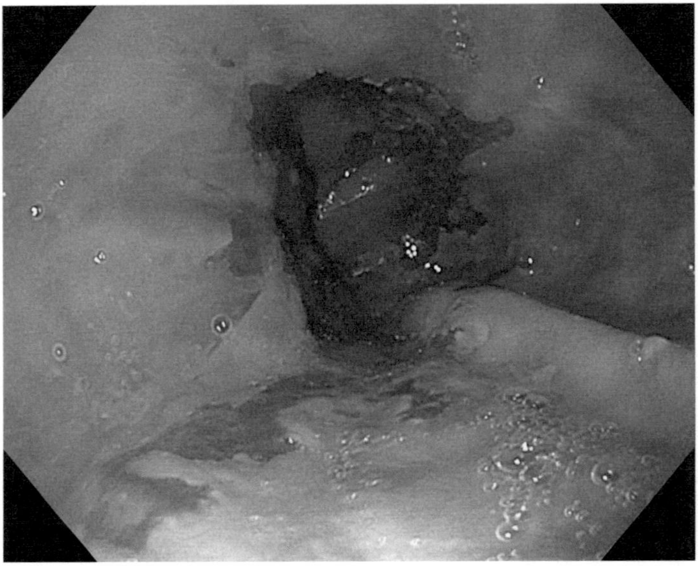

Fig. 29.1 Epithelial injury as a result of GERD as seen on endoscopy

History

Norman Barrett is credited for identifying reflux changes within the distal esophagus in 1950 [6]. However, his initial description was that of peptic ulcers and belief that the stomach had herniated through the esophageal hiatus and the mucosal change was actually normal stomach epithelium. Looking back in history we find that Albers in 1839 also identified peptic ulcer disease within the esophagus [6]. It was in 1948 that Allison described several types of hiatal hernias. At the time, it was believed that esophageal ulcers were due to a congenital shortening of the esophagus. However, Allison believed that a short esophagus was actually acquired due to sliding hiatal hernias causing incompetence of the gastric cardia and resulting in recurrent gastric reflux. In 1950, Barrett described circumferential and longitudinal strictures of the distal esophagus associated with reflux esophagitis [6]. In 1953, Allison and Johnstone described a segment of columnar epithelium lining the esophagus between the squamocolumnar junction and the stomach in an article titled "The Oesophagus Line with Gastric Mucous Membrane" [7]. This description of gastric mucosa within the esophagus was thought to be heterotopic and not normal, but it was not understood that this change was acquired and metaplastic. In this paper, Barrett's ulcers are described as chronic esophageal ulcers within the gastric mucosa of the esophagus. These ulcers were more likely to bleed and/or perforate than peptic ulcers of the esophagus. Additionally, one patient died of gastric cancer and there is a description of cardiac mucosa within the esophagus with goblet cells. Later in 1957, Barrett wrote "The Lower Esophagus Lined by Columnar Epithelium." It was this paper where he suggests the term "columnar epithelium", but the etiology was still thought to be congenital and due to "the result of a failure of the embryonic lining of the gullet to achieve normal maturity." [8]. By defining the columnar epithelium within the esophagus, Barrett's ulcers were then known as Barrett's esophagus. By the 1960s, Barrett and Allison recognized that the columnar epithelium was due to gastric reflux. In 1961, Hayward wrote an editorial describing the transformation of squamous into columnar epithelium and felt this was metaplastic [9]. The important aspects of this paper are as follows: (1) He defines the esophagogastric junction anatomically, as the end of the tube (2). He advocates for eliminating the vague anatomic term "cardia." (3) He recognizes that during normal swallowing the mucosa can slide approximately 2 cm (4). He proposes that columnar epithelium between the squamous and oxyntic mucosa was a normal and necessary transition to protect between the acid-producing gastric mucosa and the esophageal squamous mucosa. This location was determined to be the "junctional" epithelium. In patients with reflux it was noted that the junction became more proximal due to the acid causing injury to the squamous epithelium which then would heal in a metaplastic fashion. Hayward felt the proximalization of the junctional mucosa had the following implications: (1) Carcinoma of the cardia should be considered an esophageal cancer variant (2). Reflux injury leads to the proximalization of the junctional epithelium and this is not congenital ectopic tissue (3). Congenital ectopic tissue should involve resection; however, if the tissue was acquired, surgery to correct reflux might lead to regression of the junctional epithelium. In 1970, Cedric Bremner surgically created an incompetent lower esophageal sphincter causing reflux in dogs. This resulted in proof that the columnar lined esophagus could be acquired and was related to gastric reflux [10]. Back in 1951, Bosher and Tayler were the first to describe goblet cells within the columnar esophageal mucosa [11]. In 1952, Morson and Belcher described an esophageal adenocarcinoma surrounded by intestinal epithelium with goblet cells [12].

Then in 1976, Paul used esophageal manometry to determine the location of the lower esophageal sphincter. He then took biopsies of this location and found three different mucosal types: (1) Specialized columnar epithelium with a villiform surface and mucous glands, (2) Cardiac mucosa (Hayward's junctional mucosa) composed of strictly mucus cells, (3) Gastric fundic epithelium with parietal cells and mucus. If the specialized columnar epithelium was present, it was always the most proximal and the most distal was the gastric fundic epithelium [13]. Going forward, endoscopy became more prevalent and Barrett's esophagus was being diagnosed via endoscopy rather than surgical resection. Biopsies could not differentiate between normal gastric mucosa and metaplastic esophageal epithelium until deeper biopsies were taken. The deeper biopsies were able to pick up the defining characteristics of the esophagus (submucosal glands, circular and longitudinal muscularis, and less/lack of serosa).

Initially, in order to avoid a high false positive rate, a minimum of 3 cm of columnar-lined esophagus was needed to diagnose Barrett's esophagus [14]. Endoscopists would not routinely biopsy the columnar epithelium if it were less than 3 cm, nor would they biopsy the columnar epithelium in patients without severe symptoms of GERD [15]. The 3 cm rule was challenged by Spechler in 1994 and his group found 18% rate of intestinal metaplasia in the columnar-lined epithelium [16]. Patients without signs and symptoms of GERD who had developed the columnar metaplasia also appeared to be at risk and this was studied by multiple other investigators [17–19]. Following this discovery, the concept of short segment <3 cm and long segment >3 cm Barrett's esophagus was accepted. Barrett's esophagus then became associated with any increased acid exposure which resulted in Barrett's esophagus being diagnostic for pathologic GERD without pH testing [20]. Lastly, in 1997, Nandurkar standardized the use of Alcian blue because the stain is able to better identify goblet cells. After changing to Alcian blue, it was found that 50% of Barrett's would have been missed by standard H&E staining [21].

Epidemiology/Demographics

The mean age of diagnosis of Barrett's esophagus is 55 years and Barrett's is normally discovered during endoscopy [22, 23]. Barrett's esophagus is two to threefold more common in men than in women [24]. Approximately 5.6% of adults in the United States have BE. However, the prevalence of BE in the general population varies from 0.4% to greater than 20% depending on the population studied and what criteria are used to establish the diagnosis [25–29]. In Western populations, the prevalence is highest in Caucasians with Hispanics and Asians being affected at lower rates and African-Americans being affected the least [30, 31]. Short segment BE is more prevalent than long segment BE [32, 33]. In 1999, Wong studied 889 patients undergoing upper endoscopy who had biopsies taken at the gastroesophageal junction. He found that 13.2% of patients had specialized intestinal metaplasia. He also found the prevalence of short-segment BE to be 6.4% and long-segment BE to be 1.6% [25].

Risk Factors

GERD is an independent risk factor for BE, conferring a fivefold increased risk of the development of Barrett's at 5-year follow-up studies [34]. There is debate as to whether a peptic stricture increases the prevalence of BE; however, the prevalence of intestinal metaplasia appears to be similar in patients with and without a stricture [35]. Obesity, and specifically central obesity, is another risk factor for GERD as well as BE [36, 37]. Patients with a BMI

>30 have a small increased risk of developing BE based on a meta-analysis in 2009 [36]. When looking specifically at abdominal obesity, which is measured by waist-to-hip ratio, males with ratios ≥0.9 and females with ratios ≥0.85 have increased risk of BE [37–40]. Smoking also increases the risk of BE. In matched patients with GERD, smokers are 1.6 times more likely to develop BE than nonsmokers [41]. Lastly, family history appears to play a part in the development of BE. Twenty-eight percent of first-degree relatives of patients with esophageal adenocarcinoma have been found to have BE [42–44]. Currently, it is unclear if this association is due to common environmental exposures or an inherited mutation. There are several germline mutations (MSR1, ASCC1, CTHRC1 genes) that confer a risk of BE and esophageal adenocarcinoma [45]. Also, when looking at the genomes, genetic variants have been identified at chromosomes 6p21 and 16q24 with association to BE [46]. H. pylori infection appears to be protective in the esophagus and protects against the development of BE. This is especially true in H. pylori strains that express the cytotoxin-associated gene A (cagA) [47, 48]. It should also be noted that certain medications have been shown to reduce the risk of progression of BE which include proton-pump inhibitors, aspirin, nonsteroidal-anti-inflammatory agents, and statins [49–51].

Pathogenesis

Barrett's esophagus is secondary to chronic insult to the distal esophagus secondary to gastroesophageal reflux of acid and other noxious agents including nitrous compounds as well as bile [52]. Multiple physiologic abnormalities have been proposed which contribute to chronic gastroesophageal reflux in patients with Barrett's esophagus. This includes gastric acid hypersecretion, markedly low lower esophageal sphincter pressures, ineffective esophageal motility, duodenogastric reflux, decreased salivary secretion of epidermal growth factor, and decreased esophageal pain sensitivity [22]. Individual patients may have any, all, or none of these factors. Patients with normal gastric acid secretions have been found to have long segment Barrett's esophagus. Many

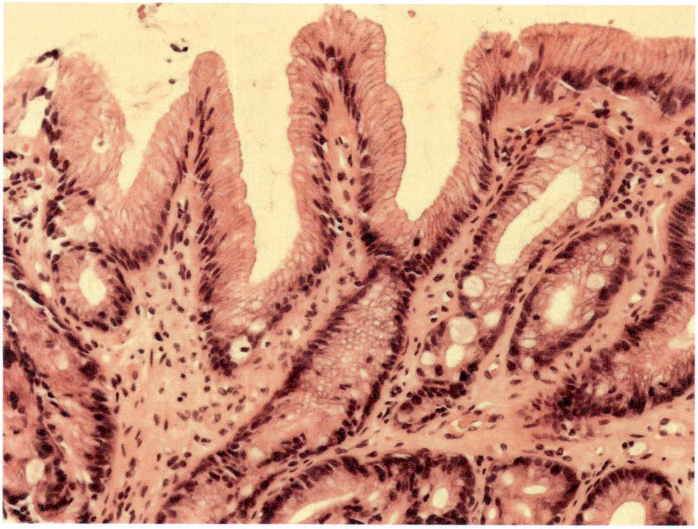

Fig. 29.2 Intestinal metaplasia as seen in Barrett's esophagus (squamous epithelium is replaced with columnar cells which can be seen at the periphery of the pathologic specimen)

patients without GERD symptoms have been shown to have Barrett's esophagus. Barrett's develops through the process of intestinal metaplasia; this occurs when gastric secretions damage the distal esophageal squamous epithelium resulting in replacement with metaplastic columnar cells which appear to be more resistant to reflux-induced injury (Fig. 29.2). Unfortunately, esophageal columnar metaplasia predisposes to the development of adenocarcinoma [53].

Dysplasia

Dysplasia is the morphologic change in Barrett's cells before they become malignant. It is a constellation of histologic abnormalities indicating genetic and epigenetic damage that renders Barrett's cells neoplastic and predisposed to malignancy [54]. Multiple cytological and architectural abnormalities are characteristic of dysplasia. These include nuclear changes, loss of cytoplastic maturation, and crowding of tubules and villiform surfaces [55]. Based on the severity of these changes, dysplasia is categorized as low grade or high grade. The diagnosis of dysplasia in Barrett's can be challenging. Interobserver agreement is better in high-grade dysplasia as compared to low grade, but any diagnosis of dysplasia should be confirmed by a second pathologist who has expertise in esophageal pathology [56]. Overall incidence of development of cancer in patients with low-grade dysplasia is approximately 0.5% per year [57]. In high-grade dysplasia, the rate is anywhere from 4–8% per year.

Diagnosis

The diagnosis of BE is confirmed with the presence of columnar lined intestinal metaplasia within the distal esophagus. This diagnosis is achieved by obtaining biopsies of the salmon-colored mucosa that extends at least 1 cm proximal to the gastroesophageal junction during endoscopy. In patients with suspected BE, the endoscopist should obtain biopsies from four circumferential quadrants starting at the 1 cm mark proximal to the GEJ. This technique should be continued through the extent of the visual changes on the esophagus with an additional biopsy on what appears to be normal esophageal squamous mucosa [58]. Additionally, the endoscopist should report the location of the diaphragmatic hiatus, GEJ, and squamocolumnar junction (Z-line). Barrett's esophagus that is ≥3 cm is termed long segment Barrett's, whereas a segment that is ≤3 cm is termed short segment Barrett's esophagus [59]. Lastly, the endoscopist should report the extent of the metaplastic changes within the esophagus using the Prague classification [60]. The Prague classification was first presented in 2006 and is the standard for measuring the length of BE [60]. First the true position of the GEJ is identified. Next, the circumferential Barrett's segment (C) is measured proximally from the GEJ. Lastly, the longest tongue of metaplastic change

(M) plus the circumferential segment is measured from the GEJ. If the circumferential segment is 2 cm and the tongue is an additional 2 cm, it would be reported as C2M4 via the Prague classification. Assessment of the extent of Barrett's esophagus on endoscopy is clinically important as multiple studies have shown that more extensive disease is associated with a higher risk of dysplasia and progression to esophageal adenocarcinoma.

Surveillance

Despite the risk of progression to esophageal adenocarcinoma, the American College of Gastroenterology does not recommend screening the general population for BE [61]. Screening should be done in patients with risk factors for esophageal adenocarcinoma including hiatal hernia, age ≥ 50, male sex, chronic GERD, caucasian race, central obesity, tobacco use, and confirmed history of Barrett's esophagus or esophageal adenocarcinoma in a first degree relative [62, 63]. After initial diagnosis is made, management and surveillance is performed based on presence or absence of degree of dysplasia. If no dysplasia is recognized, surveillance is recommended every 3–5 years. The American College of Gastroenterology recommends that if biopsies are initially indefinite for dysplasia, patients should be placed on medical anti-reflex therapy and endoscopy repeated after waiting at least 3 months [64]. Repeat endoscopy should not be delayed beyond 6 months. Patients with low-grade dysplasia may undergo surveillance every 12 months unless endoscopic therapy has been performed in which case endoscopy should be performed every 6 months for 1 year. Patients with high-grade dysplasia require surveillance every 3 months in the first year following endoscopic therapy, followed by every 6 months in the second year and annually thereafter. Endoscopic surveillance is done using the Seattle biopsy sampling protocol with four quadrant biopsies every 2 cm in patients without dysplasia and 1 cm intervals in patients with known or suspected dysplasia.

Medical Treatment

General management involves control of acid reflux with proton pump inhibitors, even in asymptomatic patients. Multiple studies suggest aggressive anti-reflux therapy may prevent cancer and hence, PPI therapy is usually indefinite [50, 65–67]. In a meta-analysis of nine studies including over 5700 patients with BE, the use of PPI's was associated with a trend toward lower risk of esophageal adenocarcinoma [68]. The recommended dose of PPI is pantoprazole 40 mg twice daily or lansoprazole 30 mg twice daily. Gashi, in 2018, published a prospective study, monitoring 50 patients with BE over 2 years. He found that the length of BE was influenced by PPI therapy and noted that the extent/lengths of short segment and long segment Barrett's esophagus were significantly improved following treatment with twice daily PPI [69]. There is some evidence that nonsteroidal anti-inflammatory medications, including aspirin, can decrease the risk of esophageal adenocarcinoma in patients with Barrett's esophagus [70]. However, there is potential of side effects and a low absolute risk of cancer precludes their regular use.

Endoscopic Management

Radiofrequency Ablation

Most cases of BE do not progress to dysplastic changes; however, when high-grade dysplasia is present, there is a significant risk of progression to esophageal adenocarcinoma. There is controversy in the use of RFA versus surveillance alone in the setting of low-grade dysplasia. However, some studies have shown a benefit to RFA in low-grade dysplasia and have noted successful eradication and lower progression rates when compared to surveillance [71, 72]. Radiofrequency ablation has become the standard of care for high-grade dysplasia [73–79]. Ablation has a high rate of eradication of dysplasia. Endoscopic mucosal resection plays a role in the ability for RFA to be successful. If there are any visible raised lesions, they must be addressed with EMR prior to ablation as ablation is only successful if the ablation can reach the muscularis mucosae. Postoperatively, it is important to place the patient on acid suppressive medications (PPI) and sucralfate suspension can also be added. Typically, patients are on a full liquid diet for 24 h followed by a regular diet as tolerated. RFA is well tolerated and a common side effect is postoperative chest pain. A feared complication is a post RFA stricture, which have been reported from 0–8% postoperatively [73, 77–80]. Strictures post-RFA are managed with dilation. Additional complications include bleeding and perforation, but these complications are rare.

Endoscopic Mucosal Resection

RFA is extremely effective and safe for treating flat lesions in the esophagus. However, one of the limitations of RFA is the inability to retain histology and provide staging information for neoplastic tissue. RFA is also not effective for deeper mucosa or submucosal lesions and can lead to inadequate treatment. Lesions that involve the submucosa have a 20–25% risk of harboring lymph node metastasis in patients with high-grade dysplasia [81, 82]. It is important to remember that if patients undergo RFA for deeper lesions and the lesion is treated inadequately, there is risk for squamous overgrowth of the submucosal cancer [83]. Deeper lesions are better treated with endoscopic mucosal resection (EMR). EMR is also able to provide adequate T staging and has been highly effective in eradicating early mucosal adenocarcinoma in the esophagus [84]. The combination of RFA and EMR is extremely effective in the management of dysplastic Barrett's esophagus and has eradication rates of >90% [85]. The technique of EMR involves identifying the lesion in question which can be added with optical enhancement in the form of chemical chromoendoscopy (methylene blue) or optical chromoendoscopy (NBI). The NBI was recently validated and can assess dysplastic areas with 85% accuracy [86]. The technique of EMR involves the process of capturing mucosal tissue into a pseudopolyp configuration and then snaring the pseudopolyp. The goal of the procedure is to remove the mucosa and a portion of the submucosa while leaving the muscularis propria intact. One technique is the cap-assisted EMR, which fits over the endoscope and accommodates a snare. First the mucosal lesion is identified, and a submucosal injection is performed to lift the lesion. The cap is then centered over the lesion and an assistant closes the snare around the lesion (Figs. 29.3 and 29.4). Electrocautery is used to resect the pseudopolyp. An alternative option is the band-assisted EMR. The technique is similar to the cap EMR; however, a submucosal injection is not required. The lesion is centered within the cap, then completely suctioned into the cap. Next, a band is positioned around the lesion. Lastly, the snare, with electrocautery, is used to resect the pseudopolyp that was created with the band. The snare can be used above or below the band. Postoperatively, patients may complain of chest pain which is usually a result of a self-limiting iat-

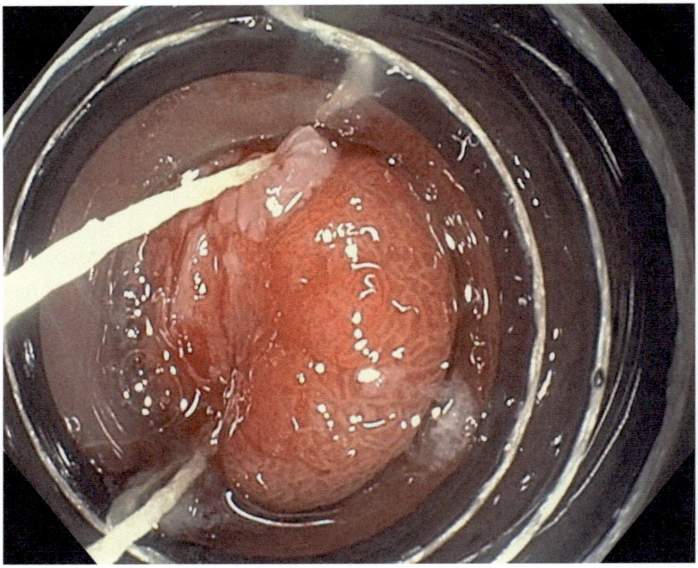

Fig. 29.3 Pseudopolyp (mucosa and submucosa only) is ensnared during endoscopic mucosal resection

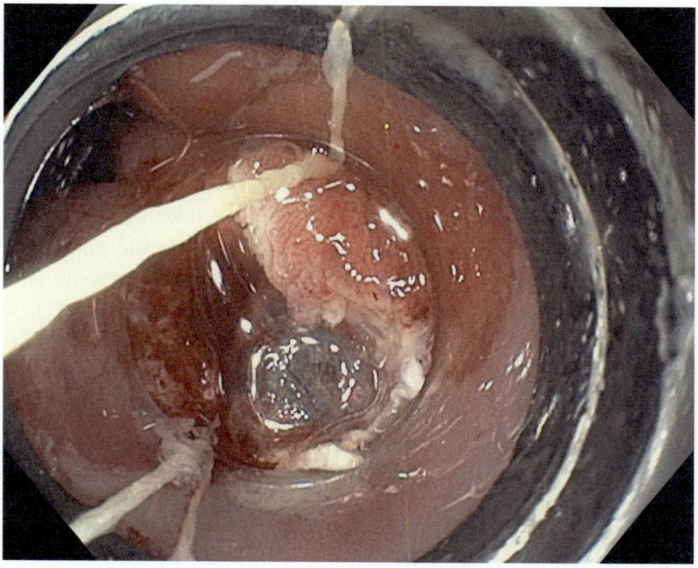

Fig. 29.4 The result of endoscopic mucosal resection

rogenic ulcer. Patients typically are on a liquid diet for 24 h followed by a soft diet for up to 1 week. After EMR, patients require follow-up endoscopy in 2 months to evaluate if additional EMR or RFA needs to be performed. The most common complication with EMR is bleeding or perforation. These risks are 1.1% and 0.2%, respectively [85]. Immediate bleeding is treated by using the cap and hemostatic forceps to coagulate the vessel. Perforation is a much more severe complication and can lead to mediastinitis and rapid decompensation. Perforations can be managed with hemostatic clips, over the scope clips, or endoscopic suturing devices. If the perforation is large, an esophageal stent is also an option. The most common late complication is stricture which is reported in up to 10% of patients. Strictures typically occur in patients with EMR sites that take up >50% of the esophageal circumference. Most strictures are amenable to dilation techniques.

Phototherapy

Less commonly utilized than the previously described modalities, photodynamic therapy (PDT) uses laser light and a photosensitizing agent (sodium porfimer) to selectively destroy tissue. The photosensitizing agent is given 48–72 h prior to endoscopy and hypermetabolic cells will preferentially take up the agent. During endoscopy, a laser light is used to activate the photosensitizing agent. The agent then reacts with oxygen to create free radicals that induce cell membrane death and apoptosis [87]. A cohort study of 100 patients with Barrett's esophagus and dysplasia was treated with phototherapy and followed for 51 months [88]. The mean reduction in length of Barrett's mucosa was 7 cm. Fifty-four percent of patients had complete resolution of BE. Ninety-three percent of patients with low-grade dysplasia, 78% of patients with high-grade dysplasia, and 48% of patients with early cancer all had complete remission. Any small areas that remained were treated with Nd:YAG laser thermal ablation and the study concluded that PDT followed by Nd:YAG was effective in patients with Barrett's esophagus with dysplasia [88]. An additional study compared PDT with omeprazole vs omeprazole therapy alone and found a significantly higher incidence of complete ablation of dysplasia in the PDT plus omeprazole group (77% vs. 39%) [89]. These patients were followed for 5 years and the response was similar, with an increased rate of complete ablation in the PDT group [87, 90–92]. Complications associated with PDT include photosensitivity in 69% of patients, esophageal strictures in 36% of patients, and vomiting in 32% of patients [89]. Other common complications reported were odynophagia and fever. Additionally, there is a concern for "buried" Barrett's esophagus which is described as residual BE hidden under the neosquamous esophagus that forms following PDT. This occurs if the PDT does not destroy all of the metaplastic epithelium. A retrospective review of 953 patients found the rate of "buried metaplasia" to be 14% [93].

Cryotherapy

Freeze-thaw cycles are used to create mucosal cellular destruction in cryotherapy. Either nitrogen or carbon dioxide is sprayed to the dysplastic area and the treatment is applied for a total of 40 s (two 20 s applications or four 10 s applications). This produces a 2 mm depth of injury [94]. The freeze-thaw cycles disrupt the cell membranes and cause tissue ischemia through vascular stasis, endothelial damage, and vascular thrombosis [95]. A multicenter retrospective study by Shaheen et al. included 98 patients undergoing cryotherapy [96]. Fifty-eight patients completed therapy and were followed for 10.5 months. Eighty-seven percent of patients had complete eradication of all dysplasia with persistent BE. Fifty-seven percent had complete eradication of all BE. Three patients developed strictures (5%). Two patients developed chest pain requiring narcotics (3%). Buried esophagus was found in two patients (3%). Another retrospective study by Gosain followed patients undergoing cryotherapy every 8 weeks until eradication of high-grade dysplasia and Barrett's esophagus was confirmed on EGD [97]. The median follow-up was 37 months. At 2 years, all 32 patients had complete resolution of their high-grade dysplasia and 84% of patients had complete resolution of their Barrett's esophagus. However, during the final follow-up, it was found that 18% of patients had developed recurrent high-grade dysplasia. One patient progressed to esophageal adenocarcinoma. Strictures were seen in 9% of patients and all were successfully dilated. As a result of the above, cryotherapy has not been adopted as a mainstay of treatment of Barrett's esophagus.

Surgical Management

The goal of medical or surgical treatment of Barrett's esophagus is to provide relief from GERD symptoms, control esophagitis, and prevent neoplastic progression of Barrett's mucosa. As mentioned in the medical management section, multiple studies suggest anti-reflux therapy may prevent the progression of cancer. There is evidence, however, that acid suppression may in fact contribute to cell proliferation and cancer development by promoting an alkaline environment which promotes bile reflux which may also contribute to neoplastic transmutation [98]. The addition of surgical therapy reduces both acid and bile reflux [99]. There is increasing evidence of surgical anti-reflux therapy causing regression of Barrett's esophagus. This includes multiple studies during the open anti-reflux surgery era as well as laparoscopic anti-reflux era [100–103]. The evidence in support of surgery reducing the risk of cancer development, however, is scarce. Surgical intervention for asymptomatic Barrett's esophagus is controversial. Patients with Barrett's associated dysplasia or carcinoma should not undergo anti-reflux surgery until the lesion is eradicated histologically by endoscopic therapy.

References

1. Shaheen NJ, Richter JE. Barrett's oesophagus. Lancet. 2009;373:850–61.
2. Sharma P, McQuaid K, Dent J, Fennerty BM, Sampliner R, Spechler S, Cameron A, Corley D, Falk G, Goldblum J, Hunter J, Jankowski J, Lundell L, Reid B, Shaheen NJ, Sonnenberg A, Wang K, Weinstein W, AGA Chicago Workshop. A critical review of the diagnosis and management of Barrett's esophagus: the AGA Chicago Workshop. Gastroenterology. 2004;127:310–30.
3. Spechler SJ, Sharma P, Souza RF, Inadomi JM, Shaheen NJ, American Gastroenterological, Association. American Gastroenterological Association technical review on the management of Barrett's esophagus. Gastroenterology. 2011;140:e18–52. quiz e13.
4. Vakil N, van Zanten SV, Kahrilas P, Dent J, Jones R, Global Consensus Group. The Montreal definition and classification of gastroesophageal reflux disease: a global evidence-based consensus. Am J Gastroenterol. 2006;101:1900–20. quiz 1943
5. Wang KK, Sampliner RE, Practice Parameters Committee of the American College of Gastroenterology. Updated Guidelines. For the diagnosis, surveillance and therapy of Barrett's esophagus. Am J Gastroenterol. 2008;2008(103):788–97.

6. Barrett NR. Chronic peptic ulcer of the oesophagus and 'oesophagitis'. Br J Surg. 1950;38:175–82.
7. Allison PR, Johnstone AS. The oesophagus lined with gastric mucous membrane. Thorax. 1953;8:87–101.
8. Barrett NR. The lower esophagus lined by columnar epithelium. Surgery. 1957;41:881–94.
9. Hayward J. The lower end of the oesophagus. Thorax. 1961;16:36–41.
10. Bremner CG, Lynch VP, Ellis FH Jr. Barrett's esophagus: congenital or acquired? An experimental study of esophageal mucosal regeneration in the dog. Surgery. 1970;68:209–16.
11. Bosher LH, Taylor FH. Heterotopic gastric mucosa in the esophagus with ulceration and stricture formation. J Thorac Surg. 1951;21:306–12.
12. Morson BC, Belcher JR. Adenocarcinoma of the oesophagus and ectopic gastric mucosa. Br J Cancer. 1952;6:127–30.
13. Paull A, Trier JS, Dalton MD, Camp RC, Loeb P, Goyal RK. The histologic spectrum of Barrett's esophagus. N Engl J Med. 1976;295:476–80.
14. Skinner DB, Walther BC, Riddell RH, Schmidt H, Iascone C, Demeester TR. Barrett's esophagus. Comparison of benign and malignant cases. Ann Surg. 1983;198:554–65.
15. Reid BJ. Barrett's esophagus and esophageal adenocarcinoma. Gastroenterol Clin N Am. 1991;20:817–34.
16. Spechler SJ, Zeroogian JM, Antonioli SA, Wang HH, Goyal RK. Prevalence of metaplasia at the gastro-oesophageal junction. Lancet. 1994;344:1533–6.
17. Rex DK, Cummings OW, Shaw M, Cumings MD, Wong RK, Vasudeva RS, Dunne D, Rahmani EY, Helper DJ. Screening for Barrett's esophagus in colonoscopy patients with and without heartburn. Gastroenterology. 2003;125:1670–7.
18. Ronkainen J, Aro P, Storskrubb T, Se J, Lind T, Bolling-Sternevald E, Vieth M, Stolte M, Talley NJ, Agreus L. Prevalence of Barrett's esophagus in the general population: an endoscopic study. Gastroenterology. 2005;129:1825–31.
19. Weston AP, Krmpotich P, Makdisi WF, Cherian R, Dixon A, McGregor DH, Banergee SK. Short segment Barrett's esophagus: clinical and histological features, associated endoscopic findings, and association with gastric intestinal metaplasia. Am J Gastroenterol. 1996;91:981–6.
20. Clark GW, Ireland AP, Peters JH, Chandrasoma P, Demeester TR, Bremner CG. Short-segment Barrett's esophagus: a prevalent complication of gastroesophageal reflux disease with malignant potential. J Gastrointest Surg. 1997;1:113–22.
21. Nandurkar S, Talley NH, Martin CJ, Ng TH, Adams S. Short segment Barrett's esophagus: prevalence, diagnosis and associations. Gut. 1997;40:710–5.
22. Spechler SJ. Barrett's esophagus. Semin Gastrointest Dis. 1996;7:51.

23. Hayeck TJ, Kong CY, Spechler SJ, et al. The prevalence of Barrett's esophagus in the US: estimates from a simulation model confirmed by SEER data. Dis Esophagus. 2010;23:451.
24. Cook MB, Wild CP, Forman D. A systematic review and meta-analysis of the sex ratio for Barrett's esophagus, erosive reflux disease, and nonerosive reflux disease. Am J Epidemiol. 2005;162:1050.
25. Hirota WK, Loughney TM, Lazas DJ, et al. Specialized intestinal metaplasia, dysplasia, and cancer of the esophagus and esophagogastric junction: prevalence and clinical data. Gastroenterology. 1999;116:277.
26. Cameron AJ, Zinsmeister AR, Ballard DJ, Carney JA. Prevalence of columnar-lined (Barrett's) esophagus. Comparison of population-based clinical and autopsy findings. Gastroenterology. 1990;99:918.
27. Ormsby AH, Kilgore SP, Goldblum JR, et al. The location and frequency of intestinal metaplasia at the esophagogastric junction in 223 consecutive autopsies: implications for patient treatment and preventive strategies in Barrett's esophagus. Mod Pathol. 2000;13:614.
28. Gerson LB, Shetler K, Triadafilopoulos G. Prevalence of Barrett's esophagus in asymptomatic individuals. Gastroenterology. 2002;123:461.
29. Ward EM, Wolfsen HC, Achem SR, et al. Barrett's esophagus is common in older men and women undergoing screening colonoscopy regardless of reflux symptoms. Am J Gastroenterol. 2006;101:12.
30. Abrams JA, Fields S, Lightdale CJ, Neugut AI. Racial and ethnic disparities in the prevalence of Barrett's esophagus among patients who undergo upper endoscopy. Clin Gastroenterol Hepatol. 2008;6:30.
31. Corley DA, Kubo A, Levin TR, et al. Race, ethnicity, sex and temporal differences in Barrett's oesophagus diagnosis: a large community-based study, 1994-2006. Gut. 2009;58:182.
32. Winters C Jr, Spurling TJ, Chobanian SJ, et al. Barrett's esophagus. A prevalent, occult complication of gastroesophageal reflux disease. Gastroenterology. 1987;92:118.
33. Spechler SJ. Clinical practice. Barrett's Esophagus. N Engl J Med. 2002;346:836.
34. Ronkainen J, Talley NJ, Storskrubb T, et al. Erosive esophagitis is a risk factor for Barrett's esophagus: a community-based endoscopic follow-up study. Am J Gastroenterol. 2011;106:1946.
35. Kim SL, Wo JM, Hunter JG, et al. The prevalence of intestinal metaplasia in patients with and without peptic strictures. Am J Gastroenterol. 1998;93:53.
36. Kamat P, Wen S, Morris J, Anandasabapathy S. Exploring the association between elevated body mass index and Barrett's esophagus: a systematic review and meta-analysis. Ann Thorac Surg. 2009;87:655.
37. Jacobson BC, Chan AT, Giovannucci EL, Fuchs CS. Body mass index and Barrett's oesophagus in women. Gut. 2009;58:1460.

38. Corley DA, Kubo A, Levin TR, et al. Abdominal obesity and body mass index as risk factors for Barrett's esophagus. Gastroenterology. 2007;133:34.
39. Edelstein ZR, Farrow DC, Bronner MP, et al. Central adiposity and risk of Barrett's esophagus. Gastroenterology. 2007;133:403.
40. Kramer JR, Fischbach LA, Richardson P, et al. Waist-to-hip ratio, but not body mass index, is associated with an increased risk of Barrett's esophagus in white men. Clin Gastroenterol Hepatol. 2013;11:373.
41. Cook MB, Shaheen NJ, Anderson LA, et al. Cigarette smoking increases risk of Barrett's esophagus: an analysis of the Barrett's and esophageal adenocarcinoma consortium. Gastroenterology. 2012;142:744.
42. Chak A, Lee T, Kinnard MF, et al. Familial aggregation of Barrett's oesophagus, oesophageal adenocarcinoma, and oesophagogastric junctional adenocarcinoma in Caucasian adults. Gut. 2002;51:323.
43. Verbeek RE, Spittuler LF, Peute A, et al. Familial clustering of Barrett's esophagus and esophageal adenocarcinoma in a European cohort. Clin Gastroenterol Hepatol. 2014;12:1656.
44. Juhasz A, Mittal SK, Lee TH, et al. Prevalence of Barrett esophagus in first-degree relatives of patients with esophageal adenocarcinoma. J Clin Gastroenterol. 2011;45:867.
45. Orloff M, Peterson C, He X, et al. Germline mutations in MSR1, ASCC1, and CTHRC1 in patients with Barrett esophagus and esophageal adenocarcinoma. JAMA. 2011;306:410.
46. Su Z, Gay LJ, Strange A, et al. Common variants at the MHC locus and at chromosome 16q24.1 predispose to Barrett's esophagus. Nat Genet. 2012;44:1131.
47. Erőss B, Farkas N, Vincze Á, et al. Helicobacter pylori infection reduces the risk of Barrett's esophagus: a meta-analysis and systematic review. Helicobacter. 2018;23:e12504.
48. Castro C, Peleteiro B, Lunet N. Modifiable factors and esophageal cancer: a systematic review of published meta-analyses. J Gastroenterol. 2018;53:37.
49. Singh S, Singh AG, Singh PP, Murad MH, Iyer PG. Statins are associated with reduced risk of esophageal cancer, particularly in patients with Barrett's esophagus: a systematic review and meta-analysis. Clin Gastroenterol Hepatol. 2013;11:620–9.
50. Singh S, Garg SK, Singh PP, Iyer PG, El-Serag HB. Acid-suppressive medications and risk of oesophageal adenocarcinoma in patients with Barrett's oesophagus: a systematic review and meta-analysis. Gut. 2014;63:1229–37.
51. Zhang S, Zhang XQ, Ding XW, et al. Cyclooxygenase inhibitors use is associated with reduced risk of esophageal adenocarcinoma in patients with Barrett's esophagus: a meta-analysis. Br J Cancer. 2014;110:2378–88.
52. Lijima K, Henry E, Moriya A, et. Al. Dietary nitrate generates potentially mutagenic concentrations of nitric oxide at the gastroesophageal junction. Gastroenterology. 2002;122:1248.

53. Morales CP, Souza RF, Spechler SJ. Hallmarks of cancer progression in Barrett's esophagus. Lancet. 2002;360:1587.
54. Specher SJ. Disputing dysplasia. Gastroenterology. 2001;120:1864.
55. Goldblum JR. Barrett's esophagus and Barrett's related dysplasia. Mod Pathol. 2003;16:316.
56. Shaheen NJ, Falk GW, Iyer PG, et al. ACG clinical guideline: diagnosis and management of Barrett's esophagus. Am J Gastroenterol. 2016;111:30.
57. Singh S, Marrickam P, Amin AV, et al. Incidence of esophageal adenocarcinoma in Barrett's esophagus with low-grade dysplasia: a systematic review and meta analysis. Gastroinest Endosc. 2014;79:897.
58. Shaheen NJ, Falk GW, Iyer PG, Gerson LB, American COG. ACG clinical guideline:diagnosis and management of Barrett's esophagus. Am J Gastroenterol. 2016;111:30–50. quiz 51.
59. Sharma P, Morales TG, Sampliner RE. Short segment Barrett's esophagus—the need for standardization of the definition and of endoscopic criteria. Am J Gastroenterol. 1998;93:1033.
60. Sharma P, Dent J, Armstrong D, et al. The development and validation of an endoscopic grading system for Barrett's esophagus: the Prague C & M criteria. Gastrogenterology. 2006;131:1392–9.
61. Shaheen NJ, Falk GN, Iyer PG, Genson LB. Amercain College of Gastroenterology. ACG clinical guideline: diagnosis and management of Barrett's esophagus. Am J Gastroenterol. 2016;111:30–50. quiz 51
62. Shechler SJ, Sharma P, et al. American gastroenterology association medical position statement on the management of Barrett's esophagus. Gastroenterology. 2011;140:1084.
63. Rubenstein JH, Scheiman JM, Sadeghi S, et al. Esophageal adenocarcinoma incidence in individuals with gatroesophageal reflux: synthesis and estimates from population studies. Am J Gastroenterol. 2011;106:254.
64. Qumseya B, Sullan S, et al. ASGE guideline on screening and surveillance of Barrett's esophagus. Gastrointest Endosc. 2019;90:335.
65. Kastelein F, Spaander M, Steyerberg E, et al. Proton pump inhibitors reduce the risk of neoplastic progression in patients with Barrett's esophagus. Clin Gastroenterol Hepatol. 2013;11:382.
66. El-Serag HB, Aguirre TV, Davis S, et al. Proton pump inhibitors are associated with reduced incidence of dysplasia in Barrett's esophagus. Am J Gastroenterol. 2004;99:1877–83.
67. Nguyen DM, El-Serag HB, Henderson L, et al. Medication usage and the risk of neoplasia in patients with Barrett's esophagus. Clin Gastroenterol Hepatol. 2009;7:1299–304.
68. Hu G, Sun TT, Hong J, et al. Proton pump inhibitors do not reduce the risk of esophageal adenocarcinoma in patients with Barrett's esophagus: a systematic review and meta-analysis. PLoS One. 2017;12:eo169691.

69. Gashi Z, Bahtiri E, Gashi A, Sherifi F. Proton pump inhibitors diminish Barrett's Esophagus length: our experience. Open Access Maced J Med Sci. 2018;6:1041–5.
70. Omer ZB, Ananthakrishnan AN, Nattinger KJ, Cole EB, Lin JJ, Kong CY, Hur C. Aspirin protects against Barrett's esophagus in a multivariate logistic regression analysis. Clin Gastroenterol Hepatol. 2012;10:722–7.
71. Small AJ, Araujo JL, Leggett CL, Mendelson AH, Agarwalla A, Abrams JA, Lightdale CJ, Wang TC, Iyer PG, Wang KK, Rustgi AK, Ginsberg GG, Forde KA, Gimotty PA, Lewis JD, Falk GW, Bewtra M. Radiofrequency ablation is associated with decreased neoplastic progression in patients with Barrett's esophagus and confirmed low-grade dysplasia. Gastroenterology. 2015;149(3):567–576.e563. quiz e513–564.
72. Phoa KN, van Vilsteren FG, Weusten BL, Bisschops R, Schoon EJ, Ragunath K, Fullarton G, Di Pietro M, Ravi N, Visser M, Offerhaus GJ, Seldenrijk CA, Meijer SL, ten Kate FJ, Tijssen JG, Bregman JJ. Radiofrequency ablation vs endoscopic surveillance for patients with Barrett's esophagus and low-grade dysplasia: a randomized clinical trial. JAMA. 2014;311(12):1209–17.
73. Shaheen NJ, Sharma P, Overholt BF, Wolfsen HC, Sampliner RE, Wang KK, Galanko JA, Bronner MP, Goldblum JR, Bennett AE, Jobe BA, Eisen GM, Fennerty MB, Junter JG, Fleischer DE, Sharma VK, Hawes RH, Hoffman BJ, Rothstein RI, Gordon SR, Mashimo H, Chang KJ, Muthusamy VR, Edmundowwicz SA, Spechler SJ, Siddiqui AA, Souza FR, Infantolino A, Falk GW, Kimmey MB, Madanick RD, Chak A, Lightdate CJ. Radiofrequency ablation in Barrett's esophagus with dysplasia. N Engl J Med. 2009;360(22):2277–88.
74. Overholt BF, Lightdate CJ, Wang KK, Canto MI, Burdick S, Haggitt RC, Bronner MP, Taylor SL, Grace MG, Depot M, Esophagus IPGfH-GDiBs. Photodynamic therapy with porfimer sodium for ablation of high-grade dysplasia in Barrett's esophagus: international, partially blinded, randomized phase III trial. Gastrointest Endosc. 2005;62(4):488–98.
75. Overholt BF, Wang KK, Burdick JS, Lightdate CJ, Kimmey M, Nava HR, Sivak MV, Nishioka N, Barr H, Marcon N, Pedrosa M, Bronner MP, Grace M, Depot M, Esophagus IPGfH-GDiBs. Fiver-year efficacy and safety of photodynamic therapy with Photofrin in Barrett's high-grade dysplasia. Gastrontest Endosc. 2007;66(3):460–8.
76. Orman ES, Li N, Shaheen NJ. Efficacy and durability of radiofrequency ablation for Barrett's esophagus: a systemic review and meta-analysis. Clin Gastroenterol Hepatol. 2013;11(10):1245–55.
77. Ganz A, Overholt BF, Sharma VK, Fleischer DE, Shaleen NJ, Lightdale CJ, Freeman SR, Fruitt RE, Urayama SM, Gress F, Pavey DA, Branch MS, Savides TJ, Chang KJ, Muthusamy VR, Bohorfoush AG, Pace SC,

DeMeester SR, Eysselein VE, Panjehpour M, Triadafilopoulos G, Registry USM. Circumferential ablation of Barrett's esophagus that contains high-grade dysplasia: a U.S. multicenter registry. Gastroinest Endosc. 2008;68(1):35–40.
78. Sharma VK, Jae Kim H, Das A, Wells CD, Nguyen CC, Fleischer DE. Circumferential and focal ablation of Barrett's esophagus containing dysplasia. Am J Gastroenterol. 2009;104(2):310–7.
79. Velanowich V. Endoscopic endoluminal radiofrequency ablation of Barrett's esophagus: initial results and lessons learned. Surg Endosc. 2009;23(10):2175–80.
80. Shaleen NJ, Overholt BF, Sampliner RE, Wolfsen HC, Wang KK, Fleischer DE, Sharma VK, Eisen GM, Fennerty BM, Hunter JG, Bronner MP, Goldblum JR, Bennett AE, Mashimo H, Rothstein RI, Gordon SR, Edmundowicz SA, Madanick RD, Perry AF, Muthusamy VR, Chang KJ, Kimmey MB, Spechler SJ, Siddiqui AA, Souza RF, Infantolino A, Dumot JA, Falk GW, Galanko JA, Jobe BA, Hawes RH, Joffman BJ, Sharma P, Chak A, Lightdale CJ. Durability of radiofrequency ablation in Barrett's esophagus with dysplasia. Gastroenterology. 2011;14(2):460–8.
81. Rice TW, Zuccaro G Jr, Adelstein DJ, et al. Esophageal carcinoma: depth of tumor invasion is predictive of regional lymph node status. Ann Thorac Surg. 1998;65:787–92.
82. Stein JH, Feith M, Bruecher BL, et al. Early esophageal cancer: pattern of lymphatic spread and prognostic factors for long-term survival after surgical resection. Ann Surg. 2005;242:566–73. discussion 573–5.
83. Spechler SJ, Sharma P, Souza FR, et al. American gastroenterological association technical review on the management of Barrett's esophagus. Gastroenterology. 2011;140:e18–52. quiz e13.
84. Pech O, May A, Manner H, et al. Long-term efficacy and safety of endoscopic resection for patients with mucosal adenocarcinoma of the esophagus. Gastroenterology. 2014;146:652–660.e1.
85. Desai M, Saligram S, Gupta N, et al. Efficacy and safety outcomes of multimodal endoscopic eradication therapy in Barrett's esophagus=related neoplasia: a systematic review and pooled analysis. Gastrointest Endosc. 2016;85(3):482–495.e4.
86. Sharma P, Bergman JJ, Goda K, et al. Development and validation of a classification system to identify high-grade dysplasia and esophageal adenocarcinoma in Barrett's esophagus using narrow-band imaging. Gastroenterology. 2016;150:591–8.
87. Overholt BF, et al. Five-year efficacy and safety of photodynamic therapy with Photofrin in Barrett's high-grade dysplasia. Gastrointest Endosc. 2007;66(3):460–8.
88. Overholt BF, Panjehpour M, Haydek HM. Photodynamic therapy for Barrett's esophagus: follow-up in 100 patients. Gastrointest Endosc. 1999;49(1):1–7.

89. Overholt BF, et al. Photodynamic therapy with porfimer sodium for ablation of high-grade dysplasia in Barrett's esophagus: international, partially blinded, randomized phase III trial. Gastrointest Endosc. 2005;62(4):488–98.
90. Wang KK, Kim JY. Photodynamic therapy in Barrett's esophagus. Gastrointest Endosc Clin N Am. 2003;12(3):483–9.
91. Wolfsen HC, et al. Clinical experience of patients undergoing photodynamic therapy for Barrett's dysplasia or cancer. Aliment Pharmacol Ther. 2004;20(10):1125–31.
92. Wolfsen HC, Woodward TA, Raimondo M. Photodynamic therapy for dysplastic Barrett's esophagus and early esophageal adenocarinoma. Mayo Clin Proc. 2002;77(11):1176–81.
93. Gray NA, Odze RD, Spechler SJ. Buried metaplasia after endoscopic ablation of Barrett's esophagus: a systematic review. Am J Gastroenterol. 2011;106(11):1899–908. Quiz 1909.
94. Azarm A, et al. Endoscopic management of Barrett's esophagus: advances in endoscopic techniques. Dig Dis Sci. 2012;57(12):3055–64.
95. Greenwald BD, Dumot JA. Cryotherapy for Barrett's esophagus and esophageal cancer. Curr Opin Gastroenterol. 2011;27(4):363–7.
96. Shaheen NJ, et al. Safety and efficacy of endoscopic spray cryotherapy for Barrett's esophagus with high-grade dysplasia. Gastrointest Endosc. 2010;71(4):680–5.
97. Gosain S, et al. Liquid nitrogen spray cryotherapy in Barrett's esophagus with high-grade dysplasia: long-term results. Gastrointest Endosc. 2013;78(2):260–5.
98. Vaezi MF, Richter JE. Role of acid and duodenogastroesophageal reflux in gastroesophageal reflux disease. Gastroenterology. 1996;111:1192–9.
99. Stein HJ, Kauer WK, Feussner H, Siewert JR. Bile reflux in benign and malignant Barrett's esophagus: effect of medical acid suppression and nissen fundoplication. J Gastrointest Surg. 1998;4:333–41.
100. Ortiz A, Martinez de Haro LF, Parrilla P, Morales G, Molina J, Bermejo J, Liron R, Aguilar J. Conservative treatment versus antireflux surgery in Barrett's oesophagus: long-term results of a prospective study. Br J Surg. 1996;83:274–8.
101. Hofstetter WL, Peters JH, DeMeester TR, Hagen JA, DeMeester SR, Crookes PF, Tsai P, Banki F, Bremner CG. Long-term outcomes of antireflux surgery in patients with Barrett's esophagus. Ann Surg. 2001;234:532–9.
102. DeMeester SR, Campos GM, DeMeester TR, Bremner CG, Hagen JA, Peters JH, Crookes PF. The impact of an antireflux procedure on intestinal metaplasia of the cardia. Ann Surg. 1998;228:547–56.
103. Bowers SP, Mattar SG, Smith CD, Waring JP, Hunter JG. Clinical and histologic follow-up after antireflux surgery for Barrett's esophagus. J Gastrointest Surg. 2002;6:532–9.

30 Diagnostic Tests for Gastroesophageal Reflux Disease

Hope T. Jackson and Ivy N. Haskins

Introduction

Gastroesophageal reflux disease (GERD) is defined as symptoms or mucosal damage produced by abnormal reflux of gastric contents into the esophagus, oral cavity, or lungs [1, 2]. Gastroesophageal reflux disease is prevalent in the United States and affects at least 10% of our adult population [1, 2]. Patients with GERD symptoms are typically evaluated first by primary care physicians and gastroenterologists. Nevertheless, a surgeon should never assume that a patient seen in their office for GERD has medical refractory symptoms or that they have undergone a thorough evaluation for their GERD symptoms. Herein, we detail the common tests used for the evaluation of GERD and their utility with respect to patient management and surgical planning.

H. T. Jackson (✉)
Department of Surgery, The George Washington University School of Medicine and Health Sciences, Washington, DC, USA
e-mail: htjacks@med.umich.edu

I. N. Haskins
Esophageal Swallowing Center, MIS/Bariatric, Foregut, and Hernia Surgery, Omaha, NE, USA
e-mail: ivhaskins@unmc.edu

A. D. Patel et al. (eds.), *The SAGES Manual of Physiologic Evaluation of Foregut Diseases*,
https://doi.org/10.1007/978-3-031-39199-6_30

Evaluation

A meticulous medical history is critical to the workup of a patient with GERD symptoms. Typical symptoms include heartburn and regurgitation. Atypical symptoms include cough, chest pain, hoarseness, and dental erosions. Dysphagia can also be commonly seen in patients with GERD, but should prompt workup for other serious diagnoses such as esophageal cancer. The goals of diagnostic studies in the workup of GERD are to establish abnormal esophageal exposure, identify any anatomical and functional abnormalities secondary to reflux, and to correlate symptoms to reflux events. The following studies are the most commonly used in the evaluation of GERD (Table 30.1).

Table 30.1 Summary of diagnostic tests for gastroesophageal reflux disease

Test	Indication	Common Findings
Barium esophagram	Preoperative planning for anti-reflux (i.e., fundoplication) surgery	• Hiatal hernia or shortened esophagus • Reflux may be present, but cannot differentiate physiologic from pathologic reflux in this setting • Peptic stricture
EGD	1. Typical GERD symptoms refractory to medical management 2. Alarming GERD symptoms 3. Suspicion for Barrett's esophagus	• Normal esophageal and gastric mucosa most common findings • Esophagitis, Barrett's esophagus, gastritis, hiatal hernia or stricture.

Table 30.1 (continued)

Test		Indication	Common Findings
pH monitoring	24 h or 48 h pH monitoring	1. Failure of medical therapy 2. Preoperative Evaluation 3. Atypical symptoms 4. Symptoms without endoscopic evidence of esophagitis 5. Recurrence of symptoms following anti-reflux surgery	Abnormal score based on • Frequency of reflux episodes • Duration of longest reflux episode • Number of episodes longer than 5 min • Total time pH less than 4.0 in supine and standing position
	Impedance	1. Refractory symptoms 2. Atypical or extraesophageal symptoms	Normal impedance values include • total reflux events ≤73 • acid reflux events ≤55 • weakly acid reflux events ≤26 • weakly alkaline reflux ≤1
Esophageal manometry		Preoperative planning for anti-reflux (i.e., fundoplication) surgery	• Normal or abnormal esophageal function • If low DCI (≤500 mmHg/s/cm), consideration for partial fundoplication

Barium Esophagram

Barium esophagram is a key study in the workup of GERD; however, it should not be performed with the goal of establishing the diagnosis of GERD. In contrast to a 24 or 48-h pH study, an esophagram only allows for evaluation of reflux during a 10-min time period. The esophagram has a relatively low diagnostic sensitivity and specificity for GERD (40% and 85%, respectively) [3]. Even when reflux is demonstrated, the short duration of the study does not allow a differentiation between physiologic and abnormal reflux. Esophageal motility can be assessed with an esophagram; however, manometry will provide a more in-depth and descriptive analysis of esophageal motility. We believe the value of the esophagram lies in providing information about the length and diameter of the esophagus, the presence and morphology of a hiatal hernia, and the presence of a peptic stricture or Schatzki ring.

Esophagogastroduodenoscopy (EGD)

Esophagogastroduodenoscopy (EGD) is the standard modality used in the evaluation of the esophageal mucosa in patients with GERD symptoms [1]. For patients with typical GERD symptoms, which include heartburn and/or regurgitation, a trial of medical therapy with an antacid, histamine-receptor blocker, or proton pump inhibitor medication is typically the first intervention [1, 2]. Evaluation of the esophagus and stomach in a patient with typical GERD symptoms is not recommended as first-line treatment due to the high specificity of heartburn (89%) and regurgitation (97%) with GERD [1]. Nevertheless, it is important to remember that a small subset of patients may have endoscopic evidence of GERD in the absence of any GERD symptoms [1].

In general, the recommendations for EGD in a patient with GERD symptoms are:

1. A patient with typical GERD symptoms refractory to medical therapy.
2. A patient with atypical or alarming GERD symptoms, such as dysphagia, odynophagia, anemia or acute blood loss, and unintentional weight loss [1, 4].
3. Suspicion for mass, stricture, or ulcer as seen on other imaging studies, including barium esophagram or computed tomography scan.
4. As an adjunct for proper placement of pH probe as part of a preoperative workup for fundoplication or other surgical management of GERD.

When performing an EGD in a patient with GERD symptoms, in addition to evaluation of the esophageal and gastric mucosa, it is important to perform random biopsies of both the esophagus (near the Z-line) and the stomach (near the antrum) to evaluate for esophagitis, Barrett's esophagus, and associated dysplasia, gastritis, and Helicobacter pylori. Further, it is important to note any anatomical abnormalities found on EGD, including hiatal hernia, peptic stricture, gastric mass, etc., which may be contributing to the patient's symptoms. Finally, it is important to remember that most patients with typical GERD symptoms have no abnormalities on EGD and that a normal EGD does not rule out GERD [1, 2, 4].

Esophageal Manometry

The performance of esophageal manometry is not part of the routine workup for GERD unless a patient is being considered for anti-reflux surgery [1]. In the case of preoperative surgical evaluation, esophageal manometry is used to evaluate the overall function of the esophagus, to rule out severe motility disorders, including achalasia and scleroderma, which are contraindications to fundoplication, and to assist with placement of transnasal pH probes [1]. There is no pathognomonic manometry tracing for GERD. When reviewing manometry, the important values to review are the location and length of the lower esophageal sphincter (LES), the resting and residual LES pressures, the percent peristalsis of wet swallows, and the distal contractile integral (DCI).

pH Monitoring

pH monitoring is the gold standard for the diagnosis of GERD. 24- or 48-h pH monitoring objectively establishes the presence of pathologic reflux and allows for correlation between the symptoms reported by the patient and episodes of reflux. pH monitoring provides information on the frequency of reflux episodes, duration of the longest episode of reflux, the number of episodes longer than 5 min, and the total time the pH is less than 4.0 in the supine and standing position. These components make up the composite score (DeMeester score) that defines normal and abnormal reflux (greater than 14.7 indicates pathologic reflux) [5]. An abnormal score is also an important predictive factor in the success of anti-reflux surgery. A multivariate analysis by Campos et al. of patients who received a laparoscopic nissen fundoplication found that the 24-h pH monitoring score was the greatest predictor of a good or excellent outcome [6]. The study similarly showed that 25% of patients with normal pH scores who had typical symptoms and responsiveness to medication had only a fair or poor outcome following surgery [6].

Forty-eight hours wireless esophageal pH monitoring (BRAVO probe) can avoid the discomfort, embarrassment, and changes in daily activity and diet that patients may experience with the 24-h nasal probe [7]. Limitations of the BRAVO study include that it only records the pH of the lower esophagus; in contrast to the 24 h probe, early detachment of the probe into the stomach can lead to false positive results (Fig. 30.1).

Impedance pH Monitoring is another helpful study that can be used in the workup for patients with GERD. The study measures the flow of liquid and gas across the gastroesophageal junction independently of the pH of the reflux contents. It provides details

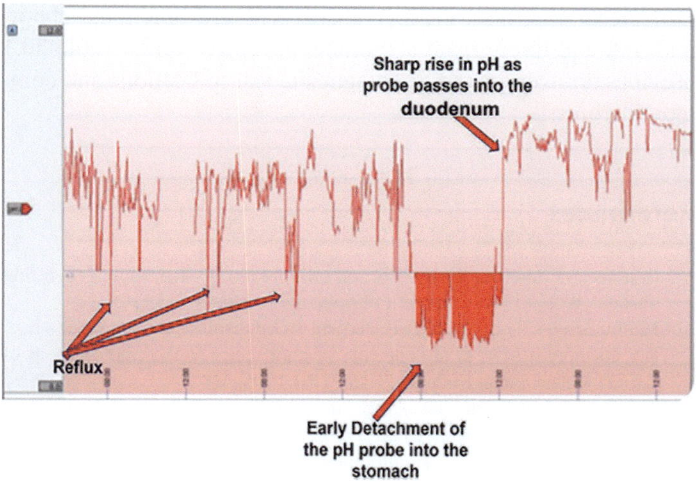

Fig. 30.1 BRAVO study tracing demonstrating reflux, early detachment of the probe from the esophagus into the stomach that can lead to false positive results, and the typical subsequent tracing as the probe travels into the duodenum

regarding the characteristics of the refluxate (gas, liquid, mixed), the pH (acid, weakly acid, alkaline) [8]. This study is typically recommended in patients with symptoms refractory to proton pump inhibitors or atypical symptoms such as cough. Mainie et al. showed that patients with refractory symptoms can have successful outcomes following anti reflux surgery when impedance-pH monitoring shows a correlation between symptoms and reflux episodes regardless of pH [9]. Normal impedance values include: total reflux events ≤73, acid reflux events ≤55, weakly acid reflux events ≤26, and weakly alkaline reflux ≤1 [10].

Summary

Accurately establishing a diagnosis of GERD is of paramount importance prior to offering surgical management. Diagnostic studies in the workup of GERD serve to establish abnormal esophageal exposure, identify anatomical and functional abnormalities, and to correlate symptoms to reflux events. Table 30.1 provides an overview of the diagnostic test indications and common findings.

References

1. Badillo R, Francis D. Diagnosis and treatment of gastroesophageal reflux disease. World J Gastrointest Pharmacol Ther. 2014;5(3):105–12.
2. Muthusamy VR, Lightdale JR, Acosta RD, Chandrasekhara V, Chathadi KV, Eloubeidi MA, et al. The role of endoscopy in the management of GERD. Gastrointest Endosc. 2015;81(6):1305–10.
3. Streets CG, DeMeester TR. Ambulatory 24-hour esophageal pH monitoring: why, when, and what to do. J Clin Gastroenterol. 2003;37(1):14–22.
4. Smith L. Updated ACG guidelines for diagnosis and treatment of GERD. Am Fam Physician. 2005;71(12):2376–82.
5. Jamieson JR, Stein HJ, DeMeester TR, Bonavina L, Schwizer W, Hinder RA, Albertucci M. Ambulatory 24-h esophageal pH monitoring: normal values, optimal thresholds, specificity, sensitivity, and reproducibility. Am J Gastroenterol. 1992;87:1102.
6. Campos GM, Peters JH, DeMeester TR, Öberg S, Crookes PF, Tan S, DeMeester SR, Hagen JA, Bremner CG. Multivariate analysis of factors predicting outcome after laparoscopic Nissen fundoplication. J Gastrointest Surg. 1999;3(3):292–300.
7. Håkanson BS, Berggren P, Granqvist S, Ljungqvist O, Thorell A. Comparison of wireless 48-h (Bravo) versus traditional ambulatory 24-h esophageal pH monitoring. Scand J Gastroenterol. 2009;44(3):276–83.
8. Blonski W, Vela MF, Castell DO. Comparison of reflux frequency during prolonged multichannel intraluminal impedance and pH monitoring on and off acid suppression therapy. J Clin Gastroenterol. 2009;43(9):816–20.
9. Mainie I, Tutuian R, Agrawal A, Adams D, Castell DO. Combined multichannel intraluminal impedance–pH monitoring to select patients with persistent gastro-oesophageal reflux for laparoscopic Nissen fundoplication. Br J Surg. 2006;93(12):1483–7.
10. Cho YK. How to interpret esophageal impedance pH monitoring. J Neurogastroenterol Motil. 2010;16(3):327.

Laryngopharyngeal Reflux

31

Charles Hill, Stephanie Doggett, and Francis P. Buckley III

Introduction

Gastroesophageal reflux disease (GERD) develops when gastric refluxate causes troublesome symptoms or complications [1]. This defines a diagnosis of GERD as one founded on patient symptoms and includes both liquid and gaseous refluxate which can be acidic, weakly acidic, or weakly alkaline. The typical GERD symptoms include heartburn and regurgitation and can result in esophageal injury. Additional extraesophageal symptoms, including chronic cough, hoarseness, asthma, throat clearing, globus sensation, and post nasal drip, fall under the broad category of laryngopharyngeal reflux (LPR). These reflux-related symptoms occur throughout the day and are associated with an upright posture. While there is a clear association between LPR and GERD, the symptoms of LPR can occur independently and proving a causative relationship is difficult [2]. For this chapter, we will focus on the presentation, diagnosis, and management of LPR as an extraesophageal manifestation of underlying GERD. The Montreal Definition of LPR refers to established

C. Hill (✉) · S. Doggett · F. P. Buckley III
Dell Medical School, University of Texas at Austin, Austin, TX, USA
e-mail: Charles.hill2@ascension.org

A. D. Patel et al. (eds.), *The SAGES Manual of Physiologic Evaluation of Foregut Diseases*,
https://doi.org/10.1007/978-3-031-39199-6_31

associations of reflux cough, laryngitis, and asthma which require careful investigation to eliminate the numerous multifactorial aggravating cofactors before the treatment can begin.

Epidemiology

The true incidence of LPR is difficult to establish due to the lack of gold standard diagnostics and complex patient presentations. The CDC estimates that cough, throat symptoms, and asthma encompass over 12% of chief complaints for primary care visits each year. A hidden prevalence likely exists within this estimate in patients presenting with isolated LPR, but because LPR is also found in up to 70% of patients with GERD, the true effect has yet to be determined [3, 4]. Because many of the primary symptoms are nonspecific, the subsequent workup can involve multiple specialty consults, procedures, diagnostic tests, and medication prescriptions. Annual healthcare costs attributed to GERD management have been estimated to be $9–12 billion [5, 6]. A recent cost analysis of Medicare patients undergoing LPR management found an average per patient cost of over $5,000/year, which is 5.6 times than that of GERD [7]. By this estimation, the healthcare burden of LPR would be over $50 billion annually. Additionally, 86% of the per patient cost was related to medication purchases, of which 61% was directly attributed to proton-pump inhibitor (PPI) usage.

Pathophysiology

There are multiple physiologic barriers to reflux that can be disrupted by independent patient factors. The lower esophageal sphincter (LES), located at the gastroesophageal junction roughly 40 cm from the incisors, functions to prevent stomach acid and food from flowing retrograde into the esophagus during gastric peristalsis with a resting pressure of 10–45 mmHg. The upper esophageal sphincter's (UES) baseline tonic contraction of 30–50 mmHg prevents air from entering the esophagus during respiration as well as reflux into the pharynx during swallowing. The UES is augmented by increased esophageal pressure during swallowing, but both physiologic sphincters can be compromised by excessive intra-abdominal pressure, incompetent resting tone, and anatomic distortions such as a hiatal hernia [8]. Inherent reflexes of glottis closure, coughing, and swallowing also aid in preventing airway exposure to harmful gastroesophageal reflux.

Direct exposure, and indirect neurogenic interactions have proposed mechanisms for upper airway injury during LPR. The reflux theory proposes that the inherent reflux barriers are overwhelmed causing a direct tissue exposure of the upper airway tissues to gastric acid, refluxate, pepsin, and bile acids. The laryngeal mucosa lacks the protective alkaline mucous secreting cells of the stomach that buffer the acidic fluid, leading to injury with exposure to the caustic secretions. The mucosal injury causes swelling, mucous hypersecretion, and an inflammatory reaction. Pepsin, the primary enzyme for protein degradation which can be present in the gastric refluxate, is most active at a pH <2 and generally inactive at a pH >6.5. Although the minimum acid exposure duration needed to produce symptoms is unknown, esophageal and laryngeal damage due to refluxed pepsin can be seen at any pH below 8.6. Regarding indirect neurogenic interactions, the reflex theory proposes a vagally-mediated mechanism of bronchoconstriction in response to esophageal-bronchial neural cough reflex. This neurogenic inflammation of the lung mimics the response of the tracheobronchial tree to micro-aspirations of gastric contents, releasing inflammatory mediators and disrupting normal tissue [9].

Diagnosis

As the constellation of symptoms associated with LPR is nonspecific, several other differential diagnoses must first be considered and evaluated before proceeding with treatment. In all patients, a history and physical should be performed with special attention to alarm symptoms such as stridor, recent surgery, recent intubation, a history of head and neck radiation, or history of smoking. Any of these would prompt a more urgent specialist evaluation to rule out malignancy. For patients presenting with a chronic cough for more than 8 weeks, the American College of Chest Physicians recommends an empiric PPI therapy only after excluding the more frequent causes like smoking, post-nasal drip, asthma, bronchitis, and acetylcholinesterase inhibitor usage [10]. Another common primary complaint is hoarseness, frequently explained by excessive voice usage, throat clearing, allergies, infection, and smoking history. The American Academy of Otolaryngology recommends that these possible etiologies be ruled out, followed by the confirmation of LPR by the combination of a validated patient reported symptom index and laryngoscopic findings of injury prior to initiating empiric PPI therapy [11]. Adult onset asthma is frequently implicated as LPR, especially in those with concomitant GERD. An expert panel report for the management of asthma supports an empiric PPI trial in all asthma patients with GERD and in those with poorly controlled asthma despite maximum medical therapy [12].

An empiric trial of double-dose PPIs has been favored as a diagnostic and therapeutic approach for LPR and is based on the assumption that LPR is caused by GERD. Furthermore, it is believed to be less expensive and less time-consuming than invasive testing, although the economic impact on long-term PPI usage is not insignificant. Multiple RCT comparing PPIs to placebo however has only shown a modest (<50%) improvement in LPR symptoms, with little to no impact on endoscopic esophageal or laryngeal injury [9, 13–15]. As a diagnostic tool for LPR, the patient-reported symptoms alone have a sensitivity and specificity of 49% and 79%, respectively, and there is no improvement in the diagnostic yield when considering the response to PPI therapy [14, 16]. When symptoms of LPR remain despite full PPI therapy, subsequent workup is recommended to rule out GERD and identify other possible etiologies.

Lacking a gold standard diagnostic test, patient symptoms have become a necessary diagnostic tool. Patient reported outcome (PRO) measures are designed to evaluate disease-specific symptom severity and their impact on quality of life. The laryngopharyngeal reflux symptom index (RSI) is the most commonly used questionnaire, which was validated by Belfasky et al. in patients with esophageal double pH probe confirmed LPR [17]. This nine-question survey uses a five-point severity scale for common LPR symptoms with a cutoff of >13 considered to be diagnostic. The RSI score can be followed overtime to monitor treatment outcomes and direct clinical decision-making [18]. Conventionally, the diagnosis of LPR has been defined by a positive RSI combined with specific findings on laryngoscopy.

Laryngoscopy is used by Otolaryngologists to evaluate the upper respiratory tract for signs of injury and malignancy and can be performed in an office setting. Common findings of laryngeal irritation include edema or hyperemia of larynx, cobblestoning of posterior pharynx, contact ulcers, polyps, interarytenoid changes, granulomas, and subglottic stenosis. In an effort to standardize findings that support a diagnosis of LPR, the Reflux Finding Score (RFS) was developed by Belafsky et al. [19]. Although the validation study for the eight item rating scale reported excellent inter-relator reliability, the subsequent studies have failed to support this correlation. Laryngeal irritation has been identified in 80–90% of normal healthy volunteers without symptoms, and the rating scale is highly subjective [9, 20]. Evaluation of the posterior larynx especially, traditionally thought to be a primary site of injury, is consistently the most difficult to rate and assess with poor inter-rater correlation [21]. Given its low specificity for LPR, the focus of laryngoscopy has shifted instead towards ruling out malignancy and has been supplanted by instruments that direct measure esophageal and pharyngeal pH and pressures.

Distal esophageal pH measurements reported as a cumulative DeMeester score have long been the gold standard for diagnosis of GERD, but studies have shown poor correlation between PPI responders and distal esophageal acid exposure [22]. To measure oropharyngeal pH changes, a single oropharyngeal probe was designed to be placed proximal to the UES. Unfortunately, clinical trials determined up to 43% of healthy volunteers may have abnormal hypopharyngeal pH, and these instruments failed to clearly differentiate between healthy volunteers and those with LPR and GERD [9, 23, 24]. Pharyngeal pH measurements also fail to measure nonacid events which likely contributes to the poor diagnostic yield. Multichannel intraluminal impedance (MII) probes are placed in the esophagus to measure the physiologic reflux events by detecting changes in the intraluminal pressure. Combined with a distal and proximal pH probes (MII/pH), these instruments are able to differentiate between composition (liquid, gas, or mixed) and acid content of refluxate. Subsequent studies have shown that MII/pH can detect LPR episodes, but the cutoff values for refluxate pH and exposure times, and proximal probe position in relation to the UES varies greatly between studies [13, 15, 25]. In an effort to establish correlation of distal esophageal reflux events with LPR, several studies have compared the findings from oropharyngeal pH probes to MII/pH probes in select patients. Results were inconclusive, as oropharyngeal pH probes detected only acidic events and MII/pH detected both acid and nonacid events, but 90% of the oropharyngeal findings were independent of MII/pH events without any obvious correlation found [2]. The use of MII/pH probes in LPR patients lacking common GERD symptoms provides a diagnostic yield of 40–50% for detecting associated GERD and improves patient selection for surgery [13]. Currently, these instruments provide the most complete picture of the reflux burden in LPR, but their clinical utility for determining the treatment response is limited to those patients with objective confirmation of GERD.

Another area of research involves the detection of upper airway pepsin exposure. Techniques for the specimen collection vary, with some studies performing laryngeal/pharyngeal biopsies and others using salivary samples to run rapid monoclonal antibody tests or quantitative ELISA PCR studies [26–28]. Pepsin levels vary depending on time of day, as higher levels are found on waking and directly after reflux events. Oropharyngeal pepsin can be found in healthy controls, but the concentration is noticeably lower compared to GERD and LPR patients, thus favoring a quantitative study for a diagnostic value. Studies have shown that pepsin at pathologic levels in the upper airway can be considered a marker for LPR but have failed to differentiate between GERD-related and non-GERD-related LPR. A recent systematic review concluded that current evidence lacks appropriate standardization of specimen collection location, collection timing, and cutoff values, thus limiting its utility as a tool to identify potential treatment responders [29].

Treatment

As in the treatment of GERD, lifestyle and dietary modifications can have a meaningful impact on disease burden for patients with LPR. The recommendations are similar, with lifestyle changes such as weight loss, cessation of smoking and alcohol usage, and refraining from supine positioning directly following a meal. Dietary changes incorporate a low fat (<45 g/day) diet, small meal size, and the elimination of coffee, tea, carbonated, and caffeinated soft drinks, chocolate, and citrus [3, 8]. A systematic review of the RCT of medical therapy for LPR treatment showed that the dietary changes were associated with a significant improvement of symptoms in both PPI responders and nonresponders [15].

The initial medical therapy for LPR has also mirrored GERD with the empirical usage of PPIs, although a mounting evidence shows a poor response rate compared to placebo. Although these studies are primarily RCT comparing PPI usage to placebo, the limitations are significant and due in large part to the poor diagnostic criteria for LPR as well as failure to standardized reported outcomes. In studies reporting a benefit from PPI usage over placebo, the studied cohort included patients with LPR who either had common GERD symptoms or objective evidence of GERD [9, 30, 31]. Of these studies, some responders reported an improvement in mean RSI scores, but investigators found no objective improvement by laryngoscopy or endoscopy [11]. The inconsistent therapeutic rate of empiric PPIs is likely multifactorial, as non-responders may have non-acid refluxate episodes or may not even have GERD. Overall, the current literature indicates that a positive response to the empiric therapy is the best indicator for eventual symptom resolution, but failure to continue the maintenance therapy carries a high risk of symptom recurrence [32, 33]. Analyses supporting anti-reflux interventions have promising long-term results but rely greatly on the appropriate workup with MII/pH identifying underlying GERD.

Endoluminal anti-reflux interventions have garnered recent attention with successful outcomes comparable to surgery. The transoral incisionless fundoplication (TIF) is performed endoscopically and creates and 270° anterior fundoplication secured with H-shaped fasteners. Cessation of daily PPI usage is reported in 70–80% of patients and was more likely in patients with poor symptom control despite maximum PPI therapy and in those with objective evidence of GERD on MII/pH or endoscopy [34–36]. Additionally, up to 60% of patients report resolution of LPR symptoms postoperatively. Recent meta-analysis show decreased efficacy with time; however, raising concern for the durability of the endoscopically reinforced LES [37]. Relatively well tolerated with a low adverse event profile, TIF is a reasonable treatment modality for the extraesophageal manifestations of GERD and should be considered in patients unable or unwilling to undergo surgery.

Anti-reflux surgery (ARS) is a highly successful treatment with excellent long-term outcomes in select patients with GERD, but predicting success in patients with concomitant and/or pure LPRD has been difficult. ARS is performed laparoscopically in the majority of cases and involves hiatal dissection, cruroplasty, and fundoplication for static reinforcement of the LES. Recent comparisons of patients undergoing ARS vs PPI therapy revealed a higher rate of symptom improvement by mean RSI (84% vs 50%), a higher proportion of patient satisfaction (63% vs 44%), and higher percentage of patients able to discontinue PPI therapy (44% vs 7%) at long-term follow-up [38, 39]. Patients with confirmed reflux asthma report a decrease in asthma symptoms and medication usage following ARS [40]. An alternative to fundoplication, magnetic sphincter augmentation (MSA) using the LINX device (Torax Medical, Shoreview, MN) provides a dynamic augmentation to the LES. Outcomes of ARS with MSA are comparable to standard fundoplication, with up to 85% of patients reporting discontinuation of PPIs and resolution of LPR symptoms [39, 41–43]. Interestingly, the frequency or severity of proximal reflux events on pharyngeal pH or MII/pH have not been shown to be predictive of therapy response. Although these outcomes are promising, the preoperative evaluation for LPR patients should include extensive counseling explaining that resolution of extraesophageal symptoms is less reliable than the response rate of typical symptoms.

Conclusion

LPR represents a significant healthcare burden as a result of complex diagnostic criteria lacking gold standard testing and poor treatment response in a significant number of patients. Further study is needed to establish the best diagnostic test for LPR, which is complicated by the lack of standardization in reporting both preoperative findings and postoperative outcomes. Treatment efficacy is thereby difficult to establish, although subjective symptom resolution may be the most important measurable outcome to patients. Using symptom resolution and cessation of PPIs as measures of treatment success, endoscopic and surgical treatments appear to have better short- and long-term results compared to medical therapy alone. However, predicting treatment responses remains a challenge, and extensive preoperative counseling is necessary prior to any intervention.

Acknowledgements None.

Conflicts of Interest There are no conflicts of interest to disclose and no funding for this study.

Author Contributions Literature review: CH.
Writing: CH, SD, FPB.
Critical revision: CH, SD, FPB.

References

1. Vakil N, Van Zanten SV, Kahrilas P, Dent J, Jones R. The Montreal definition and classification of gastroesophageal reflux disease: a global evidence-based consensus. Am J Gastroenterol. 2006;101(8):1900–20.
2. Ummarino D, Vandermeulen L, Roosens B, Urbain D, Hauser B, Vandenplas Y. Gastroesophageal reflux evaluation in patients affected by chronic cough: Restech versus multichannel intraluminal impedance/pH metry. Laryngoscope. 2013;123(4):980–4.
3. Sidwa F, Moore AL, Alligood E, Fisichella PM. Surgical treatment of extraesophageal manifestations of gastroesophageal reflux disease. World J Surg. 2017;41(10):2566–71.
4. Ward MA, Ebrahim A, Kopita J, Arviso L, Ogola GO, Buckmaster B, et al. Magnetic sphincter augmentation is an effective treatment for atypical symptoms caused by gastroesophageal reflux disease. Surg Endosc. 2019;2019:1–7.
5. Sandler RS, Everhart JE, Donowitz M, Adams E, Cronin K, Goodman C, et al. The burden of selected digestive diseases in the United States. Gastroenterology. 2002;122(5):1500–11.
6. Everhart JE, Ruhl CE. Burden of digestive diseases in the United States part I: overall and upper gastrointestinal diseases. Gastroenterology. 2009;136(2):376–86.
7. Francis DO, Rymer JA, Slaughter JC, Choksi Y, Jiramongkolchai P, Ogbeide E, et al. High economic burden of caring for patients with suspected extraesophageal reflux. Am J Gastroenterol. 2013;108(6):905–11.
8. Brown J, Shermetaro C. Laryngopharyngeal reflux. In: StatPearls. Treasure Island: StatPearls Publishing; 2020.
9. Hom C, Vaezi MF. Extra-esophageal manifestations of gastroesophageal reflux disease: diagnosis and treatment. Drugs. 2013;73(12):1281–95.
10. Irwin RS. Chronic cough due to gastroesophageal reflux disease: ACCP evidence-based clinical practice guidelines. Chest. 2006;129(1): 80S–94S.
11. Schwartz SR, Cohen SM, Dailey SH, Rosenfeld RM, Deutsch ES, Gillespie MB, et al. Clinical practice guideline: hoarseness (dysphonia). Otolaryngology. 2009;141(1):1–31.
12. National AE, Prevention P. Expert Panel Report 3 (EPR-3): guidelines for the diagnosis and management of asthma-summary report 2007. J Allergy Clin Immunol. 2007;120(5 Suppl):S94.
13. Lee BE, Kim GH, Ryu DY, Kim DU, Cheong JH, Lee DG, et al. Combined dual channel impedance/pH-metry in patients with suspected laryngopharyngeal reflux. J Neurogastroenterol Motil. 2010;16(2):157.
14. Jobe BA, Richter JE, Hoppo T, Peters JH, Bell R, Dengler WC, et al. Preoperative diagnostic workup before antireflux surgery: an evidence

and experience-based consensus of the Esophageal Diagnostic Advisory Panel. J Am Coll Surg. 2013;217(4):586–97.

15. Lechien JR, Saussez S, Schindler A, Karkos PD, Hamdan AL, Harmegnies B, et al. Clinical outcomes of laryngopharyngeal reflux treatment: a systematic review and meta-analysis. Laryngoscope. 2019;129(5):1174–87.
16. Wood JM, Athanasiadis T, Allen J. Laryngitis. BMJ. 2014;349:g5827.
17. Belafsky PC, Postma GN, Koufman JA. Validity and reliability of the reflux symptom index (RSI). J Voice. 2002;16(2):274–7.
18. Francis DO, Patel DA, Sharda R, Hovis K, Sathe N, Penson DF, et al. Patient-reported outcome measures related to laryngopharyngeal reflux: a systematic review of instrument development and validation. Otolaryngol Head Neck Surg. 2016;155(6):923–35.
19. Belafsky PC, Postma GN, Koufman JA. The validity and reliability of the reflux finding score (RFS). Laryngoscope. 2001;111(8):1313–7.
20. Vaezi MF. Benefit of acid-suppressive therapy in chronic laryngitis: the devil is in the details. Clin Gastroenterol Hepatol. 2010;8(9):741–2.
21. Branski RC, Bhattacharyya N, Shapiro J. The reliability of the assessment of endoscopic laryngeal findings associated with laryngopharyngeal reflux disease. Laryngoscope. 2002;112(6):1019–24.
22. Richter J, Pandolfino J, Vela M, Kahrilas P, Lacy B, Ganz R, et al. Utilization of wireless pH monitoring technologies: a summary of the proceedings from the Esophageal Diagnostic Working Group. Dis Esophagus. 2013;26(8):755–65.
23. Wiener GJ, Tsukashima R, Kelly C, Wolf E, Schmeltzer M, Bankert C, et al. Oropharyngeal pH monitoring for the detection of liquid and aerosolized supraesophageal gastric reflux. J Voice. 2009;23(4):498–504.
24. Yuksel E, Slaughter J, Mukhtar N, Ochieng M, Sun G, Goutte M, et al. An oropharyngeal pH monitoring device to evaluate patients with chronic laryngitis. Neurogastroenterol Motil. 2013;25(5):e315–e23.
25. Górecka-Tuteja A, Jastrzębska I, Składzień J, Fyderek K. Laryngopharyngeal reflux in children with chronic otitis media with effusion. J Neurogastroenterol Motil. 2016;22(3):452.
26. Yadlapati R, Adkins C, Jaiyeola D-M, Lidder AK, Gawron AJ, Tan BK, et al. Abilities of oropharyngeal pH tests and salivary pepsin analysis to discriminate between asymptomatic volunteers and subjects with symptoms of laryngeal irritation. Clin Gastroenterol Hepatol. 2016;14(4):535–42. e2
27. Komatsu Y, Kelly LA, Zaidi AH, Rotoloni CL, Kosovec JE, Lloyd EJ, et al. Hypopharyngeal pepsin and Sep70 as diagnostic markers of laryngopharyngeal reflux: preliminary study. Surg Endosc. 2015;29(5):1080–7.
28. Na SY, Kwon OE, Lee YC, Eun YG. Optimal timing of saliva collection to detect pepsin in patients with laryngopharyngeal reflux. Laryngoscope. 2016;126(12):2770–3.

29. Calvo-Henríquez C, Ruano-Ravina A, Vaamonde P, Martínez-Capoccioni G, Martín-Martín C. Is pepsin a reliable marker of laryngopharyngeal reflux? A systematic review. Otolaryngology. 2017;157(3):385–91.
30. Lee B, Woo P. Chronic cough as a sign of laryngeal sensory neuropathy: diagnosis and treatment. Ann Otol Rhinol Laryngol. 2005;114(4):253–7.
31. Reichel O, Dressel H, Wiederänders K, Issing WJ. Double-blind, placebo-controlled trial with esomeprazole for symptoms and signs associated with laryngopharyngeal reflux. Otolaryngology. 2008;139(3):414–20.
32. Schindlbeck N, Klauser A, Berghammer G, Londong W, Müller-Lissner S. Three year follow up of patients with gastrooesophageal reflux disease. Gut. 1992;33(8):1016–9.
33. Vigneri S, Termini R, Leandro G, Badalamenti S, Pantalena M, Savarino V, et al. A comparison of five maintenance therapies for reflux esophagitis. N Engl J Med. 1995;333(17):1106–10.
34. Trad KS, Barnes WE, Simoni G, Shughoury AB, Mavrelis PG, Raza M, et al. Transoral incisionless fundoplication effective in eliminating GERD symptoms in partial responders to proton pump inhibitor therapy at 6 months: the TEMPO randomized clinical trial. Surg Innov. 2015;22(1):26–40.
35. Testoni PA, Testoni S, Mazzoleni G, Vailati C, Passaretti S. Long-term efficacy of transoral incisionless fundoplication with Esophyx (Tif 2.0) and factors affecting outcomes in GERD patients followed for up to 6 years: a prospective single-center study. Surg Endosc. 2015;29(9):2770–80.
36. Wendling MR, Melvin WS, Perry KA. Impact of transoral incisionless fundoplication (TIF) on subjective and objective GERD indices: a systematic review of the published literature. Surg Endosc. 2013;27(10):3754–61.
37. Huang X, Chen S, Zhao H, Zeng X, Lian J, Tseng Y, et al. Efficacy of transoral incisionless fundoplication (TIF) for the treatment of GERD: a systematic review with meta-analysis. Surg Endosc. 2017;31(3):1032–44.
38. Zhang C, Hu Z-W, Yan C, Wu Q, Wu J-M, Du X, et al. Nissen fundoplication vs proton pump inhibitors for laryngopharyngeal reflux based on pH-monitoring and symptom-scale. World J Gastroenterol. 2017;23(19):3546.
39. Ayazi S, Zheng P, Zaidi AH, Chovanec K, Salvitti M, Newhams K, et al. Clinical outcome and predictors of favorable result after laparoscopic magnetic sphincter augmentation: single institution experience with over 500 patients. J Am Coll Surg. 2020;230(5):733–43.
40. Vakil NB, Halling K, Becher A, Ryden A. Systematic review of patient-reported outcome instruments for gastroesophageal reflux disease symptoms. Eur J Gastroenterol Hepatol. 2013;25(1):2–14.

41. Buckley F, Bell RC, Freeman K, Doggett S, Heidrick R. Favorable results from a prospective evaluation of 200 patients with large hiatal hernias undergoing LINX magnetic sphincter augmentation. Surg Endosc. 2018;32(4):1762–8.
42. Louie BE, Smith CD, Smith CC, Bell RC, Gillian GK, Mandel JS, et al. Objective evidence of reflux control after magnetic sphincter augmentation: one year results from a post approval study. Ann Surg. 2019;270(2):302–8.
43. Saino G, Bonavina L, Lipham JC, Dunn D, Ganz RA. Magnetic sphincter augmentation for gastroesophageal reflux at 5 years: final results of a pilot study show long-term acid reduction and symptom improvement. J Laparoendosc Adv Surg Tech. 2015;25(10):787–92.

32 Esophagitis

Federico Serrot

Introduction

Gastroesophageal reflux disease (GERD) is a chronic and highly prevalent disorder. A recent systematic review showed that the prevalence of GERD is 18.1–27.8% in North America, 8.8–25.9% in Europe, 2.5–7.8% in East Asia, 8.7–33.1% in the Middle East, 11.6% in Australia, and 23.0% in South America [1].

According to the published practice guidelines of the American College of Gastroenterology, a presumptive diagnosis of GERD can be made on the basis of typical symptoms, such as heartburn, regurgitation, epigastric pain, and sleep disturbance. An improvement of reflux symptoms on empiric medical therapy with a proton pump inhibitor (PPI) ideally confirms this symptom-based diagnosis (so-called PPI test). Upper gastrointestinal endoscopy is only recommended in the presence of lack of improvement of symptoms as well as screening of patients at high risk for complications [2, 3].

F. Serrot (✉)
Department of Surgery, Emory University, Atlanta, GA, USA

A. D. Patel et al. (eds.), *The SAGES Manual of Physiologic Evaluation of Foregut Diseases*,
https://doi.org/10.1007/978-3-031-39199-6_32

Endoscopic Features and Classification of Esophagitis

The endoscopic assessment of esophageal mucosal changes in patients with reflux symptoms is important to diagnose patients at various degrees of severity. It is well known that the endoscopic severity of esophagitis correlates with the likelihood of responding to certain treatments and with the risk of developing complications. Gastroesophageal reflux disease with endoscopically identifiable lesions (erosions, stricture, and Barrett's esophagus) is defined as erosive gastroesophageal reflux disease (GERD). Fewer than 50% of patients with typical GERD symptoms have endoscopically recognizable mucosal lesions [4]. On the other hand, non-erosive reflux disease (NERD) is characterized by the presence of reflux symptoms, abnormal pH monitoring, and absence of endoscopically visible lesions, but with the histological changes consistent with microscopic esophagitis [5]. NERD patients account for up to 60% of all patients with reflux symptoms [6]. For this reason, an early diagnosis of GERD is crucial because the chronic reflux esophagitis is a key risk factor for the development of Barrett's esophagus, which is a precursor lesion for esophageal adenocarcinoma.

A diagnosis of erosive reflux esophagitis is established when there are patchy, striated, or circular and confluent epithelial defects (erosions) in the mucosa in the distal esophagus. Nearly all of the guidelines on the diagnosis and treatment of reflux disease recommend that reflux esophagitis should be classified endoscopically. The European guidelines also recommend that findings such as stenosis, ulcer, Schatzki ring, metaplasia as well as the presence of hiatal hernia should be documented [7].

Due to its ease of use and very minor interindividual variability in the assessment, the Los Angeles (LA) classification should be used. The LA classification system was published in its final form back in 1999 (Table 32.1) [8].

It was developed by the International Working Group for the Classification of Esophagitis, supported by the World Organization of Gastroenterology, and was first proposed in 1994. It was first

Table 32.1 Los Angeles classification of esophagitis (adapted from Lundell et al. [8])

Grade	Characteristics	Diagram
A	One (or more) mucosal break no longer than 5 mm that does not extend between the tops of two mucosal folds.	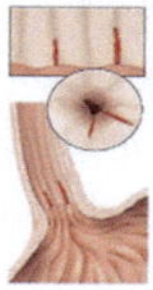
B	One (or more) mucosal break more than 5 mm long that does not extend between the tops of two mucosal folds.	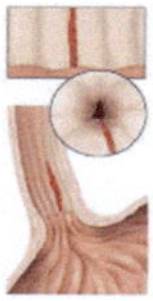
C	One (or more) mucosal break that is continuous between the tops of two or more mucosal folds involving less than 75% of the circumference.	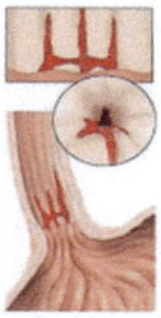
D	One (or more) mucosal break which involves at least 75% of the esophageal circumference.	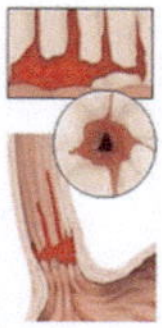

presented at the Los Angeles World Congress of Gastroenterology, and hence the name of the classification. It is the most validated classification system. Furthermore, it has been consistent at predicting the outcome of acid reflux therapy, correlates well with other tests of acid reflux such as 24-h pH monitoring studies, and when compared with other grading systems, it was the most reproducible and practical [8].

Although the clinical significance and accuracy of other findings are not included in the LA classification, such as minimal mucosal changes, it is needed to be validated rigorously before incorporating them into the classification system. Advances in endoscopic imaging techniques have allowed the visualization of these changes and could potentially in the future become relevant at the time of evaluation of patients with GERD.

It is imperative to obtain an adequate mucosal visualization. Meticulous washing with mucolytic and antifoaming agents as well as the use of high-definition endoscope are an important aspect of the technique.

Accurate endoscopic assessment of reflux esophagitis presence and severity is vital in making accurate decisions about patients' management and prognosis. Different types of therapy will be indicated depending on the extent and severity of the reflux esophagitis seen on endoscopic evaluation as well as on the extent of the symptoms.

Patients with mild cases of esophagitis, LA grade A/B (Fig. 32.1) should be treated with a PPI at the standard dosage for

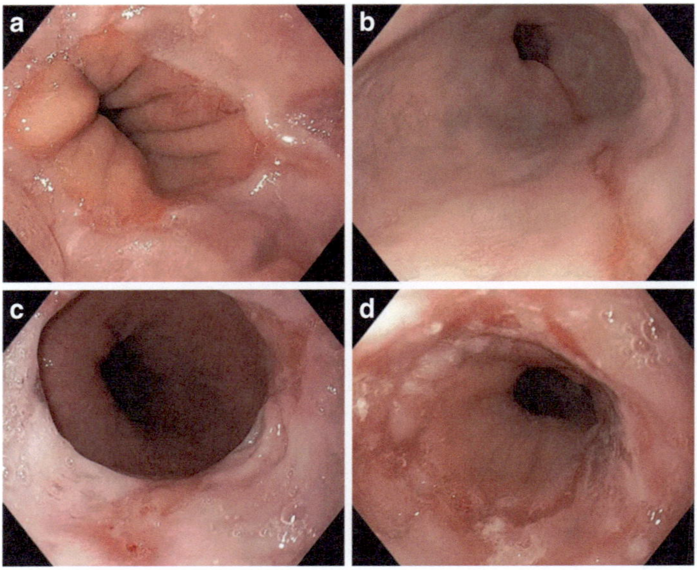

Fig. 32.1 Los Angeles (LA) classification is the endoscopic scoring system most commonly used to grade the severity of reflux esophagitis. The LA system divides reflux esophagitis into four categories (**a**–**d**) based on the extent of esophageal mucosal breaks

around 4 weeks. Most cases improve their symptoms as well as endoscopic features. On the other hand, patients with severe cases, LA grade C/D (Fig. 32.1) should receive 8 weeks of PPI at the standard dosage. These patients with more severe esophagitis are at greater risk of local complications, cannot afford PPI step down, and often require anti-reflux surgery [9].

Once diagnosis of reflux esophagitis has been made and treatment indicated, a decision has to be made regarding the need of follow-up endoscopy. Evidence shows that repeat endoscopy is not usually indicated for the control of healing of esophagitis. The absence of symptoms is a relatively sensitive indication of adequate treatment. Symptom recurrence should be taken as an indication for the need of intensification of therapy rather than endoscopy [10].

Lack of symptom improvement with PPI therapy, patients with severe grades of esophagitis as well as the need to perform further tissue sampling to clarify or confirm diagnosis of complications such as Barrett's metaplasia masked by erosive esophagitis are some indications of follow-up endoscopy.

The Histopathology of Esophagitis

The esophagus is lined by nonkeratinizing, stratified squamous epithelium, and the stomach by columnar epithelium, respectively. The border between the stomach and the esophagus, that is the GEJ, contains the lower esophageal sphincter, which is characterized as a variable zone of 2–4 cm in length and a pressure of approximately 10–26 mmHg, which is well above both intragastric and intra-esophageal pressures [11].

Upon endoscopy, the GEJ is the point where the tubular esophagus meets the gastric mucosal folds, also known as the "Z-line". In "normal" individuals, the GEJ is identical with the squamocolumnar junction (SCJ), the histological transition point between esophageal squamous and gastric columnar epithelium (Fig. 32.2).

In patients with GERD, the SCJ moves proximally as a result of metaplastic changes. Thus, the histological SCJ is located above the anatomical GEJ (Fig. 32.3). Changes related to acute

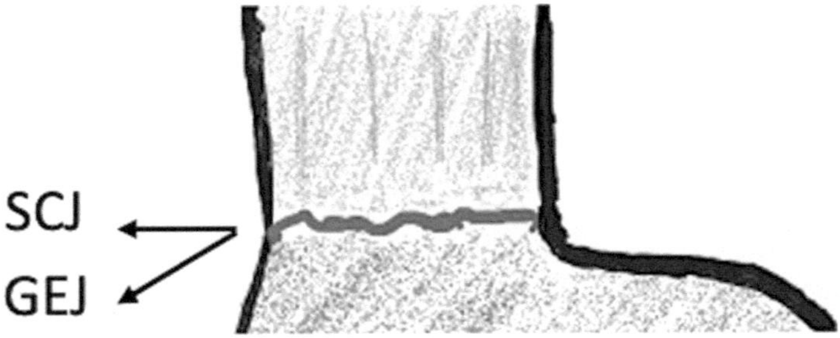

Fig. 32.2 The anatomy of the gastroesophageal junction (GEJ) and the squamocolumnar junction (SCJ). In normal individuals, the SCJ is located directly at the proximal margin of the gastric folds which corresponds to the anatomic GEJ

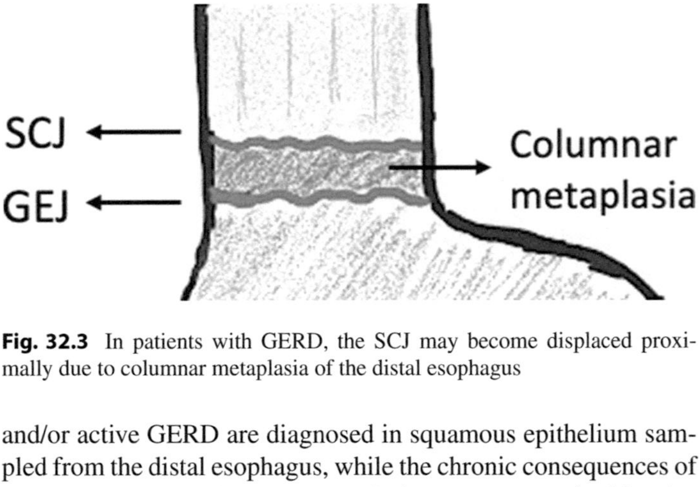

Fig. 32.3 In patients with GERD, the SCJ may become displaced proximally due to columnar metaplasia of the distal esophagus

and/or active GERD are diagnosed in squamous epithelium sampled from the distal esophagus, while the chronic consequences of GERD, such us columnar metaplasia, are present in biopsies sampled immediately below the SCJ. GERD is the major cause of inflammation and mucosal breaks of the squamous epithelium in the distal esophagus. As a consequence, the reparative capacity of the native squamous epithelium may be unable to tolerate the acidic and/or proteolytic nature of persistent reflux, and it adapts to the damaging stimuli by converting into metaplastic columnar epithelium.

The histological diagnosis of GERD is generally believed to be a tool of limited value [12]. The sensitivity and specificity of the histological GERD diagnosis are generally believed to be low. Several studies have, however, demonstrated that histology, if systematically applied, may render important diagnostic clues (Fig. 32.4). This holds particularly true for individuals with NERD, of whom approximately two-thirds have histological evidence of esophageal injury [13].

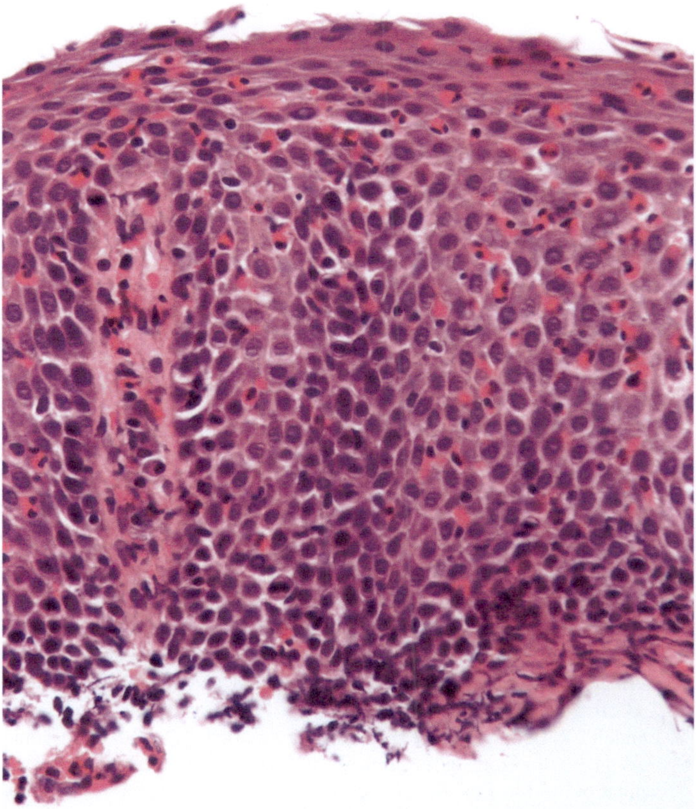

Fig. 32.4 Active reflux esophagitis with basal cell layer hyperplasia and elongation of stromal papillae

In summary, GERD continues to be a burden to healthcare systems around the world. The diagnosis is mainly clinical. There are specific indications for endoscopic evaluation of patients with GERD such as failure of medical management with PPI. An accurate endoscopic assessment of reflux esophagitis presence and severity is vital in making accurate decisions about patients' management and prognosis. Los Angeles endoscopic classification is the most validated, reproducible, and accurate in this setting, and it should uniformly be used among endoscopists performing upper gastrointestinal endoscopy procedures.

References

1. El-Serag HB, Sweet S, Winchester CC, Dent J. Update on the epidemiology of gastro-oesophageal reflux disease: a systematic review. Gut. 2014;63:871–80. https://doi.org/10.1136/gutjnl-2012-304269.
2. Katz PO, Gerson LB, Vela MF. Guidelines for the diagnosis and management of gastroesophageal reflux disease. Am J Gastroenterol. 2013;108:308–28.
3. Krugmann J, Neumann H, Vieth M, Armstrong D. What is the role of endoscopy and oesophageal biopsies in the management of GERD? Best Pract Res Clin Gastroenterol. 2013;27:373–85.
4. Fass R, Ofman JJ. Gastroesophageal reflux disease–should we adopt a new conceptual framework? Am J Gastroenterol. 2002;97(8):1901–9.
5. Vakil N, van Zanten SV, Kahrilas P, Dent J, Jones R, Global Consensus Group. The Montreal definition and classification of gastroesophageal reflux disease: a global evidence-based consensus. Am J Gastroenterol. 2006;101:1900–20.
6. Modlin IM, Hunt RH, Malfertheiner P, Moayyedi P, Quigley EM, et al. Diagnosis and management of non-erosive reflux disease–the Vevey NERD Consensus Group. Digestion. 2009;80:74–88.
7. Koop H, Fuchs KH, Labenz J, Lynen Jansen P, Messmann H, et al. S2k guideline: gastroesophageal reflux disease under the leadership of the German Society for Gastroenterology, Digestive and Metabolic Diseases. Z Gastroenterol. 2014;52(11):1299–346.
8. Lundell LR, Dent J, Bennett JR, Blum AL, Armstrong D, et al. Endoscopic assessment of oesophagitis: clinical and functional correlates and further validation of the Los Angeles classification. Gut. 1999;45(2):172–80. https://doi.org/10.1136/gut.45.2.172.
9. Dent J. Management of reflux disease. Gut. 2002;50(V):17–20.

10. Richter JE, Peura D, Benjamin SB, Joelsson B, Whipple J. Efficacy of omeprazole for the treatment of symptomatic acid reflux disease without esophagitis. Arch Intern Med. 2000;160:1810–6.
11. Odze RD. Unraveling the mystery of the gastroesophageal junction: a pathologist's perspective. Am J Gastroenterol. 2005;100:1853–67.
12. Takubo K, Honma N, Aryal G, Sawabe M, Arai T, et al. Is there a set of histologic changes that are invariably reflux associated? Arch Pathol Lab Med. 2005;129:159–63.
13. Dent J. Microscopic esophageal mucosal injury in nonerosive reflux disease. Clin Gastroenterol Hepatol. 2007;5:4–16.

Eosinophilic Esophagitis 33

Tayler J. James
and Nikolai A. Bildzukewicz

Pathophysiology and Epidemiology

Eosinophilic esophagitis (EoE) is an allergic condition of the esophagus caused by antigens that trigger an immune response in susceptible individuals. As with other allergic conditions, a number of environmental and genetic factors are suspected to play a role in a patient's susceptibility to EoE [1].

The incidence of EoE in the United States is increasing, with the current prevalence estimated between 0.5 and 1 case per 1000 [2]. EoE preferentially affects white males and young adults, although all ages can be affected [3, 4].

Most patients diagnosed with EoE have a personal or family history of atopic disorders such as atopic dermatitis, asthma, or allergic conjunctivitis [5]. Seasonal variation patterns seen in EoE suggest a role of aeroallergens in addition to food allergens as potential triggers of the response [6, 7].

T. J. James · N. A. Bildzukewicz (✉)
University of Southern California, Los Angeles, CA, USA
e-mail: Tayler.james@med.usc.edu; Nikolai.bildzukewicz@med.usc.edu

A. D. Patel et al. (eds.), *The SAGES Manual of Physiologic Evaluation of Foregut Diseases*,
https://doi.org/10.1007/978-3-031-39199-6_33

Presentation

EoE affects both children and adults, and symptoms vary with age. Younger children can present with feeding difficulties such as gagging and refusal of solid food, whereas older children more commonly present with abdominal pain, vomiting, and/or dysphagia [8, 9]. The most common symptom in adults is dysphagia to solid foods [4]. Other symptoms in adults include food impaction, chest and/or abdominal pain, and GERD-like symptoms such as heartburn and regurgitation [2, 4, 5].

The relationship between EoE and GERD is complex and differentiating between the two can be difficult. Historically, EoE was thought to be solely a manifestation of GERD. However, not all patients with suspected EoE were found to respond to antireflux treatment, thus suggesting EoE as its own clinical entity [10]. This led to a 2007 consensus definition to include "the absence of pathological GERD" in the diagnostic criteria for EoE, but this qualifier was later eliminated due to a number of overlapping features between the two [11, 12].

Heartburn and dysphagia are symptoms common in both GERD and EoE. Eosinophils can be present in biopsies of both, although patients with GERD typically have <7 eosinophils per high power field compared to >15 that is diagnostic of EoE [3]. It has been suggested that GERD can predispose at-risk patients to EoE by increasing the permeability of the esophageal mucosa, allowing food antigens to penetrate the esophageal wall and incite the allergic response [13]. Additionally, EoE may contribute to the development of GERD, as eosinophils produce substances that can relax the lower esophageal sphincter and induce tissue remodeling seen in GERD [14, 15]. In summary, while it appears that EoE is a separate clinical entity from GERD, the pathophysiology and clinical presentations of the two are closely intertwined.

Diagnosis

The diagnosis of EoE, as determined by a 2018 expert panel, requires the following: symptoms of esophageal dysfunction, at least 15 eosinophils per high power field on esophageal biopsy, and the exclusion of other causes of esophageal eosinophilia such as a parasite infection or allergic vasculitis [16].

Patients with suspected EoE are evaluated by endoscopy. Characteristic endoscopic findings of EoE include exudates, mucosal edema, linear furrows, rings, and strictures (Figs. 33.1 and 33.2)

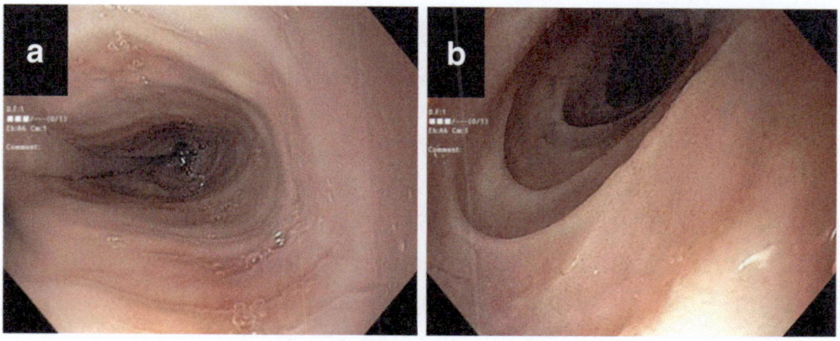

Fig. 33.1 Panels (**a**) and (**b**) show stacked, circular rights on endoscopy in a patient with eosinophilic esophagitis giving a trachea-like appearance

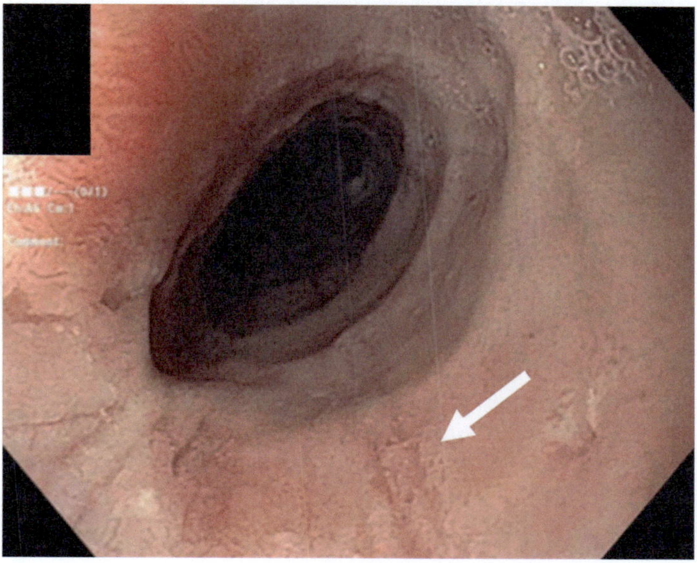

Fig. 33.2 Vertical lines termed "linear furrows" (arrow) on endoscopy in a patient with eosinophilic esophagitis

[3, 17]. The stacked, circular esophageal rings give the esophagus the appearance of a trachea. "Crepe paper esophagus," where the esophageal mucosa appears thin and fragile, has also been described in patients with EoE [17]. An endoscopic reference score (EREFS) assessing the characteristic endoscopic findings of EoE has been developed and validated to standardize diagnosis and grade disease severity (Table 33.1) [17].

During endoscopy, biopsies should be obtained from the proximal, mid, and distal esophagus. The sensitivity of biopsies for diagnosis of EoE increases with number of biopsies taken, with sensitivity reaching 100% when five or more biopsies are obtained [18, 19]. A threshold of 15 or more eosinophils per high power field is required for diagnosis (Fig. 33.3) [11].

Contrast imaging is a useful adjunct to endoscopy in the diagnosis of EoE. While not a diagnostic modality alone, barium esophagography can reveal ring-like stricturing and esophageal narrowing that may be missed on endoscopy (Fig. 33.4) [20].

Table 33.1 The endoscopic reference score (EREFS) classification system developed by Hirano et al. to standardize EoE diagnosis and disease severity

	Grade 0	Grade 1	Grade 2	Grade 3
Exudates	None	Mild (lesions involving <10% of esophageal surface area)	Severe (lesions involving >10% of esophageal surface area)	
Rings	None	Mild (subtle circumferential ridges)	Moderate (distinct rings that do not impair passage of a diagnostic endoscope)	Severe (distinct rings that do not permit passage of a diagnostic endoscope)
Edema	Absent	Mild (loss of clarity of vascular markings)	Severe (absence of vascular markings)	
Furrows	Absent	Mild (vertical lines present without visible depth)	Severe (vertical lines with mucosal depth)	
Strictures	Absent	Present		

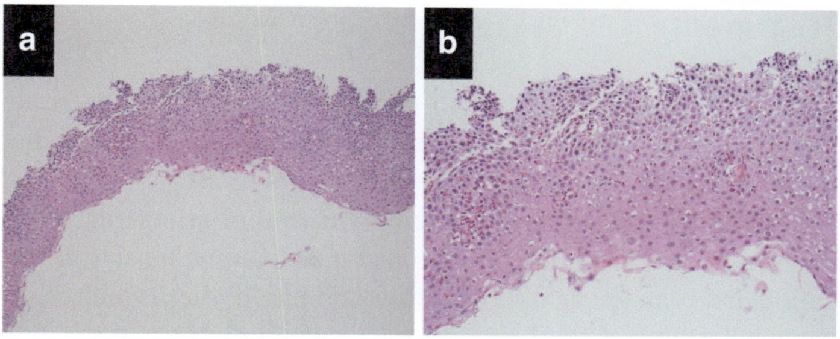

Fig. 33.3 Low-power (**a**) and high-power (**b**) view of esophageal mucosa with increased number of eosinophils in a patient with eosinophilic esophagitis

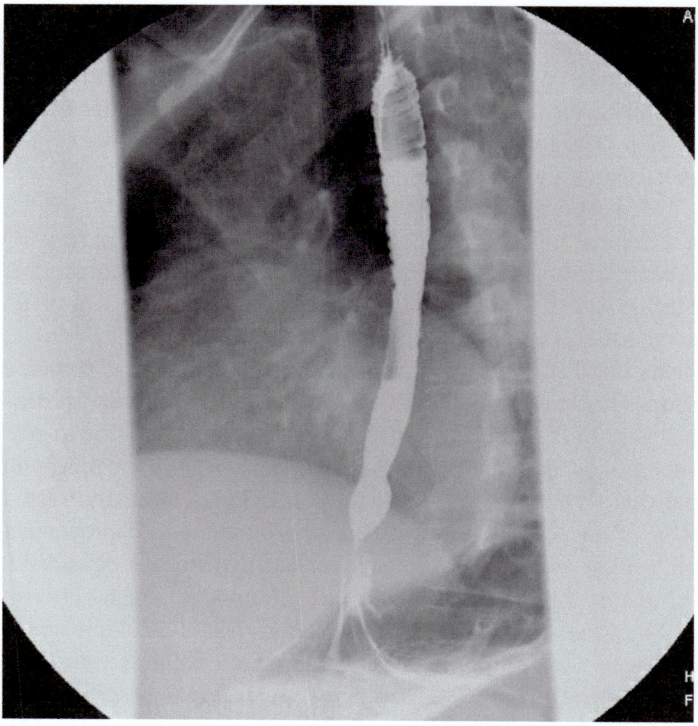

Fig. 33.4 Ring-like stricturing demonstrated on barium esophagogram in a patient with eosinophilic esophagitis

Treatment

Treatment goals of EoE are to control symptoms and decrease inflammation. The three treatment modalities for EoE are diet modification, medication, and esophageal dilation.

Dietary modification involves elimination of allergenic foods that can trigger EoE. The original and most comprehensive elimination diet is an elemental (or amino acid based) diet, which eliminates all potential food allergens. Elemental diets are restrictive and often difficult to follow, thus more selective elimination diets have been developed for better patient satisfaction and compliance. Two common diets are the “6-food elimination diet” and the “4-food elimination diet,” selectively eliminating foods that have been identified as the most commonly allergenic (namely, wheat, milk, soy, nuts, eggs, and seafood) [21–23]. Allergen testing such as radioallergosorbent testing, skin-prick testing, and atopy-patch testing have aided in the development of more personalized elimination diets for patients with EoE [24]. Disease relapse is common upon trigger food reintroduction [25].

Medications for EoE include proton pump inhibitors (PPIs) and topical glucocorticoids. Patients with EoE were previously thought to not respond to PPIs, under the assumption that the sole mechanism of PPI was gastric acid suppression [11]. However, some patients with EoE were noted to have symptomatic improvement with PPIs, and this population was termed “PPI-responsive esophageal eosinophilia” [26]. Further research into the mechanisms of PPIs found anti-inflammatory effects in addition to acid suppression, proposing a potential mechanism of treatment in patients with EoE [27]. Patients with EoE are typically treated with full-dose PPI and evaluated for symptomatic improvement after eight weeks. If symptoms persist, patients are considered refractory to PPI and are trialed with different treatment options.

In addition to PPIs, topical glucocorticoids (GCs) have been shown to successfully manage symptoms in patients with EoE, but their use is not yet FDA-approved. Histological response to GCs in patients with EoE can be seen by decreased eosinophil counts [28]. The two GCs used for EoE are fluticasone and budesonide. Fluticasone is administered via a metered dose inhaler, and budesonide is a swallowed liquid. Patients typically respond to GCs within several days, but relapse is common when the treatment is stopped [29]. The dose is titrated while monitoring symptoms to identify a maintenance dose that is individualized to the patient.

Endoscopic dilation is usually reserved for patients who have failed conservative therapy. Dilation can temporarily relieve symptoms caused by esophageal remodeling, but it has no effect on the underlying inflammatory process of the disease [30]. Dilation is typically performed gradually over multiple sessions, limiting each dilation to 3 mm due to the risks of mucosal tear (around 9%) or perforation (around 1%) [31]. Techniques to help mitigate perforation include assessing for resistance when passing the endoscope or dilators and subsequently inspecting the esophagus prior to dilation [30]. Patients can experience chest pain and bleeding after esophageal dilation [30].

Investigational treatments for EoE include monoclonal antibodies against EoE-specific cytokines and prostaglandin D2 receptor antagonists [32, 33].

Follow-up

EoE is not pre-malignant [34]. Some providers choose to perform surveillance endoscopy in EoE patients annually to assess treatment response and/or disease progression.

Conclusion

In summary, EoE is a chronic immune disorder characterized by eosinophil-mediated esophageal dysfunction. EoE affects both children and adults and can present similarly to GERD. Diagnosis is made by characteristic endoscopic findings and >15 eosinophils per high power field on esophageal biopsy. Treatment includes dietary modification to eliminate trigger foods, medication including PPIs and topical glucocorticoids, and endoscopic dilation for symptom management.

References

1. Furuta GT, Katzka DA. Eosinophilic esophagitis definition and differential diagnosis. N Engl J Med. 2016;373:1640–8.
2. Dellon ES. Epidemiology of eosinophilic esophagitis. Gastroenterol Clin N Am. 2014;43:201–18.
3. Dellon ES, Gibbs WB, Fritchie KJ, Rubinas TC, Wilson LA, Woosley JT, Shaheen NJ. Clinical, endoscopic, and histologic findings distinguish eosinophilic esophagitis from gastroesophageal reflux disease. Clin Gastroenterol Hepatol. 2009;7:1305–13.
4. Kapel RC, Miller JK, Torres C, Aksoy S, Lash R, Katzka DA. Eosinophilic esophagitis: a prevalent disease in the United States that affects all age groups. Gastroenterology. 2008;134:1316–21.
5. Chehade M, Jones SM, Pesek RD, et al. Phenotypic characterization of eosinophilic esophagitis in a large multicenter patient population from the consortium for food allergy research. J Allergy Clin Immunol Pract. 2018;6:1534–44.
6. Ram G, Lee J, Ott M, Brown-Whitehorn TF, Cianferoni A, Shuker M, Wang ML, Verma R, Liacouras CA, Spergel JM. Seasonal exacerbation of esophageal eosinophilia in children with eosinophilic esophagitis and allergic rhinitis. Ann Allergy Asthma Immunol. 2015;115:224–228.e1.
7. Reed CC, Iglesia EGA, Commins SP, Dellon ES. Seasonal exacerbation of eosinophilic esophagitis histologic activity in adults and children implicates role of aeroallergens. Ann Allergy Asthma Immunol. 2019;122:296–301.
8. Falk GW. Eosinophilic esophagitis. Gastroenterol Clin N Am. 2014;43:13.
9. Mukkada VA, Haas A, Maune NC, et al. Feeding dysfunction in children with eosinophilic gastrointestinal diseases. Pediatrics. 2010;126(3):e672–7. https://doi.org/10.1542/peds.2009-2227.
10. Attwood SEA, Smyrk TC, Demeester TR, Jones JB. Esophageal eosinophilia with dysphagia. Dig Dis Sci. 1993;38:109–16.
11. Furuta GT, Liacouras CA, Collins MH, Gupta SK, Justinich C, Putnam PE, Bonis P, Hassall E, Straumann A, Rothenberg ME. Eosinophilic esophagitis in children and adults: a systematic review and consensus recommendations for diagnosis and treatment. Gastroenterology. 2007;133:1342–63.
12. Cheng E, Souza RF, Spechler SJ. Eosinophilic esophagitis: interactions with gastroesophageal reflux disease. Gastroenterol Clin N Am. 2014;43:243–56.
13. Tobey NA, Hosseini SS, Argote CM, Dobrucali AM, Awayda MS, Orlando RC. Dilated intercellular spaces and shunt permeability in nonerosive acid-damaged esophageal epithelium. Am J Gastroenterol. 2004;99:13–22.

14. Cheng L, Harnett KM, Cao W, Liu F, Behar J, Fiocchi C, Biancani P. Hydrogen peroxide reduces lower esophageal sphincter tone in human esophagitis. Gastroenterology. 2005;129:1675–85.
15. Cheng E, Souza RF, Spechler SJ. Tissue remodeling in eosinophilic esophagitis. Am J Physiol Gastrointest Liver Physiol. 2012;303(11):G1175–87. https://doi.org/10.1152/ajpgi.00313.2012.
16. Dellon ES, Liacouras CA, Molina-Infante J, et al. Updated international consensus diagnostic criteria for eosinophilic esophagitis: proceedings of the AGREE conference. Gastroenterology. 2018;155:1022–33.
17. Hirano I, Moy N, Heckman MG, Thomas CS, Gonsalves N, Achem SR. Endoscopic assessment of the oesophageal features of eosinophilic oesophagitis: validation of a novel classification and grading system. Gut. 2013;62:489–95.
18. Gonsalves N, Policarpio-Nicolas M, Zhang Q, Rao MS, Hirano I. Histopathologic variability and endoscopic correlates in adults with eosinophilic esophagitis. Gastrointest Endosc. 2006;64:313–9.
19. Shah A, Kagalwalla AF, Gonsalves N, Melin-Aldana H, Li BUK, Hirano I. Histopathologic variability in children with eosinophilic esophagitis. Am J Gastroenterol. 2009;104:716–21.
20. Gentile N, Katzka D, Ravi K, Trenkner S, Enders F, Killian J, Kryzer L, Talley NJ, Alexander J. Oesophageal narrowing is common and frequently under-appreciated at endoscopy in patients with oesophageal eosinophilia. Aliment Pharmacol Ther. 2014;40:1333–40.
21. Kagalwalla AF, Sentongo TA, Ritz S, Hess T, Nelson SP, Emerick KM, Melin-Aldana H, Li BUK. Effect of six-food elimination diet on clinical and histologic outcomes in eosinophilic esophagitis. Clin Gastroenterol Hepatol. 2006;4:1097–102.
22. Kagalwalla AF, Wechsler JB, Amsden K, et al. Efficacy of a 4-food elimination diet for children with eosinophilic esophagitis. Clin Gastroenterol Hepatol. 2017;15:1698–707.
23. Wang R, Hirano I, Doerfler B, Zalewski A, Gonsalves N, Taft T. Assessing adherence and barriers to long-term elimination diet therapy in adults with eosinophilic esophagitis. Dig Dis Sci. 2018;63:1756–62.
24. Arias Á, González-Cervera J, Tenias JM, Lucendo AJ. Efficacy of dietary interventions for inducing histologic remission in patients with eosinophilic esophagitis: a systematic review and meta-analysis. Gastroenterology. 2014;146:1639–48.
25. Markowitz J. Elemental diet is an effective treatment for eosinophilic esophagitis in children and adolescents. Am J Gastroenterol. 2003;98:777–82.
26. Liacouras CA, Furuta GT, Hirano I, et al. Eosinophilic esophagitis: updated consensus recommendations for children and adults. J Allergy Clin Immunol. 2011;128:3–20.e6.

27. Wolf WA, Dellon ES. Eosinophilic esophagitis and proton pump inhibitors: Controversies and implications for clinical practice. Gastroenterol Hepatol. 2014;10:427–32.
28. Konikoff MR, Noel RJ, Blanchard C, et al. A randomized, double-blind, placebo-controlled trial of fluticasone propionate for pediatric eosinophilic esophagitis. Gastroenterology. 2006;131:1381–91.
29. Alexander JA. Steroid treatment of eosinophilic esophagitis in adults. Gastroenterol Clin N Am. 2014;43:357–73.
30. Schoepfer AM, Gonsalves N, Bussmann C, Conus S, Simon HU, Straumann A, Hirano I. Esophageal dilation in eosinophilic esophagitis: effectiveness, safety, and impact on the underlying inflammation. Am J Gastroenterol. 2010;105:1062–70.
31. Jung KW, Gundersen N, Kopacova J, et al. Occurrence of and risk factors for complications after endoscopic dilation in eosinophilic esophagitis. Gastrointest Endosc. 2011;73:15–21.
32. Hirano I, Dellon ES, Hamilton JD, et al. Efficacy of dupilumab in a phase 2 randomized trial of adults with active eosinophilic esophagitis. Gastroenterology. 2020;158:111–22.
33. Straumann A, Hoesli S, Bussmann C, et al. Anti-eosinophil activity and clinical efficacy of the CRTH2 antagonist OC000459 in eosinophilic esophagitis. Allergy Eur J Allergy Clin Immunol. 2013;68:375–85.
34. Lipka S, Keshishian J, Boyce HW, Estores D, Richter JE. The natural history of steroid-naïve eosinophilic esophagitis in adults treated with endoscopic dilation and proton pump inhibitor therapy over a mean duration of nearly 14 years. Gastrointest Endosc. 2014;80:592–8.

Paraesophageal Hernias 34

Isaac R. Kriley, Shaoxu Bing,
and Ruchir Puri

Introduction

Definition, Incidence, Prevalence, and Risk Factors

Hiatal hernias occur when intraabdominal organs pass through the esophageal hiatus, which is formed by the right and left diaphragmatic crura. Hiatal hernias are classified as four types: (1) sliding hernias, in which the GEJ migrates above the diaphragm and the gastric fundus remains below the diaphragm; (2) the GEJ remains in its normal anatomic location, but some portion of the gastric fundus herniates above the diaphragm; (3) both the GEJ and the gastric fundus herniate above the diaphragm; and (4) hernias that include organs besides the stomach, such as omentum, colon, or small bowel [1]. Type I hiatal hernias represent over 95% of hiatal hernias, while paraesophageal hernias (PEH) account for <5%, and more than 90% of PEH are type III. The true incidence and prevalence of PEH are unknown as most are asymptomatic and never come to clinical attention. Risk factors for PEH include body mass index, sex, and age [2]. There is a direct relationship

I. R. Kriley · S. Bing · R. Puri (✉)
Department of Surgery, UF Health Jacksonville, Jacksonville, FL, USA
e-mail: ruchir.puri@jax.ufl.edu

A. D. Patel et al. (eds.), *The SAGES Manual of Physiologic Evaluation of Foregut Diseases*,
https://doi.org/10.1007/978-3-031-39199-6_34

between increasing body mass index (BMI) and PEH; those with a BMI greater than 25 kg/m^2 have 1.93 odds of having a PEH compared to people with BMI less than 25 kg/m^2. Men are more likely to have PEH (odds ratio 1.36), and those over 50 years old are more likely to have PEH (odds ratio 2.17). This chapter focuses on the evaluation and management of hiatal hernia types II–IV, PEH.

Etiology

The etiology of paraesophageal hernias is somewhat elusive. The crura and ligaments of the hiatus have been investigated on microscopic, ultrastructural, and molecular levels for characteristics associated with PEH. In the elderly, the inferior leaf of the phrenoesophageal ligament is attenuated or absent, which might explain the prevalence of PEH among older patients [3]. Elastin is an extracellular matrix protein that allows tissues to be temporarily deformed and was found to be reduced by 50% in the phrenoesophageal ligament among patients with hiatal hernias [3, 4]. Collagen is a protein that provides strength to tissue. Conflicting results about the quantity of collagen in the phrenoesophageal ligament have been reported [5, 6]. Supporting the role of collagen in PEH and suggesting a genetic component is the observation of a single nucleotide polymorphism in *COL3A1* that is associated with hiatal hernias among male patients. *COL3A1* codes for type III collagen and mutations in the gene cause types III and IV Ehlers-Danlos syndrome [7]. Though a causative gene was not identified, a genetic component of PEH is further supported by the observation that 23 of 38 family members over five generations in Ireland had radiographic evidence of a hiatal hernia and the mode of inheritance was autosomal dominant [8]. Structural deficiencies of the crura have been observed by light and electron microscopy among patients with hiatal hernia and include dilation of the intermyofibrillar spaces, swelling of the sacrotubular structures, focal degeneration of myofibrils, extended disruption-degeneration of the muscles, reduced muscle fibers, increased inflammatory cell infiltrate, and increased interstitial spaces [9, 10].

Presentation and Evaluation

Presentation

Patient evaluation begins with a thorough history and physical exam. Many PEH are asymptomatic or have subclinical or unrecognized symptoms. Foregut and upper respiratory symptoms predominate, and their frequency will vary by clinical practice. Patients present in their 7th and 8th decades with heartburn (30–65%), chest pain (19–48%), dysphagia (5–48%), early satiety (7–50%), dyspnea (48%), and cough (14%) [11, 12]. Detailed investigation might identify more insidious symptoms such as avoiding particular foods (14%), decreased meal size (18%), and avoiding an evening meal (10%) [11]. Anemia is often observed among patients undergoing hiatal hernia repair (23–41%), but it is also common among patients in their 7th and 8th decades without a hiatal hernia [11–13]. As the proportion of intrathoracic stomach increases, there is a stronger association with symptoms of early satiety, anemia, dyspnea, and decreased meal size [11].

Physical exam is commonly nonspecific. However signs of weight loss, respiratory disease, and previous abdominal surgery should be noted. All patients undergoing elective surgery should be assessed for fitness and optimized if necessary.

Rarely do patients present with signs and symptoms of acute gastric volvulus, including epigastric pain, dry retching, and inability to pass a nasogastric tube, known as Borchardt's triad. Hill provides a good description of gastric volvulus with the observation of regurgitation of saliva, substernal chest pain, and complete inability to swallow liquids or solids in addition to Borchardt's triad [14].

Evaluation

Radiography

Chest X-ray may reveal a gastric bubble or other hollow viscous above the diaphragm or a nasogastric tube coiled above the diaphragm but will not provide detailed anatomic information.

Barium esophagram provides more detailed information than chest X-ray regarding the relationship between the GEJ and the diaphragmatic hiatus and can differentiate type II and III hiatal hernias. However, it is less sensitive and specific than endoscopy for the type of PEH [15]. On the other hand, barium esophagram has been shown to be superior to endoscopy in diagnosing type I hiatal hernias in morbidly obese patients [16]. Esophagram can also identify esophageal dilatation (Fig. 34.1) or achalasia, findings which will change management and are important since manometry cannot be performed in all patients with PEH [17, 18]. Gastric volvulus (Fig. 34.2), esophageal stricture, and esophageal diverticulum (Fig. 34.3) and a short esophagus are other findings possible on esophagram. Gastric volvuli can be organo-axial or mesentero-axial with organo-axial being more common. The

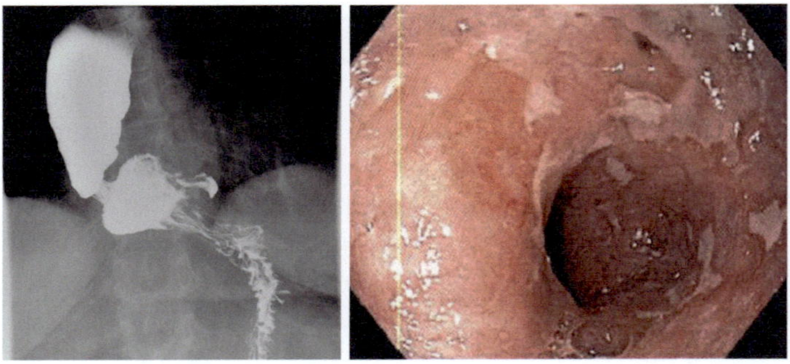

Fig. 34.1 Dilated esophagus in a patient with aperistalsis and a moderate-sized PEH, EGD showing LA D Esophagitis. The patient is a 64-year-old female that underwent a laparoscopic hiatal hernia repair and a partial fundoplication due to absent motility. She experienced complete relief of GERD symptoms and no post-operative dysphagia

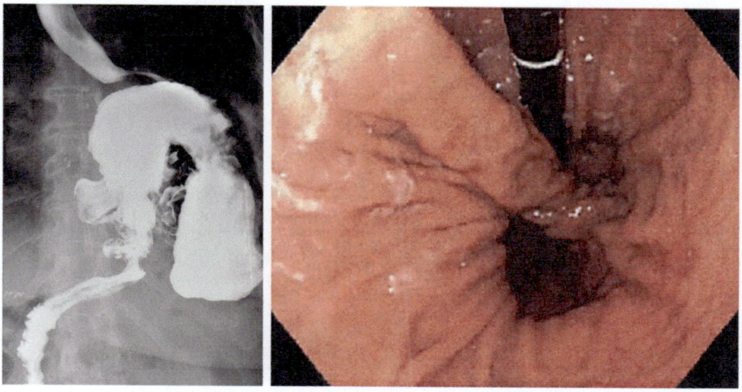

Fig. 34.2 Organoaxial gastric volvulus on esophagram and appearance on EGD. The patient is a 68-year-old female who presents to the clinic with a longstanding history of worsening chest pain, progressive dysphagia, and reflux. She underwent an uncomplicated robotic-assisted paraesophageal hernia repair with mesh and a Toupet fundoplication with good response

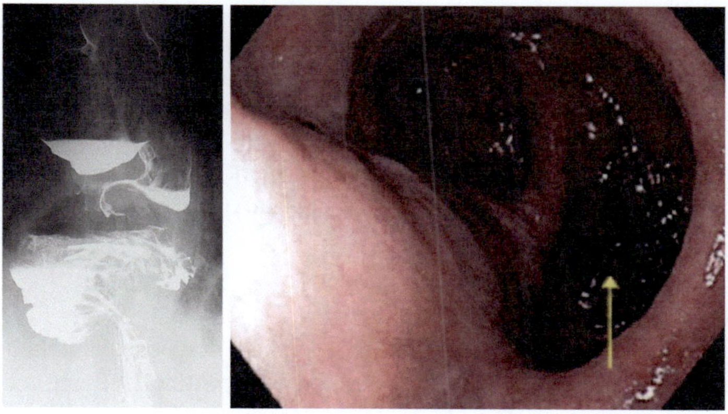

Fig. 34.3 Large PEH and an epiphrenic diverticulum. The patient is a 57-year-old female with longstanding dysphagia. A laparoscopic PEH repair with a Heller myotomy/Toupet fundoplication was performed. The diverticulum was mid esophageal and could not be reached laparoscopically and was not excised. The patient experienced complete resolution of symptoms postoperatively

organo-axial volvulus appears in a “C” configuration with the greater curvature of the stomach lying superiorly [19].

Computed tomography provides the most detailed anatomic information for hiatal hernias including the position of the GEJ in relation to the diaphragm, the degree of gastric herniation, and the presence of other abdominal organs in the hernia sac. CT scan is utilized selectively if a complicated or a “giant” PEH is suspected or to evaluate for other intraabdominal pathology.

Endoscopy

Esophagogastroduodenoscopy (EGD) should be performed preoperatively in patients with PEH. In patients with PEH, no gastroesophageal flap valve is present, and the esophageal lumen is wide open and easily visualized (Hill grade IV) [20]. A type III PEH can be distinguished from a type II PEH by observing the squamocolumnar junction 2 cm proximal to the crural indentation on the gastric lumen, comparing the relationship of the squamocolumnar junction to the hiatus on retroflexion, and assessing whether or not the fundus is herniated alongside the endoscope [21]. EGD can also identify intraluminal pathologies such as esophagitis, Barrett’s esophagus, Cameron’s ulcers, and malignancy. Difficulty or inability to reach the duodenum in the presence of a large hiatal hernia is diagnostic for a volvulus [1]. Assessment of the size of the hernia on the EGD can be misleading. The best measure of the size of the PEH may be its intraoperative assessment [22].

Manometry and pH Monitoring

High-resolution manometry (HRM) can help diagnose hiatal hernias based on the degree of separation between the LES and the crural diaphragm (Fig. 34.4). HRM however does not alter the management of PEH if an esophagram has been performed. Passing the manometry probe beyond the GEJ into the stomach can be challenging in most patients, limiting the data that can be reliably obtained. If the catheter can be advanced, the findings of abnormal motility and esophagogastric junction (EGJ) outflow obstruction are common; however, hiatal hernias have not been

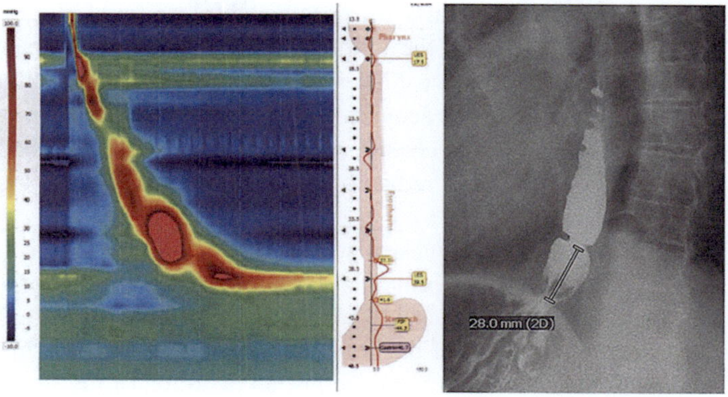

Fig. 34.4 A 2.7 cm hiatal hernia diagnosed on HRM (white arrow) and size confirmed on esophagram. The patient is a 52-year-old female with classic symptoms of GERD and high distal esophageal acid exposure who responded well to a Nissen fundoplication

shown to be an independent risk factor for esophageal dysmotility [23, 24]. Pre-operative HRM results are not associated with symptomatic outcomes after surgery [25]. Those with abnormal manometry results report similar degrees of dysphagia to those with normal manometry results after PEH repair. Omitting manometry does not lead to more dysphagia regardless of whether a total or partial fundoplication is performed [26]. Preoperative dysphagia is usually the best predictor of postoperative dysphagia in these patients. Testing pH is not routinely performed since the problem is anatomic, and it does not change the management.

Treatment

Indications for Surgery

Surgery is indicated for symptomatic PEH. In the last century, elective repair was advocated to prevent acute volvulus. An analytic model, reported in 2002, of a hypothetical cohort of patients with asymptomatic or minimally symptomatic PEH (belching or heartburn) compared elective repair to watchful waiting [27, 28]. The model revealed that the mortality of emergent PEH repair was overestimated (5% vs 17% reported in the literature), the annual rate of developing acute symptoms requiring surgery was 1.16%, and the policy of elective repair for patients greater than 65 years old resulted in a reduction of quality adjusted life years (10.78 vs 10.65).

Rarely, a patient will present with acute volvulus, which is a surgical emergency. The principles of treatment include decompression of the stomach via a nasogastric tube, intravenous fluid resuscitation, reduction of the volvulus, repair of the underlying condition predisposing to the volvulus, and fixation of the stomach via gastropexy. The patient's age, frailty, and comorbidities should also be taken into consideration as a majority of cases occur in the elderly population [29]. In frail patients, endoscopy to reduce the volvulus and gastropexy with percutaneous endoscopic gastrostomy (PEG) may be sufficient [30, 31]. When acute gastric volvulus is secondary to a PEH, as are the majority of cases, the laparoscopic technique has been shown to be safe and feasible and follows the standard technique for PEH repair including a fundoplication as a point of fixation for the stomach [29, 32–34] (Fig. 34.5).

Surgical Technique

Minimally invasive repairs of PEH are well established and are associated with decreased intraoperative injury, decreased hospital mortality (0.6% vs 3%), decreased wound healing, bleeding, urinary, septic, respiratory, and cardiac complications, and decreased length of stay (4.2 vs 8.5 days) compared to an open approach [35]. Presently, over 90% of PEH repairs are performed by a minimally invasive approach with an open approach most often reserved for emergent or difficult and re-operative cases [36]. The patient is placed in a split leg position and a five-trocar approach for a foregut operation is utilized. Basic principles of

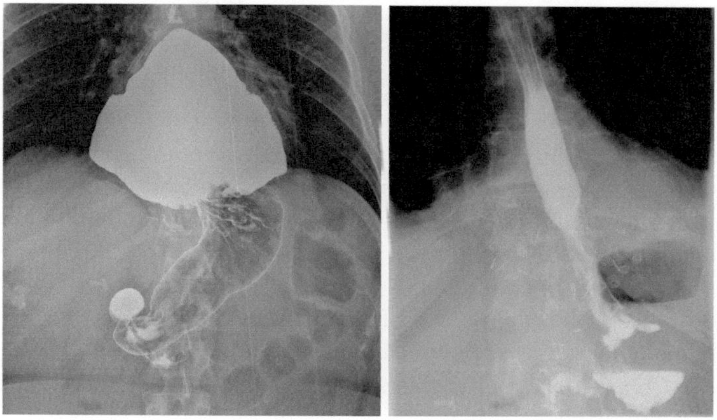

Fig. 34.5 Pre- and post-operative esophagram of a patient with a redo paraesophageal hernia repair. The patient is a 49-year-old female with two prior paraesophageal hernia repairs with mesh/Nissen fundoplication who presented with dysphagia. Pre-op esophagram shows a triangular configuration of the incarcerated proximal stomach. Intraoperatively dense adhesions were found in the mediastinum along with a short esophagus. A paraesophageal hernia repair was performed along with a Collis gastroplasty and conversion to a Roux-en-Y gastric bypass. Post-operative course was complicated by a pulmonary embolism but complete resolution of foregut symptoms

repair include reduction of hernia contents, complete sac excision, high mobilization of the esophagus to obtain 2–3 cm. of intraabdominal length, tension-free crural approximation with selective mesh reinforcement, and finally the addition of an anti-reflux procedure.

Post-Operative Care

Nausea and cough should be prevented aggressively [37]. A liquid diet can be started on the first post-operative day and should be continued for 1–2 weeks. Routine contrast esophagram in asymptomatic patients is not necessary but often performed to assess post-operative anatomy.

Robot Vs Laparoscopy

While robotic platforms are increasingly being utilized no randomized control trials have compared laparoscopic and robotic approaches to PEH repair. Recent large retrospective experiences comparing laparoscopic and robotic PEH repair have been published with differing conclusions [38, 39]. A group in New York reported on PEH repairs for 128 patients, including 84 laparoscopic and 44 robotic hiatal hernia repairs with no advantage observed in hospital length of stay, 30-day readmission, 30-day reoperation rate, and complication rates [39]. In contrast, a report from Texas included 293 patients, including 151 laparoscopic and 142 robotic hiatal hernia repairs observed reduced mean operative time (158 min, range 132–188, vs 186 min, range 152–232), fewer complications (9[6.3%] vs 29[19.2%]), and shorter length of stay (1.3 vs 1.8 days) for those undergoing robotic surgery [38]. In both studies, the robotic repair groups had higher proportions of patients who were undergoing surgery for recurrent PEH, suggesting that surgeons perceive an advantage to the robotic approach in more difficult cases.

Mesh

With recurrence rates ranging from 10–72% after cruroplasty there is a significant interest in reducing recurrences [40]. Mesh reinforcement of cruroplasty for PEH repair has been investigated in several randomized trials [40–42]. Well-designed and conducted randomized trials with long-term follow-up and rigorous objective anatomic and symptomatic evaluation did not demonstrate a reduced recurrence rate with mesh reinforcement [41–43]. Large, randomized trials reported recurrence rates of 50–54% with mesh and 39.3–59% without mesh in long-term follow-up. Neither group was shown to be significantly different [41, 42]. Both trials, using validated questionnaires to assess symptoms, found that symptoms were improved in both groups, with the exceptions of higher dysphagia and chest pain scores, greater frequency of diarrhea, and greater likelihood of adopting dietary restrictions among people who received absorbable mesh [42].

Major complications related to both absorbable and non-absorbable mesh include intraluminal esophageal erosion, hiatal stenosis, dense fibrosis, and cardiac tamponade [44–47]. Even in the absence of major complications, mesh placement can make revisional surgery more difficult and increase the rate of major resections from 4.4% to 30%, especially in cases where mesh was placed at the initial operation [48]. Given a lack of reproducible benefit, evidence of worse dysphagia, and numerous reports of major complications related to mesh placement at the hiatus, routine mesh reinforcement of cruroplasty in PEH repair is not supported by the literature. There may be a role for selective mesh placement, but this strategy is not yet defined. Mesh placement should be considered on a case-by-case basis.

Antireflux Procedure

A total or partial fundoplication is routinely performed during PEH repair. Even in the absence of heartburn, most patients with type II PEH have elevated esophageal acid exposure [49, 50]. Patients with PEH report improvement in heartburn symptoms after PEH repair with an antireflux procedure. Omitting an antireflux procedure could put patients at risk for reflux esophagitis [51, 52]. Recent reports show good outcomes with the use of magnetic sphincter augmentation in lieu of a fundoplication in conjunction with PEH repair [53, 54].

Gastropexy

The addition of gastropexy to help reduce the rate of recurrence of PEH has also yielded mixed results. A French group reported a retrospective analysis of PEH repair with and without anterior abdominal wall suture gastropexy [55]. The rate of recurrence was higher among the patients who did not undergo gastropexy (50% vs 10.8%), but the group who did not undergo gastropexy was small (11 patients), follow-up was limited (65.2% of patients were objectively evaluated for recurrence), and the study was not randomized. Diaz et al evaluated 116 patients who underwent PEH repair with or without gastropexy with similar recurrence rates [56]. In emergent cases in frail patients, hernia reduction with gastropexy with a gastrostomy tube may be the safest and most appropriate approach.

Short Esophagus

The importance of mediastinal dissection to obtain adequate esophageal length is well recognized. A subset of patients have a short esophagus despite its existence being controversial and its presence definitively determined only after mediastinal dissection is complete. Some surgeons rarely perform esophageal lengthening procedures while others perform them frequently [18, 19]. If 2–3 cm of intraabdominal esophagus cannot be achieved with mediastinal dissection alone, an esophageal lengthening procedure should be performed.

Outcomes

With long-term follow-up, PEH recur at a rate of 50% [40, 41, 57]. Despite the high rate of hernia recurrence, most patients enjoy an improvement in symptom severity and quality of life. Prior to repair, 30–90% of patients presented with heartburn [11, 12, 58]. After repair, the rates of heartburn decreased to 22.9%, which was sustained after 5 years of follow-up. Some investigators reported up to 93% of patients enjoying an improvement in heartburn [11, 41, 46]. Others have reported significant and sustained improvement in symptom severity and reflux-related quality of life, but liberation from antacid medication is not guaranteed [12, 58]. Other common symptoms associated with PEH, such as dysphagia, regurgitation, early satiety, chest pain, dyspnea, and bloating, also improved after repair [11, 57–60]. Resolution of anemia after PEH repair was more common among those with symptomatic anemia and those with esophagogastric erosions or ulcers [13].

Complications

Prior to the widespread adoption of minimally invasive approaches, open approaches were associated with higher mortality among uncomplicated PEH repairs (0.57% vs 1.34%, $p < 0.001$) [61]. Current analyses of the National Surgical Quality Improvement Program database reveal 30-day mortality rates of 0.6% vs 3.0% for minimally invasive vs open approaches [35, 62]. General complications of abdominal surgery (wound infection, urinary tract infections, pneumonia, cardiac complications, bleeding requiring transfusion, and renal complications) occur in less than 8% of patients with each type of complication occurring in less than 2% of patients [35, 62].

Specific complications of PEH repair include pneumothorax (2.4–5.6%), esophageal or gastric perforation (1.6–1.8%), acute hernia recurrence (3.2%) (Fig. 34.6), tight hiatal repair (2.4%), and splenic injury (0.8–0.9%) [42, 63]. Acute reherniations require immediate surgery to reduce the hernia. It is important to resect ischemic tissue, re-approximate the crura, and may require

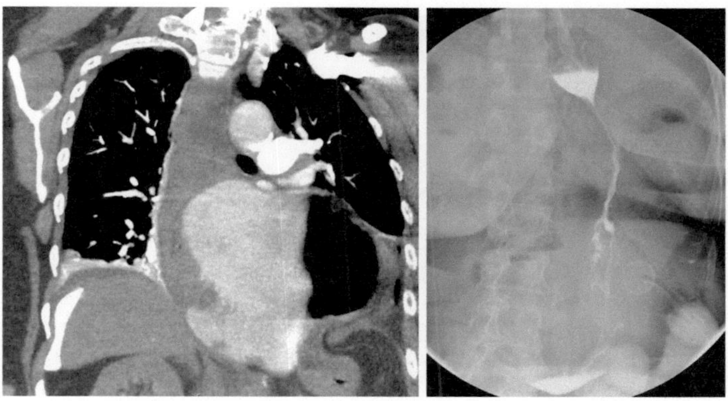

Fig. 34.6 Pre-op CT chest and post-op esophagram of a patient with a large PEH. The patient is a 67-year-old female with dysphagia that underwent a robotic repair of a giant PEH. POD#2 she developed tachycardia and emesis. CT chest revealed the stomach re-herniated into the chest. She underwent an emergent return to the OR and PEH repair with a mesh and Gastrostomy tube placement. Post-operative recovery was slow but uneventful

a gastropexy with or without gastrostomy tube placement. Perforations can be managed with either esophageal stents or with surgery.

Conclusion

Symptomatic PEH is a disease of the elderly, and good outcomes can be expected with a minimally invasive approach. The cornerstone of diagnostic workup is an upper endoscopy and contrast esophagram. While controversies exist regarding the best operative platform and ways to mitigate high anatomic recurrence rates, the risk of symptom recurrence and reoperations remains relatively low.

Editors' Note

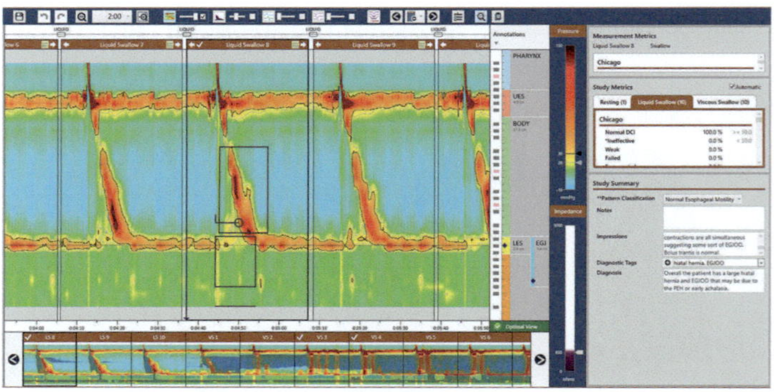

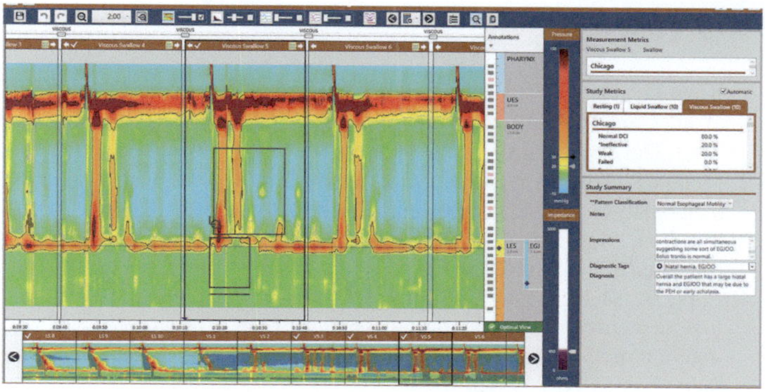

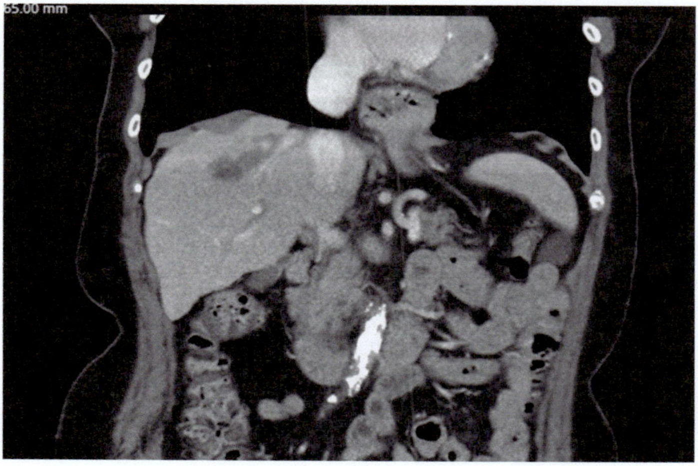

Seventy-five years female presenting with dysphagia, belching, bloating and early satiety.

Manometry is as follows: EGJOO in a patient with a large paraesophageal type hiatal hernia. The study of the LES reveals a normal length and a large hiatal hernia. The LES pressure is high at 46 mmHg and does not relax completely. The esophageal body study does demonstrate peristalsis, however there is pressurization with many swallows. With viscous swallows the contractions are all simultaneous suggesting some sort of EGJOO. Bolus transit is normal. Overall the patient has a large hiatal hernia and EGJOO that may be due to the PEH or early achalasia.

References

1. Kohn GP, Price RR, DeMeester SR, Zehetner J, Muenster OJ, Awad Z, et al. Guidelines for the management of hiatal hernia. Surg Endosc. 2013;27(12):4409–28.
2. Menon S, Trudgill N. Risk factors in the aetiology of hiatus hernia: a meta-analysis. Eur J Gastroenterol Hepatol. 2011;23(2):133–8.
3. Kwok H, Marriz Y, Al-Ali S, Windsor JA. Phrenoesophageal ligament re-visited. Clin Anat. 1999;12(3):164–70.
4. Curci JA, Melman LM, Thompson RW, Soper NJ, Matthews BD. Elastic fiber depletion in the supporting ligaments of the gastroesophageal junction: a structural basis for the development of hiatal hernia. J Am Coll Surg. 2008;207(2):191–6.
5. von Diemen V, Trindade EN, Trindade MR. (2016) Hiatal hernia and gastroesophageal reflux: study of collagen in the phrenoesophageal ligament. Surg Endosc. 2016;30(11):5091–8.
6. Brown SR, Melman L, Jenkins E, Deeken C, Frisella MM, Brunt LM, et al. Collagen type I: III ratio of the gastroesophageal junction in patients with paraesophageal hernias. Surg Endosc. 2011;25(5):1390–4.
7. Asling B, Jirholt J, Hammond P, Knutsson M, Walentinsson A, Davidson G, et al. Collagen type III alpha I is a gastro-esophageal reflux disease susceptibility gene and a male risk factor for hiatus hernia. Gut. 2009;58(8):1063–9.
8. Carre IJ, Johnston BT, Thomas PS, Morrison PJ. Familial hiatal hernia in a large five generation family confirming true autosomal dominant inheritance. Gut. 1999;45(5):649–52.
9. Ardeleanu V, Rumina Chebac G, Georgescu C, Vesa D, Francu L, Frincu D, et al. The modifications suffered by the peri-esophageal anatomical structures in the hiatal hernia disease: a qualitative and quantitative microanatomic study. Romanian J Morphol Embryol. 2010;51(4):765–70.
10. Fei L, Gianluca R, Allaria A, Conzo G, Sampaolo S, Moccia F, et al. Laparoscopic hiatal hernia repair Is the mesh hiatoplasty justified. Ann Ital Chir. 2014;85(1):38–45.
11. Carrot PW, Hong J, Kuppusamy M, Koehler RP, Low DE. Clinical ramifications of giant paraesophageal hernias are underappreciated: making the case for routine surgical repair. Ann Thorac Surg. 2012;94(2):421–6.
12. Oelschlager BK, Petersen RP, Brunt LM, Soper NJ, Sheppard BC, Rohrmann C, et al. Laparoscopic paraesophageal hernia repair: defining long-term clinical and anatomic outcomes. J Gastrointest Surg. 2012;16(3):453–9.
13. Haurani C, Carlin AM, Hammoud ZT, Velnovich V. Prevalence and resolution of anemia with paraesophageal hernia repair. J Gastrointest Surg. 2012;16(10):1817–20.

14. Hill LD, Tobias JA. Paraesophageal hernia. Arch Surg. 1968;96(5):735–44.
15. Linke GR, Borovicka J, Schneider P, Zerz A, Warschkow R, Lange J, et al. Is a barium swallow complementary to endoscopy essential in the preoperative assessment of laparoscopic antireflux and hiatal hernia surgery. Surg Endosc. 2008;22(1):96–100.
16. Fornari F, Gurski RR, Navarini D, Thiesen V, Mestriner LH, Madalosso CA. Clinical utility of endoscopy and barium swallow X-ray in the diagnosis of sliding hiatal hernia in morbidly obese patients: a study before and after gastric bypass. Obes Surg. 2010;20(6):702–8.
17. Levine MS, Rubesin SE. Diseases of the esophagus: diagnosis with esophagography. Radiology. 2005;237(2):414–27.
18. Maziak DE, Todd TR, Pearson FG. Massive hiatus hernia: evaluation and surgical management. J Thorac Cardiovasc Surg. 1998;115(1):53–60.
19. Rashid F, Thangarajah T, Mulvey D, Larvin M, Iftikhar SY. A review article on gastric volvulus: a challenge to diagnosis and management. Int J Surg. 2010;8:18–24.
20. Hansdotter I, Bjor O, Andreasson A, et al. Hill classification is superior to the axial length of a hiatal hernia for assessment of the mechanical anti-reflux barrier at the gastroesophageal junction. Endosc Int Open. 2016;4:E311–7.
21. Siegal SR, Dolan JP, Hunter JG. Modern diagnosis and treatment of hiatal hernias. Langenbeck's Arch Surg. 2017;402(8):1145–51.
22. Kahrilas PJ, Kim HC, Pandolfino JE. Approaches to the diagnosis and grading of hiatal hernia. Best Pract Res Clin Gastroenterol. 2008;22(4):601–16. https://doi.org/10.1016/j.bpg.2007.12.007.
23. Roman S, Kahrilas PJ, Kia L, Luger D, Soper N, Pandolfino JE. Effects of large hiatal hernias on esophageal peristalsis. Arch Surg. 2012;147(4):352–7. https://doi.org/10.1001/archsurg.2012.17.
24. Conrado LM, Gurski RR, da Rosa AR, Simic AP, Callegari-Jacques SM. Is there an association between hiatal hernia and ineffective esophageal motility in patients with gastroesophageal reflux disease? J Gastrointest Surg. 2011;15(10):1756–61.
25. Wirsching A, Zhang Q, McCormick SE, Hubka M, Low DE. Abnormal high-resolution manometry findings and outcomes after paraesophageal hernia repair. J Am Coll Surg. 2018;227(2):181–8.
26. Zevin B, Jones EL, Martin del Campo SE, Perry KA. Omission of preoperative esophageal manometry does not alter operative approach or postoperative dysphagia following laparoscopic paraesophageal hernia repair. Dis Esophagus. 2017;30(7):1–6.
27. Stylopoulos N, Gazelle GS, Rattner DW. Paraesophageal hernias: operation or observation. Ann Surg. 2002;236(4):492–500.
28. Jung JJ, Naimark DM, Behman R, Grantcharov TP. Approach to asymptomatic paraesophageal hernia: watchful waiting or elective laparoscopic hernia repair. Surg Endosc. 2018;32(2):864–71.

29. Light D, Links D, Griffin M. The threatened stomach: management of the acute gastric volvulus. Surg Endosc. 2016;30(5):1847–52.
30. Jamil LH, Haung BL, Kunkel DC, Jayaraman V, Soffer E. Successful gastric volvulus reduction and gastropexy using a dual endoscopic technique. Case Rep Med. 2014;2014:136381. https://doi.org/10.1155/2014/136381.
31. Ghosh S, Palmer KR. Double percutaneous endoscopic gastrostomy fixation: an effective treatment for recurrent gastric volvulus. Am J Gastroenterol. 1993;88(8):1271–2.
32. Teague WJ, Ackroyd R, Watson DI, Devitt PG. Changing patterns in the management of gastric volvulus over 14 years. Br J Surg. 2000;87(3):358–61.
33. Hosein S, Carlson T, Flores L, Rodrigues Armijo P, Oleynikov D. Minimally invasive approach to hiatal hernia repair is superior to open, even in emergent setting: a large national database analysis. Surg Endosc. 2020;35(1):423–8. https://doi.org/10.1007/s00464-020-07404-y.
34. Channer LT, Squires GT, Price PD. Laparoscopic repair of gastric volvulus. JSLS. 2000;4(3):225–30.
35. McLaren PJ, Hart KD, Hunter JG, Dolan JP. Paraesophageal hernia repair outcomes using minimally invasive approaches. JAMA Surg. 2017;152(12):1176–8.
36. Schlosser KA, Maloney SR, Prasad T, Augenstein VA, Heniford BT, Colavita PD. Mesh reinforcement of paraesophageal hernia repair: trends and outcomes from a national database. Surgery. 2019;166(5):879–85.
37. Iqbal A, Kakarlapudi GV, Awad Z, Haynatzki G, Turaga KK, Karu A, et al. Assessment of diaphragmatic stressors as risk factors for symptomatic failure of laparoscopic Nissen fundoplication. J Gastrointest Surg. 2006;10(1):12–21.
38. Soliman BG, Nguyen DT, Chan EY, Chihara RK, Meisenbach LM, Graviss EA, et al. Robot-assisted hiatal hernia repair demonstrates favorable short-term outcomes compared to laparoscopic hiatal hernia repair. Surg Endosc. 2020;34(6):24952502.
39. Howell RS, Liu HH, Petrone P, Anduaga MF, Servide MJ, Hall K, et al. Short-term outcomes in patients undergoing paraesophageal hiatal hernia repair. Sci Rep. 2020;10(1):7366. https://doi.org/10.1038/s41598-020-61566-2.
40. Frantzides CT, Madan AK, Carlson MA, Stavropoulos GP. A prospective, randomized trial of laparoscopic polytetrafluoroethylene (PTFE) patch repair vs simple cruroplasty for large hiatal hernia. Arch Surg. 2002;137(6):649–52.
41. Oelschlager BK, Pellegrini CA, Hunter JG, Brunt ML, Soper NJ, Sheppard BC, et al. Biologic prosthesis to prevent recurrence after laparoscopic paraesophageal hernia repair: long-term follow-up from a multicenter, prospective, randomized trial. J Am Coll Surg. 2011;213(4):461–8.

42. Watson DI, Thompson SK, Devitt PG, Aly A, Irvine T, Woods SD, et al. Five year follow-up of a randomized controlled trial of laparoscopic repair of very large hiatus hernia with sutures versus absorbable versus nonabsorbable mesh. Ann Surg. 2019;272(2):241–7. https://doi.org/10.1097/SLA.0000000000003734.
43. Watson DI, Thompson SK, Devitt PG, Smith L, Woods SD, Aly A, et al. Laparoscopic repair of very large hiatus hernia with sutures versus absorbable mesh versus nonabsorbable mesh: a randomized controlled trial. Ann Surg. 2015;261(2):282–9.
44. Stadlhuber RJ, El Sherif A, Mittal SK, Fitzgibbons RJ, Brunt LM, Hunter JG, et al. Mesh complications after prosthetic reinforcement of hiatal closure: a 28-case series. Surg Endosc. 2009;23(6):1219–26.
45. Tatum RP, Shalhub S, Oelschlager BK, Pellegrini CA. Complications of PTFE mesh at the diaphragmatic hiatus. J Gastrointest Surg. 2008;12(5):953–7.
46. Nandipati K, Bye M, Yamamoto SR, Pallati P, Lee T, Mittal SK. Reoperative intervention in patients with mesh at the hiatus is associated with high incidence of esophageal resection – a single-center experience. J Gastrointest Surg. 2013;17(12):2039–44.
47. Tam V, Luketich JD, Levy RM, Christie NA, Awais O, Shende M, et al. Mesh cruroplasty in laparoscopic repair of paraesophageal hernias is not associated with better long-term outcomes compared to primary repair. Am J Surg. 2017;214(4):651–6.
48. Parker M, Bowers SP, Bray JM, Harris AS, Belli EV, Pfluke JM, et al. Hiatal mesh is associated with major resection at revisional operation. Surg Endosc. 2010;24(12):3095–101.
49. Walther B, DeMeester TR, Lafontaine E, Courtney JV, Little AG, Skinner DB. Effect of paraesophageal hernia on sphincter function and its implication on surgical therapy. Am J Surg. 1984;147(1):111–6.
50. Fuller CB, Hagen JA, DeMeester TR, Peters JH, Ritter M, Bremmer CG. The role of fundoplication in the treatment of type II esophageal hernia. J Thorac Cardiovasc Surg. 1996;111(3):655–61.
51. Furnee EJ, Draaisma WA, Gooszen HG, Hazebroek EJ, Smout AJ, Broeders IA. Tailored or routine addition of an antireflux fundoplication in laparoscopic large hiatal hernia repair: a comparative cohort study. World J Surg. 2011;35(1):78–84.
52. Mark LA, Okrainec A, Ferri LE, Feldman LS, Mayrand S, Fried GM. Comparison of patient-centered outcomes after laparoscopic Nissen fundoplication for gastroesophageal reflux disease or paraesophageal hernia. Surg Endosc. 2008;22(2):343–7.
53. Guidozzi N, Wiggins T, Ahmed AR, Hanna GB, Markar SR. Laparoscopic magnetic sphincter augmentation versus fundoplication for gastroesophageal reflux disease: systematic review and pooled analysis. Dis Esophagus. 2019;32(9):31.

54. Warren HF, Reynolds JL, Lipham JC, et al. Multi-institutional outcomes using magnetic sphincter augmentation versus Nissen fundoplication for chronic gastroesophageal reflux disease. Surg Endosc. 2016;30(8):3289–96.
55. Poncet G, Robert M, Roman S, Boulez JC. Laparoscopic repair of large hiatal hernia without prosthetic reinforcement: late results and relevance of anterior gastropexy. J Gastrointest Surg. 2010;14(12):1910–6.
56. Diaz S, Brunt LM, Klingensmith ME, Frisella PM, Soper NJ. Laparoscopic paraesophageal hernia repair, a challenging operation: medium-term outcome of 116 patients. J Gastrointest Surg. 2003;7(1):59–67.
57. Dallemagne B, Kohnen L, Perretta S, Weerts J, Markiewicz S, Jehaes C. Laparoscopic repair of paraesophageal hernia. Long-term follow-up reveals good clinical outcome despite high radiological recurrence rate. Ann Surg. 2011;253(2):291–6.
58. Hall T, Warnes N, Kuchta K, Novak S, Hedberg H, Linn JG, et al. Patient-centered outcomes after laparoscopic paraesophageal hernia repair. J Am Coll Surg. 2018;227(1):106–14.
59. Luketich JD, Nason KS, Christie NA, Pennathur A, Jobe BA, Landreneau RJ, et al. Outcomes after a decade of laparoscopic giant paraesophageal hernia repair. J Thorac Cardiovasc Surg. 2010;139(2):395–404.
60. Aly A, Munt J, Jamieson GG, Ludemann R, Devitt PG, Watson DI. Laparoscopic repair of large hiatal hernias. Br J Surg. 2005;92(5):648–53.
61. Fullum TM, Oyetunji TA, Ortega G, Tran DD, Woods IM, Obayomi-Davies O, et al. Open versus laparoscopic hiatal hernia repair. JSLS. 2013;17(1):23–9.
62. Mungo B, Molena D, Stem M, Feinberg RL, Lidor AO. Thirty-day outcomes of paraesophageal hernia repair using the NSQIP database: should laparoscopy be the standard of care. J Am Coll Surg. 2014;219(2):229–36.
63. Oelschlager BK, Pellegrini CA, Hunter J, Soper N, Brunt M, Sheppard B, et al. Biologic prosthesis reduces recurrence after laparoscopic paraesophageal hernia repair: a multicenter, prospective, randomized trial. Ann Surg. 2006;244(4):481–90.

35 Primary Dysphagia: A Case-Based Approach to Diagnosis and Treatment

Matthew W. Romine and Abhishek D. Parmar

Case 1

Clinical Vignette: A 29-year-old female presents to the clinic with progressive difficulty swallowing. Initially, she noted difficulty in swallowing solid food but has since progressed to difficulty swallowing liquids as well. She describes effortless regurgitation of undigested food substances with a foul smell and heartburn. In addition, she reports a 15-pound unintentional weight loss. A primary care physician started a proton pump inhibitor for complaints of heartburn. She has no significant past medical history. Her surgical history is notable for a cesarean section at age 25.

M. W. Romine
Department of Surgery, East Carolina University Hospital System, Greenville, NC, USA
e-mail: matthew.romine@ecuhealth.org

A. D. Parmar (✉)
Department of Surgery, University of Alabama at Birmingham, Birmingham, AL, USA
e-mail: aparmar@uabmc.edu

A. D. Patel et al. (eds.), *The SAGES Manual of Physiologic Evaluation of Foregut Diseases*,
https://doi.org/10.1007/978-3-031-39199-6_35

She is a nonsmoker and currently works as an accountant. Vital signs are within normal limits. Labs including a basic metabolic panel and CBC are notable only for mild anemia.

Elements of this patient's history are instructive of a progressively worsening primary dysphagia. Her progressive dysphagia to solids and then liquids is suggestive of a mechanical cause for her dysphagia that is slowly worsening over time. In addition, her history of regurgitation of undigested food particles suggests a mechanical obstruction of her esophagus. Finally, her complaints of a foul odor to her emesis and heartburn are suggestive of longstanding stasis of undigested food debris in her distal esophagus [1]. In many cases, the retained, static food debris can become fermented and masquerade as symptoms of conventional reflux. In reality, these symptoms stem from a longstanding obstruction and not a laxity in the lower esophageal sphincter.

In general, the first step in evaluating a patient presenting with primary dysphagia is to obtain a barium swallow. Advantages of a barium swallow include easy attainability, low cost, and its noninvasive nature. A barium swallow can provide critical information on the structure and function of the esophagus. For patients with symptoms of dysphagia to solids, a solid phase agent such as a tablet, bread, or marshmallow can be added to the swallow protocol to elicit the patient's specific symptoms ("provocative" study). Most barium swallow protocols also allow for the performance of delayed imaging to characterize emptying of the distal esophagus. Delayed imaging usually performed at 1, 3, and 5 min can capture presence or absence of a column, suggesting an outlet obstruction. Results from the barium swallow can help the clinician select appropriate additional tests to perform next, including esophagogastroduodenoscopy, high-resolution manometry, or pH testing.

Clinical Vignette continued: The patient undergoes a barium swallow (Fig. 35.1). The study demonstrates an enlarged diameter esophagus with smooth tapering to a point in a classic "bird's beak" appearance. During the live portion of the swallow, there is an absence of peristalsis. The five-minute delayed image demonstrates a persistent column of 50% remaining contrast.

The barium swallow above demonstrates a classic "bird's beak" appearance of achalasia, with delayed imaging demonstrat-

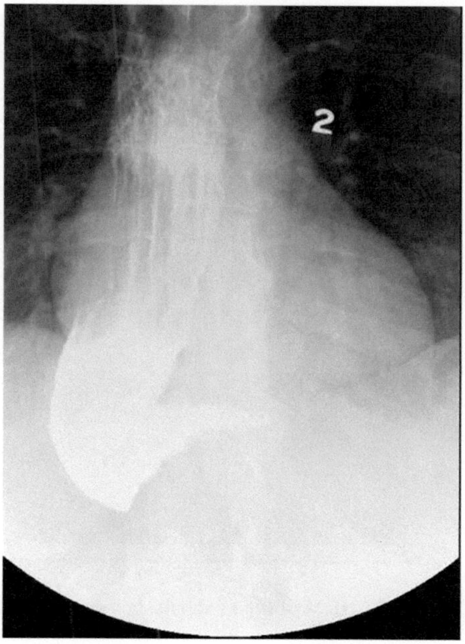

Fig. 35.1 Picture of classic achalasia barium swallow with bird's beak appearance. Image courtesy of James Callaway, MD

ing persistence of a column after 5 min. Following the barium swallow, further testing is indicated in the form of an esophagogastroduodenoscopy to assess for pseudoachalasia and high-resolution manometry to confirm pathologic motility. High-resolution manometry provides the gold standard of diagnosis and is useful for differentiating the types of achalasia from one another (Fig. 35.2) [2]. The Chicago Classification for diagnosis of achalasia includes an IRP >15 and the absence of peristalsis in type I achalasia.

Clinical Vignette continued: The patient undergoes high-resolution manometry which demonstrates an IRP of 19 and absence of peristalsis consistent with type I achalasia. The patient undergoes an EGD demonstrating retained food particles in the esophagus as well as LA grade B esophagitis. The EGD passes through the LES with some difficulty and characteristic "pop" through the distal esophagus.

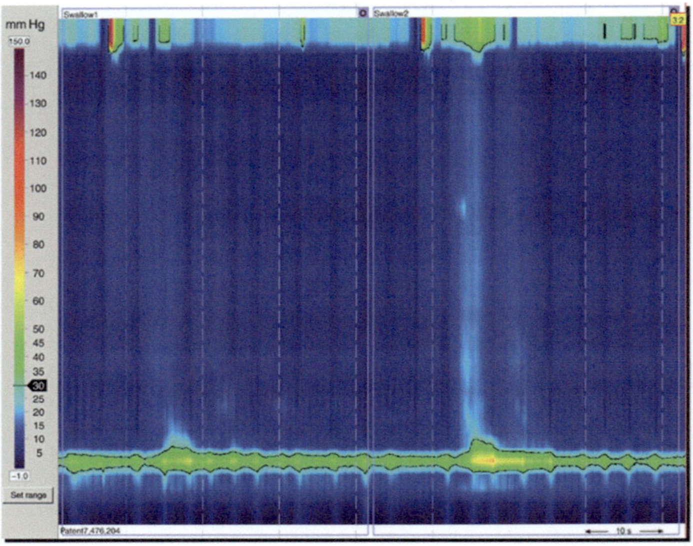

Fig. 35.2 HRM of type I achalasia. Image courtesy of James Callaway, MD

Treatment for achalasia includes surgical and nonsurgical interventions. Nonsurgical options include use of botox injections at the lower esophageal sphincter and endoscopic dilation. Surgical interventions include a laparoscopic Heller myotomy and per oral endoscopic myotomy (POEM) [3].

The definitive treatment of type I achalasia is Heller myotomy or POEM. Both procedures are safe and provide excellent palliation of symptoms [4]. The choice of procedure to perform includes patient preference, equipment and technical ability to perform POEM, and degree of esophagitis. All POEM patients should be consented for the possibility of conversion to a laparoscopic Heller myotomy as complications may arise during POEM.

Clinical Vignette conclusion: The patient elects to undergo POEM for treatment of her type I achalasia. She is discharged home on postoperative day 1 with improvement in her symptoms on a pureed diet. She returns to the clinic three weeks later reporting continued improvement in her swallowing function with no further dysphagia symptoms.

Case 2

Clinical Vignette: A 63-year-old female presents to the emergency department after experiencing squeezing chest pain during dinner in which she was drinking red wine. She reports the pain was so severe that she regurgitated undigested food. The pain is midsternal, and she reports the pain resolved spontaneously shortly after arrival to the emergency room. She reports similar episodes of pain in the past which resolved quickly and were less intense. Her past medical history is notable for hypertension, anxiety, depression, and gastroesophageal reflux disease. Family history is notable for a grandmother who had a myocardial infarction at age 66. A cardiac work-up in the emergency department is negative. While drinking a cold glass of water in the emergency room, she begins having the same pain again.

This patient has classic symptoms of both angina and diffuse esophageal spasm (DES). Differentiating diffuse esophageal spasm from angina can be challenging for clinicians and patients alike, as the symptoms and patient population can be similar between the two diagnoses. Pain from DES can be quite intense, substernal and can last anywhere from several minutes to several hours. However, in contrast to classic angina, the pain with DES typically resolves spontaneously. DES is also typically identified in patients between the ages of sixty to eighty, who may also be at risk for cardiac disease. Ultimately, based on this significant overlap in clinical symptoms, all patients with these symptoms should be promptly evaluated for myocardial infarction, especially in those with established cardiac risk factors.

In the above patient, there are several historical features that are suggestive of an esophageal, and not cardiac, etiology. In prior instances of the patient's pain, her pain began following the ingestion of food and/or drink. Classic triggers of DES include ingestion of hot and cold substances as well as alcoholic beverages; in particular, red wine. For this patient, she has additional comorbidities of gastroesophageal reflux disease, anxiety, depression, and hypertension, all of which predispose her to DES. Finally, this patient's history of regurgitation of food during or after the episode of pain is another clinical feature that is suggestive of

DES. These associations with enteral intake would be atypical of cardiac disease and is also a useful distinguishing clinical symptom between DES and hypercontractile (jackhammer) esophagus.

Clinical Vignette continued: Suspecting an esophageal disorder, a barium swallow is obtained as seen in Fig. 35.3.

Diagnostic evaluation of DES is typical for the work-up of other esophageal motility disorders. A barium swallow is the most useful first test, followed by high-resolution manometry (HRM). The barium swallow in Fig. 35.3 demonstrates the classic "corkscrew" or "rosary bead" appearance seen in patients with diffuse esophageal spasm. While this barium swallow demonstrates the classic appearance, less than 5% of patients will have these findings on barium swallow [5]. The Chicago Classification crite-

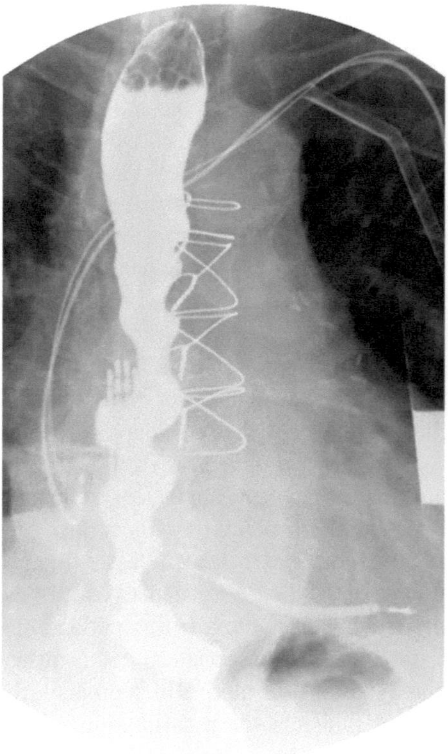

Fig. 35.3 Barium esophagram demonstrating corkscrew appearance classically seen in Diffuse Esophageal Spasm. Image courtesy of James Callaway, MD

ria for the diagnosis of DES includes a normal IRP and a shortened distal latency (≥20% of swallows are premature, for example, distal latency <4.5 s). Figure 35.4 demonstrates the classic HRM findings of DES. A screening esophagogastroduodenoscopy should also be performed to rule out malignancy, take biopsies if indicated, and evaluate for other pathology.

The mainstay of treatment of DES is medical management, with surgical intervention rarely required. Agents used include calcium channel blockers, phosphodiesterase inhibitors, and

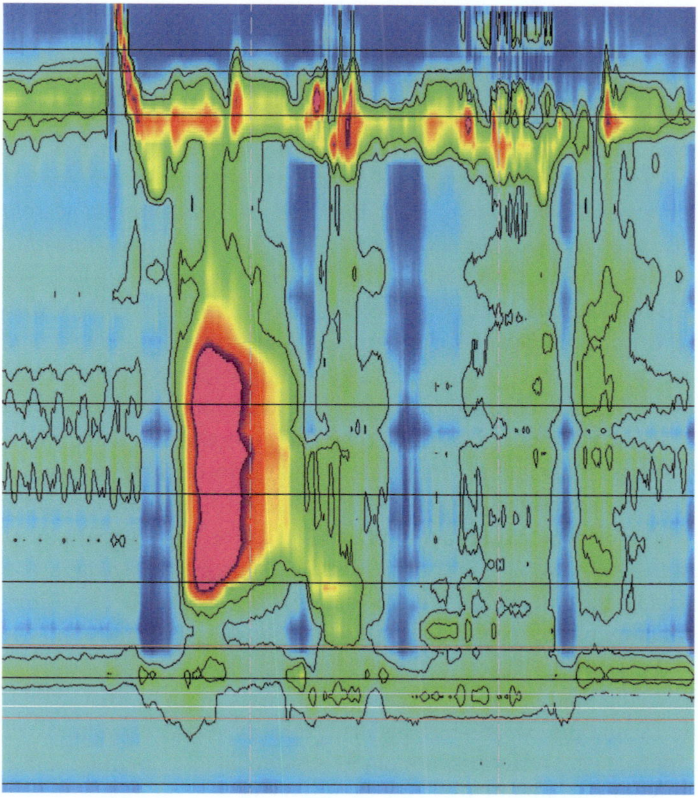

Fig. 35.4 Classic HRM findings of diffuse esophageal spasm. Image courtesy of James Callaway, MD

botox. Treatment of underlying or associated conditions such as reflux and anxiety can also aid in the treatment of DES. Surgical therapy such as POEM for DES is reserved for medically refractory disease, but there are few long-term studies documenting the durable effect of surgical therapy on DES [6].

Clinical Vignette conclusion: The patient undergoes HRM confirming DES. She is subsequently started on calcium channel blockers and a proton pump inhibitor with improvement in her symptoms.

Case 3

Clinical Vignette: A 74-year-old male with Parkinson's disease for the last 5 years presents to the clinic with complaints of difficulty swallowing. He reports it is difficult to initiate a swallow and feels a lump in the back of his throat with swallowing. He has associated symptoms of coughing and an unintentional weight loss of 15 pounds. He has been hospitalized for pneumonia within the past month. Currently, he lives in a nursing home.

Dysphagia is a relatively common problem in the elderly with an estimated prevalence of greater than 30% in nursing home patients [7]. The initiation of swallowing is a complex process, involving the coordination of greater than 30 muscles of the oropharynx and neck. Understanding the components of the swallowing process is critical to characterizing disorders of swallowing. Briefly, the swallowing process is broken down into three components: (1) the oral preparation phase, (2) the pharyngeal phase, and (3) the esophageal phase [8]. Oropharyngeal dysphagia is a broad term that encompasses a large variety of disease conditions affecting phases one and two of the swallowing process.

This patient has difficulty transferring food from the oral cavity to the pharynx and a globus sensation than can be characteristic symptoms of oropharyngeal dysphagia. Other symptoms of oropharyngeal dysphagia include odynophagia, coughing, and a choking sensation. Clinicians should be aware that globus sensation can be a diagnosis on its own, but has specific diagnostic criteria including the sensation of a nonpainful lump or foreign body within the throat in the absence of other esophageal motility disorders, GERD, or anatomical abnormality [9]. Patients frequently localize symptoms to the throat. Symptoms can occur with both solids and liquids and usually occur with most swallowing attempts. In severe cases, patients may need to extend their neck to aid with bolus transfer or digitally insert the bolus into their throat.

Oropharyngeal dysphagia can begin in the oral preparation phase. The oral phase involves bolus preparation in the swallow process and involves chewing and bolus formation with the hard palate and tongue. As this phase is the voluntary phase in the swallowing process, a wide variety of conditions can affect this phase of swallowing. Disease processes such as poor dentition, cerebrovascular disease affecting voluntary mastication and neuromotor function, inability to produce saliva, and disease conditions resulting in oropharyngeal mucosal breakdown can all affect the oral preparation phase.

The pharyngeal phase is largely reflexive and involves complex neuromuscular coordination to propel the bolus into the pharynx, relax the upper esophageal sphincter, and elevate the larynx to thereby close at the epiglottis to prevent aspiration. As this is a complex neuromuscular event, neuromuscular diseases tend to affect the pharyngeal phase. This patient's history of Parkinson's disease places him at risk for disorders with the pharyngeal phase of swallowing. Amyotrophic lateral sclerosis (ALS), myasthenia gravis, and other neurodegenerative diseases can affect the pharyngeal phase of swallowing. Mechanical obstructions such as tumors, osteophyte formation, and diverticular formation affect this phase as well.

As the differential diagnosis of oropharyngeal dysphagia is quite broad, the work-up and management varies based on the etiology. A careful history can help guide the work-up. The presence of a globus sensation, odynophagia, halitosis, coughing, gagging, timing of symptoms in relation to a meal, and regurgitation is strongly suggestive on history to be related to oropharyngeal dysphagia. In addition, a past medical history of cerebrovascular or neurodegenerative disease should raise the specter of this disease.

Clinical Vignette: Based on this patient's history of Parkinson's and symptoms, he undergoes videofluoroscopy to assess for swallowing abnormalities. This confirmed oropharyngeal dysphagia with aspiration.

The initial work-up of oropharyngeal dysphagia should include videofluoroscopy due to the ability to observe a dynamic swallow from oropharynx to the stomach. Videofluoroscopy can evaluate for silent aspiration, presence of failed swallows, and help guide the need for further testing. Fiberoptic endoscopic evaluation of swallowing (FEES) is also helpful in evaluating oropharyngeal dysphagia but is more invasive. FEES can detect aspiration, impairment of pharyngeal swallowing, and evaluate for mechanical obstructions or mucosal lesions that may affect swallow function. Treatment of oropharyngeal disease varies depending on the underlying etiology, thus making accurate diagnosis the most important part of the management process.

Clinical Vignette: Ultimately, due to the progressive nature of his Parkinson's disease, the patient underwent placement of a percutaneous endoscopic gastrostomy tube for feeding access and nil per os to help prevent future aspiration events.

References

1. Pandolfino JE, Gawron AJ. Achalasia: a systematic review. JAMA. 2015;313(18):1841. https://doi.org/10.1001/jama.2015.2996.
2. Vaezi MF, Pandolfino JE, Yadlapati RH, Greer KB, Kavitt RT. ACG clinical guidelines: achalasia. Am J Gastroenterol. 2020;115(9):1393–411. https://doi.org/10.14309/ajg.0000000000000731.
3. Kahrilas PJ, Bredenoord AJ, Fox M, et al. The Chicago classification of esophageal motility disorders, v3.0. Neurogastroenterol Motil. 2015;27(2):160–74. https://doi.org/10.1111/nmo.12477.
4. Werner YB, Hakanson B, Martinek J, et al. Endoscopic or surgical myotomy in patients with idiopathic achalasia. N Engl J Med. 2019;381(23):2219–29. https://doi.org/10.1056/NEJMoa1905380.
5. Almansa C, Heckman MG, DeVault KR, Bouras E, Achem SR. Esophageal spasm: demographic, clinical, radiographic, and manometric features in 108 patients: esophageal spasm features in 108 patients. Dis Esophagus. 2012;25(3):214–21. https://doi.org/10.1111/j.1442-2050.2011.01258.x.

6. Filicori F, Dunst CM, Sharata A, et al. Long-term outcomes following POEM for non-achalasia motility disorders of the esophagus. Surg Endosc. 2019;33(5):1632–9. https://doi.org/10.1007/s00464-018-6438-z.
7. Roy N, Stemple J, Merrill RM, Thomas L. Dysphagia in the elderly: preliminary evidence of prevalence, risk factors, and socioemotional effects. Ann Otol Rhinol Laryngol. 2007;116(11):858–65. https://doi.org/10.1177/000348940711601112.
8. Christmas C, Rogus-Pulia N. Swallowing disorders in the older population. J Am Geriatr Soc. 2019;67(12):2643–9. https://doi.org/10.1111/jgs.16137.
9. Aziz Q, Fass R, Gyawali CP, Miwa H, Pandolfino JE, Zerbib F. Esophageal disorders. Gastroenterology. 2016;150(6):1368–79. https://doi.org/10.1053/j.gastro.2016.02.012.

Persistent Dysphagia After Prior Anti-Reflux Procedure

36

Jennifer F. Preston
and Nathaniel J. Soper

Introduction

The incidence of dysphagia following anti-reflux procedures is widely variable in the literature [1]. Dysphagia in the early postoperative period is common and can usually be managed with dietary modifications and allowing time for inflammation and swelling to decrease [2]. Persistent dysphagia, defined as dysphagia that is still present 3 months after an anti-reflux procedure, can have multiple etiologies and requires a calculated, algorithmic approach to evaluation. In this chapter, we will outline the approach to evaluation of persistent dysphagia for surgical fundoplication and magnetic sphincter augmentation.

There is limited literature on dysphagia following transoral incisionless fundoplication (TIF). In fact, persistent dysphagia following TIF has not been documented in the literature [3–5]. Therefore, TIF will not be included in this chapter as reporting an evidence-based approach to evaluation is not possible at this time.

J. F. Preston (✉) · N. J. Soper
College of Medicine Phoenix, University of Arizona, Phoenix, AZ, USA
e-mail: Jennifer.preston@bannerhealth.com; Sopern@email.arizona.edu

A. D. Patel et al. (eds.), *The SAGES Manual of Physiologic Evaluation of Foregut Diseases*,
https://doi.org/10.1007/978-3-031-39199-6_36

Surgical Fundoplication

Persistent dysphagia following surgical fundoplication is reported in 5–12% of patients [6–9]. Although persistent dysphagia may be seen in fewer patients following partial compared to complete fundoplication, the etiology and evaluation of persistent dysphagia in partial fundoplication is similar to complete fundoplication [10–12]. Therefore, for the purpose of this chapter, partial and complete fundoplication will not be differentiated except in reporting normal post-fundoplication manometry findings.

The etiology for persistent dysphagia can be grouped into three main categories such as problems with the hiatal closure, which includes both intrathoracic migration of the wrap and crural stenosis, complications of the wrap itself, including a tight, twisted or slipped wrap, and motility disorders [7, 8, 13, 14]. The primary diagnostic studies which help to identify the underlying etiology include barium esophagography, endoscopy and, in some cases, esophageal manometry [7, 13].

Barium Esophagography

A barium esophagram provides essential information in evaluating patients with persistent dysphagia as it provides the best global assessment of anatomic problems and physiologic abnormalities contributing to dysphagia. This is because with appropriate positioning and swallowing procedures, information can be obtained regarding overall patterns of esophageal motility and emptying. Initially the patient should be positioned upright and asked to ingest a small amount of low-density barium. Normal post-fundoplication images will reveal narrowing of the distal esophagus with a gentle curve as contrast passes through the fundoplication. There may also be a minor delay of contrast passage through the wrap [15]. If there is a significant delay in contrast passing through the wrap, a timed swallow study should be performed with interval images at 2 and 5 min. This will identify

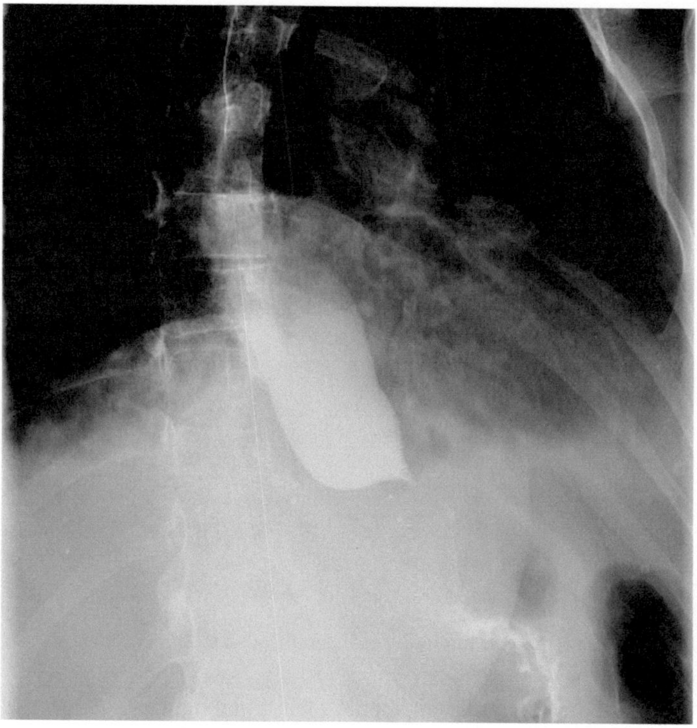

Fig. 36.1 Tight fundoplication

patients who have crural stenosis, a tight wrap or a motility disorder such as achalasia early in the examination (Fig. 36.1). In patients with a crural stenosis or a tight wrap, there will be smooth narrowing of the distal esophagus proximal to the wrap with dilatation of the proximal esophagus. If a timed study is not needed, the study should continue with an air-contrast phase to help define the anatomy of the fundoplication. The patient should be moved through several positions including upright, supine, left decubitus and right anterior oblique. Several spot films should be taken during this process. In the right anterior oblique position, the patient should be asked to ingest additional contrast with continuous fluo-

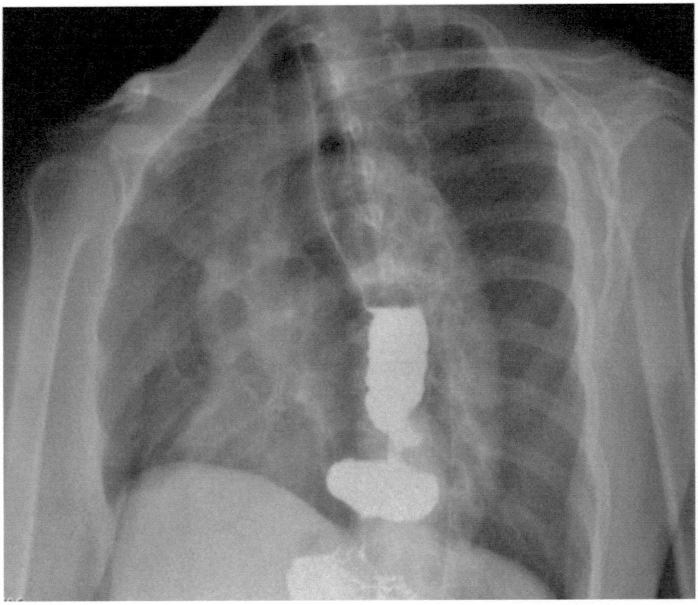

Fig. 36.2 Intrathoracic migration of fundoplication with crural stenosis

roscopy. These maneuvers should clearly define the location and anatomy of the gastroesophageal junction, the level of the diaphragm and the position and morphology of the wrap. Intrathoracic migration of the wrap (Fig. 36.2), crural stenosis (Fig. 36.2), slippage of the proximal stomach through the wrap (Fig. 36.3) and twisting or loosening of the wrap should be identifiable (Fig. 36.3). Motility can be assessed using the standard five swallows. If motility is intact but there is an issue with a tight fundoplication, peristalsis will be normal to the level of the epiphrenic ampulla which may balloon out, indicating a higher pressure gradient across the wrap than in the peristaltic wave. The rapid drinking phase is also important in determining the location of the wrap, integrity and length of the wrap, the lumen of the wrap, and intrathoracic migration of the wrap [15, 16].

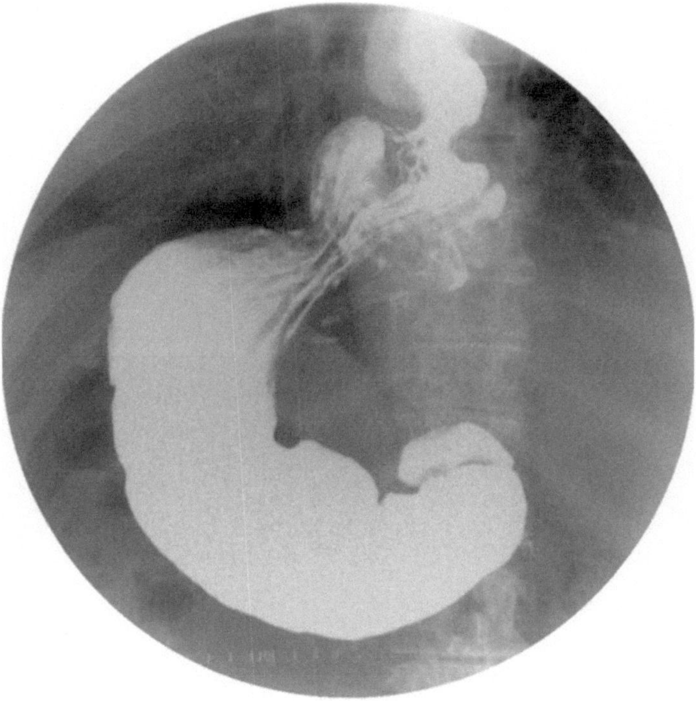

Fig. 36.3 Intrathoracic migration of the wrap with slippage onto the stomach and loosening of the wrap

Endoscopy

Endoscopy is an important diagnostic tool in evaluating patients with post-fundoplication dysphagia as it is particularly sensitive in identifying structural abnormalities of the wrap itself. Key endoscopic features that can be seen in patients with dysphagia include a slipped, twisted, disrupted or tight wrap, intrathoracic migration of the wrap and/or esophageal pathology such as esophagitis. In patients with a slipped wrap, the squamocolumnar junction will be located more than 1 cm proximal to the proximal

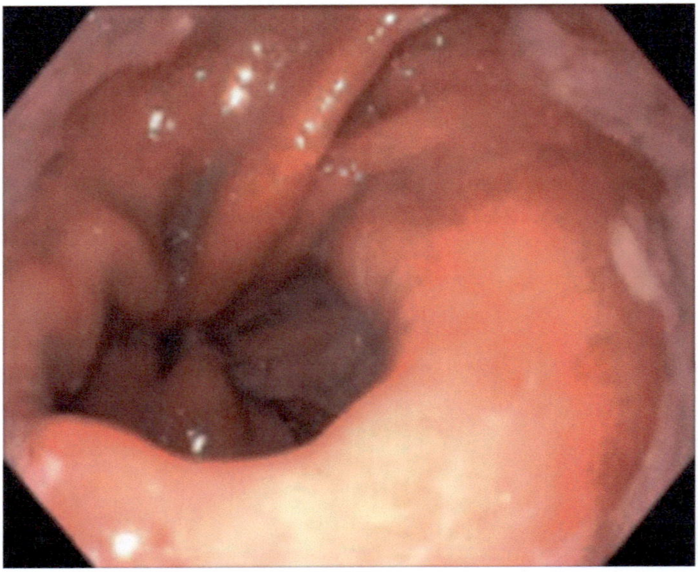

Fig. 36.4 Squamocolumnar junction noted proximal to wrap

margin of the wrap (Fig. 36.4). A disrupted wrap will appear loose or twisted on retroflexion (Fig. 36.5). A tight wrap may cause resistance to endoscopic passage into the stomach, although esophagography has been shown to be more sensitive at detecting a tight fundoplication than endoscopy. With intrathoracic migration of the wrap, the fundoplication may appear intact, but the hiatal pinch will be noted distal to the fundoplication (Fig. 36.6). Lastly, esophageal mucosal abnormalities, such as esophagitis from recurrent reflux or eosinophilic esophagitis, can also be detected endoscopically. Eosinophilic esophagitis is considered if classic concentric rings are present, as well as possible exudates, plaques or furrows. This diagnosis is confirmed on biopsies that demonstrate more than 15 eosinophils per high power field [7, 17].

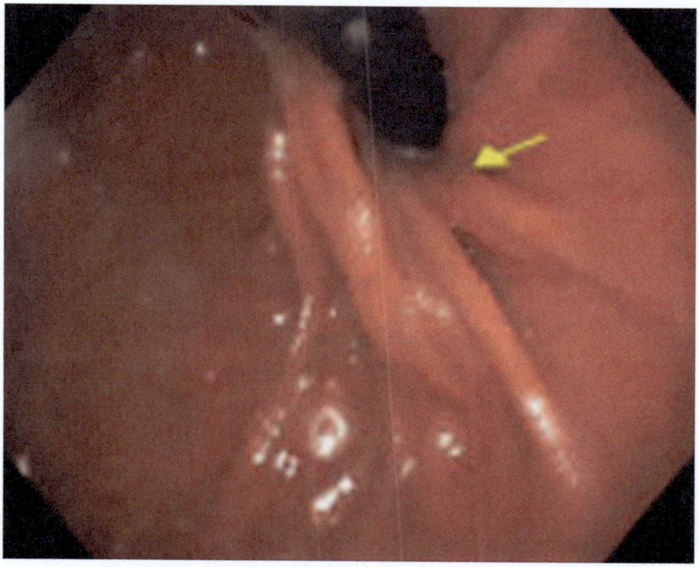

Fig. 36.5 Loosened fundoplication

Esophageal Manometry

High-resolution esophageal manometry can be helpful in patients with significant dysphagia who appear to have normal post-fundoplication anatomy on esophagography and endoscopy. In order to interpret manometry findings correctly in symptomatic patients, however, it is important to understand the normal manometric values following fundoplication in asymptomatic patients. There are also some differences between postoperative manometry following complete and partial fundoplication. In the following sections, the normal post-fundoplication findings, as described in the Chicago Classification System, will be outlined first, followed by results in patients with dysphagia.

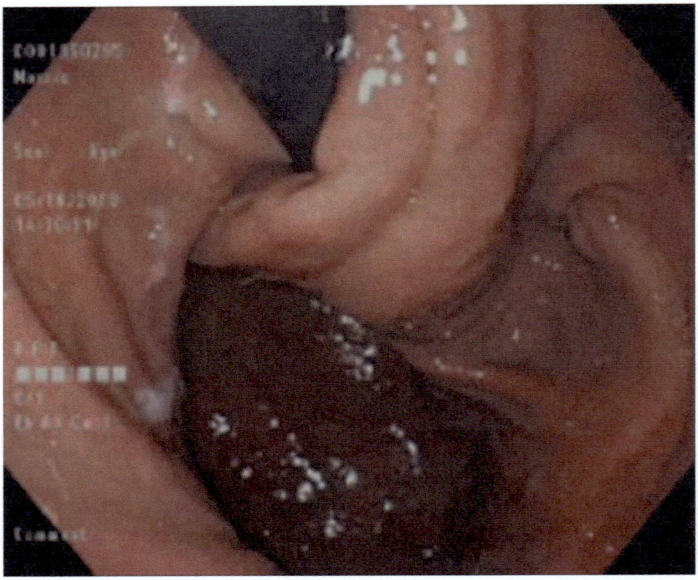

Fig. 36.6 Intrathoracic migration of fundoplication

Esophagogastric Junction Parameters

For asymptomatic patients, the mean intra-abdominal esophagogastric junction (EGJ) length is similar between Nissen (2.7 cm ± 1.1 cm) and Toupet fundoplication (2.7 cm ± 0.8 cm). The mean Integrated Relaxation Pressure (IRP) is higher for Nissen (13 ± 5.1 mmHg) than for Toupet (7.4 ± 2.9 mmHg) but both fall within the normal range (<14.7 mmHg). The same is true for the EGJ resting pressure for Nissen and Toupet (19 ± 8.3 mmHg and 12.7 ± 5.7 mmHg, respectively, $p < 0.01$) with the normal range being 5–31.6 mmHg [18].

For patients with dysphagia, the Lower Esophageal Sphincter (LES) resting pressure is commonly within the normal range. The mean IRP with wet swallows will be abnormally elevated in 15–34% of patients indicating EGJ outflow obstruction [19–21]. With the addition of a solid meal, the percentage of patients with an abnormal IRP will increase to 40.7% [19]. When directly comparing IRP in patients with dysphagia to asymptomatic patients, the mean IRP is higher in patients with dysphagia, even though for a majority of patients, the IRP value will still be within normal range [22, 23]. Achalasia is a rare finding on post-fundoplication manometry [20, 21].

The average maximal intrabolus pressure during the swallow window in asymptomatic patients is similar between Toupet and Nissen (13.7 ± 3.4 mmHg and 15.2 ± 3.6 mmHg, respectively), with slightly higher upper limits of normal for both procedures compared to the Chicago Classification (<15 mmHg) [18]. This is true for patients with dysphagia as well [19]. When post-fundoplication patients with and without dysphagia are directly compared, there does not appear to be a significant difference in intrabolus pressure between these groups, with both being elevated [22, 24].

The bolus transit time after fundoplication is significantly longer with liquids (6.8 ± 0.9 s compared to 9.8 ± 1 s, $p < 0.01$) and solids (2.8 ± 0.5 s compared 5.8 ± 0.8 s, $p < 0.01$) for all patients post-fundoplication indicating a decreased EGJ transit efficacy. This is likely a result of decreased EGJ compliance post-fundoplication limiting EGJ opening. There is a significant positive correlation with increasing bolus transit times and symptoms of dysphagia [24].

Esophageal Body Contraction Parameters/Peristalsis

In asymptomatic patients, the distal contractile integral (DCI) is significantly higher for Nissen than Toupet (2037 ± 1154 mmHg vs 845 ± 538 mmHg, respectively, $p < 0.01$); however, the upper limits of normal for both fall within the normal range (448–4721 mmHg) [18]. When comparing patients post-fundoplication with and without dysphagia, there does not appear to be a significant difference in DCI [22, 23].

The contraction amplitude in the proximal, middle and distal esophagus has been shown to be significantly higher after Nissen (63.9 ± 29.5 mmHg, 91.2 ± 42.3 mmHg, and 111.9 ± 41.6 mmHg, respectively) compared to Toupet (42.4 ± 23.3 mmHg, 62 ± 31.5 mmHg, and 64.5 ± 27 mmHg, respectively) ($p < 0.05$ for proximal and middle, $p < 0.01$ for distal) with the upper limits for Nissen being higher than the 95th percentile in Chicago Classification

(102.1, 146.4, and 146.4, respectively). However, there does not appear to be a significant difference in contraction amplitude pre- and post-fundoplication specifically in patients with dysphagia [25, 26]. The mean contractile velocity and mean distal contraction latency are similar between both Nissen and Toupet and fall within the normal range of the Chicago Classification [18]. When patients post-fundoplication with and without dysphagia are compared, the distal contraction latency and contractile velocity are not statistically different [22, 25].

There does not appear to be a significant difference in ineffective peristalsis patterns in post-fundoplication patients with and without dysphagia. There is a statistically significant increase in percentage of patients with incomplete bolus clearance with dysphagia compared to patients without dysphagia (61% vs 32%, respectively, $P = 0.01$) [27].

Manometry Summary

An increased mean IRP in the setting of dysphagia likely indicates an issue with the wrap. Increased bolus transit time and/or incomplete bolus clearance may indicate either an issue with the wrap or with crural stenosis. LES resting pressure, intrabolus pressure, DCI, contraction amplitude and peristaltic patterns do not appear to be significantly different between patients with and without dysphagia, making these parameters less useful in identifying causes for dysphagia.

Functional Luminal Imaging Probe (FLIP)

The functional luminal imaging probe is a balloon-based catheter that uses impedance planimetry to measure diameter, cross-sectional area and distensibility of the EGJ in response to volume-controlled distension. Over the past few years, this technology has been used to evaluate and better understand EGJ distensibility following fundoplication. When compared to controls, patients post-fundoplication exhibit reduced EGJ distensibility and reduced EGJ compliance during deglutitive relaxation and a longer segment of reduced distensibility [28]. The feasibility of utilizing this technology intraoperatively to aid in decision-making and to understand postoperative outcomes is still being explored, but recent studies have shown this to be a promising technology. Su et al. published a series of 226 patients in which FLIP was utilized intraoperatively [29]. During the final year of that series, the number of procedures in which management was changed based on FLIP measurements was recorded. During that year, management was changed based on high or low intraoperative FLIP distensibility indices (DI) in 12 of 52 patients. The changes recorded included additional crural sutures (high DI after closure) and change in type of fundoplication based on high (changed to Nissen) or low DI (changed to Toupet) [29]. In a subsequent follow-up series, that group demonstrated patients with a final intraoperative DI < 2 $mm^2/mmHg$ experienced significantly more dysphagia at 1 year compared to those patients with a DI ≥ 2 $mm^2/mmHg$. This difference became even larger at 2 years [30].

Magnetic Sphincter Augmentation (MSA)

Persistent moderate to severe dysphagia following MSA ranges from 1–15% in the literature and is the most common indication for device removal [31–34]. The etiologies for persistent dysphagia include recurrent hiatal hernia, migration of the device, device erosion, outflow resistance from either crural stenosis or an undersized device, and inadequate intake of bulky food allowing the device to be encapsulated by scar tissue in the 'closed' position. Other patients experience dysphagia of unknown etiology, defined as patients with normal testing but persistent symptoms [31, 33–37]. With a recurrent hiatal hernia, migration of the device, and device erosion, there will often be a symptom-free interval prior to representation with dysphagia. The primary investigations to identify the underlying etiology include barium esophagography and endoscopy [31, 33, 34, 36–39]. Esophageal manometry has not been shown to be different in patients with dysphagia compared to patients without dysphagia. For thoroughness of this chapter, the expected manometry findings following MSA will be described.

Barium Esophagography

The initial scout film taken during a barium esophagram can give important information regarding device migration. A device located above the level of the diaphragm indicates either proximal migration or a recurrent hiatal hernia [36, 37]. If there is an early postoperative comparison image, change in position of the device can be evaluated. This is particularly useful if there is distal migration of the device (Fig. 36.7) [38]. With the addition of barium, the contour and function of the esophagus can be evaluated. Dilation of the esophagus may indicate outflow obstruction [31, 37]. In addition, recurrence of the hiatal hernia can be evaluated with a similar technique utilized for post-fundoplication esophagram (Fig. 36.8) [36, 37]. There are no routinely noted changes on barium esophagram associated with device erosion [37–40]. In one case study involving an eroded device, a slight delayed transit of contrast was noted with mild distal esophageal dilation [38]. Utilization of barium esophagram for evaluating the opening/closing function of the device in the setting of dysphagia has not

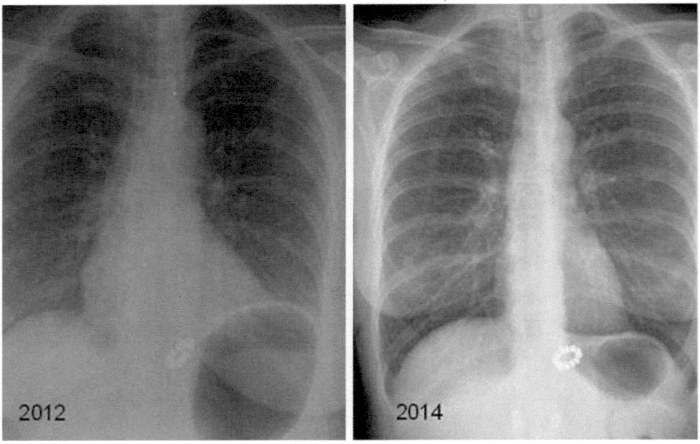

Fig. 36.7 Chest X-ray from 2012 and 2014, respectively, showing distal migration of the LINX device. Image used with permission [38]

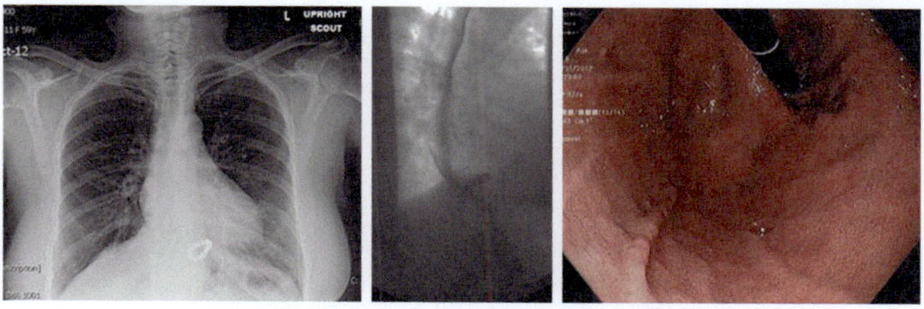

Fig. 36.8 Recurrent hiatal hernia with proximal migration of MSA device. Image used with permission [36]

been documented in the literature but might be an interesting topic for future research, particularly for patients with an unknown etiology for persistent dysphagia.

Endoscopy

Endoscopy is vital for evaluating patients with persistent dysphagia following MSA. This allows identification of device erosion by intraluminal visualization of device beads (Fig. 36.9). Endoscopy can also be therapeutic in this setting as endoscopic removal of eroded devices has been well documented in the literature [33–35, 37–39]. Migration of the device, either proximal or distal, can also be seen on endoscopy. Outflow obstruction may be indicated by a dilated esophagus with or without fluid retention (Fig. 36.10) [31, 36, 38]. Lastly, a recurrent hiatal hernia can also be diagnosed endoscopically, including the location of the GE junction and device in relation to level of the diaphragmatic hiatus (Fig. 36.7) [36]. Endoscopic dilation may also help resolve dysphagia if caused by scarring around the MSA device [31].

Manometry

When compared to preoperative manometry, there are several documented changes noted in high-resolution manometry following MSA. The total (2.8 ± 1 cm, $p = 0.002$) and intra-abdominal

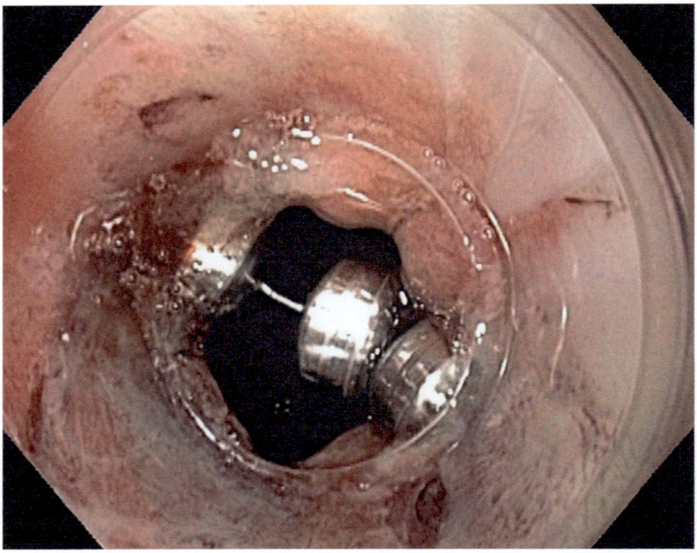

Fig. 36.9 Endoscopic view of full-thickness MSA erosion. Image used with permission [33]

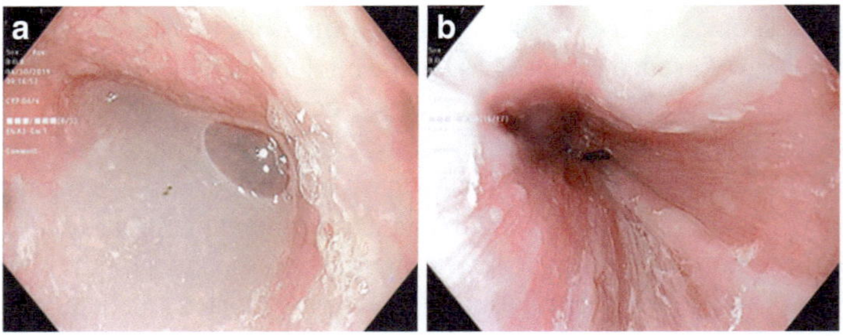

Fig. 36.10 Patient with severe dysphagia and significant fluid retention above the GE junction (**a**) and esophageal lining changes suggestive of retention esophagitis (**b**). Image used with permission [31]

(1.2 ± 1.4 cm, $p = 0.001$) LES length increases significantly after surgery [40]. Resting LES has been reported as both increased and unchanged, but these values remained within normal range in Chicago Classification [40, 41]. IRP is significantly increased following MSA, but only 13% of patients will have an IRP above normal level (10.2 ± 5.1 mmHg $p < 0.001$, normal <14.7 mmHg). Intrabolus pressure (IBP) has also been shown to be increased after surgery with 56% of patients having an IBP above normal level (17.7 ± 7.3 mmHg $p < 0.001$, normal <15 mmHg) [40, 41]. Further studies are needed to understand whether peristalsis patterns are affected by MSA. In one series, peristaltic patterns were not routinely altered by MSA [41]. In another series, 64% of patients with preoperative ineffective esophageal motility (IEM) were noted to have no change in peristaltic pattern and 36% had resolution of IEM. In that series, 14% developed de novo IEM [40]. DCI is noted to significantly increase following MSA but remain within a normal range (1175 ± 1708 mmHg $p < 0.001$, normal 448–4721 mmHg). In patients with persistent dysphagia, there is no documented difference in resting LES pressure, IRP, IBP, DCI or peristaltic patterns compared to asymptomatic patients [40, 41].

Editors Note

Persistent dysphagia after prior anti-reflux procedure

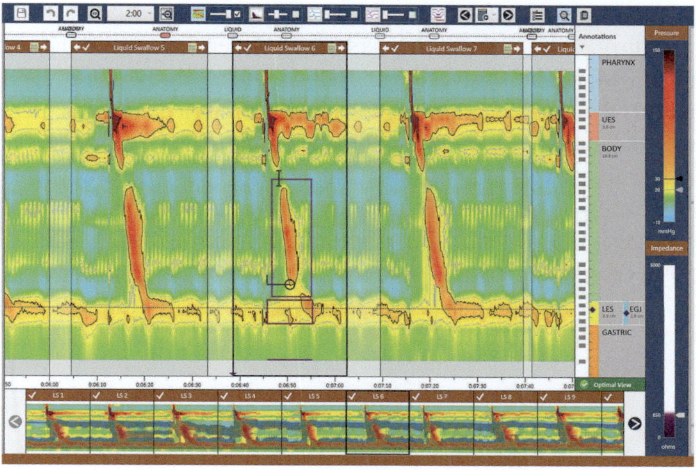

Patient is a 47 years male post Nissen with persistent dysphagia. On manometry, the read was as follows: the study of the LES reveals a normal length and intraabdominal component. The LES pressure is normal at 20 mmHg but does not relax completely. The IRP fluctuates from 12–16 indicating some EGJ outflow obstruction. The esophageal body demonstrates normal peristalsis and contraction amplitudes. Bolus transit is normal. Overall this is consistent with EGJ outflow obstruction post Nissen.

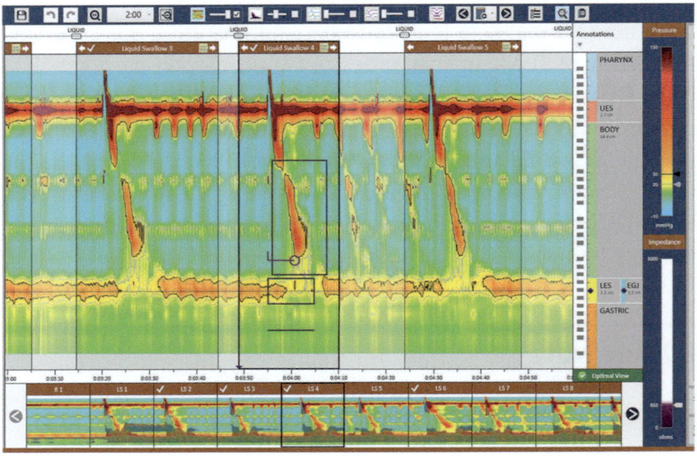

Thirty years female 2 years post Nissen and hiatal hernia repair. Manometry reveals the following: the study of the LES reveals a normal length post nissen and there is a distal high pressure indicating a possible small hiatal hernia. The LES pressure is higher than expected post nissen at 44 mmHg and does not relax completely. The esophageal body study demonstrates normal peristalsis and contraction amplitudes. Bolus transit is low at 50%. Overall the patient has a tight nissen and hiatal hernia.

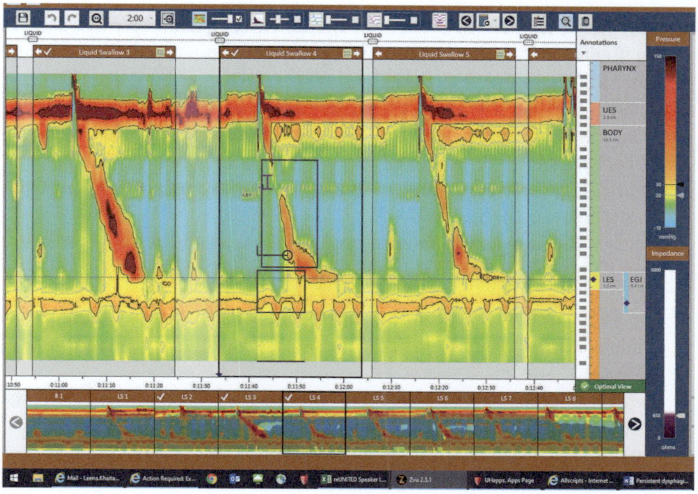

Sixty-six years female 2 years post Nissen fundoplication with symptoms of dysphagia and heartburn. Manometric reading as follows: the study of the LES reveals shortened length and a recurrence of her hiatal hernia with the plication sitting below the LES. The LES pressure is 5 mmHg and relaxes adequately. The esophageal body study demonstrates normal peristalsis and contraction amplitudes. IRP is high due to slip of the plication. Higher pressure is seen between the LES and hiatus. Bolus transit is decreased at 60%. Overall the patient has a hypotensive LES with a slip of the plicaiton and hiatal hernia leading to an elevated IRP.

Interestingly in the second example, the patient's IRP was not elevated.

References

1. Wills VL, Hunt DR. Dysphagia after antireflux surgery. Br J Surg. 2001;88:486–99.
2. Yadlapati R, Hungness ES, Pandolfino J. Complications of antireflux surgery. Am J Gastroenterol. 2018;113:1137–47.

3. Bell RCW, Barnes WE, Cater BJ, Sewell R, et al. Transoral incisionless fundoplication: 2-year results from prospective multicenter U.S. Study. Am Surg. 2014;80:1093–105.
4. Rinsma N, Smeets F, Bruls D, Kessing BF, et al. Effect of transoral incisionaless fundoplication on reflux mechanisms. Sug Endosc. 2014;28:941–9.
5. Trad KS. Transoral incisionless fundoplication: current status. Curr Opin Gastroenterol. 2016;32:338–43.
6. Pessauz P, Arnaud JP, Delatarre JF, et al. Laparoscopic antireflux surgery: five-year results and beyond in 1340 patients. Arch Surg. 2005;140:946–51.
7. Lin DC, Chun CL, Triadafilopoulos G. Evaluation and management of patients with symptoms after anti-reflux surgery. Dis Esophagus. 2015;28:1–10.
8. Soper NJ, Dunnegan D. Anatomic fundoplication failure after laparoscopic antireflux surgery. Ann Surg. 1999;299:669–77.
9. Herron DM, Swanstrom LL, Ramzi N, Hansen PD. Factors predictive of dysphagia after laparoscopic nissen fundoplication. Surg Endosc. 1999;13:1180–3.
10. Fein M, Seyfried F. Is there a role for anything other than a Nissen's operation? J Gastrointest Surg. 2010;14(Suppl 1):S67–74.
11. Broeders JAJL, Mauritz FA, Ahmed Ali U, et al. Systematic review and meta-analysis of laparoscopic Nissen versus Toupet fundoplication for gastro-oesophageal reflux disease. Br J Surg. 2010;97:1318–30.
12. Tan G, Yang Z, Wang Z. Meta-analysis of laparoscopic total versus posterior fundoplication for gastro-oesophageal reflux disease based on randomized clinical trials. ANZ J Surg. 2011;81:246–52.
13. Wo J, Trus T, Richardson WS, Hunter JG, et al. Evaluation and management of postfundoplication dysphagia. Am J Gastreoentol. 1996;91:2318–22.
14. Hunter JG, Smith CD, Branum GD, Waring JP, et al. Laparoscopic fundoplication failures: patterns of failure and response to fundoplication revision. Ann Surg. 1999;230:595–606.
15. Carbo AI, Kim RH, Gates T, D'Agostino HR. Imagins findings of successful and failed fundoplication. RadioGraphics. 2014;34:1873–84.
16. Baker M, Einstein D. Barium esophagram: does it have a role in gastroesophageal reflux disease? Gastroenterol Clin N Am. 2014;43:47–68.
17. Jailwala J, Massey B, Staff D, Shaker R, Hogan W. Post-fundoplication symptoms: the role for endoscopic assessment of fundoplication integrity. Gastrointest Endosc. 2001;54:351–6.
18. Weijenborg PW, Savarino E, Kessin BF, Roman S, et al. Normal values of esophageal motility after antireflux surgery; a study using high-resolution manometry. Neurogastroenterol Motil. 2015;27:929–35.
19. Wang YT, Tai LF, Yazaki E, Jafari J, et al. Investigation of dysphagia after antireflux surgery by high-resolution manometry: Impact of multiple

water swallows and a solid test meal on diagnosis, management and clinical outcome. Clin Gastroenterol. 2015;13:1575–83.
20. Peixoto A. Role of high resolution manometry in the diagnostic and therapeutic approach to post fundoplication dysphagia. Gastroenterol Hepatol. 2019;42:488–9.
21. Carlson DA, Kahrilas PJ, Ritter K, Lin Z, Pandolfino JE. Mechanisms of repetitive retrograde contractions in response to sustained esophageal distension: a study evaluating patients with postfundoplication dysphagia. Am J Physiol Gastrointest Liver Physiol. 2018;314:G334–40.
22. Marjoux S, Roman S, Juget-Pietu F, Robert M, et al. Impaired postoperative EGJ relaxation as a determinant of post laparoscopic fundoplication dysphagia: a study with high-resolution manometry before and after surgery. Surg Endosc. 2012;26:3642–9.
23. Yamamoto SR, Akimot S, Hoshino M, Mittal SK. High-resolution manometry findings in symptomatic post-Nissen fundoplication patients with normal endoscopic configuration. Dis Esophagus. 2016;29:967–70.
24. Scheffer RCH, Samsom M, Haverkamp A, Oors J, et al. Impaired bolus transit across the esophagogastric junction in postfundoplication dysphagia. Am J Gastroenterol. 2005;100:1677–84.
25. Genio G, Tolon S, Genio F, D'Allesandro A, et al. Impact of total fundoplication on esophageal transit; analysis of combined multichannel intraluminal impedance and manometry. J Clin Gastroenterol. 2012;46:e1–5.
26. Lindeboom MYA, Ringers J, Straathof WA, Van Rijn PJJ, et al. The effect of laparoscopic partial fundoplication on dysphagia, esophageal and lower esophageal sphincter motility. Dis Esophagus. 2007;20:63–8.
27. Yigit T, Quiroga E, Oelschlager B. Multichannel intraluminal impedance for the assessment of post-fundoplication dysphagia. Dis Esophagus. 2006;19:382–8.
28. Kwiatek M, Kahrilas P, Soper N, Bulsiewicz WJ. Esophagogastric junction distensibility after fundoplication assessed with a novel functional luminal imaging probe. J Gastrointest Surg. 2010;14:268–76.
29. Su B, Callahan Z, Kuchta K, Linn JG, et al. Use of impedence planimetry (Endoflip) in foregut surgery practice: experience in more than 400 cases. J Am Coll Surg. 2020;231:160–71.
30. Su B, Novak S, Callahan Z, Kuchta K, et al. Using impedance planimetry (EndoFLIP) in the operating room to assess gastroesophageal junction distensibility and predeict patient outcomes following fundoplication. Surg Endosc. 2020;34:1761–8.
31. Ayazi S, Zheng P, Zaidi A, Chovanec K, et al. Magnetic sphincter augmentation and postoperative dysphagia: characterization, clinical risk factors, and management. J Gastrointest Surg. 2020;24:39–49. https://doi.org/10.1007/s11605-019-04331-9.
32. Warren H, Reynolds J, Lipham J, Zehetner J, et al. Multi-institutional outcomes using magnetic sphincter augmentation verses Nissen

fundoplication for chronic gastroesophageal reflux disease. Surg Endosc. 2016;30:3289–96.

33. Tatum J, Alicuben E, Bildzukewicz N, Samakar K, et al. Removing the magnetic sphincter augmentation device: operative management and outcomes. Surg Endosc. 2019;33:2663–9. https://doi.org/10.1007/s00464-018-6544-y.
34. Asti E, Siboni S, Lazzari V, Bonitta G, et al. Removal of the magnetic sphincter augmentation device: Surgical technique and results in a single-center cohort study. Ann Surg. 2017;265:941–5.
35. Lipham JC, Taiganides PA, Louie BE, Ganz A, et al. Safety analysis of the first 1000 patients treated with magnetic sphincter augmentation for gastroesophageal reflux disease. Dis Esophagus. 2015;28:305–11.
36. Ayazi S, Chowdhury N, Zaidi A, Chovanec K, et al. Magnetic sphincter augmentation in patients with hiatal hernia: clinical outcome and patterns of recurrence. Surg Endosc. 2020;34:1835–46. https://doi.org/10.1007/s00464-019-06950-4.
37. Alicuben E, Bell R, Jobe B, Buckley FP III, et al. Worldwide experience with erosion of the magnetic sphincter augmentation device. J Gastrointest Surg. 2018;22:1442–7.
38. Bauer M, Meining A, Kranzfelder M, Jell A, et al. Endoluminal perforation of a magnetic antireflux device. Surg Endosc. 2015;29:3806–10. https://doi.org/10.1007/s00464-015-4145-6.
39. Salvador R, Costantini M, Capovilla G, Polese L, et al. Esophageal penetration of the magnetic sphincter device: history repeats itself. J Laparoendosc Adv Surg Tech A. 2017;27:834–8.
40. Riva C, Siboni S, Sozzi M, Lazzari V, et al. High-resolution manometry findings after LINX procedure for gastro-esophageal reflux disease. Neurogastroenterol Motil. 2020;32:e13750.
41. Warren H, Louie B, Farivar AS, Wilshire C, et al. Manometric changes to the lower esophageal sphincter after magnetic sphincter augmentation in patients with chronic gastroesophageal reflux disease. Ann Surg. 2017;266:99–104.

37 Persistent Dysphagia After Esophageal Myotomy

Alison Y. Haruta and Andrew S. Wright

Introduction

Achalasia is an esophageal motility disorder characterized by abnormal relaxation of the lower esophageal sphincter (LES) and lack of normal peristalsis of the esophagus. It is thought to be due to the loss of myenteric plexus ganglion cells at the distal esophagus and LES leading to unopposed excitatory signaling and thus abnormal sphincter relaxation. Clinically, most patients complain of dysphagia, reflux, regurgitation, chest pain, and epigastric pain. Occasionally, patients also experience odynophagia and respiratory symptoms. Recommended initial evaluation includes high-resolution manometry, upper endoscopy, and upper GI X-ray [1].

Achalasia is not curable at this time, so treatment is aimed at symptom relief. Management of primary achalasia is discussed in a previous chapter. Briefly, there are several interventions available including medical management (typically with smooth muscle relaxants), botulinum toxin injection, endoscopic pneumatic dilation, and myotomy [1]. Myotomy has become the standard

A. Y. Haruta · A. S. Wright (✉)
Department of Surgery, University of Washington, Seattle, WA, USA
e-mail: Awright2@uw.edu

A. D. Patel et al. (eds.), *The SAGES Manual of Physiologic Evaluation of Foregut Diseases*,
https://doi.org/10.1007/978-3-031-39199-6_37

treatment for appropriate surgical candidates, with superior long-term symptom relief compared to botulinum injection and with fewer interventions required than pneumatic dilation. Traditionally, myotomy was performed through thoracic or laparoscopic abdominal approaches (Heller myotomy) with or without addition of a fundoplication to reduce risk of post-procedural acid reflux. More recently, an endoscopic approach to myotomy has been developed and popularized (per-oral endoscopic myotomy, or POEM).

Persistent or recurrent dysphagia after intervention for achalasia occurs in about 5–15% of patients after laparoscopic myotomy [2]. Similar recurrence rates have been reported after POEM, though post-procedural reflux may be higher in this group [3]. The diagnosis and management of dysphagia following myotomy can be quite challenging and should be driven by the suspected cause of the recurrent or persistent symptoms.

Potential Etiologies of Persistent/Recurrent Dysphagia

The initial step in assessing patients with dysphagia following myotomy is determining the suspected etiology of symptoms. We first attempt to determine if the dysphagia is persistent (incomplete relief following myotomy) or recurrent (initial relief after myotomy with late development of symptoms). We define initial success of the initial operation based on whether a patient is able to eat a regular diet after the cessation of any post-operative dietary restrictions, which roughly corresponds with an Eckardt score of 3 or less. This suggests that the initial diagnosis of achalasia was correct and the myotomy relieved the symptoms at least temporarily.

Persistent dysphagia is often due to the underlying motility issues of the esophagus, as myotomy will release the LES obstruction but not affect the esophagus. Persistent symptoms are more common when the esophagus is significantly dilated and tortuous, especially when the esophagus has become so dilated that it has a sigmoid "megaesophagus" appearance.

An alternate cause of persistent dysphagia is misdiagnosis at the initial operation, with the true underlying issue being a different esophageal motility disorder such as ineffective esophageal motility, absent peristalsis, diffuse esophageal spasm, or nutcracker esophagus. Misdiagnosis can also be a missed secondary esophageal motility disorder due to systemic disease such as scleroderma causing "lead pipe" esophagus. Pseudo-achalasia can be the result of anatomic obstruction from various causes, such as esophago-gastric outlet obstruction from a para-esophageal hernia, malignancy, or reflux-induced peptic stricture at the LES. Pseudo-achalasia may also be seen following adjustable gastric band placement for obesity.

In our experience, the most common cause of both persistent and recurrent dysphagia is incomplete myotomy due to inadequate distal extension. Traditional surgical myotomy extends only 1–2 cm onto the stomach, and this is widely considered the most difficult part of the operation. The sling fibers of the LES complex actually extend 2–3 cm onto the gastric cardia, so inadequate distal myotomy can be common. We have previously shown that extension of the myotomy 3 cm onto the gastric cardia at index operation can significantly reduce the risk of persistent or recurrent dysphagia, from 17% to 3% [4], with significantly improved dysphagia and no increased risk of reflux in the extended myotomy group [5] at long-term follow-up.

Patients may also develop dysphagia due to functional obstruction due to prior fundoplication. This may be early dysphagia if the fundoplication was too tight at the time of the initial surgery, for example, in a patient who had a 360° Nissen fundoplication instead of a partial (Dor or Toupet) fundoplication. It can also present late, either due to a malformed wrap or migration of the wrap through a hiatal hernia. Occasionally, patients will develop a diverticulum at the site of a previous myotomy. The diverticulum itself can cause symptoms, and in our experience is typically associated with an inadequate distal myotomy. Rarely, patients may develop anatomic obstruction due to a de novo tumor arising after myotomy, potentially due to severe reflux causing Barrett's esophagus and eventual malignant transformation. Patients with achalasia also have an increased risk of development of a squamous esophageal cancer which can occur 10 years or more after primary treatment [1].

In our study of 43 patients requiring surgery for recurrent or persistent dysphagia after myotomy, 93% of patients were found to have an inadequate distal myotomy as the cause of their symptoms [6], with the remainder having technical issues with the prior fundoplication as the source. We found no incidence of peptic strictures or reflux-induced fibrosis in our series, perhaps because of liberal use of anti-reflux fundoplication or routine PPI use. In contrast, in a similar series of 34 patients, Smith et al. [7] found the source of dysphagia following myotomy was periesophageal/perihiatal fibrosis in 27%, obstructing fundoplication in 27%, incomplete myotomy in 20%, progression of disease in 22%, and epiphrenic diverticulum in 2%. Four patients in that series were thought to have multi-factorial issues.

Evaluation of Persistent/Recurrent Dysphagia

Evaluation of persistent/recurrent dysphagia aims to identify the underlying cause to target appropriate treatment. It should include review of the patient's presenting history and initial pre-operative studies to look for clues for an alternate diagnosis. Review of the index operative report is also important to assess for approach (laparoscopic vs thoracoscopic vs endoscopic), length of myotomy, intraoperative difficulties, areas of potential scarring, or post-operative complications that may point to a cause for dysphagia.

Repeat studies typically include upper endoscopy, manometry, and UGI series. High-resolution impedance planimetry (endoluminal functional lumen imaging probe or Endoflip, Medtronic, Minneapolis, MN) may also be used as an adjunct to evaluate the LES. Upper endoscopy can assess the previous myotomy by evaluating if the LES appears visibly closed, likely indicative of inadequate prior myotomy. It will also be able to evaluate for the presence of obstructing lesions/tumors, strictures, esophagitis, degree of esophageal dilation, diverticula, and degree of angulation or narrowing from prior fundoplication. While concurrent dilation can be performed, we often perform a diagnostic EGD 1st and then if indicated will bring the patient back for therapeutic endoscopy at a later date.

We repeat esophageal manometry in all patients in order to confirm the diagnosis and evaluate for adequacy of the myotomy or presence of an alternate motility disorder. Some authors recommend routine pH testing; however, in our experience, this is not typically helpful for dysphagia unless reflux-induced stricture is suspected. Notably, pH monitoring can be difficult to interpret in patients with achalasia as fermentation from stasis within the esophagus stasis may lead to false positives [8]. We therefore perform pH testing only selectively.

Upper GI series can more fully evaluate the location and extent of obstruction and degree of esophageal dilation, as well as look for presence of diverticula. UGI can also observe the dynamics of the LES with swallowing. It can also be used to predict success of a repeat operation based on the esophageal anatomy, with the lowest success rates in those with a sigmoid-shaped esophagus [6]. A timed barium swallow can add additional information compared to a traditional barium swallow. A conversation with the radiology team prior to the study can be helpful.

Clinical findings that should raise suspicion for underlying malignancy include short duration of symptoms <6 months, age of presentation >60, and rapid weight loss. EUS with biopsy may be helpful in these settings, especially if a submucosal tumor or tumor outside of the esophagus is suspected. CT of the chest and abdomen can be helpful if there is any concern for extrinsic compression or malignancy. CT may also be needed in the presence of diverticulum to confirm that it is a pulsion rather than traction diverticulum.

Management Algorithm for Persistent/Recurrent Achalasia

Perhaps, the most common cause of post-myotomy dysphagia is the underlying esophageal dysmotility which cannot be corrected by myotomy. This is especially the case when the esophagus is tortuous or sigmoid, which delays esophageal emptying. Fortunately, these symptoms are often mild in comparison to the initial presenting dysphagia which is partially relieved by the myotomy. In this situation, additional interventions directed to the LES are not likely to help, assuming adequate myotomy. This type of mild persistent dysphagia is typically manageable with dietary and lifestyle changes. These modifications include eating more slowly, chewing well, not eating within a few hours of lying down, and sleeping on a wedge. Some patients with a severely dilated sigmoid esophagus at the initial operation will continue to have severe PO intolerance and dysphagia and/or regurgitation even after adequate myotomy, due to anatomic distortion and stasis within the dilated esophagus. Rarely, this may require esophagectomy, as discussed below.

Some patients will have had an incorrect diagnosis before the index procedure. In these patients, treatment should be directed at the true underlying cause of dysphagia such as dysmotility (DES, Jackhammer esophagus, pseudo-achalasia, etc.)

For the majority of patients with moderate to severe persistent dysphagia, we suspect an incomplete myotomy. In these patients, we typically start with dilation. It is common that patients referred to surgery for possible redo operation have only had Savary or through-the-scope dilation. This is typically inadequate, so we recommend pneumatic dilation to 30 or 35 mm, which can be repeated if necessary. In our series of series of 115 pts with achalasia treated with laparoscopic myotomy, 12 patients required additional intervention for dysphagia and eight of these were managed with dilation alone [5]. In this series, only four patients went on to need additional surgery.

In patients with suspected incomplete myotomy who do not improve with pneumatic dilation, our preferred intervention is repeat myotomy. We previously recommended redo laparoscopic Heller myotomy as this approach gives the best access to the cardia where the prior myotomy most likely was inadequate. However, with the advent of POEM, we now recommend endoscopic myotomy if initial Heller myotomy failed and there is no concern for wrap issues or angulation due to herniation. This approach allows repeat myotomy while avoiding a re-operative abdomen. Additionally, in most redo patients, a wrap has already been performed with the initial Heller myotomy, limiting the acid reflux which is the main drawback of primary POEM. If POEM is not feasible, redo Heller myotomy remains a safe and effective treatment.

If other surgical issues are found on work up, such as a malformed or tight wrap, interventions should target the cause. In these cases, a redo laparoscopic operation should be performed to takedown and redo the wrap. If the patient has a new/recurrent PEH, it should be repaired as a possible cause of the recurrent dysphagia. In some cases, the dysphagia may be multifactorial requiring wrap takedown and PEH repair as well as myotomy extension. As previously noted, reflux in itself is a rare cause of recurrent/persistent dysphagia though if a peptic stricture is found to be the cause, PPIs and lifestyle modifications to reduce acid reflux should also be implemented. Dilation may also be helpful in these patients.

While some authors recommend esophagectomy as the main treatment for persistent dysphagia [9, 10], we feel that esophagectomy should be reserved for refractory cases of recurrent/persistent dysphagia who have failed repeat interventions, are not amenable to redo myotomy, or suffer an esophageal injury during attempted repeat myotomy that cannot be repaired safely. Patients who have a dilated and tortuous esophagus are more likely to have recurrent/persistent dysphagia, though these factors do not automatically make them poor candidates for redo myotomy. Many patients with megaesophagus will respond well to Heller myotomy [6, 11], and therefore, we will almost always try a myotomy first and reserve esophagectomy only for treatment failure after repeat myotomy. If patients continue to have ongoing symptoms and esophagectomy is pursued after myotomy, we recommend a thoracic approach for the dissection of the thoracic esophagus under direct vision, as opposed to a transhiatal approach, as in this setting, the esophagus is prone to large venous collaterals in the mediastinum due to prior inflammation.

Operative Approach to Redo Laparoscopic Heller Myotomy

We prefer a laparoscopic approach to a thoracic or thoracoscopic approach because it allows better visualization of the gastric cardia and extension of the myotomy 2–3 cm onto the stomach. The first portion of the operation involves dissection of the distal esophagus away from adhesions to the liver, diaphragm, and mediastinum. We then encircle the esophagus with a penrose drain and mobilize the distal esophagus well into the chest, straightening it out as much as possible. This can be especially important in patients with tortuous, dilated, or sigmoid esophagus. We then completely undo any previous fundoplication. This dissection can be difficult and of high risk, as the esophageal myotomy is often stuck to surrounding structures and the wall of the esophagus is already quite thin, consisting of only the mucosa and submucosa. We find that a lighted bougie (Innervision → TransIllumination System, Diversatek Healthcare) can be helpful in identifying the layers of the esophagus and facilitates this dissection.

After the dissection is complete, we then identify the old myotomy. Again, the lighted bougie can be quite helpful here. Most commonly, we do not attempt to lengthen the original myotomy, but instead start a new myotomy at least 90° away on the lateral esophagus. This allows us to work in a fresh, unscarred plane. We extend the myotomy at least 3 cm onto the gastric cardia. We prefer to do this on the patient right of the esophagus and stomach, because if the patient eventually requires salvage esophagectomy we want to preserve the fundus for the gastric conduit. We routinely then perform an intra-operative endoscopy in order to check the myotomy and confirm no inadvertent full thickness injury.

We perform a new fundoplication in only a minority of redo cases because we want to minimize anything that might be a new cause of dysphagia. Often in these patients, the esophagus is very dilated and a new fundoplication risks angulation. We will only do a new fundoplication in patients in which the esophagus is not dilated. We will typically perform a Toupet fundoplication with the exception of patients in whom we have to repair an inadvertent full thickness injury which we cover with a Dor anterior fundoplication.

Outcomes of Intervention for Recurrent/ Persistent Dysphagia

Initial Heller myotomy for achalasia has about a 90% success rate at 5-year follow-up [5, 8]. For those with recurrent/persistent dysphagia, retrospective studies and a meta-analysis have looked at success rates for repeat interventions with either pneumatic dilation, redo Heller myotomy, or POEM, though no randomized control studies were found. Pneumatic dilation was shown in several reviews to have short-term success rates up to 90%, though effectiveness decreased with time to a 64% success rate at 3 years [12]. Pneumatic dilation can therefore be an effective first-line treatment, can be repeated if necessary, and does not preclude other surgical or endoscopic treatments. In our series of 115 patients after Heller myotomy, 12 required pneumatic dilation which was successful in eight, leaving only four patients that needed redo surgery [5].

We have previously reported a series of 43 patients who required redo laparoscopic myotomy between 1994 and 2011 and found that 79% of patients reported an improvement in symptoms at median follow-up of 63 months [6]. Median satisfaction after the redo myotomy was 7 on a 10-point Likert scale. Post-surgical symptoms correlated closely with findings on pre-operative UGI. All patients with minimal to mild esophageal dilation improved, as did 75% of those with moderate dilation. One patient with moderate dilation had severe recalcitrant symptoms but was felt to be too frail for esophagectomy and was managed with G-tube placement for enteral nutrition. Of the six patients in the study with sigmoid mega-esophagus, results were dichotomous, two had complete relief while four patients had no relief of symptoms. All four of those patients went on to have esophagectomy for refractory/recurrent symptoms. In a similar series of 34 patients undergoing re-operative surgery for post-myotomy dysphagia from the University of South Florida, 75% of patients had symptom improvement [7].

Redo surgical myotomy can be very technically challenging and should only be attempted by experienced foregut surgeons. In our series of 43 patients, we had two intra-operative esophageal perforations, both of which were recognized, repaired, and covered with a Dor anterior fundoplication. There were no late complications. In the Smith et al series of 34 patients [7] (37 operations), there was a 10% rate of peri-operative complications with seven patients having major complications (septic shock secondary to esophageal perforation, mediastinitis, pneumonia, incarcerated umbilical hernia, ventral hernia, postoperative leak, and pleural effusion). One patient could not be weaned off the ventilator and died on comfort measures.

Case series at several institutions have so far shown good success of POEM after failure of Heller myotomy [12, 13]. In one series, Zhou et al. performed POEM after failed surgical myotomy in 12 patients and had success in 11/12, with a mean Eckardt score decreasing from 9.2 to 1.3, and mean LES pressure improving from 29.4 to 13.5 mmHg [14]. One patient in that series developed GERD symptoms requiring medical treatment. Fumagalli et al. have reported a case series of 15 patients requiring repeat myotomy, nine performed surgically and six endoscopically [15]. Procedure time and length of stay was slightly longer in the surgical group. Seven of the nine surgical patients and all of the POEM patients improved to an Eckardt score <3, with shorter follow-up in the endoscopic group. While these studies are promising for the role of POEM after failed myotomy, there is significant risk of selection bias and the number of reported cases is low, so the role of POEM in this setting remains unclear.

Because POEM is relatively new, outcomes of repeat intervention following failed POEM are still unclear. Li et al. have reported a series of 15 patients who underwent repeat POEM, claiming therapeutic success in all patients but with 33% clinical reflux after repeat POEM [16]. In a large multi-national study of 441 patients across three hospitals in the Netherlands, Germany, and the US, 8% of patients after POEM required retreatment [17]. Pneumatic dilation was tried in 15 patients and only successful in

20%. Redo POEM was performed in eight patients with 63% success, and laparoscopic Heller myotomy was performed in 11 patients with 45% success. Again, the effect of selection bias and small numbers makes it difficult to make definitive recommendations regarding choice between Heller myotomy and redo POEM for failed initial POEM.

Summary

Achalasia is a rare disease that leads to impaired quality of life and sometimes life-threatening complications. In the case of persistent or recurrent dysphagia, a thorough history and accurate work up is important to establish the diagnosis and suspected etiology of the patient's symptoms. Treatment can then be directed at the suspected underlying cause. Dilation alone is sufficient in some cases of persistent or recurrent dysphagia, but occasionally more aggressive interventions are needed. While redo myotomy is still recommended in cases due to incomplete myotomy, the demonstration of POEM as a safe and effective alternative to surgical myotomy provides a new endoscopic alternative to surgical myotomy which avoids the prior surgical plane and may avoid some of the morbidity of an operation. Surgical approaches are still needed if there are anatomic issues contributing to dysphagia, such as hiatal hernia or a slipped, malformed, or too-tight fundoplication. Esophagectomy should be reserved for refractory cases due to the higher morbidity and mortality compared to redo Heller myotomy or redo endoscopic myotomy.

References

1. Zaninotto G, Bennett C, Boeckxstaens G, Costantini M, Ferguson MK, Pandolfino JE, Patti MG, Ribeiro U Jr, Richter J, Swanstrom L, Tack J, Triadafilopoulos G, Markar SR, Salvador R, Faccio L, Andreollo NA, Cecconello I, Costamagna G, da Rocha JRM, Hungness ES, Fisichella PM, Fuchs KH, Gockel I, Gurski R, Gyawali CP, Herbella FAM, Holloway RH, Hongo M, Jobe BA, Kahrilas PJ, Katzka DA, Dua KS, Liu D, Moonen A, Nasi A, Pasricha PJ, Penagini R, Perretta S, Sallum RAA,

Sarnelli G, Savarino E, Schlottmann F, Sifrim D, Soper N, Tatum RP, Vaezi MF, van Herwaarden-Lindeboom M, Vanuytsel T, Vela MF, Watson DI, Zerbib F, Gittens S, Pontillo C, Vermigli S, Inama D, Low DE. The 2018 ISDE achalasia guidelines. Dis Esophagus. 2018;31(9):71. https://doi.org/10.1093/dote/doy071. PMID: 30169645.
2. Chen Z, Bessell JR, Chew A, et al. Laparoscopic cardiomyotomy for achalasia: clinical outcomes beyond 5 years. J Gastrointest Surg. 2010;14:594–600.
3. Werner YB, Hakanson B, Martinek J, et al. Endoscopic or surgical myotomy in patients with idiopathic achalasia. N Engl J Med. 2019;381:2219–29.
4. Oelschlager BK, Chang L, Pellegrini CA. Improved out-come after extended gastric myotomy for achalasia. Arch Surg. 2003;138:490–5.
5. Wright AS, Williams CW, Pellegrini CA, Oelschlager BK. Long-term outcomes confirm the superior efficacy of extended Heller myotomy with Toupet fundoplication for achalasia. Surg Endosc. 2007;21:713–8.
6. Loviscek MF, Wright AS, Hinojosa MW, Petersen R, Pajitnov D, Oelschlager BK, Pellegrini CA. Recurrent dysphagia after Heller myotomy: is esophagectomy always the answer? J Am Coll Surg. 2013;216(4):736–43.
7. Smith KE, Saad AR, Hanna JP, et al. Revisional surgery in patients with recurrent dysphagia after heller myotomy. J Gastrointest Surg. 2020;24:991–9. https://doi.org/10.1007/s11605-019-04264-3.
8. Patti MG, Diener U, Milena D. Esophageal achalasia: preoperative assessment and postoperative follow-up. J Gastrointest Surg. 2001;5:11–2.
9. Orringer MB, Stirling MC. Esophageal resection for achalasia: indications and results. Ann Thorac Surg. 1989;47(3):340–5. https://doi.org/10.1016/0003-4975(89)90369-x. PMID: 2649031.
10. Aiolfi A, Asti E, Bonitta G, Siboni S, Bonavina L. Esophageal resection for end-stage achalasia. Am Surg. 2018;84(4):506–11. PMID: 29712597.
11. Sweet MP, Nipomnick I, Gasper WJ, et al. The outcome of laparoscopic Heller myotomy for achalasia is not influenced by the degree of esophageal dilatation. J Gastrointest Surg. 2008;12:159–65.
12. Fernandez-Ananin S, Fernández AF, Balagué C, Sacoto D, Targarona EM. What to do when Heller's myotomy fails? Pneumatic dilatation, laparoscopic remyotomy or peroral endoscopic myotomy: a systematic review. J Minim Access Surg. 2018;14(3):177–84. https://doi.org/10.4103/jmas.JMAS_94_17. PMID: 29319024; PMCID: PMC6001296.
13. Vigneswaran Y, Yetasook AK, Zhao JC, Denham W, Linn JG, Ujiki MB, et al. Peroral endoscopic myotomy (POEM): feasible as reoperation following Heller myotomy. J Gastrointest Surg. 2014;18:1071–6.

14. Zhou PH, Li QL, Yao LQ, Xu MD, Chen WF, Cai MY, et al. Peroral endoscopic remyotomy for failed Heller myotomy: a prospective single-center study. Endoscopy. 2013;45:161–6.
15. Fumagalli U, Rosati R, De Pascale S, Porta M, Carlani E, Pestalozza A, Repici A. Repeated surgical or endoscopic myotomy for recurrent dysphagia in patients after previous myotomy for achalasia. J Gastrointest Surg. 2016;20(3):494–9. https://doi.org/10.1007/s11605-015-3031-9. Epub 2015 Nov 20. PMID: 26589525.
16. Li QL, Yao LQ, Xu XY, Zhu JY, Xu MD, Zhang YQ, Chen WF, Zhou PH. Repeat peroral endoscopic myotomy: a salvage option for persistent/recurrent symptoms. Endoscopy. 2016;48(2):134–40. https://doi.org/10.1055/s-0034-1393095. Epub 2015 Sep 8. PMID: 26349067.
17. van Hoeij FB, Ponds FA, Werner Y, Sternbach JM, Fockens P, Bastiaansen BA, Smout AJPM, Pandolfino JE, Rösch T, Bredenoord AJ. Management of recurrent symptoms after per-oral endoscopic myotomy in achalasia. Gastrointest Endosc. 2018;87(1):95–101. https://doi.org/10.1016/j.gie.2017.04.036. Epub 2017 May 3. PMID: 28478028.

Recurrent Reflux After Prior Fundoplication

38

Tanuja Damani and Justin Henning

Introduction

Fundoplication was first described by Rudolph Nissen in 1956 as an antireflux operation. The advent of laparoscopic surgery in 1991 led to an exponential increase in the number of patients undergoing fundoplications to treat severe and/or refractory gastroesophageal reflux disease. Excellent symptomatic and functional results with patient satisfaction rates of 85–96% after fundoplication have been demonstrated by several studies [1–3].

Fundoplication failure rates of 3–30% have been reported in the literature [1, 3–7]. There is no standard definition of what constitutes failure of antireflux surgery. It may be defined subjectively as return of symptoms, resumption of antacids, and patient dissatisfaction. It may be objective with evidence of anatomic or

T. Damani (✉)
NYU Grossman School of Medicine, New York, NY, USA

Center for Esophageal Health, NYU Langone Health, New York, NY, USA
e-mail: Tanuja.damani@nyulangone.org

J. Henning
Center for Esophageal Health, NYU Langone Health, New York, NY, USA

NYU Langone Health, New York, NY, USA

A. D. Patel et al. (eds.), *The SAGES Manual of Physiologic Evaluation of Foregut Diseases*,
https://doi.org/10.1007/978-3-031-39199-6_38

physiologic failure of antireflux barrier with recurrent hiatal hernias, wrap disruption, and/or recurrent reflux disease. Failure of a fundoplication has been attributed to one of the following causes: wrong indications for the operation, wrong preoperative work-up, and failure to execute the proper technical steps [8]. Failure to recognize esophageal shortening and failure of crural repair either from excessive tension or weak crural pillars without preservation of the peritoneal lining are the two commonly identified technical failures. Errors in construction of fundoplication, injury to the vagus nerves causing gastroparesis, and pseudoachalasia after a tight Nissen fundoplication would be other anatomic causes of failure. There are also patient-specific factors that can contribute to surgical failure including morbid obesity, atypical symptoms, lack of response to medications, chronic coughing, retching, preoperative poor esophageal peristalsis, larger hiatal hernia, female gender, or age older than 50 years [9–12].

Early symptoms after primary fundoplication can include transient bloating and mild dysphagia, and they typically improve in the first six weeks. Other chronic symptoms such as those of gas bloat can be managed conservatively. Mild recurrent typical or atypical symptoms of reflux can be managed nonoperatively; however, revisional surgery is needed in 3–6% of patients [5, 6]. The most common indications for reoperation after a primary fundoplication are recurrent reflux with symptoms of heartburn and regurgitation, paraesophageal hernia usually with wrap herniation or disruption, and dysphagia [4, 5, 7, 13, 14].

Diagnostic Work-Up

A thorough evaluation is required in patients with recurrent symptoms after antireflux surgery. A careful review of a patient's original symptoms before the primary antireflux operation, symptom improvement after surgery, previous response to medical therapy, and prior test results is important to identify an underlying esophageal motility disorder or undiagnosed gastrointestinal disorder.

Review of the operative report is critical with attention to specific technical details regarding esophageal dissection and length, identification and preservation of the vagus nerves, type of crural repair, division of short gastric vessels, use and size of bougie during fundoplication, and technique used for fundoplication. Assessment of patient's body mass index prior to the initial surgery and any significant weight gain since is important in deciding the kind of revisional operation after a failed antireflux surgery.

A comprehensive diagnostic work-up is essential for recurrent symptoms after fundoplication and should include esophagogastroduodenoscopy (EGD), barium esophagram, pH testing, and esophageal manometry. A nuclear medicine gastric emptying study should be strongly considered and is essential for symptoms of nausea, bloating, or vomiting. Recent studies also suggest possible utility of Functional Lumen Imaging Probe (FLIP) in some patients with symptoms post-fundoplication to assess GE junction distensibility, although further evidence is needed [15].

EGD

Endoscopic assessment of the failed fundoplication is instrumental in diagnosis and surgical management. A thorough endoscopic evaluation noting esophageal dilation, evidence of esophagitis or Barrett's, the gastroesophageal junction and its relation to fundoplication, ease of traversing the fundoplication, crural impression, symmetry and competence of fundoplication, and evidence of recurrent hiatal hernia is important [16]. Recognition of the type of failure, (disruption, herniation, slippage, and twisting) of fundoplication on retroflexion views is important for management planning (Fig. 38.1).

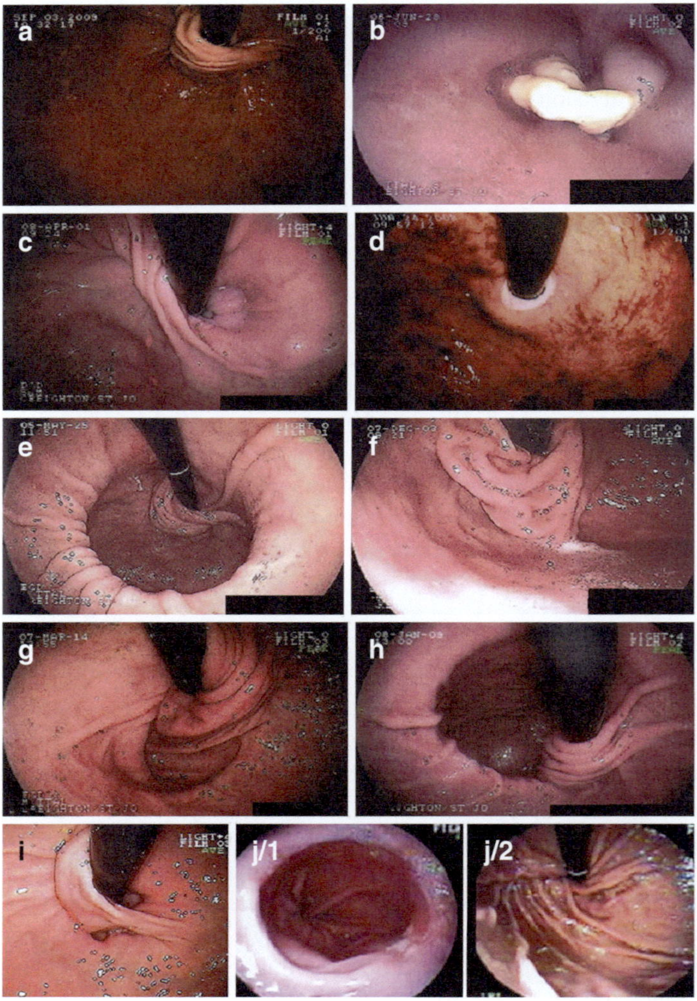

Fig. 38.1 Endoscopic views of main alterations after a failed fundoplication. (**a**) normal fundoplication; (**b**) mesh erosion; (**c**) partially disrupted fundoplication; (**d**) near completely disrupted fundoplication; (**e**) recurrent hiatal hernia with intrathoracic fundoplication; (**f**) slipped fundoplication; (**g**) twisted fundoplication; (**h**) two-compartment stomach; (**i**) partially disrupted fundoplication with recurrent paraesophageal hernia; (**j**) slipped fundoplication (*J*/1: antegrade view; *J*/2: retroflexed view). (*From* Juhasz A, Sundaram A, Hoshino M, Lee TH, Filipi CJ, Mittal SM. Endoscopic assessment of failed fundoplication: A case for standardization. Surg Endosc 2011;25:2761-66; with permission)

Barium Esophagram

Esophagram gives excellent anatomic delineation of the gastroesophageal junction and can show hiatal/paraesophageal hernia, and causes of failure such as intrathoracic migration, and slipped, disrupted or malpositioned wrap. Several patterns of recurrence have been described [17, 18] (Fig. 38.2). pH testing and manometry may not be absolutely necessary when there is a clear anatomic failure noted on barium esophagram, explaining the patient's symptoms.

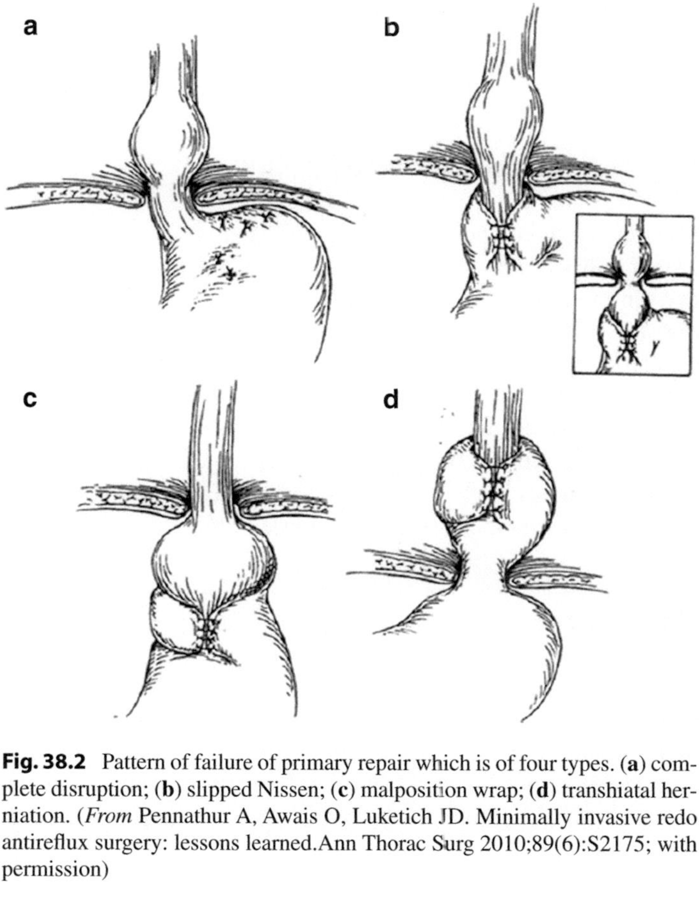

Fig. 38.2 Pattern of failure of primary repair which is of four types. (**a**) complete disruption; (**b**) slipped Nissen; (**c**) malposition wrap; (**d**) transhiatal herniation. (*From* Pennathur A, Awais O, Luketich JD. Minimally invasive redo antireflux surgery: lessons learned.Ann Thorac Surg 2010;89(6):S2175; with permission)

Ambulatory pH Monitoring

Symptoms of heartburn after a fundoplication are assumed to be due to failure of surgery, and acid suppressing medications are often prescribed. However, several studies have shown that when patients with recurrent heartburn are tested by ambulatory pH monitoring, pathologic esophageal acid exposure is present in only 23–39% [19–21]. Normal results on pH testing may point to a diagnosis of functional heartburn or non-acidic reflux that may require additional testing with multichannel impedance pH. Documentation of recurrent reflux with objective evidence should be obtained prior to any revisional anti-reflux surgery, especially in the absence of an anatomic failure on upper endoscopy or esophagram.

High-Resolution Manometry (HRM)

Manometry should be performed in all cases of recurrent or persistent reflux to rule out underlying esophageal motility disorder, even in the absence of significant dysphagia. It has been shown that 1.2% of patients who fail anti-reflux surgery actually carry achalasia as a primary diagnosis [5]. In addition to providing valuable information about esophageal peristalsis and pressure and relaxation of the lower esophageal sphincter, some studies have also shown the presence of a dual high-pressure zone on HRM in patients after fundoplication to be a strong predictor of recurrent gastroesophageal reflux disease [22].

Management

Transthoracic herniation of the wrap, essentially a recurrent hiatal hernia, has been reported to be the most common cause of failure of a prior antireflux operation, followed by wrap disruption [5, 7, 23]. Two well-recognized factors potentially playing a role in recurrent hiatal hernia are short esophagus creating longitudinal tension on the fundoplication and mode of crural closure. A short esophagus has been identified in about 40% of patients in a large series of patients that underwent reoperative antireflux surgery [23].

Satisfaction rates after revisional antireflux surgery are lower than primary surgery but still remain high at about 80% in most studies [23–25]. Similarly, objective outcomes assessed by normal acid exposure on pH monitoring and lack of esophagitis on endoscopy are noted to be about 80% after reoperative antireflux surgery [5, 23, 25]. It is important to note that positive outcomes have been shown to decrease by approximately 20% with each redo operation, partly due to the higher failure rate associated with each subsequent redo operation [7, 25]. Also intraoperative and postoperative complication rates are higher with revisional antireflux surgery as expected, reported in the range of 15–20% with laparoscopic surgery [5]. The most common intraoperative complication rates reported in large studies are esophageal or gastric injury followed by pneumothorax, hemorrhage, and splenectomy. The most frequent postoperative complications reported are infectious, pulmonary, and cardiac complications. Recent data using the robotic approach for reoperative antireflux surgery have shown a much lower complication rate as well as length of stay compared to the laparoscopic cohorts, hypothesized to be due to improved ergonomics and visualization [26].

The typical approach to reoperative antireflux surgery is a minimally invasive transabdominal approach. Occasionally, if there have been multiple prior abdominal operations and concern for a hostile abdomen, then a transthoracic approach may be indicated. Significant adhesions around the hiatus are typically encountered during revisional hiatal surgery, and care must be taken to avoid injury to the esophagus or stomach. A complete hernia sac dissection and reduction should be performed. It is important to completely take down the prior fundoplication with the fundus returned to its normal position and restoration of the normal anatomy. Once normal anatomy has been re-established, assessing the intra-abdominal esophageal length is critical. There should be 2.5–3 cm of tension-free intra-abdominal esophagus with complete circumferential mobilization in the mediastinum. If this is not successful, a Collis gastroplasty should be performed. Recent studies reviewing robotic approaches to paraesophageal hernia repair have shown an exceedingly low rate of a Collis gastroplasty, hypothesized to be secondary to extensive mediastinal dissection and esophageal mobilization facilitated by the robotic approach [27].

Crural repair is then undertaken and should be performed with permanent braided sutures on robust crural pillars with preserved peritoneum. If the closure requires more than 3 sutures, there is any tension on the closure, or the crural pillars are attenuated or devoid of peritoneum, then an absorbable synthetic mesh should be used to reinforce the repair, as it has been shown to be associated with lower anatomic recurrence rates [28]. The fundus is then delivered posterior to the stomach and a floppy Nissen or Toupet fundoplication performed on the distal esophagus.

In patients with BMI greater than 35, a Roux-en-Y gastric bypass (RYGB) is considered the preferred operation in both resolving GERD as well as managing morbid obesity and associated comorbidities. A RYGB effectively ameliorates GERD by diverting the flow of acid and bile away from the esophagus, and avoids the potential for dysphagia from an esophageal outflow obstruction as may occur with a reoperative fundoplication. Roux-en-Y reconstruction with a smaller pouch containing only gastric cardia to eliminate any parietal cell mass and thus acid production has also been shown to have superior symptom outcomes in patients with two or more previous antireflux surgeries, esophageal dysmotility and delayed gastric emptying [29, 30].

There are some small studies showing favorable subjective outcomes after radiofrequency energy delivery to the lower esophageal sphincter (Stretta) in patients with failed fundoplication without herniation as a minimally invasive alternative to revisional antireflux surgery or PPI dependence [31, 32]. Transoral fundoplication has also been reported in small series of similar patients with failed fundoplication without herniation with symptomatic improvement of GERD [33]. While both these endoscopic options do not have the associated morbidity of a revisional operation, more robust studies are needed prior to recommending these options for recurrent reflux after failed fundoplication.

Summary

Fundoplication has a high success rate in patients with gastroesophageal reflux disease. Recurrent reflux after fundoplication can be secondary to a variety of patient and technical factors. A thorough patient evaluation and work-up is essential before proceeding with revisional antireflux surgery. Attention to technical details during reoperative surgery, especially short esophagus and crural closure, is essential. Reoperative antireflux surgery has high patient satisfaction rates, albeit inferior to those of primary surgery, with a higher complication rate. Overall excellent outcomes have been reported in high-volume surgeons and with robotic approach. Conversion to RNY anatomy should be performed in patients with multiple failed reoperative antireflux surgeries or those with morbid obesity.

References

1. Dallemagne B, et al. Clinical results of laparoscopic fundoplication at ten years after surgery. Surg Endosc. 2006;20(1):159–65.
2. Kellokumpu I, et al. Quality of life following laparoscopic Nissen fundoplication: assessing short-term and long-term outcomes. World J Gastroenterol. 2013;19(24):3810–8.
3. Lafullarde T, et al. Laparoscopic Nissen fundoplication: five-year results and beyond. Arch Surg. 2001;136(2):180–4.
4. Carlson MA, Frantzides CT. Complications and results of primary minimally invasive antireflux procedures: a review of 10,735 reported cases. J Am Coll Surg. 2001;193(4):428–39.
5. Furnee EJ, et al. Surgical reintervention after failed antireflux surgery: a systematic review of the literature. J Gastrointest Surg. 2009;13(8):1539–49.
6. Hunter JG, et al. Laparoscopic fundoplication failures: patterns of failure and response to fundoplication revision. Ann Surg. 1999;230(4):595–604; discussion 604-6.

7. Smith CD, et al. When fundoplication fails: redo? Ann Surg. 2005;241(6):861–9; discussion 869-71.
8. Patti MG, Allaix ME, Fisichella PM. Analysis of the causes of failed antireflux surgery and the principles of treatment: a review. JAMA Surg. 2015;150(6):585–90.
9. Broeders JA, et al. Predictors of objectively identified recurrent reflux after primary Nissen fundoplication. Br J Surg. 2011;98(5):673–9.
10. Jackson PG, et al. Predictors of outcome in 100 consecutive laparoscopic antireflux procedures. Am J Surg. 2001;181(3):231–5.
11. Morgenthal CB, et al. Who will fail laparoscopic Nissen fundoplication? Preoperative prediction of long-term outcomes. Surg Endosc. 2007;21(11):1978–84.
12. Power C, Maguire D, McAnena O. Factors contributing to failure of laparoscopic Nissen fundoplication and the predictive value of preoperative assessment. Am J Surg. 2004;187(4):457–63.
13. Dallemagne B, et al. Long-term results after laparoscopic reoperation for failed antireflux procedures. Br J Surg. 2011;98(11):1581–7.
14. van Beek DB, Auyang ED, Soper NJ. A comprehensive review of laparoscopic redo fundoplication. Surg Endosc. 2011;25(3):706–12.
15. Carlson DA, Hirano I. Application of the functional lumen imaging probe to esophageal disorders. Curr Treat Options Gastroenterol. 2017;15(1):10–25.
16. Juhasz A, et al. Endoscopic assessment of failed fundoplication: a case for standardization. Surg Endosc. 2011;25(12):3761–6.
17. Hinder RA, et al. Management of the failed antireflux operation. Surg Clin North Am. 1997;77(5):1083–98.
18. Pennathur A, Awais O, Luketich JD. Minimally invasive redo antireflux surgery: lessons learned. Ann Thorac Surg. 2010;89(6):S2174–9.
19. Galvani C, et al. Symptoms are a poor indicator of reflux status after fundoplication for gastroesophageal reflux disease: role of esophageal functions tests. Arch Surg. 2003;138(5):514–8; discussion 518-9.
20. Lord RV, et al. Absence of gastroesophageal reflux disease in a majority of patients taking acid suppression medications after Nissen fundoplication. J Gastrointest Surg. 2002;6(1):3–9. discussion 10
21. Thompson SK, et al. Recurrent heartburn after laparoscopic fundoplication is not always recurrent reflux. J Gastrointest Surg. 2007;11(5):642–7.
22. Tatum RP, et al. High-resolution manometry in evaluation of factors responsible for fundoplication failure. J Am Coll Surg. 2010;210(5):611–7, 617-9.
23. Awais O, et al. Reoperative antireflux surgery for failed fundoplication: an analysis of outcomes in 275 patients. Ann Thorac Surg. 2011;92(3):1083–9; discussion 1089-90.
24. Coelho JC, et al. Late laparoscopic reoperation of failed antireflux procedures. Surg Laparosc Endosc Percutan Tech. 2004;14(3):113–7.

25. Khajanchee YS, et al. Laparoscopic reintervention for failed antireflux surgery: subjective and objective outcomes in 176 consecutive patients. Arch Surg. 2007;142(8):785–901; discussion 791-2.
26. Elmously A, et al. Robotic reoperative anti-reflux surgery: low perioperative morbidity and high symptom resolution. World J Surg. 2018;42(12):4014–21.
27. Gerull WD, et al. Robotic approach to paraesophageal hernia repair results in low long-term recurrence rate and beneficial patient-centered outcomes. J Am Coll Surg. 2020;231(5):520–6.
28. Abdelmoaty WF, et al. Combination of surgical technique and bioresorbable mesh reinforcement of the crural repair leads to low early hernia recurrence rates with laparoscopic paraesophageal hernia repair. J Gastrointest Surg. 2020;24(7):1477–81.
29. Yamamoto SR, et al. Long-term outcomes of reintervention for failed fundoplication: redo fundoplication versus Roux-en-Y reconstruction. Surg Endosc. 2014;28(1):42–8.
30. Weber CE, et al. Roux-en-Y gastric bypass as a salvage procedure in complicated patients with failed fundoplication(s). Surg Endosc. 2019;33(3):738–44.
31. McClusky DA, et al. Radiofrequency energy delivery to the lower esophageal sphincter (Stretta procedure) in patients with recurrent reflux after antireflux surgery: can surgery be avoided? Surg Endosc. 2007;21(7):1207–11.
32. Noar M, Squires P, Khan S. Radiofrequency energy delivery to the lower esophageal sphincter improves gastroesophageal reflux patient-reported outcomes in failed laparoscopic Nissen fundoplication cohort. Surg Endosc. 2017;31(7):2854–62.
33. Bell RC, et al. Revision of failed traditional fundoplication using EsophyX transoral fundoplication. Surg Endosc. 2013;27(3):761–7.

39 Reflux After Myotomy

Mohsen Alhashemi, Abdulaziz Karam Ali, and Mohammed Al Mahroos

Reflux After Myotomy

There are multiple modalities for the treatment of achalasia, however, the most effective treatment to date is a cardio-myotomy, in which the longitudinal and circular muscles of the lower esophageal sphincter (LES) are transected, leaving only the mucosa, to relieve the high pressure at the LES. Currently, myotomy can be achieved by two techniques: either surgically, whether through a trans-peritoneal or a trans-thoracic approach, or endoscopically through a relatively new technique called peroral endoscopic myotomy (POEM). However, this deliberate obliteration of the

M. Alhashemi (✉)
Department of Surgery, College of Health Sciences, Kuwait University, Kuwait, Kuwait
e-mail: mohsen.alhashemi@ku.edu.kw

A. K. Ali
Department of Surgery, McGill University, Montreal, QC, Canada

Montreal General Hospital, Montreal, QC, Canada

Department of Surgery, College of Health Sciences, Kuwait University, Kuwait, Kuwait

M. Al Mahroos
Department of Surgery, McGill University, Montreal, QC, Canada
e-mail: mohammed.almahroos@mail.mcgill.ca

A. D. Patel et al. (eds.), *The SAGES Manual of Physiologic Evaluation of Foregut Diseases*,
https://doi.org/10.1007/978-3-031-39199-6_39

LES causes the esophagus to lose its main anti-reflux mechanism, thereby leaving the patient at risk of developing postoperative gastro-esophageal reflux (GER) [1]. In this chapter, we will discuss the incidence, causes, treatment, and implications of GER after surgical or endoscopic myotomy.

Reflux After Surgical Myotomy

Heller described the first cardio-myotomy in 1913 as a treatment for achalasia, which consisted of anterior and posterior myotomies done through an abdominal approach [2]. This technique was revised later with a single anterior myotomy [3]. Heller's myotomy has since been recognized as the gold-standard procedure for the surgical treatment of achalasia. Another modification was introduced later in which the myotomy was done through an open thoracic approach [4]. However, since the introduction of minimal-invasive techniques (laparoscopic and thoracoscopic), a transabdominal laparoscopic approach is most commonly used due to improved outcomes both in terms of dysphagia and postoperative gastro-esophageal reflux (GER) [5, 6].

The incidence of GER after Heller's myotomy alone, without fundoplication, varies in the literature, and is likely affected by multiple factors including the length of myotomy, the extent of myotomy extension into the gastric mucosa, the assessment tools for GER (subjective vs. objective measures), and follow-up duration. A meta-analysis by Campos et al. showed that the reported incidence of GER after laparoscopic Heller's myotomy (LHM), without fundoplication, ranged between 11 and 60%, with a mean of 31.5%. This is compared to a mean rate of 28.3% associated with a thoracoscopic approach. However, with the addition of fundoplication, the incidence of postoperative GER after LHM is reduced to 8.8%, while none of the thoracoscopic studies reported performing a fundoplication [6]. Interestingly, in a prospective analysis of 66 patients undergoing LHM without fundoplication, the incidence of postoperative GER was found to reach 60% based on objective testing with endoscopy or 24-hour pH testing.

However, 33% of these patients were asymptomatic [7]. Therefore, the true incidence of postoperative GER may be higher than reported in the literature due to a known lack of correlation between subjective symptoms and objective findings in this population of patients [8].

Choice of Antireflux Procedure (ARP)

Due to the reported high rates of postoperative GER after LHM, the use of fundoplication as an anti-reflux measure has been advocated and shown to reduce the risk of postoperative GER [6]. However, controversy still exists as to which type of APR is the best—complete (Nissan's) vs. partial (Toupet or Dor) fundoplication. In particular, performing a complete 360° Nissen's fundoplication is controversial due to fear of postoperative dysphagia in patients with aperistaltic esophagus. Nonetheless, multiple studies reported performing Nissen's fundoplication after LHM with varying degrees of success. A study reporting 10 years' experience included 48 patients that underwent a "floppy" Nissen's fundoplication, with only two patients reported to have post-operative dysphagia (4%). The wrap was done over a 50 Fr bougie and was made loose enough to fit a 1 cm instrument between the wrap and the esophagus. The authors attributed the dysphagia in one of the patients due to incomplete myotomy and a tight wrap in the other patient. Only one patient had postoperative GER based on symptoms in this study [9]. A small randomized controlled trial (RCT) comparing open Heller's myotomy alone versus the addition of "floppy" Nissen's fundoplication included 10 patients in each arm, and showed a significantly higher incidence of postoperative GER when an ARP was not performed, without increasing the risk of dysphagia even with the addition of Nissen's fundoplication [10]. However, another RCT compared the addition of "floppy" Nissen's vs. Dor's (partial, 180°, anterior) fundoplication after LHM with 72 patients in each group with 5 years follow-up, showing a significant increase in the rate of postoperative dysphagia with Nissen's compared to Dor's fundoplication (15%

vs. 2.8%), with 40% patients in Nissen's group requiring endoscopic dilatation postoperatively. Postoperative GER was more frequent in Dor's group (5.6% vs. 0) based on clinical criteria, while pH studies were abnormal in only 2 patients (2.8%). There was no evidence of esophagitis on endoscopy in either patient [11].

Due to these findings of comparable efficacy between a partial and complete fundoplication in the control of post-operative GER, and the possible higher incidence of post-operative dysphagia after a complete myotomy, a partial fundoplication gained more popularity. Dor's fundoplication is a particularly common choice. In a RCT by Richard et al. that included 43 patients, the addition of Dor's fundoplication after Heller's myotomy decreased the incidence of pathological GER on pH study from 47.6% to 9.1% compared to Heller alone, without a significant difference in surgical outcomes and dysphagia scores [12]. Similar lower rates of GER reduction after Dor's fundoplication have been also reported in other long-term studies and systematic reviews [6, 13]. However, the long-term durability of Dor's fundoplication has been questioned in recent studies. Doubova et al. reported a progressive increase in the incidence of GER symptoms after LHM and Dor's fundoplication with an 11 year follow-up, with 88.2% of the patients requiring anti-reflux medications at 8–11 years postoperatively despite initial improvement in GER symptoms in the first year after surgery. This is in comparison to a 58.8% rate of anti-reflux medications used preoperatively [14]. A long-term follow-up of the RCT by Richard et al. also noted a worsening of the incidence of GER at a mean of 11-year follow-up compared to the immediate postoperative period (69% vs. 9.1%, respectively) with no difference in the outcomes between patients who underwent LHM + Dor's vs. those who underwent LHM alone. Moreover, a study with long-term data (up to >20 years) reported the development of esophageal squamous cell carcinoma in 3 out of 67 patients who underwent LHM with Dor's fundoplication [15], signifying a possible deleterious effect secondary to prolonged pathological acid exposure. This lack of long-term durability of the anti-reflux effect of Dor's fundoplication is reported in multiple other studies, and can be due to the deterioration of

Dor's itself, but can also be attributed to the natural progressive nature of the disease [15] or food stagnation and acid production rather than true acid reflux [16], and not necessarily related to the integrity of the fundoplication.

Another commonly used ARP after cardio-myotomy is Toupet's fundoplication (partial, 270°, posterior), with multiple studies reporting on the efficacy of Toupet's in controlling GER after Heller myotomy. Wright et al. report long-term results of a comparison of two techniques; an extended myotomy (>3 cm on gastric side) with Toupet's fundoplication vs. patients undergoing short myotomy (1–2 cm on the gastric side) with Dor's fundoplication, and showed improved dysphagia scores with the extended myotomy and no worsening in postoperative GER regardless of difference in the ARP performed [17]. A RCT comparing Toupet's (19 patients) vs. Dor's (24 patients) fundoplication at 1 year after LHM showed evidence of GER in 21.1% and 41.7% of patients on pH studies, respectively. However, the difference did not reach statistical significance, likely due to the small number of patients who underwent postoperative pH studies [18]. On the other hand, another RCT comparing Dor's vs. Toupet's fundoplication with 2 years follow-up showed a higher incidence of abnormal acid reflux on pH studies in Toupet's group at 6 months (34% vs. 6.9%), however, at 24 months, although still a higher percentage of patients in Toupet's group had abnormal acid exposure (31.5% vs. 10.5%), the difference did not reach statistical significance [19].

Nonetheless, in a similar fashion observed after Dor's fundoplication, the incidence of postoperative reflux increases with time, with up to 13.9% and 24% of patients undergoing Heller's myotomy with Toupet's fundoplication having evidence of acid reflux subjectively and on pH studies, respectively, 15 years after the surgery [20].

To further address the question of whether Dor's or Touept's fundoplication is superior than the other, a meta-regression analysis of objective postoperative GER and dysphagia in published RCTs and observational studies by Kurian et al. showed a similar incidence of reflux after a myotomy with an anterior fundoplication (14.3%) compared to a posterior fundoplication (15.8%), while an anterior fundoplication was associated with a higher incidence of dysphagia requiring intervention (10.1% vs. 5.9%) [21]. However, two more recent meta-analysis showed no difference in postoperative reflux or dysphagia between the two groups [22, 23].

Therefore, based on the currently available evidence, there seems to be similar short- and long-term outcomes between a partial-anterior or posterior fundoplication after myotomy, and the choice of the APR is left to the surgeon's discretion and expertise until more data are available. This is in-line with the recommendations of the Society of American Gastrointestinal and Endoscopic Surgeons (SAGES) which recommends performing a partial fundoplication ARP with LHM in the treatment of achalasia, while avoiding a complete fundoplication for the risk of increased post-operative dysphagia, however, no recommendation is made whether an anterior or posterior fundoplication is preferred [24]. Nonetheless, a Dor fundoplication may be an attractive option in the case of inadvertent mucosal perforation, and to avoid a more extensive posterior dissection of the esophagus.

Predictors of Reflux After Heller's Myotomy

In an attempt to elucidate factors associated with increased incidence of GER after LHM, Carter et al. [25] reported the outcomes of 165 patients who underwent LHM and Dor's fundoplication, with follow-up reaching more than 5 years, and could not identify predictors of postoperative GER from the preoperative disease and patient characteristics, or operative variables. Nonetheless, there are still areas of ongoing controversies with regard to the risk of GER after LHM.

One area of controversy has been the extent of the myotomy, particularly on the length of the myotomy on the gastric side. Extending the myotomy beyond the gastro-esophageal junction (GEJ) leads to the obliteration of the sling fibers, which are important in the integrity of the anti-reflux mechanism. The current accepted length of the myotomy is 6–8 cm in total length, with

2–3 cm being on the gastric side [26–28]. A retrospective study by El Nakeeb et al. reviewed the outcomes of 3 groups of patients who underwent LHM with Dor's fundoplication with different myotomy extension on the gastric side: <1.5 cm, 1.5–2.5 cm, and >2.5 cm, and found a significantly increased incidence of recurrent achalasia when the myotomy was <1.5 cm, while patients who had a myotomy >2.5 cm on the gastric side had a significantly higher incidence of GER on pH studies [29]. Nonetheless, a previous study by Oelschlager et al. comparing their outcomes after a myotomy with short (1.5 cm) extension on the stomach with Dor's fundoplication vs outcomes after a long (3 cm) extension on the stomach with Toupet's fundoplication showed improved relieve of dysphagia in the latter group without an increase in the risk of GER on pH studies done 3–6 months postoperatively. However, whether these outcomes are purely due to the change in the fundoplication or the extent of the myotomy is not entirely clear [28]. Another study by Salvador et al. similarly compared outcomes after a short myotomy (1.5–2 cm) vs. long myotomy (2.5–3 cm) on the gastric side, with Dor's fundoplication, and showed no difference in the incidence of GER or dysphagia either symptomatically or on pH and manometric studies. It is therefore not clear whether the extent of the myotomy would significantly affect the incidence of GER, however, an overly short extension of the myotomy on the gastric side is consistently associated with an increase in the risk of treatment failure, and should be avoided.

Another area of controversy is the extent of dissection of the hiatus and the phreno-esophageal membrane as it may potentially further disturb the natural anti-reflux mechanisms. Bonavina et al. [30] published a study in 1992 and reported the incidence of GER to be 8.6% (7 patients from 81 in total) on pH studies after open Heller's myotomy and Dor fundoplication. The majority of patient in the study underwent limited phreno-esophageal dissection, just enough to expose the anterior wall of the esophagus, while the posterior and lateral attachments were kept intact. Interestingly, in 4 of the 7 patients who had documented GER, the esophagus was circumferentially dissected. The results of this study suggested that complete mobilization of the esophagus may indeed be contributing to the incidence of GER after myotomy. More recently, a RCT with a 3 years follow-up comparing 3 groups of patients undergoing LHM was published in 2010 with a total of 84 patients included in the study; the first group underwent complete hiatal dissection and mobilization of the GEJ, a myotomy and Dor's fundoplication, the second group underwent limited anterior phreno-esophageal mobilization with a myotomy and Dor's fundoplication, and the third group underwent anterior mobilization with a myotomy, but no fundoplication was done. The study showed significantly higher DeMeester scores in the first group compared to the second and third groups, and there was a higher incidence of hiatal hernia occurrence in the first group with complete hiatal mobilization [31]. Although the study is limited by a small number of patients in each group and a relatively short follow-up, the incidence of GER appeared to be similar in the groups with limited phreno-esophageal dissection, regardless of whether Dor's fundoplication was performed or not. However, the results of this technique are yet to be verified by larger studies with longer follow-up.

Reflux After POEM

Since the first report of peroral endoscopic myotomy (POEM) as a treatment for achalasia in 2010, this procedure has gained great popularity due to its non-invasive nature and effectiveness [32]. Multiple studies showed that POEM is associated with high success rate in short- and long-term follow-up which is comparable, if not superior, to the gold standard procedure LHM [33–37].

However, it was noted that POEM might be associated with higher risk of GER than LHM. In a landmark RCT by Werner et al. comparing POEM vs. laparoscopic HM, POEM was found to be associated with higher risk of reflux esophagitis on endoscopy at 3 months (57% vs. 20%) and 24 months (44% vs. 29%), and higher percentage of abnormal acid exposure at 3 months on esophageal pH monitoring. In a post-hoc analysis, more patients were receiving proton-pump inhibitors in the POEM group compared to the HM group [37]. Multiple meta-analyses also showed higher risk of esophageal GER after POEM compared to HM [35, 38].

Interestingly, the incidence of subjective GER symptoms after POEM does not correlate with the incidence of objective measures of GER, similar to the findings after LHM. The incidence of symptomatic post-POEM GER is estimated to be around 8.5–19%, while the incidence of erosive esophagitis on endoscopy is 13–29.4% and the incidence of abnormal acid exposure on 24-h pH monitoring study is estimated to be 39–47.5% [35, 38, 39]. However, most of these patients respond to treatment with proton-pump inhibitors, and appear to have mild forms of erosive esophagitis on endoscopy (Los Angeles [LA] grade A or B) [40, 41]. Nonetheless, regardless of whether esophageal reflux is measured subjectively or objectively, POEM appears to be associated with a two- threefold increase in incidence compared to HM [38]. Therefore, continuous monitoring of patients post-POEM with regular endoscopy and ambulatory pH monitoring has been advocated to reduce the risk of developing complications related to long-term esophageal acid exposure, like Barret's metaplasia [41]. For refractory esophageal GER after POEM, few case series reported performing surgical or novel endoscopic fundoplication as a salvage procedure with good symptomatic relief [42, 43]. Recently, a novel procedure of concomitant POEM and endoscopic fundoplication (POEM+F) has been described as a solution to mitigate the high incidence of GER after POEM. However, long-term data on the efficacy and safety of this technique are still lacking [44].

Predictors of Reflux After POEM

Traditionally, POEM is either performed posteriorly (5 O'clock position) or anteriorly (2 o'clock position) [32, 45]. In theory, a posterior myotomy may injure the gastric sling fibers at the greater curvature of the stomach and angle of His, therefore disturbing the natural anti-reflux mechanism at the gastroesophageal junction. Therefore, an anterior myotomy may potentially reduce the risk of esophageal reflux after POEM. A randomized pilot trial by Ramchandai et al. showed comparable incidence of esophagitis between patients randomized to receive an anterior or posterior POEM, however, they found a higher incidence of esophageal acid exposure in the posterior myotomy group (37% vs. 16%) on pH study at 3 months [46]. Nonetheless, another randomized clinical trial comparing anterior vs. posterior myotomy showed no difference in the incidence of post-POEM GER between the two groups by pH studies, symptoms, or proton-pump inhibitor use at 1 year [47]. These results were confirmed by a recent meta-analysis comparing clinical outcomes after anterior vs. posterior myotomy and showed no difference in short-term clinical success or incidence of GER assessed by symptoms, pH studies, or by endoscopy, however, the authors noted that the results were limited by considerable heterogeneity between the included studies [48].

While some studies reported no association between post-POEM GER and patient, disease, procedural characteristics, or previous achalasia treatment [49–52], other studies showed that low integrated relaxation pressure [53], female sex [54], pre-operative esophagitis, and high Eckardt score [55] are associated with higher incidence of post-POEM GER. Moreover, a follow-up study of patients randomized to receive "short-myotomy" (<3 cm, using a single-scope technique) and "long-myotomy" (>3 cm, using a double-scope technique) on a gastric side showed that a long gastric myotomy was not associated with increased incidence of post-POEM reflux, but rather an increase in the severity of reflux disease (LA grade B) [56]. Similar results were found in a previous meta-analysis [39].

It is important to note that most studies reporting the incidence of post-POEM GER are retrospective in nature and include a relatively low number of patients, and there is considerable heterogeneity in the definition and diagnosis modality of post-POEM GER in the literature, which renders any pooling of data challenging and likely unreliable. Moreover, the diagnosis of post-POEM reflux disease based on pH studies has been questioned by experts. High acid-exposure time (AET) found on pH studies in Achalasia patients can be due to fermentation in a subset of patients rather than true reflux disease, and similar findings can be found in Achalasia patients even after successful treatment with a myotomy. Therefore, patients with high AET post-POEM due to fermentation may be diagnosed with reflux disease if the pH studies are not carefully and manually examined to differentiate between the two entities [57]. Given this variability in the definition of post-POEM reflux and limitations of each diagnostic modality, a consensus statement by experts in the field have called for a unified definition to standardize the assessment of GERD after POEM [58].

References

1. Boeckxstaens GE, Zaninotto G, Richter JE. Achalasia. Lancet. 2014;383(9911):83–93. https://doi.org/10.1016/s0140-6736(13)60651-0.
2. Heller E, Chir MGM. Extramukose kerkioplastic beim chronischen Kardiospasmus mit Dilation des Oesophagus. Med Chir. 1914;27:141.
3. Zaaijer JH. Cardiospasm in the aged. Ann Surg. 1923;77(5):615–7. https://doi.org/10.1097/00000658-192305000-00014.
4. Ellis FH Jr, Olsen AM, Holman CB, Code CF. Surgical treatment of cardiospasm (achalasia of the esophagus); considerations of aspects of esophagomyotomy. J Am Med Assoc. 1958;166(1):29–36. https://doi.org/10.1001/jama.1958.02990010031007.
5. Society for Surgery of the Alimentary Tract. SSAT patient care guidelines. J Gastrointest Surg. 2007;11(9):1210–2. https://doi.org/10.1007/s11605-007-0207-y.
6. Campos GM, Vittinghoff E, Rabl C, Takata M, Gadenstätter M, Lin F, et al. Endoscopic and surgical treatments for achalasia: a systematic review and meta-analysis. Ann Surg. 2009;249(1):45–57. https://doi.org/10.1097/SLA.0b013e31818e43ab.
7. Burpee SE, Mamazza J, Schlachta CM, Bendavid Y, Klein L, Moloo H, et al. Objective analysis of gastroesophageal reflux after laparoscopic heller myotomy: an anti-reflux procedure is required. Surg Endosc Other Interv Tech. 2005;19(1):9–14. https://doi.org/10.1007/s00464-004-8932-8.
8. Gholoum S, Feldman LS, Andrew CG, Bergman S, Demyttenaere S, Mayrand S, et al. Relationship between subjective and objective outcome measures after Heller myotomy and Dor fundoplication for achalasia. Surg Endosc. 2006;20(2):214–9. https://doi.org/10.1007/s00464-005-0213-7.
9. Frantzides CTMDPD, Moore REMD, Carlson MAMD, Madan AKMD, Zografakis JGMD, Keshavarzian AMD, et al. Minimally invasive surgery

for achalasia: a 10-year experience. J Gastrointest Surg. 2004;8(1):18–23. https://doi.org/10.1016/j.gassur.2003.09.021.

10. Falkenback D, Johansson J, Öberg S, Kjellin A, Wenner J, Zilling T, et al. Heller's esophagomyotomy with or without a 360° floppy Nissen fundoplication for achalasia. Long-term results from a prospective randomized study. Dis Esophagus. 2003;16(4):284–90. https://doi.org/10.1111/j.1442-2050.2003.00348.x.
11. Rebecchi F, Giaccone C, Farinella E, Campaci R, Morino M. Randomized controlled trial of laparoscopic Heller myotomy plus Dor fundoplication versus Nissen fundoplication for achalasia: long-term results. Ann Surg. 2008;248(6):1023–30. https://doi.org/10.1097/SLA.0b013e318190a776.
12. Richards WO, Torquati A, Holzman MD, Khaitan L, Byrne D, Lutfi R, et al. Heller myotomy versus Heller myotomy with Dor fundoplication for achalasia: a prospective randomized double-blind clinical trial. Ann Surg. 2004;240(3):405–15. https://doi.org/10.1097/01.sla.0000136940.32255.51.
13. Salvador R, Pesenti E, Gobbi L, Capovilla G, Spadotto L, Voltarel G, et al. Postoperative gastroesophageal reflux after laparoscopic heller-dor for achalasia: true incidence with an objective evaluation. J Gastrointest Surg. 2017;21(1):17–22. https://doi.org/10.1007/s11605-016-3188-x.
14. Doubova M, Gowing S, Robaidi H, Gilbert S, Maziak DE, Shamji FM, et al. Long-term symptom control after laparoscopic heller myotomy and dor fundoplication for achalasia. Ann Thorac Surg. 2020;111(5):1717–23. https://doi.org/10.1016/j.athoracsur.2020.06.095.
15. Csendes A, Braghetto I, Burdiles P, Korn O, Csendes P, Henríquez A. Very late results of esophagomyotomy for patients with achalasia: clinical, endoscopic, histologic, manometric, and acid reflux studies in 67 patients for a mean follow-up of 190 months. Ann Surg. 2006;243(2):196–203. https://doi.org/10.1097/01.sla.0000197469.12632.e0.
16. Tsiaoussis J, Pechlivanides G, Gouvas N, Athanasakis E, Zervakis N, Manitides A, et al. Patterns of esophageal acid exposure after laparoscopic Heller's myotomy and Dor's fundoplication for esophageal achalasia. Surg Endosc. 2008;22(6):1493–9. https://doi.org/10.1007/s00464-007-9681-2.
17. Wright AS, Williams CW, Pellegrini CA, Oelschlager BK. Long-term outcomes confirm the superior efficacy of extended Heller myotomy with toupet fundoplication for achalasia. Surg Endosc. 2007;21(5):713–8. https://doi.org/10.1007/s00464-006-9165-9.
18. Rawlings A, Soper NJ, Oelschlager B, Swanstrom L, Matthews BD, Pellegrini C, et al. Laparoscopic dor versus toupet fundoplication following Heller myotomy for achalasia: results of a multicenter, prospective, randomized-controlled trial. Surg Endosc. 2012;26(1):18–26. https://doi.org/10.1007/s00464-011-1822-y.
19. Torres-Villalobos G, Coss-Adame E, Furuzawa-Carballeda J, Romero-Hernández F, Blancas-Breña B, Torres-Landa S, et al. Dor vs toupet fun-

doplication after laparoscopic heller myotomy: long-term randomized controlled trial evaluated by high-resolution manometry. J Gastrointest Surg. 2018;22(1):13–22. https://doi.org/10.1007/s11605-017-3578-8.
20. Ortiz A, de Haro LF, Parrilla P, Lage A, Perez D, Munitiz V, et al. Very long-term objective evaluation of heller myotomy plus posterior partial fundoplication in patients with achalasia of the cardia. Ann Surg. 2008;247(2):258–64. https://doi.org/10.1097/SLA.0b013e318159d7dd.
21. Kurian AA, Bhayani N, Sharata A, Reavis K, Dunst CM, Swanström LL. Partial anterior vs partial posterior fundoplication following transabdominal esophagocardiomyotomy for achalasia of the esophagus: meta-regression of objective postoperative gastroesophageal reflux and dysphagia. JAMA Surg. 2013;148(1):85–90. https://doi.org/10.1001/jamasurgery.2013.409.
22. Siddaiah-Subramanya M, Yunus RM, Khan S, Memon B, Memon MA. Anterior dor or posterior toupet with heller myotomy for achalasia cardia: a systematic review and meta-analysis. World J Surg. 2019;43(6):1563–70. https://doi.org/10.1007/s00268-019-04945-9.
23. Aiolfi A, Tornese S, Bonitta G, Cavalli M, Rausa E, Micheletto G, et al. Dor versus toupet fundoplication after laparoscopic heller myotomy: systematic review and bayesian meta-analysis of randomized controlled trials. Asian J Surg. 2020;43(1):20–8. https://doi.org/10.1016/j.asjsur.2019.03.019.
24. Stefanidis D, Richardson W, Farrell TM, Kohn GP, Augenstein V, Fanelli RD. SAGES guidelines for the surgical treatment of esophageal achalasia. Surg Endosc. 2012;26(2):296–311. https://doi.org/10.1007/s00464-011-2017-2.
25. Carter JT, Nguyen D, Roll GR, Ma SW, Way LW. Predictors of long-term outcome after laparoscopic esophagomyotomy and dor fundoplication for achalasia. Arch Surg. 2011;146(9):1024–8. https://doi.org/10.1001/archsurg.2011.214.
26. Litle VR. Laparoscopic heller myotomy for achalasia: a review of the controversies. Ann Thorac Surg. 2008;85(2):S743–S6. https://doi.org/10.1016/j.athoracsur.2007.12.004.
27. Salvador R, Caruso V, Costantini M, Parise P, Nicoletti L, Cavallin F, et al. Shorter myotomy on the gastric site (≤2.5 cm) provides adequate relief of dysphagia in achalasia patients. Dis Esophagus. 2015;28(5):412–7. https://doi.org/10.1111/dote.12226.
28. Oelschlager BK, Chang L, Pellegrini CA. Improved outcome after extended gastric myotomy for achalasia. Arch Surg. 2003;138(5):490–7. https://doi.org/10.1001/archsurg.138.5.490.
29. El Nakeeb A, Ezzat H, Shehta A, El Gawad MA, Abou El-Magd ES, El Sorogy M, et al. Impact of the myotomy extent on gastric side on surgical outcome after Heller's cardiomotomy for achalasia. Surg Laparosc Endosc Percutan Tech. 2019;29(5):362–6. https://doi.org/10.1097/sle.0000000000000647.

30. Bonavina L, Nosadini A, Bardini R, Baessato M, Peracchia A. Primary treatment of esophageal achalasia: long-term results of myotomy and dor fundoplication. Arch Surg. 1992;127(2):222–7. https://doi.org/10.1001/archsurg.1992.01420020112016.
31. Simić AP, Radovanović NS, Skrobić OM, Raznatović ZJ, Pesko PM. Significance of limited hiatal dissection in surgery for achalasia. J Gastrointest Surg. 2010;14(4):587–93. https://doi.org/10.1007/s11605-009-1135-9.
32. Inoue H, Minami H, Kobayashi Y, Sato Y, Kaga M, Suzuki M, et al. Peroral endoscopic myotomy (POEM) for esophageal achalasia. Endoscopy. 2010;42(4):265–71. https://doi.org/10.1055/s-0029-1244080.
33. Bhayani NH, Kurian AA, Dunst CM, Sharata AM, Rieder E, Swanstrom LL. A comparative study on comprehensive, objective outcomes of laparoscopic Heller myotomy with per-oral endoscopic myotomy (POEM) for achalasia. Ann Surg. 2014;259(6):1098–103. https://doi.org/10.1097/sla.0000000000000268.
34. Podboy AJ, Hwang JH, Rivas H, Azagury D, Hawn M, Lau J, et al. Long-term outcomes of per-oral endoscopic myotomy compared to laparoscopic Heller myotomy for achalasia: a single-center experience. Surg Endosc. 2020;35(2):792–801. https://doi.org/10.1007/s00464-020-07450-6.
35. Schlottmann F, Luckett DJ, Fine J, Shaheen NJ, Patti MG. Laparoscopic heller myotomy versus peroral endoscopic myotomy (POEM) for achalasia: a systematic review and meta-analysis. Ann Surg. 2018;267(3):451–60. https://doi.org/10.1097/sla.0000000000002311.
36. Costantini A, Familiari P, Costantini M, Salvador R, Valmasoni M, Capovilla G, et al. Poem versus laparoscopic heller myotomy in the treatment of esophageal achalasia: a case-control study from two high volume centers using the propensity score. J Gastrointest Surg. 2020;24(3):505–15. https://doi.org/10.1007/s11605-019-04465-w.
37. Werner YB, Hakanson B, Martinek J, Repici A, von Rahden BHA, Bredenoord AJ, et al. Endoscopic or surgical myotomy in patients with idiopathic achalasia. N Engl J Med. 2019;381(23):2219–29. https://doi.org/10.1056/NEJMoa1905380.
38. Repici A, Fuccio L, Maselli R, Mazza F, Correale L, Mandolesi D, et al. GERD after per-oral endoscopic myotomy as compared with Heller's myotomy with fundoplication: a systematic review with meta-analysis. Gastrointest Endosc. 2018;87(4):934–43. https://doi.org/10.1016/j.gie.2017.10.022.
39. Akintoye E, Kumar N, Obaitan I, Alayo QA, Thompson CC. Peroral endoscopic myotomy: a meta-analysis. Endoscopy. 2016;48(12):1059–68. https://doi.org/10.1055/s-0042-114426.
40. Shiwaku H, Inoue H, Onimaru M, Minami H, Sato H, Sato C, et al. Multicenter collaborative retrospective evaluation of peroral endoscopic myotomy for esophageal achalasia: analysis of data from more than 1300

patients at eight facilities in Japan. Surg Endosc. 2020;34(1):464–8. https://doi.org/10.1007/s00464-019-06833-8.
41. Teitelbaum EN, Dunst CM, Reavis KM, Sharata AM, Ward MA, DeMeester SR, et al. Clinical outcomes five years after POEM for treatment of primary esophageal motility disorders. Surg Endosc. 2018;32(1):421–7. https://doi.org/10.1007/s00464-017-5699-2.
42. Nurczyk K, Farrell TM, Patti MG. Antireflux surgery for gastroesophageal reflux refractory to medical treatment after peroral endoscopic myotomy. J Laparoendosc Adv Surg Tech A. 2020;30(6):612–4. https://doi.org/10.1089/lap.2020.0106.
43. Tyberg A, Choi A, Gaidhane M, Kahaleh M. Transoral incisional fundoplication for reflux after peroral endoscopic myotomy: a crucial addition to our arsenal. Endosc Int Open. 2018;6(5):E549–52. https://doi.org/10.1055/a-0584-6802.
44. Inoue H, Ueno A, Shimamura Y, Manolakis A, Sharma A, Kono S, et al. Peroral endoscopic myotomy and fundoplication: a novel NOTES procedure. Endoscopy. 2019;51(2):161–4. https://doi.org/10.1055/a-0820-2731.
45. Cai MY, Zhou PH, Yao LQ, Xu MD, Zhong YS, Li QL, et al. Peroral endoscopic myotomy for idiopathic achalasia: randomized comparison of water-jet assisted versus conventional dissection technique. Surg Endosc. 2014;28(4):1158–65. https://doi.org/10.1007/s00464-013-3300-1.
46. Ramchandani M, Nabi Z, Reddy DN, Talele R, Darisetty S, Kotla R, et al. Outcomes of anterior myotomy versus posterior myotomy during POEM: a randomized pilot study. Endosc Int Open. 2018;6(2):E190–e8. https://doi.org/10.1055/s-0043-121877.
47. Khashab MA, Sanaei O, Rivory J, Eleftheriadis N, Chiu PWY, Shiwaku H, et al. Peroral endoscopic myotomy: anterior versus posterior approach: a randomized single-blinded clinical trial. Gastrointest Endosc. 2020;91(2):288–97. https://doi.org/10.1016/j.gie.2019.07.034.
48. Mohan BP, Ofosu A, Chandan S, Ramai D, Khan SR, Ponnada S, et al. Anterior versus posterior approach in peroral endoscopic myotomy (POEM): a systematic review and meta-analysis. Endoscopy. 2020;52(4):251–8. https://doi.org/10.1055/a-1090-0788.
49. Familiari P, Greco S, Gigante G, Calì A, Boškoski I, Onder G, et al. Gastroesophageal reflux disease after peroral endoscopic myotomy: Analysis of clinical, procedural and functional factors, associated with gastroesophageal reflux disease and esophagitis. Dig Endosc. 2016;28(1):33–41. https://doi.org/10.1111/den.12511.
50. Nabi Z, Ramchandani M, Kotla R, Tandan M, Goud R, Darisetty S, et al. Gastroesophageal reflux disease after peroral endoscopic myotomy is unpredictable, but responsive to proton pump inhibitor therapy: a large, single-center study. Endoscopy. 2020;52(8):643–51. https://doi.org/10.1055/a-1133-4354.
51. Liu ZQ, Li QL, Chen WF, Zhang XC, Wu QN, Cai MY, et al. The effect of prior treatment on clinical outcomes in patients with achalasia under-

going peroral endoscopic myotomy. Endoscopy. 2019;51(4):307–16. https://doi.org/10.1055/a-0658-5783.
52. Ngamruengphong S, Inoue H, Ujiki MB, Patel LY, Bapaye A, Desai PN, et al. Efficacy and safety of peroral endoscopic myotomy for treatment of achalasia after failed heller myotomy. Clin Gastroenterol Hepatol. 2017;15(10):1531–7. https://doi.org/10.1016/j.cgh.2017.01.031.
53. Shiwaku H, Inoue H, Sasaki T, Yamashita K, Ohmiya T, Takeno S, et al. A prospective analysis of GERD after POEM on anterior myotomy. Surg Endosc. 2016;30(6):2496–504. https://doi.org/10.1007/s00464-015-4507-0.
54. Kumbhari V, Familiari P, Bjerregaard NC, Pioche M, Jones E, Ko WJ, et al. Gastroesophageal reflux after peroral endoscopic myotomy: a multicenter case-control study. Endoscopy. 2017;49(7):634–42. https://doi.org/10.1055/s-0043-105485.
55. Arevalo G, Sippey M, Martin-Del-Campo LA, He J, Ali A, Marks J. Post-POEM reflux: who's at risk? Surg Endosc. 2020;34(7):3163–8. https://doi.org/10.1007/s00464-019-07086-1.
56. Grimes KL, Bechara R, Shimamura Y, Ikeda H, Inoue H. Gastric myotomy length affects severity but not rate of post-procedure reflux: 3-year follow-up of a prospective randomized controlled trial of double-scope per-oral endoscopic myotomy (POEM) for esophageal achalasia. Surg Endosc. 2020;34(7):2963–8. https://doi.org/10.1007/s00464-019-07079-0.
57. Bechara R, Inoue H, Shimamura Y, Reed D. Gastroesophageal reflux disease after peroral endoscopic myotomy: lest we forget what we already know. Dis Esophagus. 2019;32(12):106. https://doi.org/10.1093/dote/doz106.
58. Inoue H, Shiwaku H, Kobayashi Y, Chiu PWY, Hawes RH, Neuhaus H, et al. Statement for gastroesophageal reflux disease after peroral endoscopic myotomy from an international multicenter experience. Esophagus. 2020;17(1):3–10. https://doi.org/10.1007/s10388-019-00689-6.

GERD After Duodenal Switch

40

Filippo Filicori and D'Artagnan DeBow

Introduction

The rate of gastroesophageal reflux disease (GERD) is higher in the morbidly obese population compared to the general population [1–4]. Much has been published on the incidence of postoperative GERD following sleeve gastrectomy (SG) and Roux-en-Y gastric bypass (RYGB); however, the literature is currently lacking prospective data on the incidence of GERD following the duodenal switch (DS) procedure. SG and RYGB are the most common bariatric procedures today accounting for 61% and 17% of all cases, respectively [5]. DS has had a resurgence in popularity given the increasing incidence of super morbidly obese patients with a BMI exceeding 50 kg/m^2. Although the duodenal switch makes up approximately 1% of all bariatric procedures performed today [5], it is increasingly recognized as the most effective procedure for excess weight loss and resolution of diabetes and hyperlipidemia.

F. Filicori (✉) · D. DeBow
Division of Minimally Invasive and Bariatric Surgery, Zucker School of Medicine at Hofstra/Northwell, Lenox Hill Hospital, New York, NY, USA
e-mail: ffilicori@northwell.edu; ddebow1@northwell.edu

A. D. Patel et al. (eds.), *The SAGES Manual of Physiologic Evaluation of Foregut Diseases*,
https://doi.org/10.1007/978-3-031-39199-6_40

Significant symptomatic reflux or significant GERD found on preoperative diagnostic tests (upper endoscopy, 24-h esophageal pH monitoring) has generally been heralded as an indication to perform RYGB over sleeve gastrectomy, as the rate of postoperative reflux is significantly lower [6]. This is largely thought to be due to multiple physiologic and anatomic changes causing increased reflux with sleeve gastrectomy including decreased gastric compliance and volume leading to higher pressures, severance of the gastric sling muscle fibers which contribute to the lower esophageal sphincter compliance, blunting of the angle of His, and decreased gastric emptying.

As DS includes a sleeve gastrectomy to anatomically achieve a restrictive component to weight loss, it has been postulated it might have postoperative reflux rates that are potentially similar to SG. There are, however, physiologic and anatomical differences between the DS and SG to consider which result in improved reflux rates.

Biliopancreatic Diversion and Duodenal Switch

The biliopancreatic diversion/duodenal switch (BPD/DS) that is most commonly performed today was originally developed as a two-stage procedure, beginning with an SG, followed in 8–12 months with a duodenoileostomy [7–12]. Today it is generally done as a single-stage procedure for those with a high BMI (≥50 kg/m^2). The technique includes an SG, which is typically larger capacity than in the stand-alone SG operation. A post-pyloric anastomosis is then created with the alimentary limb in a standard Roux-en-Y configuration, with the alimentary limb commonly 250 cm in length and a 100 cm common channel. The "loop" duodenal switch is an alternative technique that has gained some popularity over the BPD-DS recently with the description of Stomach Intestinal Pylorus-Sparing (SIPS) and Single-Anastomosis Duodenal-Ileal Bypass Surgery (SADI-S). Sanchez-Pernaute and Torres described SADI-S in 2007 as a technique to avoid some complications and technical issues of the BPD-DS

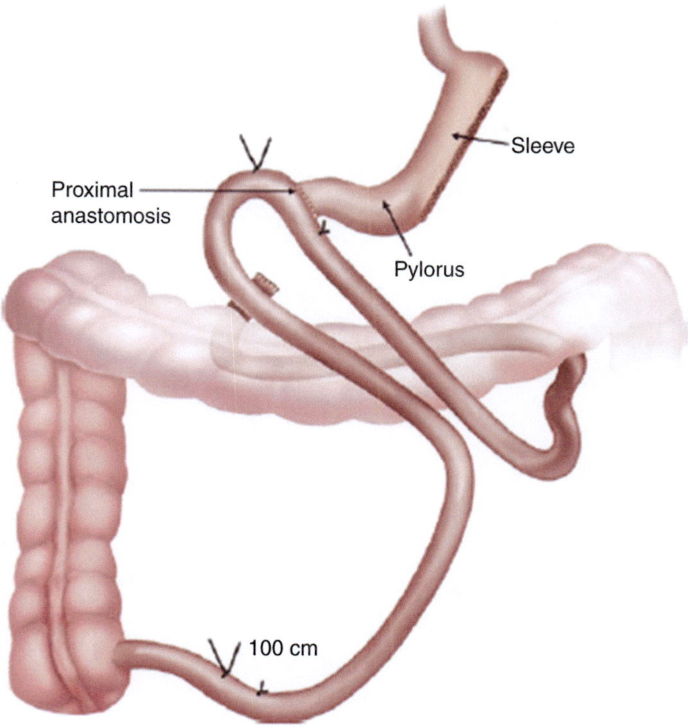

Fig. 40.1 Traditional duodenal switch. Sudan, R., Podolsky, E. Totally robot-assisted biliary pancreatic diversion with duodenal switch: single dock technique and technical outcomes. Surg Endosc 29, 55–60 (2015). Reprinted with permission from Springer Nature

(Figs. 40.1 and 40.2) [13, 14]. It involved a single duodenal-ileal end-to-side anastomosis with a 200 cm common channel. This technique was further developed by Cottam et al. and Roslin et al. by increasing the length of the common channel to 300 cm, which decreased postoperative malnutrition and diarrhea [15–19]. As the sleeve remnant is typically larger with the loop duodenal switch when compared to the stand-alone vertical sleeve gastrectomy, patients can eat a larger portion of food, therefore helping to prevent hypoproteinemia and other nutritional deficiencies.

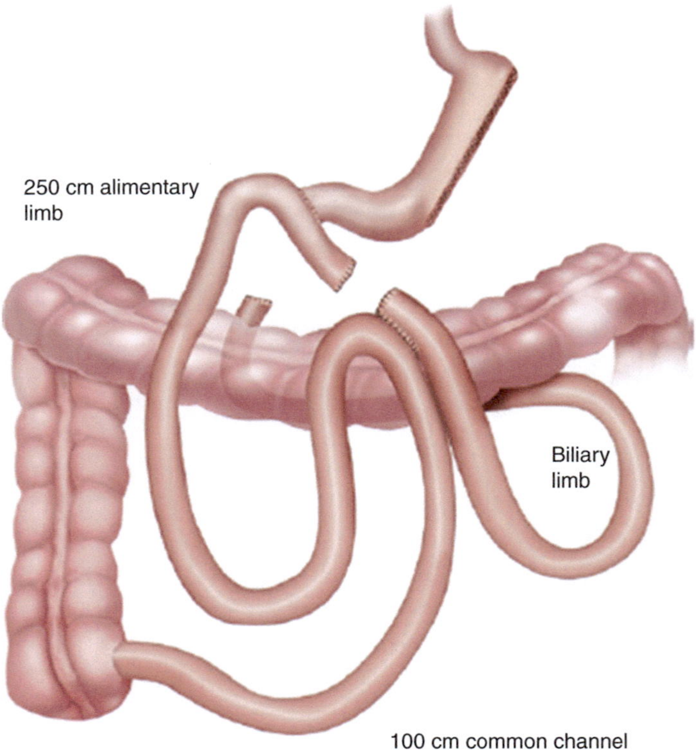

Fig. 40.2 Modified duodenal switch. Sudan, R., Podolsky, E. Totally robot-assisted biliary pancreatic diversion with duodenal switch: single dock technique and technical outcomes. Surg Endosc 29, 55–60 (2015). Reprinted with permission from Springer Nature

Preoperative GERD Workup and Considerations

Like other bariatric procedures, the preoperative decision to proceed with a duodenal switch requires an evaluation of the upper gastrointestinal anatomy and physiology. It is essential to assess the patient for reflux symptoms, as symptomatic GERD may change the extent of the preoperative evaluation. Many centers advocate for esophagogastroduodenoscopy (EGD) in all patients, especially in those undergoing an intestinal exclusion procedure (RYGB or DS). Because of the potential to increase GERD with the sleeve component of the DS and the overall increased rate of squamocolumnar metaplasia in the bariatric population, we recommend that all patients undergoing DS should undergo a preoperative EGD. If squamocolumnar metaplasia is detected, or if GERD symptoms are moderate to severe, the patient should be counseled on giving consideration to a different bariatric procedure such as RYGB.

GERD Outcomes

In patients with significant symptomatic reflux, proceeding with primary sleeve gastrectomy is discouraged and most centers recommend proceeding with a gastric bypass instead. Because the duodenal switch (BPD/DS or SIPS/SADI-S) is much less commonly performed, the majority of the data discussing the impact of DS on GERD hinges on retrospective series in centers which have extensive experience in BPD/DS.

A multi-institutional propensity matched analysis on the comparative effectiveness of bariatric operations was conducted by Sudan et al. [6] Of 130,796 patients, 57,094 underwent gastric band, 5942 underwent sleeve gastrectomy, 66,324 underwent RYGB, and 1436 underwent BPD/DS. RYGB was found to result in the best resolution rates of GERD with an odds ratio 1.5 times higher when compared to gastric banding. The odds ratio of GERD resolution was 0.87. Gastric banding was also more likely to result in GERD resolution than SG (OR = 0.87). Interestingly, the BPD/DS, despite incorporating the SG as a portion of the procedure, had an odds ratio of GERD resolution at 1.2 times higher than gastric banding.

Although the improved resolution of GERD after BPD/DS compared with SG is anecdotal and not fully understood, there are a few possible explanations. Perhaps, the larger capacity of the gastric sleeve in the duodenal switch procedure compared to the stand-alone SG may contribute to less symptomatic reflux. It is important to point out that in the modified duodenal switch with a single loop anastomosis (SIPS/SADI-S), the sleeve is typically performed over a bougie ≥40 Fr, whereas in the SG, the bougie size is 32–38 Fr in most instances [20]. Furthermore, by creating a larger remnant stomach, the sling fibers contributing to the Lower Esophageal Sphincter (LES) tension at the Angle of His are left intact and there is less chance of narrowing the stomach at the incisura angularis, which, combined with the increased gastric volume and compliance, may contribute to decreased rates of GERD postoperatively.

Conclusions

Although RYGB remains the recommended operation for bariatric patients who suffer from moderate to severe reflux disease or for those with squamocolumnar metaplasia, it is becoming more evident that the duodenal switch results in a less prominent worsening of GERD compared to SG alone. As the duodenal switch increases in popularity with increasing rates of obesity >50 kg/m^2, it is recognized that DS might offer improved long-term weight loss outcomes and resolution of comorbid conditions including diabetes and hyperlipidemia over SG or RYGB. Duodenal switch might be a reasonable option for patients with a BMI ≥ 50 kg/m^2 with mild GERD, and/or reflux due to the presence of a hiatal hernia with planned concomitant repair. More prospective data are needed to further elucidate the effects of duodenal switch on gastroesophageal physiology and long-term reflux outcomes.

References

1. Corley DA, Kubo A, Zhao W. Abdominal obesity, ethnicity and gastro-oesophageal reflux symptoms. Gut. 2007;56:756.
2. Jacobson BC, Somers SC, Fuchs CS, et al. Body-mass index and symptoms of gastroesophageal reflux in women. N Engl J Med. 2006;354:2340.
3. Pandolfino JE, El-Serag HB, Zhang Q, et al. Obesity: a challenge to esophagogastric junction integrity. Gastroenterology. 2006;130:639.

4. El-Serag HB, Ergun GA, Pandolfino J, et al. Obesity increases oesophageal acid exposure. Gut. 2007;56:749.
5. https://asmbs.org/resources/estimate-of-bariatric-surgery-numbers.
6. Sudan R, Maciejewski ML, Wilk AR, Nguyen NT, Ponce J, Morton JM. Comparative effectiveness of primary bariatric operations in the United States. Surg Obes Relat Dis. 2017;13(5):826–34.
7. Scopinaro N, Gianetta E, Civalleri D, Bonalumi U, Bachi V. Biliopancreatic bypass for obesity: 1. An experimental study in dogs. Br J Surg. 1979;66(9):613–7.
8. Demeester TR, Fuchs KH, Ball CS, et al. Experimental and clinical results with proximal end-to-end duodenojejunostomy for pathological duodenogastric reflux. Ann Surg. 1987;206:414–26.
9. Hess DS, Hess DW. Biliopancreatic diversion with a duodenal switch. Obes Surg. 1998;8(3):267–82.
10. Ren CJ, Patterson E, Gagner M. Early results of laparoscopic biliopancreatic diversion with duodenal switch: a case series of 40 consecutive patients. Obes Surg. 2000;10(6):514–23.
11. Johnston D, Dachtler J, Sue-Ling HM, King RF, Martin G. The magenstrasse and mill operation for morbid obesity. Obes Surg. 2003;13(1):10–6.
12. Marceau P, Biron S, Bourque RA, Potvin M, Hould FS, Simard S. Biliopancreatic diversion with a new type of gastrectomy. Obes Surg. 1993;3(1):29–35.
13. Sánchez-Pernaute A, Rubio Herrera MA, Pérez-Aguirre E, et al. Proximal duodenal-ileal end-to-side bypass with sleeve gastrectomy: proposed technique. Obes Surg. 2007;17(12):1614–8.
14. Sánchez-Pernaute A, Rubio MÁ, Pérez Aguirre E, Barabash A, Cabrerizo L, Torres A. Single-anastomosis duodenoileal bypass with sleeve gastrectomy: metabolic improvement and weight loss in first 100 patients. Surg Obes Relat Dis. 2013;9(5):731–5.
15. Mitzman B, Cottam D, Goriparthi R, et al. Stomach intestinal pylorus sparing (SIPS) surgery for morbid obesity: retrospective analyses of our preliminary experience. Obes Surg. 2016;26(9):2098–104.
16. Cottam A, Cottam D, Roslin M, et al. A matched cohort analysis of sleeve gastrectomy with and without 300 cm loop duodenal switch with 18-month follow-up. Obes Surg. 2016;26(10):2363–9.
17. Surve A, Zaveri H, Cottam D. A safer and simpler technique of duodenal dissection and transection of the duodenal bulb for duodenal switch. Surg Obes Relat Dis. 2016;12(4):923–4.
18. Surve A, Zaveri H, Cottam D. Retrograde filling of the afferent limb as a cause of chronic nausea after single anastomosis loop duodenal switch. Surg Obes Relat Dis. 2016;12(4):e39–42.
19. Zaveri H, Surve A, Cottam D, et al. Mid-term 4-year outcomes with single anastomosis duodenal-ileal bypass with sleeve gastrectomy surgery at a single US center. Obes Surg. 2018;28:3062–72.
20. Topart P, Becouarn G. The single anastomosis duodenal switch modifications: a review of the current literature on outcomes. Surg Obes Relat Dis. 2017;13:1306.

Sleeve Gastrectomy and Gastroesophageal Reflux Disease

41

Anna Ibele and Emily Adams

The effects of sleeve gastrectomy on gastroesophageal reflux disease (GERD) remain somewhat controversial. However, there is considerable mounting evidence to suggest that sleeve gastrectomy is a poor choice of procedure in a patient with preexisting GERD and may lead to de novo GERD symptoms and complications of GERD in certain patients [1–11].

Several retrospective studies have found an increased incidence of GERD symptoms in patients following sleeve gastrectomy. In a large retrospective review of the Bariatric Outcomes Longitudinal Database (BOLD), DuPree et al. compared the reflux outcomes of 4832 patients who underwent sleeve gastrectomy between 2007 and 2010 to 33,867 who underwent gastric bypass. Of the 44% of sleeve gastrectomy patients with preoperative reflux symptoms, 84.1% had persistent symptoms postoperatively. Nine percent of patients developed de novo reflux symptoms, while Roux-en-Y gastric bypass (RYGB) resolved GERD in the majority of patients (62.8% postoperatively). Of

A. Ibele (✉) · E. Adams
Department of Surgery, The University of Utah,
Salt Lake City, UT, USA
e-mail: anna.ibele@hsc.utah.edu; emily.adams@hsc.utah.edu

A. D. Patel et al. (eds.), *The SAGES Manual of Physiologic Evaluation of Foregut Diseases*,
https://doi.org/10.1007/978-3-031-39199-6_41

note, patients who had preoperative reflux and underwent sleeve gastrectomy had an increased need for revisional surgery compared to those who underwent sleeve gastrectomy and had no preoperative reflux symptoms (0.6% versus 0.3%, $p = 0.03$) [4]. Medication usage for the treatment of GERD has also been found to be increased following sleeve gastrectomy. Sheppard et al. found evidence for increased proton pump inhibitor (PPI) requirement following sleeve gastrectomy. They performed a retrospective review of 387 patients who underwent either laparoscopic sleeve gastrectomy (LSG) or laparoscopic RYGB over a two-year time period (2010–2012) at their institution. Preoperative proton pump inhibitor use did not differ between groups, but at one month ($p < 0.05$) and 1–2 years ($p < 0.001$) after surgery, there was significantly increased PPI use in patients who underwent LSG. Of patients who underwent sleeve gastrectomy and were on a preoperative PPI, 58% increased their dose postoperatively and 42% continued on the same dose [5].

The poor prognosis for GERD symptoms following sleeve gastrectomy has also been demonstrated prospectively. In the SM-BOSS randomized clinical trial published in 2018 comparing outcomes of LSG with RYGB, Peterli et al. found that gastroesophageal reflux remission was observed more frequently after Roux en Y gastric bypass (60.4%) than after sleeve gastrectomy (25%) and that GERD worsened after LSG more often (31.8%) than in RYGB patients (6.3%). Of concern, they found that 31.6% of sleeve gastrectomy patients developed de novo GERD symptoms 5 years out from surgery compared with 10% of gastric bypass patients. Although these authors state that most of these cases of GERD symptoms were treated successfully with pharmaceutical therapy, 10% of these patients required surgical conversion to gastric bypass [10].

In addition to an increased incidence or exacerbation of GERD symptoms following sleeve gastrectomy, sleeve has also been found to fail to improve or exacerbate the objective assessment of gastroesophageal reflux pathophysiology. In a prospective study, Del Genio et al. performed high-resolution manometry and 24-h pH impedance monitoring in 25 consecutive patients before and after laparoscopic sleeve gastrectomy. At a median follow-up of

13 months, impedance pH studies demonstrated an increase in both acid exposure of the distal esophagus and the number of non-acid reflux events in postprandial periods. Notably, manometric findings were unchanged lower esophageal sphincter function, increased ineffective peristalsis, and incomplete bolus transit [6]. In a similar prospective study by Burgerhart et al., 20 patients underwent high-resolution manometry and 24-h pH/impedance testing before and 3 months after laparoscopic sleeve gastrectomy. Preoperative and postoperative symptoms were assessed using reflux disease questionnaires. The authors found that GERD symptoms did not significantly change after sleeve gastrectomy, but other upper gastrointestinal symptoms particularly belching, epigastric pain, and vomiting increased. In contrast to the findings of Del Genio et al., manometrically, the percentage of normal peristaltic esophageal contractions remained unchanged, but the distal contractile integral decreased after LSG from 2006.0 ± 1806.3 to 1537.4 ± 1671.8 mmHg cm s ($p = 0.01$). The lower esophageal sphincter (LES) pressure decreased from 18.3 ± 9.2 to 11.0 ± 7.0 mmHg ($p = 0.02$). Esophageal acid exposure significantly increased after sleeve gastrectomy: upright from 5.1 ± 4.4 to 12.6 ± 9.8% ($p=0.003$), supine from 1.4 ± 2.4 to 11 ± 15% ($p=0.003$), and total acid exposure from 4.1 ± 3.5 to 12 ± 10.4% ($p=0.004$) [7].

Several case series have begun to emerge, demonstrating an association between sleeve gastrectomy and new-onset Barrett's esophagus (BE). Felsenreich et al. performed 24-h pH studies, manometry, upper GI endoscopy, and reflux questionnaires in 43 sleeve patients more than 10 years out from their surgery who did not have symptomatic reflux or hiatal hernia preoperatively. They note that of the 43, six patients were converted to gastric bypass for intractable reflux. Ten of the remaining patients had de novo reflux and 15% had de novo endoscopic findings of BE (compared to their preoperative endoscopies). Forty-five percent of patients developed de novo hiatal hernias postoperatively as indicated by the migration of the gastric staple line above the crural diaphragm, perhaps due to over-dissection at the base of the left crus. Nine out of 12 patients who underwent preoperative pH testing had an increase in the DeMeester Score from their preoperative baseline with an average score of 52.7 [11]. In another study of 110 patients who underwent sleeve gastrectomy after completing a GERD visual analogue scale and preoperative EGD, Genco et al. reported that at a mean of 58 months post op, the incidence of GERD symptoms, visual analogue mean GERD score, and PPI intake had significantly increased compared to preoperative values (68.1% vs 33.6%, 3 vs 1.8, and 57.2% vs 19.1%; $p < 0.05$ for all). Non-dysplastic Barrett's esophagus was newly diagnosed in 19 patients who did not have this finding on preoperative endoscopy [8]. Finally, a recent systematic review was published in February 2020 by Yeung et al. including 46 studies and 10,718 patients looking at the effects of sleeve gastrectomy and exposure of the distal esophagus to severe reflux. They found high rates of GERD and resultant sequelae of esophagitis and Barrett's esophagus to be strongly prominent in sleeve gastrectomy patients: there was a 19% increase in all reflux symptoms and a 20% rate of long-term de novo reflux, 28% occurrence rate of esophagitis, and an 8% occurrence rate of Barrett's esophagus. There did not appear to be a correlation between symptoms and esophagitis or Barrett's esophagus, implying that postoperative surveillance should be instituted in all sleeve gastrectomy patients and that these numbers likely underestimate the incidence of long-term esophageal damage following sleeve [11].

Proponents of sleeve gastrectomy in patients with GERD cite more favorable findings in competing studies [2, 12]. These studies postulate that a reduction of GERD symptoms reported by some patients could be explained by the resultant decreased gastric emptying time, decreased presence of acid-secreting parietal cells created by resection of the gastric fundus, and weight loss leading to a decreased intraabdominal pressure and thus a decreased pressure gradient across the LES [12]. For example, in 2013 Melissas et al. evaluated gastric emptying times via scintigraphy in 21 patients with morbid obesity undergoing laparoscopic sleeve gastrectomy before the procedure and 4 months following the procedure. The time for 10% gastric emptying was found to be significantly decreased after SG from 15.5 min (range, 6.5–24.2 min) preoperatively to 8.4 min (range, 3.0–22.4) 4 months postoperatively ($P < 0.05$). T gastric 50% was also found to be accelerated significantly from 61.7 min (range, 37–94.3 min) preoperatively to 49.1 min (range, 22.4–92.1 min) at 4 months postoperatively ($P < 0.05$) [12]. Despite the small sample size, this study is convincing that sleeve gastrectomy does decrease gastric emptying time. However, the remainder of the above evidence shows that this benefit does not outweigh the other anatomical disadvantages associated with this procedure, which may ultimately exacerbate reflux and reflux symptoms.

Many attribute the increased incidence of reflux as well as the exacerbation of reflux post sleeve to the anatomic changes associated with sleeve gastrectomy. The angle of His is a known antireflux mechanism under normal anatomic conditions. It creates a flap valve mechanism at the esophagogastric junction, allowing for a relative barrier between fluid and particulate matter in the stomach and the esophagus, and becomes more acutely angled with gastric filling. In the creation of the apex staple line during a sleeve gastrectomy, the surgeon obliterates this angle, therefore eliminating this natural barrier to reflux. Another anatomic consequence of the gastric sleeve operation which is conducive to reflux is the decrease in basal lower esophageal sphincter pressure after division of the gastric sling fibers during the longitudinal stomach transection [3]. Poor surgical technique resulting in a torsed staple line, narrowing the sleeve at the gastric incisura, or an overly narrow gastric tube can raise gastric pressures also contributing to reflux occurrence [3, 13]. Finally, redundant fundus left at the superior portion of the sleeve can dilate over time resulting in a dependent fundic "pouch" or "fundic diverticulum" in which food can preferentially lodge resulting in increased regurgitation [14]. Several experts have suggested that the ideal shape for a gastric sleeve is a conformation of a relatively intact antrum with attention to excision of the fundus and preservation of the angle of His [1, 13]. However, to date, the surgical technique varies, and there is no consensus on optimal techniques to avoid de novo GERD or exacerbation of GERD or its complications.

Hiatal hernia may also contribute to an increased incidence of postoperative GERD following sleeve gastrectomy. It is believed that up to 40% of patients with morbid obesity have a hiatal hernia. This is a known risk factor for GERD both in the general population and in the postoperative bariatric surgery population [15]. A systematic review was performed by Mahawar et al. in 2015 of 17 studies in which hiatal hernia repair was performed concurrent with sleeve gastrectomy including a total of 737 patients. In 16 out of 17 studies, the authors found favorable results (reduction in reflux symptoms without increased morbidity) and recommended this combination treatment option [16]. It has now become common to perform hiatal hernia repair or repair concurrently with LSG in many centers in an effort to mitigate potential postoperative GERD symptoms. However, the durability of hiatal hernia repair performed with a concurrent bariatric operation on postoperative GERD symptoms, postoperative complications, and the risk of hiatal hernia recurrence is unclear due to the variability in patient populations and surgical technique in published series. In the systematic review by Mahawar et al, a postoperative GERD rate of 12.6% in patients who underwent concurrent hiatal hernia repair and sleeve gastrectomy was found [16]. In one study included in that same review, Santonicola et al. found that reflux symptoms after surgery were comparatively worse in the sleeve gastrectomy with the hiatal hernia repair group when compared with the sleeve gastrectomy alone group [16, 17]. It is postulated that these outcomes may be due to a higher likelihood of symptomatic hiatal hernia recurrence when repair is performed with gastric sleeve as opposed to gastric bypass. A study which supports this hypothesis by Patel et al in 2014 evaluated mid-term outcomes of LSG with PEH repair in 18 patients and found that 33% had a small (<2 cm) hernia recurrence with 17% having evidence of reflux routine on postoperative UGI and GERD questionnaires with an average follow-up from surgery of 19.9 ± 16.7 months [18].

There is currently no standardized protocol in the bariatric field for the evaluation and treatment of patients presenting with new-onset or worsening GERD symptoms following a sleeve gastrectomy. Due to concerns about de novo Barrett's esophagus following sleeve gastrectomy, many have advocated for routine endoscopic surveillance post sleeve at various intervals, but to date surgical consensus on this issue is in evolution. Given the wealth of evidence supporting increased risk of GERD and complications of GERD following sleeve gastrectomy, many surgeons no longer perform sleeve gastrectomy in patients with symptomatic pathologic GERD [3]. Surgeons and their patients should be aware of and discuss the evidence indicating the potential risk of exacerbating preexisting GERD or inducing de novo GERD following sleeve gastrectomy. Surgical technique is likely a contributing factor in reflux outcomes, and attention should be paid to avoiding technical complications, such as incisural narrowing, torsion of staple lines, retained fundus, and failure to identify or address an associated hiatal hernia or over-dissection at the base of the left crus leading to postoperative hiatal hernia, which may exacerbate reflux [3].

References

1. Nadelto BF. Gastroesophageal reflux disease in the obese: pathophysiology and treatment. Surgery. 2016;159:475–86.
2. Chiu S, Shi X, et al. Effect of sleeve gastrectomy on gastroesophageal reflux disease: a systematic review. Surg Obes Relat Dis. 2011;7(4):510–5.
3. Braghetto ILE, Valladares H, Molina JC, Henriquez A. Manometric changes of the lower esophageal sphincter after sleeve gastrectomy in obese patients. Obes Surg. 2010;20:357–263.
4. Dupree CE, Martin MJ. Laparoscopic sleeve gastrectomy in patients with preexisting gastroesophageal reflux disease: a national analysis. JAMA Surg. 2014;149:328–34.
5. Sheppard CE, Karmali S, Birch DW. Rates of reflux before and after laparoscopic sleeve gastrectomy for severe obesity. Obes Surg. 2015;25:763–8.
6. Del Genio G, Brusciano L, D'Alessandro A, Docimo G, Rossetti G, Silecchia G, Iannelli A, del Genio A, del Genio F, Docimo L. Sleeve gastrectomy and development of "de novo" gastroesophageal reflux. Obes Surg. 2014;24:71–7.
7. Burgerhart JS, Smulders JF, van de Meeberg PC, Siersema PD, Smout AJ. Effect of sleeve gastrectomy of gastroesophageal reflux. Obes Surg. 2014;24(9):1436–41.
8. Felsenreich DM, Beckerhinn P, et al. Reflux, sleeve dilation, and Barrett's esophagus after laparoscopic sleeve gastrectomy: long-term follow-up. Obes Surg. 2017;27:3092–101.
9. Genco A, Maselli R, Castagneto-Gissey L, Di Lorenzo N, Basso N. Gastroesophageal reflux disease and Barrett's esophagus after laparo-

scopic sleeve gastrectomy: a possible underestimated long-term complication. Surg Obes Relat Dis. 2017;13:568–74.

10. Peterli R, Peters T, Vetter D, Kroll D, Borbely Y. Effect of laparoscopic sleeve gastrectomy vs laparoscopic roux-en-y gastric bypass on weight loss in patients with morbid obesity: the SM-BOSS randomized clinical trial. JAMA. 2018;319(3):255–65.
11. Yeung KT, Ashrafian L, Darzi A, Ashrafian H. Does sleeve gastrectomy expose the distal esophagus to severe reflux? A systematic review and meta-analysis. Ann Surg. 2020;271(2):257–65.
12. Melissas J, Perisinakis K, Koukouraki S, de Bree E, Karkavitsas N. Alterations of global gastrointestinal motility after sleeve gastrectomy: a prospective study. Ann Surg. 2013;258:976–82.
13. Daes J, Daza JC, Dennis R. Laparoscopic sleeve gastrectomy: symptoms of gastroesophageal reflux can be reduced by changes in surgical technique. Obes Surg. 2012;22:1874–9.
14. Keidar A, Elazary R, Baltasar A. Dilated upper sleeve can be associated with severe postoperative gastroesophageal dysmotility and reflux. Obes Surg. 2010;20:140–7.
15. Che F, Cohen A, Nguyen NT. Prevalence of hiatal hernia in the morbidly obese. Surg Obes Relat Dis. 2013;9(6):920–4.
16. Mahawar KK, Jennings N, Balupuri S, Small PK. Simultaneous sleeve gastrectomy and hiatus hernia repair: a systematic review. Obes Surg. 2014;25(1):159–66.
17. Santonicola A, Cutolo P, Formisano G, Iovino P. The effect of laparoscopic sleeve gastrectomy with or without hiatal hernia repair on gastroesophageal reflux disease in obese patients. Surg Obes Relat Dis. 2014;10(2):250–5.
18. Patel AD, Lytle NW, et al. Combining laparoscopic giant paraoesophageal hernia repair with sleeve gastrectomy in obese patients. Surg Endosc. 2014;29(5):1115–22.

42 Reflux After Gastric Bypass: Roux en-Y and One-Anastomosis Gastric Bypass

Gabriel Diaz Del Gobbo
and Matthew Kroh

Roux en-Y Gastric Bypass (RYGB)

It is known that the incidence of gastroesophageal reflux disease (GERD) is four times higher in patients with obesity than in those with normal body mass index (BMI) and that obesity is an independent risk factor for the development of reflux and hiatal hernia (HH) [1]. Roux en-Y gastric bypass (RYGB) is the preferred intervention to treat morbid obesity with concomitant GERD. Anatomical factors of the operation, including a small pouch disconnected from the rest of the stomach, prevent acid and biliary reflux into the esophagus, as well as fast transit of the alimentary bolus into the bowel, resulting in symptom resolution in a vast majority of patients.

Reflux after RYGB, although less common, may be produced by several pathologies and is reported in up to 22% of cases, based

G. D. Del Gobbo · M. Kroh (✉)
Cleveland Clinic Abu Dhabi, Abu Dhabi, UAE

Cleveland Clinic Lerner College of Medicine, Cleveland, Ohio, USA
e-mail: krohm@ccf.org

A. D. Patel et al. (eds.), *The SAGES Manual of Physiologic Evaluation of Foregut Diseases*,
https://doi.org/10.1007/978-3-031-39199-6_42

on different definitions [2]. In this section, we will focus on the pathophysiology, symptoms, findings of diagnostic tests, and a brief review of treatment.

Hiatal Hernia

Between 10 and 40% of patients with morbid obesity have HH. HH are more frequently discovered and repaired during a sleeve gastrectomy than RYGB (21% vs 10%) [3]. Mobilization of the stomach and dissection of the angle of His may disrupt existing anti-reflux mechanisms and weight loss after bariatric surgery may lead to proximal stomach migration through the hiatus. Both of these mechanisms may be contributory to reflux after bariatric surgery.

The incidence of hiatal hernia after RYGB is poorly documented; available data come from small case series [3]. In the largest retrospective study, hiatal hernia was found in up to 53% of patients with reflux after RYGB. Symptoms included GERD, dysphagia, abdominal pain, vomiting, and in some cases loss of appetite. In this study, an endoscopic evaluation showed that when the esophago-gastric junction was above the hiatus (Fig. 42.1), esophagitis and Barrett's epithelium are common (50% and 15%, respectively) [2]. Upper gastro-intestinal (GI) series and CT scan are commonly used imaging techniques that can also aid in the diagnosis of hiatal hernia after bariatric surgery (Fig. 42.2).

The authors describe surgical correction with complete mobilization of the gastroesophageal junction, obtaining 2–4 cm of the intra-abdominal esophagus and resection of the hernia sac. In this cohort, a posterior cruroplasty was performed with permanent sutures, pledgets, and bioabsorbable mesh. They had no recurrences at a mean follow-up of 19 months, but one patient had to resume medical therapy due to relapsed GERD [3].

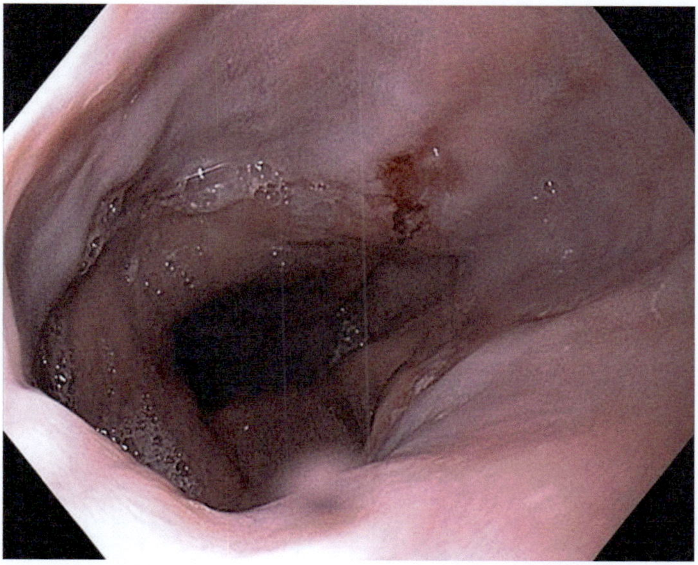

Fig. 42.1 Endoscopic view of hiatal hernia with grade A esophagitis

Marginal Ulcers

Reported incidences are highly variable with reports ranging from 0.6 to 25% [4, 5], likely determined by definition how widespread endoscopy is used in a given practice. The development of marginal ulcers (MU) is likely due to some combination of injury secondary to poor oxygenation, increased acid or bile exposure, and reaction to foreign bodies like suture material. Among the risk factors that have been described, smoking (HR 5.03), immunosuppression (HR 4.60), and preoperative NSAID use (HR 3.11) lead to a significantly increased probability of MU that requires surgical revision [5].

MU has a wide range of clinical presentations. Up to 61% of cases can be asymptomatic, while other patients present with

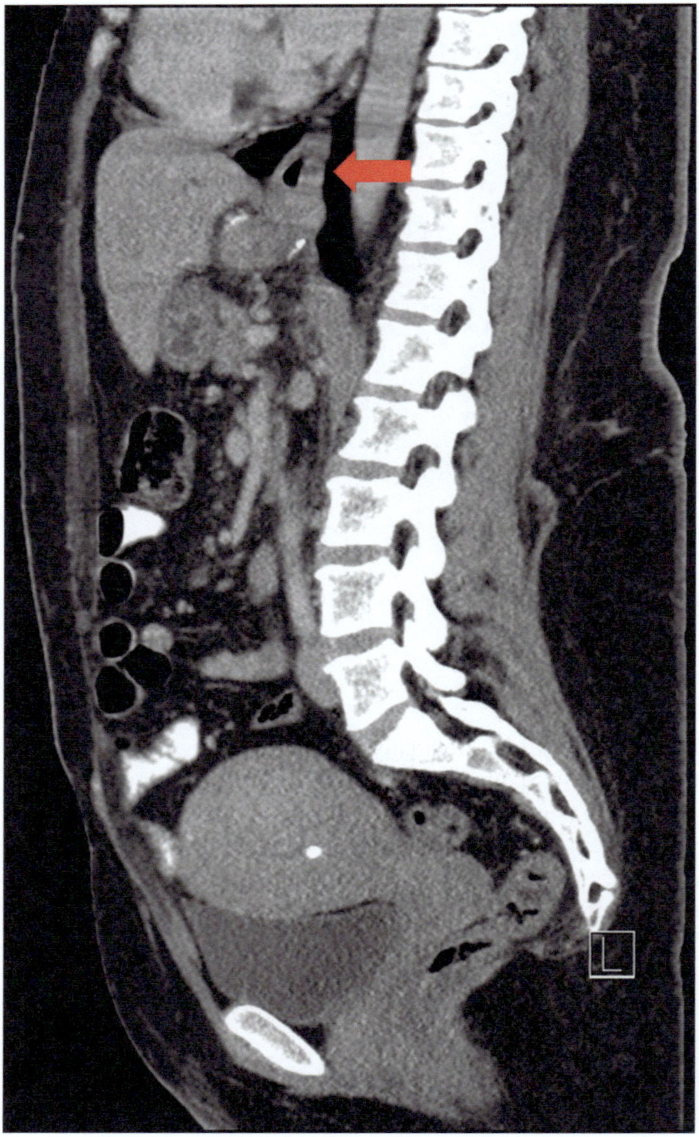

Fig. 42.2 CT chest and abdomen demonstrating mediastinal migration of the pouch (red arrow)

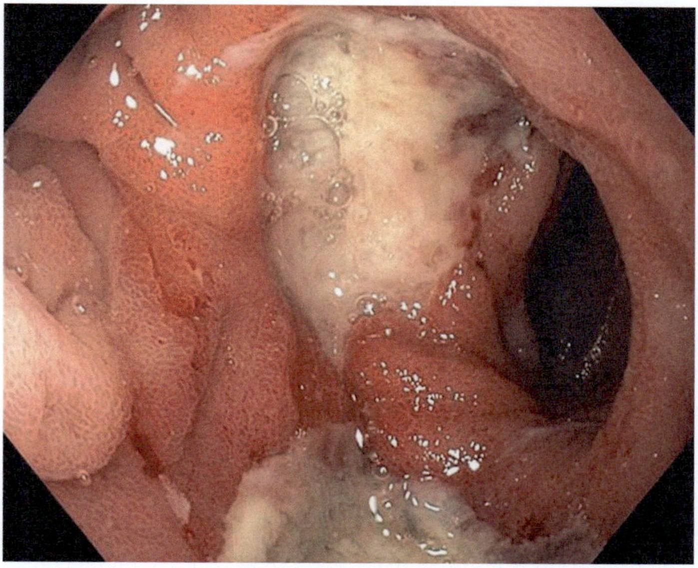

Fig. 42.3 Upper GI endoscopy showing a marginal ulcer located above the GJ anastomosis

heartburn, nausea, abdominal pain, gastrointestinal bleeding, or acute abdomen due to perforation [6]. The most effective way to evaluate a MU is an upper GI endoscopy (Fig. 42.3). Endoscopy allows for the determination of size and location of the ulcer and also permits for treatment in instances of bleeding or perforation. Upper GI series can be used to rule out gastro-gastric (GG) fistula, and often the findings of upper GI series and endoscopy can give complementary information [7]. A CT scan is less useful but can be helpful to evaluate other intra-abdominal processes and acute pathology including perforation or obstruction.

Initial treatment includes proton pump inhibitors, sucralfate, and avoidance of causative factors. Surgery is indicated when patients do not respond to medical therapy or during acute events such as perforation; this can happen in 1–9.2% of symptomatic MU. The surgical procedure may include gastro-jejunal (GJ) resection and revision, with or without truncal vagotomy. In a retrospective study that included 67 revisions, patients reported resolution of symptoms in only 36% of cases and 57% developed a recurrent ulcer [5, 6, 8].

Gastro-Jejunal Stenosis

This is a narrowing of the GJ anastomosis that occurs in a range of 3–28% after RYGB. The contributing factors including tissue ischemia, anastomotic tension, edema, foreign body reaction, and chronic GJ ulcers may lead to formation [7, 8]. A randomized control trial showed that GJ stenosis is more frequent when using a 21 mm circular stapler [9].

Typically, patients have symptoms of nausea, vomiting, reflux, progressive dysphagia, and may experience higher weight loss than expected. GJ stenosis often becomes symptomatic when the lumenal diameter is less than 10 mm. Endoscopy is the most effective tool for diagnosis and treatment simultaneously (Fig. 42.4a). Upper GI series may also reveal stenosis, showing a linear passage of contrast through the anastomosis or delayed pouch emptying [7].

Endoscopic balloon dilation constitutes the first therapeutic line (Fig. 42.4b), especially during the first 3 postoperative months. This technique allows for direct visualization and pro-

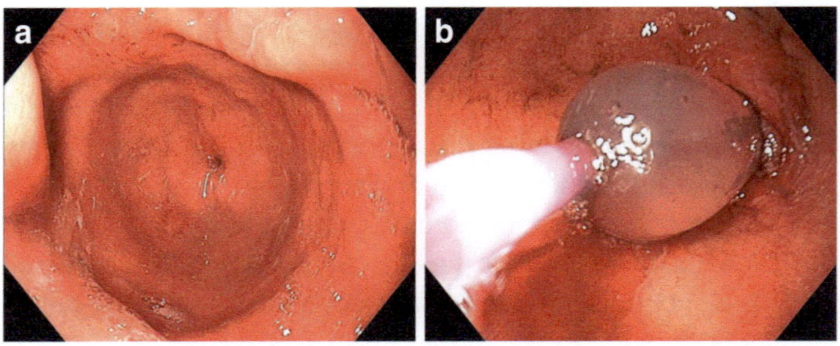

Fig. 42.4 (**a**, **b**) Endoscopic diagnosis and treatment of GJ stenosis. (**a**) Severe lumen narrowing in a patient with dysphagia after RYGB. (**b**) Balloon dilation, between 1 to 3 sessions achieve symptoms resolution

gressive dilation through radial expansion. Other endoscopic treatments such as stents represent a salvage for failed endoscopic dilation, with success rates up to 83% reported. Surgical revision is needed in less than 1% of cases and is reserved for patients with stenosis refractory to endoscopic interventions [7, 8].

Gastro-Gastric Fistula

Gastro-gastric fistula is an abnormal communication between the gastric pouch and the gastric remnant. The incidence of gastro-gastric (GG) fistula was higher in the era of non-divided gastric bypass and has decreased with complete resection of the pouch from the remnant stomach during the primary operation. Currently, this may occur in up to 1–6% of patients and is likely secondary to leak or marginal ulcer [2, 10, 11].

This anomalous track allows the passage of content into the previously disconnected stomach and rest of the gastro-intestinal tract. This can present as weight regain and reflux. An upper GI endoscopy establishes the diagnosis (Fig. 42.5a), demonstrating an orifice in the mucosa leading to the remnant stomach. Upper GI fluoroscopy is also useful, especially in smaller fistulae; reveal-

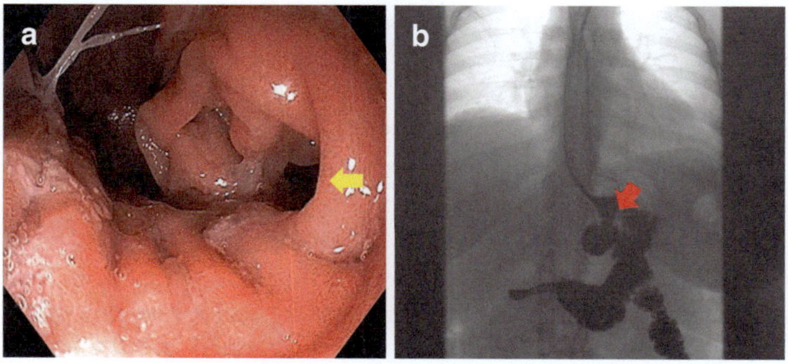

Fig. 42.5 (**a**, **b**) Gastro-gastric fistula in a patient with suboptimal weight loss and intermittent reflux after RYGB. (**a**) Endoscopy showing the track in the gastric pouch (yellow arrow). (**b**) Upper GI series demonstrating contrast flowing from the pouch into the gastric remnant (red arrow)

ing passage of contrast to the gastric remnant (Fig. 42.5b). With a large opening, the endoscope can be advanced through the fistula to evaluate the stomach and duodenum.

With a small fistula, endoscopic management has been described, though the recurrence rate is high [11]. Symptomatic patients require surgical treatment [8]. Principles of the operation include resection, typically of the remnant stomach, and often revision of the gastrojejunostomy. This approach yields success rates between 87 and 100% symptom resolution at follow-up [10, 12].

Enlarged Pouch

Usually the gastric pouch in a RYGB measures between 3 and 4 cm or less, and when enlarged may include a persistent presence of acid production from retained parietal cells, or regurgitation, especially in the presence of stenotic anastomosis [13]. Histological examination of doughnuts after circular mechanical anastomosis in patients undergoing RYGB showed reduced number of parietal cells in smaller gastric pouches (2 vs 4 cm) [14]. In previously published reports, a pouch is considered enlarged when it is longer than 5–6 cm [2, 15].

Long gastric pouches can produce GERD and suboptimal weight loss. During an upper GI endoscopy, it is possible to measure the distance from the Z-line to the level of the GJ anastomosis. Upper GI series has also been described to characterize gastric pouches using vertebrae height as a reference.

Surgical revision is mostly described in cases of weight regain or insufficient weight loss. Technical conduct of the operation for revision includes mobilization of the gastric pouch and roux limb, resection more proximal to the esophagogastric junction, and re-anastomosis. In a cohort of 25 patients that underwent this surgical technique, almost half of them reported resolution or improvement of their symptoms post-operatively [15].

Candy Cane Syndrome

Candy cane syndrome represents a constellation of symptoms caused by an enlarged blind loop in some patients with RYGB. The mechanism of development of these symptoms is thought to be secondary to bowel dysmotility that induces progressive dilation of the bowel, or creation of a long afferent limb at the time of operation [16, 17]. This enlarged blind loop gets filled after oral intake resulting in bowel distention. Authors have reported this situation in case reports and small retrospective studies [13, 14].

The syndrome presents with postprandial epigastric pain or distension that gets relief after vomiting; some patients report acid and non-acid reflux. The diagnosis is established either by upper GI endoscopy or upper GI series confirming a long afferent limb that may also contain food or bezoar. Often the endoscope and oral contrast preferentially go first into the blind loop and then into the Roux limb [16, 18].

Resection of the redundant limb is the most effective therapeutic approach, and up to 94% of patients report symptom resolution [16]. Endoscopic treatment has been attempted with limited success [18].

Bile Reflux

Although more rare, bile reflux after RYGB has been reported [13, 19]. The most common cause is a short Roux limb and reflux retrograde from the jejuno-jejunostomy or from gastro-gastric fistula [13, 20].

Patients complain of abdominal pain, GERD, or bilious vomiting. Upper GI endoscopy can confirm bile in the gastric pouch or in the esophagus causing gastritis, esophagitis, or ulcers [19, 20]. Bile reflux can be diagnosed using the Sydney scoring system after grading intestinal metaplasia, edema, chronic inflammation, and *Helicobacter pylori* status. Recently, it has been published that a tailored HIDA scan with addition of a SPECT-CT scan, ingestion of a fatty meal, and prolonged scanning duration permit bile reflux detection in patients with previous bariatric surgery [21].

Alginates can ameliorate the symptoms, but the definitive treatment is surgery by lengthening the Roux limb, usually to at least 100 cm, or by resection of the fistulous tract. Surgical correction results in high resolution of symptoms [20].

Motility Disorders

Manometry evaluation has shown that up to 20% of patients have some degree of motility disorders after RYGB. This percentage is even higher (40%) in a cohort of 47 patients with de novo or persistent reflux after bypass. Findings included, hypotensive lower esophageal sphincter (LES), 58%, 18% had absent contractility, and 20% ineffective esophageal motility or fragmented peristalsis; all in the absence of the anastomotic stricture [2].

Achalasia is rare, but few case reports and small cohorts have been published [22]. It is unknown if the condition existed before the gastric bypass or developed after the surgery. Surgical or endoscopic myotomy is the preferred treatment [23].

Others

Eosinophilic esophagitis (EoE) is an allergic disorder estimated between 10 and 50 per 100,000 persons in the United States and Europe. The eosinophilic infiltration of the esophageal mucosa produces dysphagia. EoE and GERD are linked by a non-allergic pathway that results in chronic inflammation triggered by the acid exposure. In a Japanese study of 27 cases, hiatal hernia and obesity were risk factors for EoE. Linear furrows, esophageal rings, white plaques, and mucosal edema are seen during upper GI endoscopy; the diagnosis is confirmed by biopsy that reveals esophageal intraepithelial eosinophil infiltration of ≥15 per high-power fields [2, 24].

Zollinger Ellison syndrome is a rare entity and manifests in patients as recurrent gastric ulcers induced by neuroendocrine tumors with increased gastrin production. The exact incidence after RYGB is unknown. Confirmation diagnosis can be a challenge as tumors may be located in the excluded stomach or proximal duodenum [2, 25].

Lastly, there is a group of patients that undergo a wide range of evaluations without identifying a clear diagnosis. These are presumed to have functional disorders and may represent up to 13% of patients after RYGB [2].

One Anastomosis Gastric Bypass or Mini-Gastric Bypass

A spectrum of loop gastric bypass operations have become increasingly popular worldwide. Known commonly as one anastomosis gastric bypass (OAGB) and mini-gastric bypass (MGB), there are technical differences in conduct and outcome. This operation is a modern version of loop gastric bypass described by Mason in 1967. Typically the surgery includes the construction of a long and narrow gastric pouch that measures between 15 and 18 cm with a GJ anastomosis at 200–250 cm distally from the ligament of Treitz [26, 27]. Though not currently endorsed by the American Society of Metabolic and Bariatric Surgeons (ASMBS), variations of this operation represent 4.3% of the bariatric operations performed worldwide. In the Middle East and North Africa, these operations constitute the second most common procedure after sleeve gastrectomy [28, 29]. Results have shown significant weight loss and resolution of comorbidities, as well as metabolic and mechanical complications [29–31], including reflux.

Bile Reflux

The rate of bile reflux and the implications of bile reflux after OAGB are not well documented. Bile reflux into the pouch and

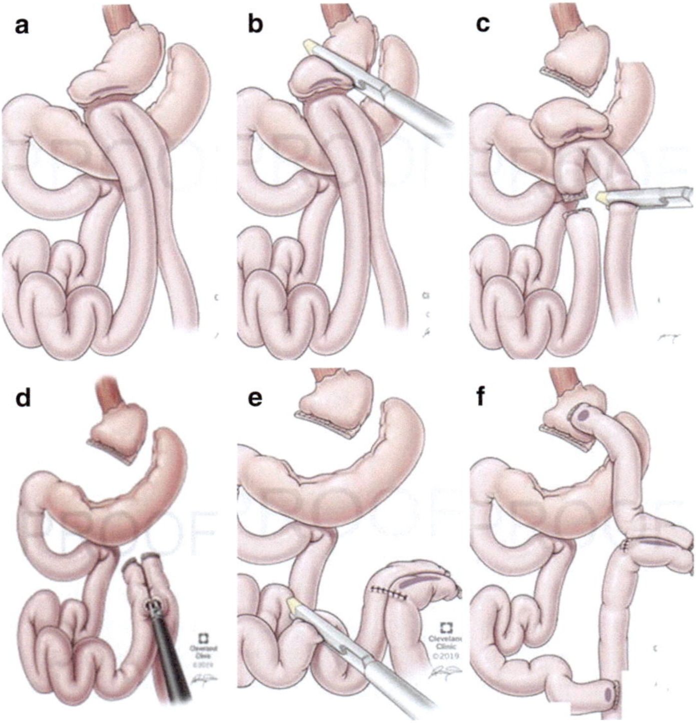

Fig. 42.6 (**a**–**f**) Step by step conversion OAGB to RYGB [27]. (**a**) OAGB configuration. (**b**) section above the previous GJ. (**c**) Section of the bowel involved in the initial anastomosis. (**d**) Bowel transit reconstruction. (**e**) Creation of the Roux limb. (**f**) New RYGB

potentially the esophagus may occur as a result of the loop anastomosis (Fig. 42.6a).

When symptomatic, bile reflux can result in epigastric pain, bilious vomiting, GERD, and loss of appetite. Upper GI endoscopy (Fig. 42.7a, b) is used to evaluate post-surgical anatomy and associated changes including stricture, ulcer, or mucosal inflammation. Several publications, including randomized control trials,

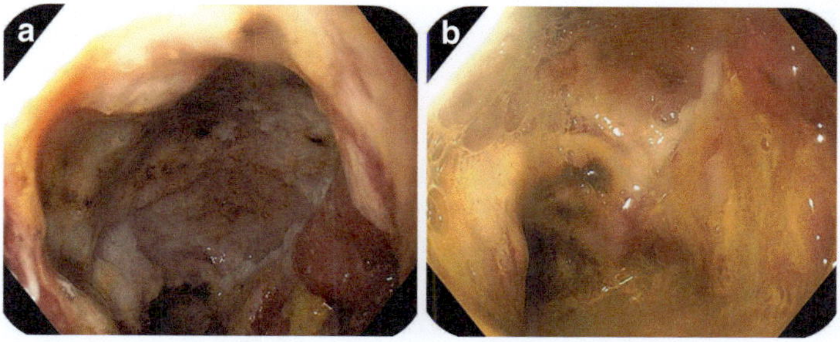

Fig. 42.7 (**a**, **b**) Bile reflux in a patient who underwent OAGB one year prior, complaining of severe abdominal pain, bilious vomiting and poor appetite. (**a**) Extensive and deep GJ ulcer. (**b**) Bile noted in the gastric pouch and esophagus

have reported bile in the esophagus or gastric pouch (6.6–18%), gastritis (19–28%), ulcers (1.65–18.8%), esophagitis (7.2–10%), and Barret's esophagus (1.72%) [27, 30, 31].

Mechanical Complications

As this is a relatively newer procedure, fewer reports of complications after OAGB are in the current literature.

Hiatal hernia has been found between 4.4% and 29.2% of cases with a significant correlation to GERD [27, 32]. Gastro-jejunal anastomosis stenosis (0.85–12.5%) and pouch torsion have also been reported after OAGB [27, 30].

Medical therapy including anti-secretory and barrier medication can be helpful as first line therapy. In refractory patients or in those with severe mechanical or malnutrition complications, conversion to RYGB has been reported with success [27]. As the number of operations performed worldwide increases, attention to rates of reflux and subsequent complications will be important to report.

Editor Note

Dysphagia after gastric bypass

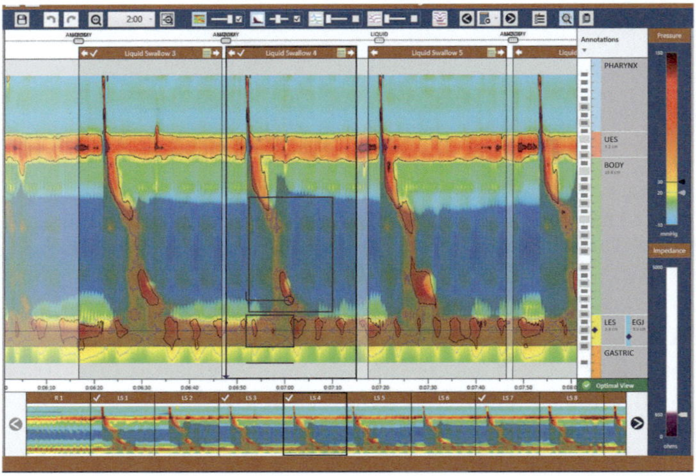

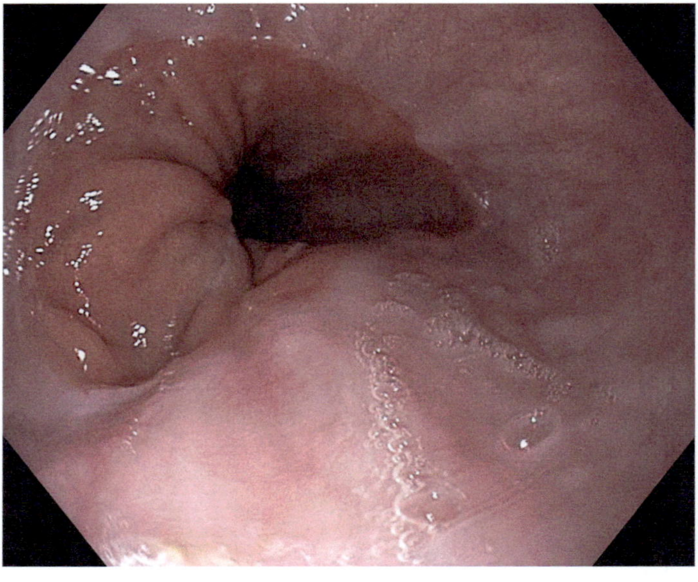

56 years female 10 years post sleeve and 5 years post conversion to bypass comes in with complaints of food sticking. The manometric tracing read as EGJOO with a small sliding hiatal hernia. Esophageal motility remains peristaltic although bolus clearance is poor. Endoscopic finding confirms a small hiatal hernia with some esophageal dilation and a small hiatal opening. After a gastric bypass, even small 1–2 cm hiatal hernias can act like a paraesophageal hernia since it can be 20% or more of the gastric pouch. Ultimately the hiatal hernia was repaired and the dysphagia symptoms resolved.

When a patient complains of dysphagia after gastric bypass, the first step is dietary counseling. However additional workup with esophagram, endoscopy and manometry may reveal other findings such as hiatal hernia causing EGJOO. Achalasia has also been seen after RYGBP.

Reflux after RYGBP

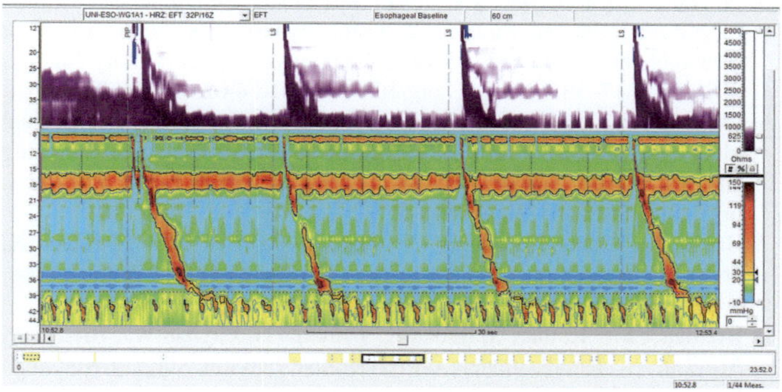

A gastric bypass procedure is an excellent drainage procedure for those with GERD, however it does not affect the LES. In this study, a patient presented with severe reflux symptoms after RYGBP. The manometry revealed a hypotensive LES and a hiatal hernia. She underwent LES augmentation utilizing magnetic beads and hiatal hernia repair. The reflux/regurgitation resolved.

References

1. Boules M, Corcelles R, Guerron AD, Dong M, Daigle CR, El-Hayek K, et al. The incidence of hiatal hernia and technical feasibility of repair during bariatric surgery. Surgery. 2015;158(4):911–8. https://doi.org/10.1016/j.surg.2015.06.036.
2. Borbély Y, Kröll D, Nett PC, Moreno P, Tutuian R, Lenglinger J. Radiologic, endoscopic, and functional patterns in patients with symptomatic gastroesophageal reflux disease after Roux-en-Y gastric bypass. Surg Obes Relat Dis. 2018;14(6):764–8. https://doi.org/10.1016/j.soard.2018.02.028.
3. Clapp B, Vo LU, Lodeiro C, Harper B, Montelongo S, Lee I, et al. Late-term hiatal hernia after gastric bypass: an emerging problem. Surg Obes Relat Dis. 2020;16(4):471–5. https://doi.org/10.1016/j.soard.2020.01.018.
4. Coblijn UK, Goucham AB, Lagarde SM, Kuiken SD, Van Wagensveld BA. Development of ulcer disease after Roux-en-Y gastric bypass, incidence, risk factors, and patient presentation: a systematic review. Obes Surg. 2014;24(2):299–309.
5. Di Palma A, Liu B, Maeda A, Anvari M, Jackson T, Okrainec A. Marginal ulceration following Roux-en-Y gastric bypass: risk factors for ulcer development, recurrence and need for revisional surgery. Surg Endosc. 2020;35:2347–53. https://doi.org/10.1007/s00464-020-07650-0.
6. Pyke O, Yang J, Cohn T, Yin D, Docimo S, Talamini MA, et al. Marginal ulcer continues to be a major source of morbidity over time following gastric bypass. Surg Endosc. 2019;33(10):3451–6. https://doi.org/10.1007/s00464-018-06618-5.
7. Boules M, Chang J, Haskins IN, Sharma G, Froylich D, El-Hayek K, et al. Endoscopic management of post-bariatric surgery complications. World J Gastrointest Endosc. 2016;8(17):591.
8. Brethauer SA, Kothari S, Sudan R, Williams B, English WJ, Brengman M, et al. Systematic review on reoperative bariatric surgery American Society for Metabolic and Bariatric Surgery Revision Task Force. Surg Obes Relat Dis. 2014;10(5):952–72. https://doi.org/10.1016/j.soard.2014.02.014.
9. Abellán I, López V, Lujan J, Abrisqueta J, Hernández Q, Frutos MD, et al. Stapling versus hand suture for gastroenteric anastomosis in Roux-en-Y gastric bypass: a randomized clinical trial. Obes Surg. 2015;25(10):1796–801.
10. Chahine E, Kassir R, Dirani M, Joumaa S, Debs T, Chouillard E. Surgical management of gastrogastric fistula after Roux-en-Y gastric bypass: 10-year experience. Obes Surg. 2018;28(4):939–44.
11. Storm AC, Thompson CC. Endoscopic treatments following bariatric surgery. Gastrointest Endosc Clin N Am. 2017;27(2):233–44. https://doi.org/10.1016/j.giec.2016.12.007.

12. Tucker ON, Szomstein S, Rosenthal RJ. Surgical management of gastro-gastric fistula after divided laparoscopic Roux-en-Y gastric bypass for morbid obesity. J Gastrointest Surg. 2007;11(12):1673–9.
13. Suter M. Gastroesophageal reflux disease, obesity, and Roux-en-Y gastric bypass: complex relationship—a narrative review. Obes Surg. 2020;30(8):3178–87.
14. Siilin H, Wanders A, Gustavsson S, Sundbom M. The proximal gastric pouch invariably contains acid-producing parietal cells in Roux-en-Y gastric bypass. Obes Surg. 2005;15(6):771–7.
15. Hamdi A, Julien C, Brown P, Woods I, Hamdi A, Ortega G, et al. Midterm outcomes of revisional surgery for gastric pouch and gastrojejunal anastomotic enlargement in patients with weight regain after gastric bypass for morbid obesity. Obes Surg. 2014;24(8):1386–90.
16. Aryaie AH, Fayezizadeh M, Wen Y, Alshehri M, Abbas M, Khaitan L. "Candy cane syndrome:" an underappreciated cause of abdominal pain and nausea after Roux-en-Y gastric bypass surgery. Surg Obes Relat Dis. 2017;13(9):1501–5. https://doi.org/10.1016/j.soard.2017.04.006.
17. Dallal RM, Cottam D. "Candy cane" Roux syndrome-a possible complication after gastric bypass surgery. Surg Obes Relat Dis. 2007;3(3):408–10.
18. Granata A, Cicchese N, Amata M, De Monte L, Bertani A, Ligresti D, et al. Candy cane syndrome: a report of a mini-invasive endoscopic treatment using OverStitch, a novel endoluminal suturing system. Endoscopy. 2019;51(1):E16–7.
19. Keleidari B, Mahmoudieh M, Davarpanah Jazi AH, Melali H, Nasr Esfahani F, Minakari M, et al. Comparison of the bile reflux frequency in one anastomosis gastric bypass and Roux-en-Y gastric bypass: a cohort study. Obes Surg. 2019;29(6):1721–5.
20. Swartz DE, Mobley E, Felix EL. Bile reflux after Roux-en-Y gastric bypass: an unrecognized cause of postoperative pain. Surg Obes Relat Dis. 2009;5(1):27–30. https://doi.org/10.1016/j.soard.2008.10.009.
21. Eldredge TA, Bills M, Myers JC, Bartholomeusz D, Kiroff GK, Shenfine J. HIDA and seek: challenges of scintigraphy to diagnose bile reflux post-bariatric surgery. Obes Surg. 2020;30(5):2038–45.
22. Boules M, Corcelles R, Zelisko A, Batayyah E, Froylich D, Rodriguez J, et al. Achalasia after bariatric surgery. J Laparoendosc Adv Surg Tech A. 2016;26(6):428–32.
23. Casas MA, Schlottmann F, Herbella FAM, Buxhoeveden R, Patti MG. Esophageal achalasia after Roux-en-Y gastric bypass for morbid obesity. Updat Surg. 2019;71(4):631–5. https://doi.org/10.1007/s13304-019-00688-3.
24. Tanaka F, Fukumoto S, Morisaki T, Otani K, Hosomi S, Nagami Y, et al. Obesity and hiatal hernia may be non-allergic risk factors for esophageal eosinophilia in Japanese adults. Esophagus. 2019;16(3):309–15. https://doi.org/10.1007/s10388-019-00662-3.

25. Court I, Zissman P, Rosenthal RJ. Diagnosis and treatment of Zollinger Ellison syndrome in a morbidly obese patient after Roux-en-Y gastric bypass. Surg Obes Relat Dis. 2010;6(6):714–7. https://doi.org/10.1016/j.soard.2010.06.009.
26. Deitel M. History of the MGB and OAGB operations. Int J Surg. 2019;66:79–83. https://doi.org/10.1016/j.ijsu.2019.04.018.
27. Landreneau JP, Barajas-Gamboa JS, Strong AT, Corcelles R, Kroh MD. Conversion of one-anastomosis gastric bypass to Roux-en-Y gastric bypass: short-term results from a tertiary referral center. Surg Obes Relat Dis. 2019;15(11):1896–902. https://doi.org/10.1016/j.soard.2019.09.059.
28. Angrisani L, Santonicola A, Iovino P, Vitiello A, Higa K, Himpens J, et al. IFSO worldwide survey 2016: primary, endoluminal, and revisional procedures. Obes Surg. 2018;28(12):3783–94.
29. Haddad A, Fobi M, Bashir A, Al Hadad M, ElFawal MH, Safadi B, et al. Outcomes of one anastomosis gastric bypass in the IFSO Middle East North Africa (MENA) region. Obes Surg. 2019;29(8):2409–14.
30. Pizza F, D'Antonio D, Lucido FS, Tolone S, Dell'Isola C, Gambardella C. Postoperative clinical-endoscopic follow-up for GERD and gastritis after one anastomosis gastric bypass for morbid obesity: how, when, and why. Obes Surg. 2020;30(11):4391–400.
31. Robert M, Espalieu P, Pelascini E, Caiazzo R, Sterkers A, Khamphommala L, et al. Efficacy and safety of one anastomosis gastric bypass versus Roux-en-Y gastric bypass for obesity (YOMEGA): a multicentre, randomised, open-label, non-inferiority trial. Lancet. 2019;393(10178):1299–309.
32. Kermansaravi M, Kabir A, Mousavimaleki A, Pazouki A. Association between hiatal hernia and gastroesophageal reflux symptoms after one-anastomosis/mini gastric bypass. Surg Obes Relat Dis. 2020;16(7):863–7. https://doi.org/10.1016/j.soard.2020.03.011.

43 Pediatric and Adolescent Foregut Motility

Stefan Scholz, Vibha Sood, and Elizabeth Sharbaugh

Gross Development of the Foregut

The gastrointestinal (GI) tract is a complex physiological system consisting of the hollow organs of the digestive system (pharynx, esophagus, stomach, intestine, and colon) and the GI tract derivatives (thyroid, thymus, parathyroid, lungs, liver, and pancreas).

S. Scholz (✉)
Department of Surgery, University of Pittsburgh School of Medicine, Pittsburgh, PA, USA

Division of Pediatric General and Thoracic Surgery, UPMC Children's Hospital of Pittsburgh, Pittsburgh, PA, USA
e-mail: stefan.scholz@chp.edu

V. Sood
Department of Pediatrics, University of Pittsburgh School of Medicine, Pittsburgh, PA, USA

Division of Pediatric Gastroenterology, Hepatology, and Nutrition, UPMC Children's Hospital of Pittsburgh, Pittsburgh, PA, USA
e-mail: vibha.sood@chp.edu

E. Sharbaugh
Department of Surgery, University of Pittsburgh Medical Center, Pittsburgh, PA, USA
e-mail: paceek@upmc.edu

A. D. Patel et al. (eds.), *The SAGES Manual of Physiologic Evaluation of Foregut Diseases*,
https://doi.org/10.1007/978-3-031-39199-6_43

Each region of the gut exists as a sophisticated multi-layered system consisting of a mucosal layer, neural plexuses, and several muscle layers with all three germ layers participating in their development. The endoderm forms the epithelial layers, the mesoderm forms the muscle layers, and the ectoderm forms the submucosal (Meissner's) and the myenteric (Auerbach's) plexuses. These neural plexuses are present throughout the GI tract and are suitably termed "the enteric nervous system". Disruptions of the enteric nervous system, either congenitally during embryogenesis or organogenesis (e.g. esophageal atresia) or acquired later in life (e.g. achalasia), are primarily responsible for the various motility disorders of the gut.

During embryogenesis, the gut develops as a result of cephalocaudal and lateral embryo folding and incorporation of the endoderm-lined yolk sac. This leads to the formation of two blind-ending endodermal invaginations at the anterior and posterior ends of the embryo, which fuse to give rise to the primitive gut. This primitive gut structure subsequently undergoes significant patterning along the anterior–posterior axis and is delineated into three main areas: the foregut (esophagus and stomach), midgut (small intestine), and hindgut (colon) [1, 2].

Anatomically, the foregut can further be divided into two portions, the anterior and posterior foregut, with the former giving rise to the esophagus, trachea, and lungs and the latter to the stomach, pancreas, and liver. During the development of the foregut, both the digestive and respiratory systems share a common embryonic origin despite their differing functions, and both derive from the developing anterior foregut. During weeks 4–6 in human gestation, a compartmentalization process takes place with the formation of the respiratory diverticulum (lung buds) from the ventral anterior foregut endoderm and the gradual separation of the ventral respiratory diverticulum from the dorsal anterior foregut by the esophagotracheal septum. Two independent and separate systems that progress to form the trachea and the esophagus develop, but molecular processes that drive compartmentalization are not fully understood. The most accepted model of foregut development, the separation model, suggests that lateral ridges of thickening epithelium, along the dorsoventral midline, make contact across the lumen and fuse together, forming the esophagotracheal septum. This septum moves rostrally to separate the trachea and the esophagus. Definitive affirmation of this model, however, has been hampered by the paucity of data on the development of the lateral ridge [3, 4].

Esophageal dysmotility is a well-recognized disorder in children born with esophageal atresia. Lemoine et al. performed high-resolution esophageal manometry in newborns before surgical repair and demonstrated abnormal esophageal motility likely caused by loss, disruption, and/or dysfunction of the intrinsic innervation of the esophagus [5]. The entire enteric nerve system is principally derived from a population of vagal neural crest cells, which enter the foregut at approximately week 4 and migrate in a rostrocaudal fashion starting from the presumptive esophagus to colonize the entire gut by approximately week 7. To enable full gut colonization during embryogenesis, the neural crest cell population displays significant proliferative capacity. This proliferative capacity is tightly coordinated by Ret/GDNF signaling, while SOX10 and endothelin 3 signaling have been shown to be critical in the maintenance of multilineage enteric nervous system progenitors.

Two concentric plexuses form the enteric nervous system. The inner submucosal plexus in the submucosa (Meissner) and the outer myenteric plexus (Auerbach), which is present between the circular and longitudinal muscle layers along the length of the GI tract. In the normal esophagus, the enteric nervous system is largely present in the myenteric plexus; the submucosal plexus is absent or sparsely present. Nakazato et al. showed that the myenteric (Auerbach) plexus of infants with esophageal atresia (EA) is deficient. A lower amount of neural tissue was present in the distal esophagus compared to the proximal end of untreated esophageal atresia patients and control patients [6].

More recently, Boleken et al. suggested that the expression of neuronal markers, such as neurofilaments, specifically found in neuronal cells, and synaptophysin, a calcium-binding protein present in the presynaptic vesicles of neurons, was significantly reduced in the affected part of the esophagus while S100 expression, a marker of glial cells, was increased in the muscular layers and the myenteric plexus. GDNF expression, an important neurotrophic factor for neural cells, was significantly reduced in these esophageal atresia patients, suggesting a possible signaling deficiency, which could account for the observed intrinsic innervation deficits [7].

Challenges Unique to the Pediatric Population

Unique challenges are encountered when performing and interpreting motility evaluations in the pediatric population. Many important aspects of the development and maturation of the infant and pediatric gastrointestinal system are still being elucidated. After birth, motor processes of the foregut begin to mature until they develop adult characteristics. Research efforts have included the determination of necessary factors and the accurate timeline of enteric nervous system maturation, as well as contractile patterns of the foregut musculature. Congenital anomalies, such as esophageal atresia or esophageal stricture, can lead to subsequent secondary esophageal motor disorders, which add additional complexity in regard to growth and development as well as long-term dysmotility patterns [8, 9].

With increasing overall survival rates of preterm infants, pharyngeal, and gastrointestinal motility disorders, their roles in causing swallowing and feeding difficulties in infants are becoming exceedingly important. Preterm and small gestational age neonates have the greatest risk of developing motility problems. Infants can have congenital and developmental pharyngeal and/or gastrointestinal motility disorders, many of which are also seen in adults. These disorders might limit nutritional intake, leading to failure to thrive, and might manifest clinically as gastroesophageal reflux symptoms, feeding difficulties and/or refusal, choking episodes, and airway changes secondary to micro- or overt aspiration [10].

The ability to swallow develops in utero and contributes to the maintenance of homeostasis of the amniotic fluid volume and composition. Swallowing activity appears at 10–14 weeks gestation as one of the first motor responses in the pharynx. Real sucking (defined by a dominant posterior–anterior movement of the tongue) begins to develop at the gestational age of 18–24 weeks, which corresponds with the timing of myelination of the brain stem. Between weeks 26 and 29, sucking does not likely mature substantially further. Feeding behavior in neonates born prematurely improves up to 36 weeks postmenstrual age (PMA), in concert with full maturation of the suck–swallow–breathe cycle. By week 34 gestational age, most of the healthy neonates seem to be capable of successful oral feeding [11].

Although reported lower esophageal sphincter (LES) resting pressures vary widely between studies, a trend toward higher LES pressures with increasing PMA can be identified during this maturation process (resting pressure between 10 and 25 mmHg). Maturation of the propagation of peristalsis along the esophagus and at the lower esophageal sphincter (LES) also continues throughout the infant/toddler period before reaching an adult peristaltic pattern. In addition to LES relaxation in response to swallowing, transient LES relaxations (TLESRs) occur, which are independent of both swallowing and the primary peristaltic activity of the esophagus. These TLESRs are known to be the predominant mechanism underlying gastroesophageal reflux (GER). Healthy premature infants born at >28 weeks PMA demonstrate TLESRs with characteristics similar to those described in adults [12, 13].

Advancing technology, in addition to the development of variable-sized equipment, enables improved insight into the pathophysiology of gastrointestinal motility disorders. With the increase of our pathophysiologic knowledge, the next challenge will be the development of treatment options that are specific to the age and disorder of the patient in order to improve the prognosis of children with upper gastrointestinal motility disorders.

Reliable interpretation of diagnostic evaluations in children of different ages can be challenging since child-control data are sparse. The majority of "normal" values have been derived either from the adult literature or from pediatric populations, which were retrospectively characterized as "normal." This is relevant especially for more invasive studies, such as antro-duodenal manometry, and for the pediatric age groups outside neonates and late adolescents. Analysis of studies is commonly not straightforward due to the lack of child-specific information, and care must be taken to avoid overinterpretation as certain patterns deemed to be abnormal in adults may in fact be normal in children [14, 15].

The pediatric provider faces unique technical challenges when performing manometry or other invasive motility studies in the pediatric population. Especially younger children may not cooperate with the examiner and the study, and communication may be a challenge. There are limitations with regard to the available equipment, such as catheter size and the amount and type of fluid, which can be used in perfusion systems. Prolonged perfused manometry may be contraindicated in young children due to the risk of water intoxication. Advances in silicon tubing have allowed the creation of smaller catheters with sleeves, which have permitted the study of premature infants, which provides information on developmental processes. In the case of solid-state catheters, transducer size and cost often present a limiting step to the reduction of catheter diameter [9, 10].

Children typically show varying levels of cognition and cooperation, which adds to the challenge and difficulty of performing pediatric motility evaluations. We always try to use age- and developmentally appropriate techniques to minimize patient anxiety. The anxiety of the patient may influence the observed motility patterns, and results may be difficult or impossible to interpret due to artifacts caused by crying or with movement. In pediatric practice, studies are commonly performed by physicians or nurses, not technicians, who must be familiar with the interpretation of the nuances of the studies and with the basic aspects of cognitive infant and childhood development. Parents of patients are often present and may even help with the study to allow for the best level of cooperation. Parent–child interactions should be observed to study the pattern of a specific behavior, which may be of importance for interpreting the study. It is common to evaluate children who are unable to understand what is asked of them or refuse to cooperate with parts of the study, such as swallowing on command. Particularly in young children, sedation may be necessary to place and perform esophageal manometry. Midazolam and chloral hydrate are two substances that do not significantly affect gastrointestinal motility. For some esophageal and antro-duodenal manometry evaluations, the catheter is often placed under general anesthesia, and the study is started the next day after the effect of the general anesthesia has worn off [16–18].

Approach to the Pediatric Patient with Suspected Motility Disorder, Diagnostic Imaging, and Interventional Studies

After a careful history and physical examination for the signs and symptoms pertaining to motility disorders, anatomical abnormalities as well as mucosal and/or metabolic disorders should be excluded.

Diagnostic Imaging

Exclusion of anatomical problems as an initial step should be undertaken in all patients. Plain radiographs and contrast studies have a role to detect congenital and acquired structural GI abnormalities, such as the presence or absence of hiatal hernia, duodenal stenosis, malrotation, achalasia, esophageal atresia, stricture, and situs anomalies. An upper GI contrast study is not a reliable test to diagnose gastroesophageal reflux, and it has a sensitivity of 42.8% and a negative predictive value of 24%. Timed barium esophagograms are utilized to assess esophageal emptying, particularly helpful in the follow-up of patients with achalasia. A Computerized Tomography (CT) Scan or a Magnetic Resonance Imaging (MRI) imaging using luminal and intravenous contrast provides spatial resolution and tissue differentiation to detect malformations, inflammation, the presence of adhesions, or postoperative complications [15, 19, 20].

Esophago-Gastro-Duodenoscopy (EGD)

Diagnostic endoscopy in conjunction with laboratory examinations should be performed to exclude mucosal or metabolic disorders in patients presenting with symptoms of dysphagia, odynophagia, oropharyngeal dysphagia, regurgitation/vomiting, intractable gastroesophageal reflux disease (GERD), abdominal pain, early satiety, anorexia, and weight loss. Therapeutic EGD indications include control of GI bleeding (hematemesis and hematochezia), ingestions (foreign body and caustic), stricture dilation, and varices treatment.

Gastrointestinal Manometry

Measurement of the contractile activity of the GI tract has been increasingly used as a diagnostic tool in children to evaluate gastrointestinal motility [14, 21–23]. Manometry testing allows assessment of neuropathic or myopathic processes affecting the GI motility. High resolution manometry has replaced standard manometry as the "gold standard" test for the evaluation of gastrointestinal motility.

High Resolution Esophageal Manometry (HREM)

HREM assesses peristalsis by measuring the shape, amplitude, and duration of the esophageal contractions. HREM utilizes an increased number of recording sites with decreased spacing between them and specialized software, which transforms the data into contour plots. The addition of impedance measurements to HREM provides additional information if the peristaltic abnormalities are impairing the esophageal bolus transit. HREM evaluates dysphagia, chest pain, and intractable regurgitation, and it is used to diagnose different subtypes of achalasia. HREM is helpful in patients with post esophageal atresia repair presenting with recurrent dysphagia and respiratory infections with or without a

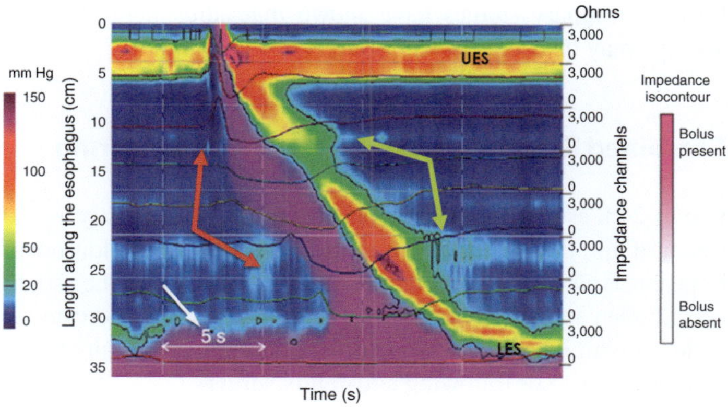

Fig. 43.1 Normal swallow with high resolution esophageal manometry combined with impedance. White arrow: normal sphincter relaxation; green arrow: peristaltic wave; and red arrow: impedance waves showing normal bolus transit after a saline swallow

fundoplication [24, 25]. Both water-perfused and solid-state catheters can be used for high-resolution manometry.

The solid-state manometry catheter contains up to 36 pressure sensors distributed 1 cm apart. These sensors provide spatiotemporal, topographic maps of the propagating motor patterns by simultaneously measuring the pressures in the entire esophagus and its sphincters (Fig. 43.1). When impedance sensors are added, the interrelationship between bolus flow, peristalsis, and sphincter opening can be studied.

The performance of motility studies in the pediatric population can be challenging due to lack of cooperation, inability to use sedation, and catheter size. The availability of small caliber silicon rubber catheters has improved the tolerability and performance of motility testing in children [26–28]. The normal values and patterns have not been established in children; often, the values are determined based on the comparison with adult patterns. It is important to correlate clinical findings and avoid overinterpretation. Chicago classification incorporates parameters for analysis of high-resolution esophageal manometry (HREM) for adults

[26]. Preliminary studies have shown that adjustments for size and age may be needed in children.

Combined Esophageal pH/Impedance Monitoring

Use of 24 h esophageal pH-Impedance testing is currently a gold standard for the detection of reflux episodes. The addition of impedance with pH testing detects bolus transit within the esophageal lumen and reflux events independent of pH. It is indicated in children with incomplete or lack of response to acid suppression therapy, prior to or following anti-reflux surgery [29, 30].

Antro-duodenal Manometry

The propulsion of luminal contents and absorption of nutrients take place due to organized motor activity in the fasting and postprandial periods in the small intestine [31]. The fasting period is characterized by a sequence of three main phases of motor activity with an average duration of about 100 min known as migrating motor complex (MMC) [32]. Phase three of the MMC, which is the most distinctive pattern of gastrointestinal motor activity, is a hallmark of normal small bowel motility [33]. Antro-duodenal

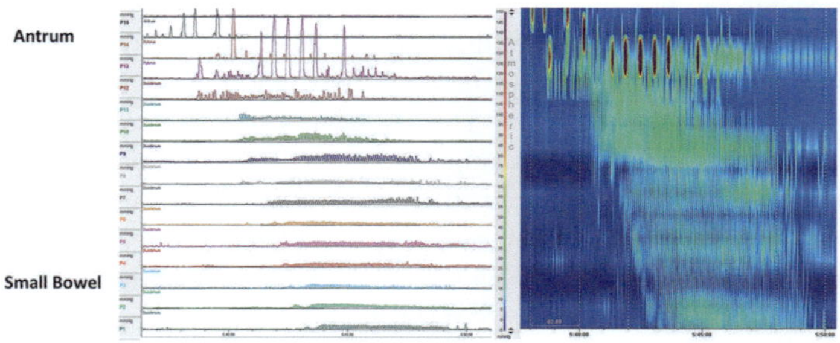

Fig. 43.2 Conventional vs high resolution ADM tracings (normal fasting manometry tracing) HRM tracing patterns: Antrum(red) and small bowel (green/yellow)

manometry studies assess gastric and duodenal motilities and are useful in the diagnosis of intestinal pseudo-obstruction and enteric dysmotility. HRM has also become the standard for antro-duodenal studies (Fig. 43.2).

Wireless Motility Capsule (WMC)

WMC is an alternative method to observe small bowel motility. It consists of a capsule with an inbuilt radio transmitter and receiver, as well as sensors for pH, pressure, and temperature (SmartPill Corporation, Buffalo, NY, USA). WMC non-invasively provides information on gastric emptying (the pH rises abruptly when the capsule passes to the duodenum), total gut transit time, and contractility by simultaneously measuring intraluminal pressure, pH, and temperature in a well-tolerated and ambulatory manner [34–36].

Specific Foregut Motility Disorders in Children

This section focuses on more common foregut motility disorders, which offer a unique perspective on children and represent important problems in daily practice. An overview of the complete spectrum of esophageal motor disorders in children is outlined in Table 43.1.

Esophageal Atresia

Esophageal atresia (EA) represents one of the most common and severe developmental disorders of the foregut affecting approximately 1 in 3500 live births. The digestive and the respiratory systems, two very diverse functional entities, share a common origin, and EA appears to result from incomplete separation of the ventral and dorsal parts of the foregut during development. This results in disruption of esophageal anatomy and a frequent association with tracheo-esophageal fistulas. However, the precise

Table 43.1 Spectrum of esophageal motor disorders in children (adapted from [17])

1. Striated muscle predominant disorders
(a) Oropharyngeal problems
(b) Cricopharyngeal dysfunction
(c) Abnormalities of resting tone
(d) Abnormalities in relaxation
(e) Neuromuscular disorders
(f) Neurologic disorders
(g) Muscular disorders
(h) Neuromuscular disorders
(i) Structural lesions
(j) Central nervous system malformations
2. Smooth muscle predominant disorders
(a) Primary esophageal motor disorders
Achalasia
Diffuse esophageal spasm
Ineffective peristalsis
Nutcracker esophagus
(b) Secondary esophageal motor disorders
Gastrointestinal disorders
Congenital malformations (e.g. esophageal atresia)
Eosinophilic esophagitis
Collagen vascular disease
Neuromuscular disorders
Graft-versus-host disease
Infectious diseases
Exogenous factors (e.g. medications and caustic ingestions)
Iatrogenic disorders
Other

etiopathogenesis of EA in human patients has yet to be determined.

Not surprisingly, and likely inherent to EA, associated abnormalities are seen in components of the enteric neuromusculature and ultimately loss of esophageal functional integrity. Surgical correction aims at reconstituting gut continuity and disrupting the connection between the digestive and respiratory systems. Despite considerable surgical advanced expertise, including minimally invasive approaches, the prognosis often remains guarded, and quality of life throughout childhood and adolescence can be severely affected.

From a surgical perspective, EA can be differentiated into two main groups according to the distance of separation between the two esophageal pouches: long gap EA and non-long gap EA. A commonly used definition of long gap EA is a gap length greater than four vertebral bodies or 4–6 cm in length, while others have defined this as the inability of joining the esophagus at the first surgery. Surgeons from the International Network of Esophageal Atresia have proposed that either Gross' classification type A or B EA that has no intra-abdominal air on initial abdominal radiograph should be considered as long-gap, accounting for up to 10% of all cases [37]. It is therapeutically important to distinguish long gap EA since surgical repair can present a significant challenge due to the lack of adequate esophageal length for a straightforward primary anastomosis.

Multiple techniques for connection have been proposed and attempted. More recently, closure of the gap by mechanical lengthening via external (Foker technique) or internal traction has been described and successfully employed for some of these complex patients [38]. These techniques follow the paradigm that the native esophagus is the best and most functional intra-thoracic conduit for transporting food from the mouth to the stomach. Khan et al. reported preservation of the mural layers of the esophagus and its thickness after external traction treatment and subsequent successful anastomosis, but functional motility studies defining outcomes are lacking [39].

For some patients with minimal native esophageal length or failed previous attempts of esophageal lengthening or anastomosis, esophageal replacement becomes necessary. Gastric transposition (gastric pull-up), jejunal, or colonic interpositions all are being used in different centers. During the gastric pull-up procedure, either the entire stomach is used or a tubular esophageal substitute is created from the larger curvature of the stomach, trans-positioned into the chest, and anastomosed to the well-perfused upper esophageal pouch. In other cases, either the jejunum or colon is used as a substitute, and these intestinal substitutions are relocated with their own vascular supply into the chest. Motility of the "neo-esophagus" as well as short- and long-term outcomes are mixed and often poor, especially with colonic substitutes. The intra-thoracic conduit relies most heavily on gravity due to a lack of adequate motility and significant dilation in the negative-pressure environment of the thorax over time.

A definitive therapy for EA has yet to be developed. Such efforts have been halted by a failure in determining the precise etiopathogenesis of EA in human patients and the challenging genetics of EA, which is frequently associated with malformations in other organs, especially congenital defects of the heart and other endodermal organs. The VACTERL syndrome is characterized by the involvement of defects in at least three body systems, including the Vertebral, Anorectal, Cardiovascular, Tracheal, Esophageal, Renal, and Limb systems. Tracheo-esophageal fistula (TEF) has been reported to be variably associated with this syndrome in up to 80% of cases. There is, however, emerging evidence of an important role of genetic factors in the molecular specification of foregut development. Significant evidence has been garnered from multiple transgenic animal models, which are beginning to shed light on possible dysfunctional mechanisms resulting in EA and associated TEF, which may have translational consequences for clinical diagnostics in human EA [2].

With surgical treatment, the survival rate of EA is well above 90% in dedicated centers but surgical complications and long-term esophageal morbidities are common. Post-EA repair complications can be categorized as either early or late. Early complications include esophageal anastomotic leakage, esophageal strictures, recurrent TEF, and dysphagia. Long-term complications affect 75–100% of patients and are mainly related to esophageal dysmotility and GERD. Children continue to suffer from dysphagia, esophagitis, as well as poor weight gain together with chronic respiratory infections and tracheomalacia due to aspiration, bronchial hyper-reactivity, airway damage, and decreased exercise tolerance. Esophageal strictures become less responsive to esophageal dilatation management in the presence of severe GERD. Early and late complications are more frequent in patients with long-gap atresia without fistula, patients with severe associated malformations, and patients born prematurely (<37 weeks gestational age) [40].

Long-term outpatient follow-up for EA children is considered crucial for monitoring, diagnosis, and treatment of complications. Problems continue into adolescence and adulthood with patients at an increased risk for Barrett's esophagus requiring life-long endoscopic monitoring [41].

Contributing factors for post-operative abnormal esophageal motility patterns in EA are being debated, and most likely a combination of factors share responsibility. Some authors hypothesize that dysmotility may be predominantly congenital, secondary to a malformation in the development of the innervation and the musculature of the esophagus [7]. Lower density as well as immaturity of the interstitial cells of Cajal compared with individuals without gastrointestinal pathology have been demonstrated in the proximal and distal esophagus in EA patients [42]. Supporting this approach, Lemoine et al. demonstrated abnormal esophageal motility, hypomotility with distal contraction, as well as complete aperistalsis in patients before repair of the EA [5]. Other theories point to iatrogenic causes, such as possible intrinsic or extrinsic denervation due to injury or excessive tension on the vagus nerve or due to mobilization and vascular interruption of the esophagus itself during the actual surgical repair. In addition, increased tension on the created anastomosis might cause esophageal shortening as well as an intra-thoracic cardia of the stomach or a shorter intra-abdominal esophageal segment, leading to a decrease in pressure in the lower esophagus as well as an obtuse angle of His promoting reflux.

Esophageal motility has been studied radiologically, manometrically, and with impedance and pH recordings in children with esophageal atresia, but few studies have focused on specifically investigating the upper and lower esophageal sphincters in children or adults. Mostly, the upper and lower esophageal sphincters were found to be normal but reduced resting pressure or incomplete relaxation in the lower sphincter has been described. The esophageal body, however, is almost always affected and anomalies tend to persist in adulthood. Esophageal impedance measurements after repair of EA showed considerably longer bolus and acid clearing times in comparison to children without congenital malformation. Manometric studies have identified lower mean esophageal as well as peak pressures in patients with EA compared to age-matched controls, even in patients who are not symptomatic [43, 44]. Esophageal motility in patients with EA has been evaluated with high-resolution esophageal manometry (HREM) in a multi-institutional study providing more detailed data [45]. In this study, no child had a normal peristaltic pattern. Three different major motility patterns were found during the HREM tracing analysis: complete aperistalsis (38%), pressurization (15%), and distal contraction with evidence of middle-third or distal-third esophageal contraction (47%). However, no clear correlation between clinical symptoms of patients and impaired esophageal motility could be identified.

Achalasia

Achalasia is a primary neurodegenerative esophageal motility disorder characterized by progressive symptoms of dysphagia, regurgitation, failure to thrive, and anorexia. The symptoms are caused by the absence of peristalsis, high resting pressure of the lower esophageal sphincter (LES), and failure of receptive relaxation of the LES. Achalasia of the esophagus is a very rare condition, with an estimated annual incidence of 1:100,000 cases overall, and less than 5% of those occurring in children (0.11 per 100,000 pediatric patients) before 15 years of age. The median age for diagnosis in children is about 8 years; however, infant cases have been reported. It is found to occur more frequently in males. Achalasia is often misdiagnosed due to a symptom profile overlapping with gastroesophageal reflux disease (GERD), rumination syndrome, and eating disorders. Although no cure currently exists that can reverse the underlying neuropathology, current treatments are aimed at symptom palliation [46].

The etiology of achalasia is not fully understood. Loss of ganglion cells in the distal esophagus may lead to an imbalance between inhibitory and excitatory neurotransmitters. The absence of non-adrenergic, non-cholinergic inhibitory ganglion cells causes unopposed acetylcholine and substance P action, resulting in a nonrelaxing, spastic LES. In particular, deficiency of nitric oxide releasing neurons has been implicated. In autopsy and resected specimens, signs of an inflammatory response with CD3/CD8-positive cytotoxic T cells as well as eosinophils and mast cells have been encountered in the area, suggesting a possible autoimmune phenomenon.

There is an association with Chagas disease, prevalent in South America, where circulating autoantibodies cause destruction of the myenteric plexus and aganglionosis of the LES after infection with the parasite Trypanosoma cruzi. The clinical findings mirror idiopathic achalasia.

Hereditary and familial cases of achalasia are seen in Algood's or "AAA"-syndrome (achalasia, alacrima, and adrenocorticotropic hormone (ACTH) insensitivity), pointing also to a genetic link [47].

The presentation of achalasia varies according to age. While adults and children both present with progressive dysphagia initially to solids and in some cases to liquids, the manifestations can be more variable and challenging to diagnose in children. In a review of 475 pediatric achalasia cases, 80% presented with vomiting, 76% with dysphagia, 61% with weight loss, 44% with respiratory symptoms, 38% with thoracic pain, 31% with growth failure, and 21% with nocturnal regurgitation [17].

Many pediatric patients, especially those younger than 7 years, commonly present with difficulty eating and progressive weight loss and will be treated for failure to thrive as well as gastroesophageal reflux disease (GERD) due to vomiting and regurgitation, since those conditions are much more prevalent. Proton pump inhibitors, histamine receptor blockers, and prokinetics are used to mask the actual diagnosis, which may not be correctly made for years. Some children are treated for feeding aversion due to the inability to eat foods with certain textures from progressive dysmotility and dysphagia. Regurgitation of food, typically undigested food, in achalasia patients is brought up without gastric contents or evidence of mixing, as opposed to severe GERD. Nocturnal cough is an important presenting feature in children and is caused by chronic aspiration of esophageal contents when lying flat. Older children may present with chest pain from dilation or acid exposure. A chest X-ray done for chronic cough may reveal the outline of a dilated esophagus with an air–fluid level that can hint at the diagnosis. As in adults, the dysphagia is often gradual and progressive, initially involving solids and progressing toward intermittent liquid involvement.

The diagnostic work-up in children is similar to adults; however, malignancy and pseudoachalasia are usually not part of the differential diagnosis. After a chest X-ray, many clinicians start with an esophagogram, which can show a dilated esophagus tapering into the LES with a characteristic "bird's beak" appearance. A timed barium esophagram, which quantifies time to esophageal clearance, can be useful to assess the peristaltic activity and the degree of LES hypertension. An upper endoscopy is useful to evaluate the mucosa and potentially estimate the degree of LES hypertension. Biopsies should be performed to rule out other pathologies, such as severe GERD. The definite diagnosis of achalasia requires esophageal manometry. High-resolution esophageal manometry (HRM) with intraluminal impedance monitoring is considered the gold standard to confirm and subtype achalasia with defined pediatric parameters [48].

During HRM, a catheter is placed to measure the impedance during swallowing. HRM creates a topographical pressure map of the esophagus, which can document the lack of esophageal peristalsis, an increased LES pressure, as well as partial or incomplete relaxation of the LES, although some heterogeneity is found in kids in comparison to adults. Three subtypes are defined in the recent adult Chicago Classification, which all require a mean integrated relaxation pressure above 15 mmHg. Type I is defined as minimal esophageal contractility, type II as intermittent compartmentalized pressurizations with no peristalsis, and type III with spastic distal contractions. HRM is also employed to assess therapy response and to evaluate recurrent symptoms. Intraoperative HRM can guide the length and completeness of the myotomy [49].

Like for adults, the Eckardt score has been found to be helpful in older children to grade the symptoms of dysphagia, regurgitation, chest pain, and weight loss from 0 to 3 on a Likert-scale. Scores can range from 0 to 12 and allow monitoring of successful therapy as well as standardizing outcomes [50].

Untreated patients and up to 5% of treated patients develop end-stage disease of achalasia with an extremely dilated and tortuous esophagus termed mega-esophagus. Patients may suffer from severe symptoms. At this stage, traditional treatment modalities are unsuccessful, and esophagectomy with reconstruction remains the only option with reasonable outcomes. The mega esophagus is unlikely to occur in the pediatric age group; however, it may happen with long-term follow-up of patients treated as children.

The treatment algorithm of choice for pediatric achalasia remains somewhat controversial since available long-term data are lacking, and recommendations are often extrapolated from the adult literature. To date, there is no prospective randomized pediatric data available. All management goals are palliative since achalasia has no definitive cure. Treatments target improvement of esophageal emptying by reducing pressure at the gastroesophageal junction to improve dysphagia during swallowing. Dietary modifications, such as more liquid or soft consistency in combination with frequent small meals, are usually part of the adaptive process in children as dysphagia progressively worsens. Since there are no medications to induce more efficient esophageal peristalsis, gravity in combination with soft and frequent meals is essential to assist esophageal clearance even after lowering the LES pressure [47].

Medications, such as calcium channel blockers, nitroglycerin, and sildenafil targeting relaxation of the LES, have shown minimal efficacy and should only be tried as a short-term bridge to more definitive therapy. Treatment modalities have evolved over the past two decades from balloon dilation and botulinum toxin injection to open and then laparoscopic Heller myotomy (LHM) and endoscopic myotomy.

Pneumatic dilation of the LES is one of the oldest therapies for achalasia and works by stretching and tearing the circular muscle fibers resulting in incompetence and reduction of LES resting pressure. Pneumatic dilation has been used extensively using 30–35 mm diameter balloons for children usually older than 8 years. Multiple pediatric studies have reported the immediate reduction of dysphagia symptoms in children with low complication rates of perforation, chest pain, and GERD. At long-term follow-up, up to half of the patients needed further dilations, which is consistent with the adult literature [51, 52]. In their landmark prospective study, Boeckxstaens et al. noted that younger patients below 40 years had less durable relief of symptoms with dilation versus LHM. They also noted that 25% of patients had required re-dilation at 5-year follow-up [53].

Endoscopic injection of botulinum toxin into the LES causes relaxation of the muscles by inhibition of acetylcholine release, and good initial relief of symptoms can be achieved. Unfortunately, botox is often only temporarily effective for 3–6 months, lacking long-term efficacy, and optimal dosing for children remains unclear. Botox injection is only rarely used in children since dilation and Heller myotomy are considered superior options with more durable symptom relief. The recently published guidelines of the International Society of Diseases of the Esophagus (ISDE) recommend against using botulinum toxin injection as an appropriate first-line therapy in young children with achalasia with exceptions for those children who are medically frail and at high-risk for surgical intervention [51]. In addition, surgical myotomy after botox injection as well as pneumatic dilation is considered to be more challenging due to the level of fibrosis and scarring at the LES, and a higher perforation rate has to be accepted.

Performed since the 1990s, laparoscopic Heller myotomy (LHM) is currently considered the gold standard for the treatment of achalasia. Key steps of the procedure include esophageal myotomy, which extends 5–6 cm above the gastroesophageal junction as well as up to 1–3 cm inferiorly onto the cardia of the stomach [54]. The exact length of the myotomy for pediatric patients remains controversial, especially for different age groups and very young children. Today, the procedure should be performed with concurrent endoscopy to monitor for mucosal perforation and to allow the surgeon to identify the exact location of the LES. Intraoperative manometry should be used to prevent an incomplete myotomy and confirm adequate reduction of LES pressure [49].

In children, there are no randomized studies concerning the management of achalasia. Multiple retrospective single-center reports have confirmed the safety of laparoscopic LHM as well as higher rates of long-term relief of dysphagia (up to 85%) in comparison to dilation. As discussed above, after dilation up to 100% of patients required additional dilations and up to 75% underwent subsequent surgical myotomy [47, 55, 56]. Sharp et al. compared Heller myotomy to dilation in their recent systematic review of the pediatric literature and noted that dilation had a higher failure rate, especially for younger children [57]. Reviewing the recent pediatric literature, most pediatric centers appear to have transitioned to a primary surgical approach to achalasia, especially for younger children. However, dilation can still be considered an appropriate first option with the understanding additional dilations, or surgery may become necessary for long-term success [58]. Van Lennep et al. noted, in their recent international practice survey, increased heterogeneity in the management of pediatric achalasia among different centers worldwide, necessitating well-designed intervention trials in children with achalasia. They recommended that patients should be managed in centers with access to appropriate diagnostic and treatment modalities [59].

After surgical myotomy, pathological gastroesophageal reflux can become problematic in up to 50% of cases in the adult series. In adults, many studies have focused on the inclusion of an anti-reflux procedure, such as a Dor, Toupet, or Nissen fundoplication.

Richards et al. compared LHM with LHM and Dor and found that pathologic reflux occurred in 48% versus 9% of patients [60]. Sharp et al. reported similar results, and both groups recommended adding a Dor fundoplication [61]. Other studies have found similar success in preventing post-myotomy reflux with Dor as well as Toupet fundoplication, whereas a 360-degree Nissen fundoplication prevented reflex effectively but increased the risk of recurrent dysphagia. Although there is no data specifically on children, most pediatric centers have followed the adult literature and included a fundoplication, most commonly a Dor. This is supported by a survey, in 2016, of the International Pediatric Endosurgery Group (IPEG), which showed that 95% of international pediatric surgeons perform a concurrent anti-reflux operation, 79% of which are Dor fundoplications [62].

Peroral endoscopic myotomy (POEM) was first described in adult patients by Inoue in Japan in 2010 and led to rapid and wide adoption in practice [63]. Endoscopically, a submucosal plane is developed through a 2cm mucosal incision above the LES, and the myotomy is then created across the gastroesophageal junction. Results have been favorable in long-term follow-up in adults. The procedure can be used in very advanced cases of mega-esophagus as well as in patients considered too high-risk for laparoscopic surgery. POEM has been advocated for failures of LHM as well as dilation. Inoue reported the first POEM in a pediatric patient, a 3-year old girl in 2012 [64]. Multiple small pediatric series have since confirmed safety and reported excellent early results [65–67]. Further adoption of this innovative interventional technique in pediatric centers is ongoing.

In 2018, the International Society for Diseases of the Esophagus (ISDE) published guidelines for adult and pediatric achalasia based on available evidence and expert opinion. Reviewing the pediatric literature, 96% of experts recommended that children with suspected achalasia should follow the same diagnostic work-up as adult patients with the possible exception of esophageal biopsies. A large majority of ISDE experts (80%) recommended surgical or endoscopic myotomy (as compared to dilation) as the preferred treatment for pediatric patients with idiopathic achalasia, especially for those aged 5 years or more, although the strength of this recommendation based on the GRADE (Grading of Recommendations, Assessment, Development, and Evaluations) scale was very low. Most agreed (94%) that the long-term outcome of achalasia treatment in children should be assessed by symptoms, function, physical growth, and general development.

In most patients with achalasia, myenteric ganglion cells of the esophagus and the GE junction have already disappeared at the time of diagnosis, and therefore, all existing therapies aim at palliation through the destruction of the LES. Future treatments with stem cells as gut-differentiated neural cells could target replacement of the myenteric plexus of the esophagus [68].

Eosinophilic Esophagitis

Eosinophilic esophagitis (EoE) is a chronic, antigen-immune inflammatory mediated disease caused by infiltration of eosinophils in the esophageal mucosa and is the most prevalent cause of esophagitis after GERD. EoE is characterized by symptoms of esophageal dysfunction, such as dysphagia or food impaction. Children with EoE often have other atopic diseases, such as asthma, eczema, allergic rhinitis, or food allergies. Especially in children who may not report symptoms reliably, clinical suspicion and diagnostic upper endoscopy with biopsies are paramount. The pathogenesis of EoE is complex and not completely clear. Over the last two decades, the incidence of this once rare disease has significantly increased in children [69, 70].

Untreated EoE leads to persistent symptoms and worsening inflammation. Esophageal remodeling causes fibrosis and stricture formation as well as functional abnormalities. Once EoE is diagnosed, therapy is necessary to resolve symptoms, induce remission, and prevent complications. Treatment strategies include dietary elimination of triggers as well as medications, such as a proton pump inhibitor and topical steroids. If medical therapy does not resolve symptoms and strictures have formed in severely symptomatic cases, endoscopic dilation may become necessary. Dilations can be performed safely in children with fibrostenotic EoE. In their recent large series with 68 dilations in

40 children, Menard-Katcher et al. reported no perforations or significant hemorrhage with the procedure [71].

Emerging data suggest that children with repaired esophageal atresia (EA) have a higher prevalence of eosinophilic esophagitis. In these children, symptoms are commonly attributed exclusively to GERD and not EoE, which may lead to excessive use of anti-reflux therapy and possible unnecessary interventions, such as fundoplication. EoE should be considered especially in older children with esophageal atresia who have persistent symptoms on standard anti-reflux treatment, increasing dysphagia, and recurrent strictures [72, 73]. Recently, the European Society for Pediatric Gastroenterology Hepatology and Nutrition (ESPGHAN) and the North American Society for Pediatric Gastroenterology, Hepatology and Nutrition (NASPGHAN) published joint guidelines on the long-term management of esophageal atresia. They suggested excluding EoE in all symptomatic EA patients, especially before proceeding to anti-reflux surgery [74].

Gastroesophageal Reflux Disease (GERD)

As in adults, gastroesophageal reflux (GER) is a normal physiologic process that occurs frequently in all infants. In addition, almost all infants have some physiological regurgitation, which is caused by a combination of large fluid intake and mostly supine positioning.

Increased GER can lead to esophagitis, and symptoms include feeding problems and failure to thrive in young patients. Symptoms of GERD tend to disappear spontaneously with increasing age after infancy, and most patients have resolved symptoms by 18 months of age [75].

In childhood, a wide spectrum of complex and chronic conditions predisposes patients to severe and chronic GERD. Patients with neurologic impairment, such as cerebral palsy, or congenital abnormalities, such as esophageal atresia or diaphragmatic hernia, have a very high incidence of pathological GERD. Patients with obesity as well as chronic pulmonary disease, including cystic fibrosis, are at an increased risk for reflux problems. As in adults, pediatric gastroesophageal reflux is predominantly caused by transient relaxation of the lower esophageal sphincter, which can develop into GERD due to multiple factors, such as insufficient esophageal clearance and inadequate buffering of reflux [12].

Distinguishing between physiological and pathological reflux in infants and children poses a common diagnostic challenge. In otherwise healthy and thriving infants with physiological GER, management includes parental education, guidance, and support with thickening of feedings as well as modification of feeding volume and frequency. In contrast, infants and children with GERD will need further evaluation and likely treatment. In contrast to adults, no gold standard diagnostic tool for confirming GERD in infants and children has been conclusively established. Impedance monitoring with 24-h esophageal pH measurements is the most complete investigation to quantify all GER, but its clinical utility for diagnosis and management of GER has yet to be determined. The diagnostic approach for GERD in infants and children principally depends on its presenting features, and no one combination of symptoms seems to be reliably conclusive [76].

Cow's milk protein allergy and GERD share similar symptoms, and distinguishing between the two remains challenging for the clinician. Cow's milk protein allergy is common and might be present in up to two thirds of infants with GERD. Removing cow's milk protein from an infant's diet could resolve symptoms suggestive of severe GERD [12].

When conservative measures fail for GERD, pharmacological treatment with acid suppressive therapy or prokinetics, such as low-dose erythromycin, might be considered. For most children, anti-reflux surgery, such as laparoscopic Nissen fundoplication, is often considered a treatment of last resort and is reserved for patients with intractable symptoms or recurrent apparent life-threatening events (ALTE). Patients in high-risk groups as well as children after lung transplants or with complex congenital cardiac defects routinely undergo anti-reflux procedures, often in combination with a gastrostomy feeding button. The pediatric laparoscopic Nissen fundoplication is performed in a technically different fashion than in adults. The phreno-esophageal membrane is not divided, and extensive esophageal mobilization is avoided [77]. Due to very limited data and the lack of long-term outcomes, endoluminal approaches, such as Stretta or endoluminal gastroplication techniques, cannot be recommended as surgical options for the treatment of GERD in children.

For more detailed information, updated clinical practice guidelines for pediatric gastroesophageal reflux are regularly published by pediatric specialty societies, such as the recent joint recommendations of the North American Society for Pediatric Gastroenterology, Hepatology, and Nutrition (NASPGHAN) and the European Society for Pediatric Gastroenterology, Hepatology, and Nutrition (ESPGHAN) [78].

Fundoplication and Gastrostomy Feeding Buttons

A large number of infants and children who require fundoplication also receive a gastrostomy feeding button, which is often the primary indication for the procedure. A small number of children with severe GERD and intact swallowing who are not dependent on tube feeding are candidates for fundoplication alone. In the past, most infants and children who required placement of a feeding gastrostomy would also receive a fundoplication. Today, a simultaneous fundoplication is mostly reserved for patients considered at high risk for postoperative failures, such as severely neurologically impaired children and patients with complex congenital cardiac anomalies, such as single ventricle physiology [79].

In adults, it is well established that gastric emptying is improved after fundoplication. In infants and children, evidence is sparse, and this relationship remains less clear. Pacilli et al. evaluated 11 children before and after fundoplication without gastrostomy placement with gastric emptying scintigraphy. Similar to adult studies, gastric emptying was found to significantly accelerate after surgery. Pre-operative gastric emptying did not predict post-operative outcomes in this study, suggesting that a gastric emptying study is not needed before fundoplication in children. Due to improved gastric emptying after fundoplication, a pyloroplasty or pyloromyotomy is not routinely performed for children with GERD or feeding problems [80]. The addition of these procedures is reserved for complex or neurologically impaired patients who fail fundoplication and do not tolerate gastric feedings. A more commonly offered alternative in today's practice is gastrojejunal feeding tubes, which bypass the stomach delivering enteral nutrition directly to the small bowel. These tubes, however, are not ideal as a long-term management strategy due to intermittent tube dislodgement into the stomach, inability to bolus feed, and described enteroenteric intussusceptions [79].

Smits et al. measured gastric emptying in 10 children before and after fundoplication. The four patients with post-operative dysphagia had a longer gastric emptying half time compared to the patients without dysphagia after fundoplication [81]. The pediatric literature seems inconsistent on the pathophysiology of the interaction between gastric emptying, GERD, and post-operative dysphagia and deserves further study. Conflicting results are also reported by Franken et al. and Kawahara et al. who studied gastric emptying after placement of a feeding gastrostomy tube in children. Kawahara et al. found that laparoscopic gastrostomy placement reduces GER in neurologically impaired children with pathological GERD by improving gastric emptying, although they also saw a paradoxical influence on patients without pathological GER. In contrast to this study, gastrostomy placement in children caused significant delays in gastric emptying in the study by Franken et al. Postoperative delayed gastric emptying was associated with gastroesophageal reflux and was found in most patients with postoperative feeding intolerance [82, 83].

As a last resort, children who have repeatedly failed fundoplication, especially those with severe neurologic impairment, may be candidates for total esophagogastric dissociation originally described by Adrian Bianchi in 1997. With this procedure, GERD is permanently eliminated by transecting the esophagus from the stomach. An esophagojejunal anastomosis is created, and the biliopancreatic limb is then anastomosed to the jejunal loop approximately 30 cm distal to the GE junction. Gastric feedings can still be given through a gastrostomy tube in the remnant stomach.

Future Advances

Responsible genes for intestinal motor disorders are being elucidated, and greater insight into the pathophysiology of pediatric motility disorders will continue to emerge. For example, future treatments with stem cells as gut-differentiated neural cells could target the replacement of the myenteric plexus in children with achalasia. Tissue-engineering technology could revolutionize congenital disorders, such as long-gap esophageal atresia, and improve outcomes significantly.

For small children, new technological equipment, such as micro-perfusion systems and microcatheters, will allow a more detailed study of motility processes and add new perspectives to the understanding of pediatric motility disorders.

One of the greatest challenges is the lack of specific and effective drugs for the treatment of gastrointestinal motor disorders, and new medications are needed. With continued scientific discoveries of the enteric nervous system, new treatment modalities might emerge, and the treatment and prognosis of children with primary and secondary motility disorders will improve.

Due to lower case numbers in the pediatric world, there is a significant lack of good outcome data, especially in terms of randomized prospective studies. Pediatric systematic reviews and meta-analyses are increasingly produced, evaluating available evidence. New multi-institutional and international cooperative research efforts, often sponsored by national or international societies and their members, are underway to address important clinical questions for children. Professional societies publish guidelines based on evidence and expert opinion, also for children. Wherever feasible, randomized prospective trials are being organized. With increasing amounts of new data, clear management strategies for children are further emerging and will help to guide and improve treatment by pediatric clinicians.

References

1. de Santa BP, van den Brink GR, Roberts DJ. Molecular etiology of gut malformations and diseases. Am J Med Genet. 2002;115(4):221–30.
2. Perin S, McCann CJ, Borrelli O, De Coppi P, Thapar N. Update on foregut molecular embryology and role of regenerative medicine therapies. Front Pediatr. 2017;5:91.

3. Qi BQ, Beasley SW. Stages of normal tracheo-bronchial development in rat embryos: resolution of a controversy. Develop Growth Differ. 2000;42(2):145–53.
4. Zaw-Tun HA. The tracheo-esophageal septum–fact or fantasy? Origin and development of the respiratory primordium and esophagus. Acta Anat. 1982;114(1):1–21.
5. Lemoine C, Aspirot A, Le Henaff G, Piloquet H, Lévesque D, Faure C. Characterization of esophageal motility following esophageal atresia repair using high-resolution esophageal manometry. J Pediatr Gastroenterol Nutr. 2013;56(6):609–14.
6. Nakazato Y, Landing BH, Wells TR. Abnormal auerbach plexus in the esophagus and stomach of patients with esophageal atresia and tracheo-esophageal fistula. J Pediatr Surg. 1986;21(10):831–7.
7. Boleken M, Demirbilek S, Kirimiloglu H, Kanmaz T, Yucesan S, Celbis O, et al. Reduced neuronal innervation in the distal end of the proximal esophageal atretic segment in cases of esophageal atresia with distal tracheoesophageal fistula. World J Surg. 2007;31(7):1512–7.
8. Berseth CL. Gestational evolution of small intestine motility in preterm and term infants. J Pediatr. 1989;115(4):646–51.
9. Montgomery RK, Mulberg AE, Grand RJ. Development of the human gastrointestinal tract: twenty years of progress. Gastroenterology. 1999;116(3):702–31.
10. Omari TI, Benninga MA, Barnett CP, Haslam RR, Davidson GP, Dent J. Characterization of esophageal body and lower esophageal sphincter motor function in the very premature neonate. J Pediatr. 1999;135(4):517–21.
11. Staiano A, Boccia G, Salvia G, Zappulli D, Clouse RE. Development of esophageal peristalsis in preterm and term neonates. Gastroenterology. 2007;132(5):1718–25.
12. Singendonk MMJ, Rommel N, Omari TI, Benninga MA, van Wijk MP. Upper gastrointestinal motility: prenatal development and problems in infancy. Nat Rev Gastroenterol Hepatol. 2014;11(9):545–55.
13. Jadcherla SR, Duong HQ, Hofmann C, Hoffmann R, Shaker R. Characteristics of upper oesophageal sphincter and oesophageal body during maturation in healthy human neonates compared with adults. Neurogastroenterol Motil. 2005;17(5):663–70.
14. Di Lorenzo C, Hillemeier C, Hyman P, Loening-Baucke V, Nurko S, Rosenberg A, et al. Manometry studies in children: minimum standards for procedures. Neurogastroenterol Motil. 2002;14(4):411–20.
15. Nurko S. Gastrointestinal manometry: methodology and indications. In: Pediatric gastrointestinal disease. Philadelphia: BC Decker Inc.; 2000. p. 1485–510.
16. Fung KP, Math MV, Ho CO, Yap KM. Midazolam as a sedative in esophageal manometry: a study of the effect on esophageal motility. J Pediatr Gastroenterol Nutr. 1992;15(1):85–8.

17. Nurko S. Motility disorders in children. Pediatr Clin N Am. 2017;64(3):593–612.
18. Di Lorenzo C, Flores AF, Reddy SN, Snape WJ, Bazzocchi G, Hyman PE. Colonic manometry in children with chronic intestinal pseudo-obstruction. Gut. 1993;34(6):803–7.
19. Macharia EW. Comparison of upper gastrointestinal contrast studies and pH/impedance tests for the diagnosis of childhood gastro-oesophageal reflux. Pediatr Radiol. 2012;42(8):946–51.
20. Katzka DA. A gastroenterologist's perspective on the role of barium esophagography in gastroesophageal reflux disease. Abdom Radiol N Y. 2018;43(6):1319–22.
21. Camilleri M, Bharucha AE, di Lorenzo C, Hasler WL, Prather CM, Rao SS, et al. American Neurogastroenterology and Motility Society consensus statement on intraluminal measurement of gastrointestinal and colonic motility in clinical practice. Neurogastroenterol Motil. 2008;20(12):1269–82.
22. Camilleri M, Hasler WL, Parkman HP, Quigley EM, Soffer E. Measurement of gastrointestinal motility in the GI laboratory. Gastroenterology. 1998;115(3):747–62.
23. Rodriguez L, Sood M, Di Lorenzo C, Saps M. An ANMS-NASPGHAN consensus document on anorectal and colonic manometry in children. Neurogastroenterol Motil. 2017;29(1):12944.
24. Dhawan I, O'Connell B, Patel A, Schey R, Parkman HP, Friedenberg F. Utility of esophageal high-resolution manometry in clinical practice: first. Do HRM Dig Dis Sci. 2018;63(12):3178–86.
25. Rommel N, Omari TI, Selleslagh M, Kritas S, Cock C, Rosan R, et al. High-resolution manometry combined with impedance measurements discriminates the cause of dysphagia in children. Eur J Pediatr. 2015;174(12):1629–37.
26. Bredenoord AJ, Fox M, Kahrilas PJ, Pandolfino JE, Schwizer W, Smout AJPM, et al. Chicago classification criteria of esophageal motility disorders defined in high resolution esophageal pressure topography. Neurogastroenterol Motil. 2012;24(1):57–65.
27. Rosen R, Garza JM, Tipnis N, Nurko S. An ANMS-NASPGHAN consensus document on esophageal and antroduodenal manometry in children. Neurogastroenterol Motil. 2018;30(3):13239.
28. Staiano A, Boccia G, Miele E, Clouse RE. Segmental characteristics of oesophageal peristalsis in paediatric patients. Neurogastroenterol Motil. 2008;20(1):19–26.
29. Spencer J. Prolonged pH recording in the study of gastro-oesophageal reflux. Br J Surg. 1969;56(12):912–4.
30. European Society of Pediatric Gastroenterology and Nutrition. A standardized protocol for the methodology of esophageal pH monitoring and interpretation of the data for the diagnosis of gastroesophageal reflux. J Pediatr Gastroenterol Nutr. 1992;14(4):467–71.

31. Vantrappen G, Janssens J, Hellemans J, Ghoos Y. The interdigestive motor complex of normal subjects and patients with bacterial overgrowth of the small intestine. J Clin Invest. 1977;59(6):1158–66.
32. Kellow JE, Borody TJ, Phillips SF, Tucker RL, Haddad AC. Human interdigestive motility: variations in patterns from esophagus to colon. Gastroenterology. 1986;91(2):386–95.
33. Quigley EM. Gastric and small intestinal motility in health and disease. Gastroenterol Clin N Am. 1996;25(1):113–45.
34. Kuo B, McCallum RW, Koch KL, Sitrin MD, Wo JM, Chey WD, et al. Comparison of gastric emptying of a nondigestible capsule to a radiolabelled meal in healthy and gastroparetic subjects. Aliment Pharmacol Ther. 2008;27(2):186–96.
35. Rao SSC, Kuo B, McCallum RW, Chey WD, DiBaise JK, Hasler WL, et al. Investigation of colonic and whole-gut transit with wireless motility capsule and radiopaque markers in constipation. Clin Gastroenterol Hepatol. 2009;7(5):537–44.
36. Surjanhata B, Brun R, Wilding G, Semler J, Kuo B. Small bowel fed response as measured by wireless motility capsule: comparative analysis in healthy, gastroparetic, and constipated subjects. Neurogastroenterol Motil. 2018;30(5):e13268.
37. van der Zee DC, Bagolan P, Faure C, Gottrand F, Jennings R, Laberge J-M, et al. Position paper of INoEA Working Group on long-gap esophageal atresia: for better care. Front Pediatr. 2017;5:63.
38. Foker JE, Linden BC, Boyle EM, Marquardt C. Development of a true primary repair for the full spectrum of esophageal atresia. Ann Surg. 1997;226(4):533–41; discussion 541-543.
39. Khan KM, Sabati AA, Kendall T, Foker JE. The effect of traction on esophageal structure in children with long-gap esophageal atresia. Dig Dis Sci. 2006;51(11):1917–21.
40. Comella A, Tan Tanny SP, Hutson JM, Omari TI, Teague WJ, Nataraja RM, et al. Esophageal morbidity in patients following repair of esophageal atresia: a systematic review. J Pediatr Surg. 2020;56(9):1555–63.
41. Ijsselstijn H, van Beelen NWG, Wijnen RMH. Esophageal atresia: long-term morbidities in adolescence and adulthood. Dis Esophagus. 2013;26(4):417–21.
42. Midrio P, Alaggio R, Strojna A, Gamba P, Giacomelli L, Pizzi S, et al. Reduction of interstitial cells of Cajal in esophageal atresia. J Pediatr Gastroenterol Nutr. 2010;51(5):610–7.
43. Hassan M, Mousa H. Impedance testing in esophageal atresia patients. Front Pediatr. 2017;5:85.
44. Di Pace MR, Caruso AM, Catalano P, Casuccio A, Cimador M, De Grazia E. Evaluation of esophageal motility and reflux in children treated for esophageal atresia with the use of combined multichannel intraluminal impedance and pH monitoring. J Pediatr Surg. 2011;46(3):443–51.

45. Kovesi T, Rubin S. Long-term complications of congenital esophageal atresia and/or tracheoesophageal fistula. Chest. 2004;126(3):915–25.
46. Chumpitazi B, Nurko S. Pediatric gastrointestinal motility disorders: challenges and a clinical update. Gastroenterol Hepatol. 2008;4(2):140–8.
47. Islam S. Achalasia. Semin Pediatr Surg. 2017;26(2):116–20.
48. Singendonk MMJ, Omari TI, Rommel N, van Wijk MP, Benninga MA, Rosen R, et al. Novel pressure-impedance parameters for evaluating esophageal function in pediatric achalasia. J Pediatr Gastroenterol Nutr. 2018;66(1):37–42.
49. Yu YR, Rosenfeld EH, Chiou EH, Chumpitazi BP, Fallon SC, Brandt ML. High-resolution manometric guidance during laparoscopic Heller myotomy: impact on quality of life and symptom severity for children with achalasia. J Pediatr Surg. 2019;54(5):1063–8.
50. Eckardt VF. Clinical presentations and complications of achalasia. Gastrointest Endosc Clin N Am. 2001;11(2):281–92. vi
51. Pastor AC, Mills J, Marcon MA, Himidan S, Kim PCW. A single center 26-year experience with treatment of esophageal achalasia: is there an optimal method? J Pediatr Surg. 2009;44(7):1349–54.
52. Boeckxstaens GE, Annese V, Varannes SB, Chaussade S, Costantini M, Cuttitta A, et al. Pneumatic dilation versus laparoscopic Heller's myotomy for idiopathic achalasia. N Engl J Med. 2011;364(19):1807–16.
53. Moonen A, Annese V, Belmans A, Bredenoord AJ, Bruley Varannes S, Costantini M, et al. Long-term results of the European achalasia trial: a multicentre randomised controlled trial comparing pneumatic dilation versus laparoscopic Heller myotomy. Gut. 2016;65(5):732–9.
54. Franklin AL, Petrosyan M, Kane TD. Childhood achalasia: a comprehensive review of disease, diagnosis and therapeutic management. World J Gastrointest Endosc. 2014;6(4):105–11.
55. Pacilli M, Davenport M. Results of laparoscopic Heller's myotomy for achalasia in children: a systematic review of the literature. J Laparoendosc Adv Surg Tech A. 2017;27(1):82–90.
56. van Lennep M, van Wijk MP, Omari TIM, Benninga MA, Singendonk MMJ. Clinical management of pediatric achalasia. Expert Rev Gastroenterol Hepatol. 2018;12(4):391–404.
57. Sharp NE, St Peter SD. Treatment of idiopathic achalasia in the pediatric population: a systematic review. Eur J Pediatr Surg. 2016;26(2):143–9.
58. Hung Y-C, Westfal ML, Chang DC, Kelleher CM. Heller myotomy is the optimal index procedure for esophageal achalasia in adolescents and young adults. Surg Endosc. 2019;33(10):3355–60.
59. van Lennep M, van Wijk MP, Omari TIM, Salvatore S, Benninga MA, Singendonk MMJ, et al. Clinical management of pediatric achalasia: a survey of current practice. J Pediatr Gastroenterol Nutr. 2019;68(4):521–6.

60. Richards WO, Torquati A, Holzman MD, Khaitan L, Byrne D, Lutfi R, et al. Heller myotomy versus Heller myotomy with Dor fundoplication for achalasia: a prospective randomized double-blind clinical trial. Ann Surg. 2004;240(3):405–12; discussion 412-415.
61. Sharp KW, Khaitan L, Scholz S, Holzman MD, Richards WO. 100 consecutive minimally invasive Heller myotomies: lessons learned. Ann Surg. 2002;235(5):631–8; discussion 638-639.
62. Gould JL, Rentea RM, St Peter SD. Contemporary management of achalasia by pediatric surgeons: a survey of the international pediatric endosurgical group. J Laparoendosc Adv Surg Tech A. 2016;26(7):567–9.
63. Inoue H, Minami H, Kobayashi Y, Sato Y, Kaga M, Suzuki M, et al. Peroral endoscopic myotomy (POEM) for esophageal achalasia. Endoscopy. 2010;42(4):265–71.
64. Maselli R, Inoue H, Misawa M, Ikeda H, Hosoya T, Onimaru M, et al. Peroral endoscopic myotomy (POEM) in a 3-year-old girl with severe growth retardation, achalasia, and Down syndrome. Endoscopy. 2012;44(2):285–7.
65. Nabi Z, Ramchandani M, Chavan R, Darisetty S, Kalapala R, Shava U, et al. Outcome of peroral endoscopic myotomy in children with achalasia. Surg Endosc. 2019;33(11):3656–64.
66. Tan Y, Zhu H, Li C, Chu Y, Huo J, Liu D. Comparison of peroral endoscopic myotomy and endoscopic balloon dilation for primary treatment of pediatric achalasia. J Pediatr Surg. 2016;51(10):1613–8.
67. Petrosyan M, Khalafallah AM, Guzzetta PC, Sandler AD, Darbari A, Kane TD. Surgical management of esophageal achalasia: evolution of an institutional approach to minimally invasive repair. J Pediatr Surg. 2016;51(10):1619–22.
68. Burns AJ, Goldstein AM, Newgreen DF, Stamp L, Schäfer K-H, Metzger M, et al. White paper on guidelines concerning enteric nervous system stem cell therapy for enteric neuropathies. Dev Biol. 2016;417(2):229–51.
69. Iuliano S, Minelli R, Vincenzi F, Gaiani F, Ruberto C, Leandro G, et al. Eosinophilic esophagitis in pediatric age, state of the art and review of the literature. Acta Bio-Med Atenei Parm. 2018;89(8-S):20–6.
70. Papadopoulou A, Koletzko S, Heuschkel R, Dias JA, Allen KJ, Murch SH, et al. Management guidelines of eosinophilic esophagitis in childhood. J Pediatr Gastroenterol Nutr. 2014;58(1):107–18.
71. Mark JA, Anderson BT, Pan Z, Menard-Katcher C, Kramer RE. Comparative analysis of adverse events after esophageal balloon and bougie dilations in children. J Pediatr Gastroenterol Nutr. 2019;68(5):630–4.
72. Tambucci R, Rea F, Angelino G, Malamisura M, Mennini M, Riccardi C, et al. Eosinophilic esophagitis in esophageal atresia: tertiary care experience of a "selective" approach for biopsy sampling. World Allergy Organ J. 2020;13(4):100116.

73. Krishnan U. Eosinophilic esophagitis in esophageal atresia. Front Pediatr. 2019;7:497.
74. Krishnan U, Mousa H, Dall'Oglio L, Homaira N, Rosen R, Faure C, et al. ESPGHAN-NASPGHAN guidelines for the evaluation and treatment of gastrointestinal and nutritional complications in children with esophageal atresia-tracheoesophageal fistula. J Pediatr Gastroenterol Nutr. 2016;63(5):550–70.
75. Hegar B, Dewanti NR, Kadim M, Alatas S, Firmansyah A, Vandenplas Y. Natural evolution of regurgitation in healthy infants. Acta Paediatr Oslo Nor. 2009;98(7):1189–93.
76. van der Pol RJ, Smits MJ, Venmans L, Boluyt N, Benninga MA, Tabbers MM. Diagnostic accuracy of tests in pediatric gastroesophageal reflux disease. J Pediatr. 2013;162(5):983–7.
77. Holcomb GW, St Peter SD. Error traps and safety steps when performing a laparoscopic Nissen fundoplication. Semin Pediatr Surg. 2019;28(3):160–3.
78. Rosen R, Vandenplas Y, Singendonk M, Cabana M, DiLorenzo C, Gottrand F, et al. Pediatric gastroesophageal reflux clinical practice guidelines: joint recommendations of the North American Society for Pediatric Gastroenterology, Hepatology, and Nutrition and the European Society for Pediatric Gastroenterology, Hepatology, and Nutrition. J Pediatr Gastroenterol Nutr. 2018;66(3):516–54.
79. Jackson HT, Kane TD. Surgical management of pediatric gastroesophageal reflux disease. Gastroenterol Res Pract. 2013;2013:863527.
80. Pacilli M, Pierro A, Lindley KJ, Curry JI, Eaton S. Gastric emptying is accelerated following laparoscopic Nissen fundoplication. Eur J Pediatr Surg. 2008;18(6):395–7.
81. Smits MJ, Loots CM, Benninga MA, Omari TI, van Wijk MP. New insights in gastroesophageal reflux, esophageal function and gastric emptying in relation to dysphagia before and after anti-reflux surgery in children. Curr Gastroenterol Rep. 2013;15(10):351.
82. Franken J, Mauritz FA, Stellato RK, Van der Zee DC, Van Herwaarden-Lindeboom MYA. The effect of gastrostomy placement on gastric function in children: a prospective cohort study. J Gastrointest Surg. 2017;21(7):1105–11.
83. Kawahara H, Tazuke Y, Soh H, Yoneda A, Fukuzawa M. Does laparoscopy-aided gastrostomy placement improve or worsen gastroesophageal reflux in patients with neurological impairment? J Pediatr Surg. 2014;49(12):1742–5.

Index

A. D. Patel et al. (eds.), *The SAGES Manual of Physiologic Evaluation of Foregut Diseases*,
https://doi.org/10.1007/978-3-031-39199-6

H

P

MIX
Papier aus verantwortungsvollen Quellen
Paper from responsible sources
FSC® C105338

If you have any concerns about our products,
you can contact us on
ProductSafety@springernature.com

In case Publisher is established outside the EU,
the EU authorized representative is:
Springer Nature Customer Service Center GmbH
Europaplatz 3, 69115 Heidelberg, Germany

Printed by Libri Plureos GmbH
in Hamburg, Germany